The Neuman Systems Model

Third Edition

Betty Neuman, PhD, FAAN
Theorist-Consultant
Founder/Director, Neuman Systems Model Trustee Group, Inc.
Beverly, Ohio

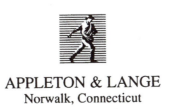

APPLETON & LANGE
Norwalk, Connecticut

95 96 97 98 99 / 10 9 8 7 6 5 4 3 2 1

Prentice Hall International (UK) Limited, *London*
Prentice Hall of Australia Pty. Limited, *Sydney*
Prentice Hall Canada, Inc., *Toronto*
Prentice Hall Hispanoamericana, S.A., *Mexico*
Prentice Hall of India Private Limited, *New Delhi*
Prentice Hall of Japan, Inc., *Tokyo*
Simon and Schuster Asia Pte. Ltd., *Singapore*
Editora Prentice Hall do Brasil Ltda., *Rio de Janeiro*
Prentice Hall, *Englewood Cliffs, New Jersey*

Library of Congress Cataloging-in-Publication Data

The Neuman systems model / [edited by] Betty Neuman. — 3rd ed.
        p.   cm.
    Includes bibliographical references and index.
    ISBN 0-8385-6701-0
    1. Nursing—Philosophy.   2. Nursing—Study and teaching.
I. Neuman, Betty M.
    [DNLM: 1. Philosophy, Nursing.   2. Models, Nursing.   3. Education,
Nursing.   WY 86 N489 1995]
    RT84.5.N474   1995
    610.73'07—dc20   **175367**
    DNLM/DLC   94-30479
    for Library of Congress   CIP

Acquistions Editor: David P. Carroll
Production Editor: Elizabeth C. Ryan
Production Service: Editorial Services of New England
Designer: Michael J. Kelly
Cover Designer: Mary Skudlarek

ISBN 0-8385-6701-0

90000

9 780838 567012

CONTENTS

CONTRIBUTORS

Kathryn Hoehn Anderson, PhD, RN
Associate Professor
School of Nursing
University of Wisconsin–Eau Claire
Eau Claire, Wisconsin

Gail Beddome, RN, MSN
Faculty of Nursing
Division of Health
Okanagan University College
Kelowna, British Columbia, Canada

Birgitta Bertilson, RN, BSc
District Nurse
Servicehuset Union
Jönköping, Sweden

Charlene E. Beynon, BScN, MScN
Assistant Professor
Faculty of Nursing
University of Western Ontario
London, Ontario, Canada

Eva Bjälming, RN, BSc, EdD
Lecturer
University College of Health Sciences
Jönköping, Sweden

Carol Bloch, MEd, MSN, RN, CTN
Master Teacher
School of Nursing
Los Angeles County and University of
    Southern California Medical Center
Los Angeles, California

Carolyn Bloch, MEd, MSN, RN, CTN
Coordinator of Recruitment, Retention and
    Educational Services
School of Nursing
Los Angeles County and University of
    Southern California Medical Center
Los Angeles, California

Diane M. Breckenridge, RN
    PhD Candidate, University of Maryland
Independent Renal Nurse Consultant and
    Instructor
School of Nursing
Abington Memorial Hospital
Abington, Pennsylvania

Maureen McCormac Bueno, PhD, RN
Director, Nursing Systems
Department of Nursing
Robert Wood Johnson University Hospital
New Brunswick, New Jersey

Sandra J. Butler, RN, C, MS
District Nursing Supervisor
Oklahoma State Department of Health
Oklahoma City, Oklahoma

Cynthia Flynn Capers, PhD, RN
Associate Professor and Director of
    Undergraduate Program
School of Nursing
La Salle University
Philadelphia, Pennsylvania

Verna Carson, PhD, RN, CS
Associate Professor
Department of Psychiatric and Community
  Health Nursing
School of Nursing
University of Maryland
Baltimore, Maryland

Julianne Cheek, PhD
Lecturer
Faculty of Nursing
University of South Australia
Adelaide, South Australia

Patricia Chiverton, EdD, RN
Assistant Professor
College of Nursing
University of Rochester
Rochester, New York

Julie G. Cox, RN, MSN
Senior Nursing/Coordinator Day Program
Department of Nursing
Friends Hospital
Philadelphia, Pennsylvania

Dorothy M. Craig, RN, BA, BScN, MScN
Associate Professor
Faculty of Nursing
University of Toronto
Toronto, Ontario, Canada

Glenn Curran, RN, RMN, BN (Hons)
Clinical Nurse Manager
Sexual Health HIV/AIDS Program
North West Health Region
Burnie, Tasmania, Australia

Margaret Damant, MPhil, BA
Educator—Community Health Nursing
Postgraduate Medical School
University of Exeter
Exeter, England

Patricia Davies, RMN, DipN, MPhil
Research Nurse
Powys NHS Trust
Post Basic Education and Research
  Department
Mid Wales Hospital
Talgarth, Brecon, Wales

Sandra I. Dunn, RN(C), BNSc, MEd
Perinatal Coordinator, Perinatal Education
  Program of Eastern Ontario, and
  Lecturer
School of Nursing
University of Ottawa
Ottawa, Ontario, Canada

Ann Estes Edgil, RN, DSN
Professor
School of Nursing
University of Alabama
Birmingham, Alabama

**Ingegerd Bergbom Engberg, RN, BSc,
  EdD, DMSc**
Lecturer
Research Department
Borås College of Health and Caring
  Sciences
Borås, Sweden

Jacqueline Fawcett, PhD, FAAN
Professor
School of Nursing
University of Pennsylvania
Philadelphia, Pennsylvania

Margot Felix, RN, BSSc, MPA
Nurse Educator/Research and
  Development
Elisabeth Bruyere Health Centre
Ottawa, Ontario, Canada

Jeanne C. Flannery, RN, DSN, CNRN, CRRN
Associate Professor
School of Nursing
Florida State University
Tallahassee, Florida

Filomena C. Flores, RN, PhD
Professor
Department of Nursing
California State University
Fresno, California

Juanzetta S. Flowers, RN, DSN
Associate Professor
School of Nursing
University of Alabama
Birmingham, Alabama

Toni D. Frioux, RNC, BSN, MS
Chief, Nursing Services
Oklahoma State Department of Health
Oklahoma City, Oklahoma

Terry T. Fulmer, RN, PhD, FAAN
Professor of Nursing Research
College of Nursing
Columbia University
New York, New York

Ruth Ann B. Fulton, RN, DNSc
Associate Professor
Nursing Program
College Misericordia
Dallas, Pennsylvania

Rita S. Glazebrook, PhD, RN, ANP, CS
Associate Professor
St. Olaf College
Director
Minnesota Intercollegiate Nursing
  Consortium
Northfield, Minnesota

Pippa Gough, RGN, HV, RM, PGCEA, MPS
Project Officer
Nursing Developments Programme
King's Fund Centre
London, England

Marilyn D. Grafton, RN, MSN
Associate Director and Dean
School of Nursing
Los Angeles County and University of
  Southern California Medical Center
Los Angeles, California

Joan S. Grant, DSN, RN, CS
Associate Professor
School of Nursing
University of Alabama
Birmingham, Alabama

Loretta J. Heyduk, MSN, RN,C
Director of Ambulatory Services
Friends Hospital
Philadelphia, Pennsylvania

Judy Willis Hileman, RN, ARNP, PhD
Clinical Instructor
School of Nursing
University of Missouri
Kansas City, Missouri

Sharon A. Hilton, RN, MS
Director and Dean
School of Nursing
Los Angeles County and University of
  Southern California Medical Center
Los Angeles, California

Cora Hinds, RN, MScN, EdD
Associate Professor
Community Health Nursing
School of Nursing
University of Ottawa
Ottawa, Ontario, Canada

Jean A. Kelley, EdD, RN, FAAN
Professor Emeritus
School of Nursing
University of Alabama
Birmingham, Alabama

Linda Campbell Klotz, PhD, RN
Associate Professor of Nursing and
    Coordinator, Graduate Program
Division of Nursing
The University of Texas
Tyler, Texas

Margaret Louis, PhD, RN
Associate Professor in Nursing
College of Health Sciences
University of Nevada
Las Vegas, Nevada

Lois W. Lowry, DNSc, RN
Associate Professor
College of Nursing
University of South Florida
Tampa, Florida

Patricia A. Maglicco, RNCS, MSN
Associate Director of Nursing
Department of Nursing
Friends Hospital
Philadelphia, Pennsylvania

Antoinette Martin, RN, MHA
Vice President, Nursing
Chronic Care Hospital
Department of Nursing
Elisabeth Bruyere Health Center
Ottawa, Ontario, Canada

**Sybil Jennifer McCulloch, RN, BEd,
    Grad Dip Ed Ad, FRCNA**
Associate Professor and Acting Dean
School of Nursing
City and Whyalla Campuses
University of South Australia
Adelaide, South Australia

Marian McGee, RN, Dr PH
Professor
School of Nursing
University of Ottawa
Ottawa, Ontario, Canada

**Afaf Ibrahim Meleis, RN, PhD,
    DrPs (Hon)**
Professor
School of Nursing
Department of Mental Health, Community
    and Administrative Nursing
University of California
San Francisco, California

Rosalie Mirenda, MSN, BSN
    DNSc Candidate, Witener University
Vice President for Academic Affairs and
    Professor, Nursing
Division of Nursing and Health Sciences
Neumann College
Aston, Pennsylvania

**Corinne Morris-Coulter, RN, BScN,
    MSc**
Clinical Nurse Specialist
Nursing Education and Research
Whitby Psychiatric Hospital
Whitby, Ontario, Canada

Betty Neuman, PhD, FAAN
Theorist-Consultant
Founder/Director, Neuman Systems Model
    Trustee Group, Inc.
Beverly, Ohio

Grace G. Newsome, RN, EdN
Grant Coordinator
Georgia Hospital Association
Marietta, Georgia

Patricia Nuttall, PhD, RN, CPNP
Associate Professor
Department of Nursing
California State University
Fresno, California

Anne Griswold Peirce, RN, PhD
Director of Doctoral Studies
College of Nursing
Columbia University
New York, New York

Victoria L. Poole, RN, DSN
Assistant Professor
School of Nursing
University of Alabama
Birmingham, Alabama

Nicholas G. Procter, RGN, RPN, BA, Grad Dip Ed
Lecturer
Faculty of Nursing
University of South Australia
Adelaide, South Australia

Harold Proctor, RMN, CPNCert
Psychiatric Nurse Coordinator
Powys NHS Trust
Ystradgynlais Mental Health Team
Ystradgynlais, Powys, Wales

Anita Gayle Roberts, RN, MS
District Nursing Supervisor—Local Health
  Services
Oklahoma State Department of Health
Oklahoma City, Oklahoma

Marion L. Rodriguez, PhD, MEd, CNA
Director, Quality Assurance and Staff
  Development
Sylvan Manor Health Care Center
Silver Spring, Maryland

Jan Russell, RN, PhD
Associate Professor
School of Nursing
University of Missouri
Kansas City, Missouri

Nena F. Sanders, RN, DNS
Associate Professor
School of Nursing
University of Alabama
Birmingham, Alabama

Nancy A. Sargent, RN, MSN
Assistant to Director of Clinical Services
Department of Nursing
Friends Hospital
Philadelphia, Pennsylvania

Beverly J. Schmoll, PhD, PT
Director and Associate Professor, Physical
  Therapy
School of Health Professions and Studies
University of Michigan
Flint, Michigan

Betty Scicchitani, RN, BSN, EdD
Director of Clinical Services
Department of Nursing
Friends Hospital
Philadelphia, Pennsylvania

Kathy Kendall Sengin, RN, MSN, CCRN, CNAA
Vice President, Nursing
Department of Nursing
Robert Wood Johnson University Hospital
New Brunswick, New Jersey

Mary K. Shannahan, RN, PhD
Associate Professor
School of Nursing
Florida State University
Tallahassee, Florida

Mary Colette Smith, RN, PhD
Professor, Graduate Programs in Nursing
School of Nursing
University of Alabama
Birmingham, Alabama

Raphella Sohier, PhD, MS, MSN, RN
Professor of Nursing
Graduate Program in Nursing and
    Community Health Nursing
MGH Institute of Health Professions at
    Massachussetts General Hospital
Boston, Massachussetts

Ann E. Sprague, RN(C), BN, MEd
Perinatal Coordinator, Perinatal Education
    Program of Eastern Ontario, and
    Lecturer
School of Nursing
University of Ottawa
Ottawa, Ontario, Canada

Eleanor M. Stittich, RN, M Litt
Professor Emeritus
Department of Nursing
California State University
Fresno, California

Victoria Strickland-Seng, PhD, RN
Chair and Associate Professor
Department of Nursing
University of Tennessee
Martin, Tennessee

Gail W. Stuart, PhD, RN, CS, FAAN
Professor, College of Nursing and
    Associate Professor, College of
    Medicine
Medical University of South Carolina
Charleston, South Carolina

Patricia Short Tomlinson, RN, MS, PhD
Professor
Health Sciences
School of Nursing
University of Minnesota
Minneapolis, Minnesota

Jane L. Toot, PhD, PT
Professor and Department Chair
Acting Director, School of Health Science
Grand Valley State University
Allendale, Michigan

Marie-Josée Trépanier, RN(C), BScN, MEd
Perinatal Coordinator, Perinatal Education
    Program of Eastern Ontario, and
    Lecturer
School of Nursing
University of Ottawa
Ottawa, Ontario, Canada

Barbara Vaughan, MSc, RGN, DipN, DANS, RNT
Program Director/Nursing Developments
Kings Fund Centre
London, England

Frans Verberk, RN, MN
Social Psychiatric Nurse
Regional Institute for the Netherlands
    Association for Out-Patient Mental
    Health Care
Hellevoetsluis, The Netherlands

Patricia Hinton Walker, PhD, RN, FAAN
Associate Professor of Clinical Nursing
Associate Dean and Director of
    Community Centered Practice
Health Systems Division, School of
    Nursing
University of Rochester
Rochester, New York

Leigh Ann Ware, RN, MSN
NICU Parent Support Coordinator
Developmental Evaluation and
    Intervention Program
Sacred Heart Hospital
Pensacola, Florida

Sister Carmen Wolfe, RN, MSc
Assistant Executive Director
Department of Nursing
Provincial Superior,
Sisters of Charity of Ottawa
Ottawa, Ontario, Canada

Lore K. Wright, PhD, RN, CS
Associate Professor
College of Nursing and Assistant Professor
College of Medicine
Medical University of South Carolina
Charleston, South Carolina

PREFACE

Since the mid 1970s, the first use of the Neuman Systems Model for nursing education and practice, the model has both led and followed evolving health care trends. During the 1980s, the model increasingly gained world-wide popularity as a valid and appropriate health care organizing structure easily crossing cultural barriers and multidisciplinary boundaries.

This third edition is expanded to further illustrate the model's relevancy for the 21st century. It is viewed as an appropriate wellness-focused organizing structure, comprehensive and flexible, allowing for creative, collaborative and cooperative interdisciplinary programming for service delivery consistent with evolving wholistic social health care trends.

This volume provides information on development and use of the model from its inception to new, in-process, initiatives for the future. Its content reflects continued model relevance for the 21st century. Each of the chapters in this book has gone through the peer review process.

Section One provides an historical look to review the past and make predictions as to the Neuman Model's role in restructuring and shaping the future of nursing. New world view perspectives and conceptualizations are provided for analyses related to the model's spiritual and sociocultural variables. Projections are made as to the role of the nurse in world catastrophic events and family health as a system.

Section Two presents specific information for curriculum development adaptable from diploma level transition to associate degree and higher education. Content reflects interdisciplinary programming, cultural diversity, curricular development process, and content utilization. Evaluation data includes a compilation of longitudinal findings from several associate degree level programs.

Section Three outlines a wide variety of nursing practice applications consistent with current and anticipated changes in health care delivery.

Section Four provides directives for the nurse administrative role and management process in keeping with newer health mandates. Content includes total quality management and futuristic organizational health care principles as well as implementations from a variety of nurse managed health services ranging from state to local level programming: state public health nursing services, community nursing centers, psychiatric inpatient facilities, pregnancy substance abuse, and geriatric continuing care.

Section Five proposes challenges, principles, and directives for future research, including projections for a research center, and a proposed "transformative world-view" for a more congruent interpretive approach to theory support for nursing. The "state-of-the-art" in model research is set forth as research abstracts. Rules are given for theory development and examples are provided of mid-range theory derived from nursing practice.

Section Six presents a wide variety of international model implementations, evaluations, proposals, and abstracts of model usage in several countries reflecting the breadth of its applicability across cultural boundaries.

Section Seven chronicles the Neuman Systems Model's development, utilization, and future potential. Its future visibility and direction will continue to be heavily influenced by the stewardship of the carefully chosen and highly valued Neuman Systems Model Trustee Group membership.

This third edition is suitable as a text for all levels of nursing education and directive for all areas of nursing practice. The Neuman Systems-based concepts are futuristic and have unlimited potential and relevance for the scientific development of nursing.

ACKNOWLEDGMENTS

The enthusiasm of world-wide pioneering Neuman Model users, and would-be users, has been a highly motivating force for development of this third edition. Many of their fine contributions will, indeed, further develop the model for the future of nursing, distinguishing each in the process.

I wish to thank all contributing authors for their important contributions and fine cooperation during manuscript preparation.

I am, indeed, grateful for the excellent support received from Neuman Trustee Group members who acted as reviewers and consultants. Their high commitment level will assure protection, preservation, and promotion of the model's integrity.

I commend my typist, a neighbor and gifted senior high school student, Rebecca Fields, for her availability and perseverance.

Special appreciation is extended to the fine Appleton & Lange editorial staff—Sally Barhydt, Editor-in-Chief; David Carroll, Senior Editor; and John Waggoner, Editorial Assistant—for their most valued support and cooperative spirit. I also extend my appreciation to Linda McLatchie, Copy Editor, and Lauren Byrne, Project Editor, of Editorial Services of New England, Inc., for their superb editorial assistance.

Lastly, I am most grateful for the love and support of my husband Kree and daughter Nancy.

Betty Neuman, PhD, FAAN

FOREWORD

Several trends characterize the development of nursing knowledge as we approach the 21st century. First is the co-existence of numerous theories that guide nursing practice, second is the structuring of existing knowledge, third is the attention needed for critical global events and their influence on health, and fourth is the need to support critical thinking and critical judgment of members of the discipline. Dr. Betty Neuman provides the reader with rich discussions to support dialogues related to each of these trends as well as to support further progress in knowledge development.

Progress in knowledge development in any discipline requires that members of the discipline construct, describe, and explain aspects of reality within that discipline through theories. Progress in knowledge development is measured by the extent to which members of the discipline are able to articulate the urgent and central questions in the discipline and the extent to which members of the discipline can systematically answer these questions. The nature of the questions changes, reflecting progress in answering previous questions. Questions that occupied nurse scholars in the past were related to creating models as overall frameworks for nursing and its practice. Other questions followed related to the utility of these models in research, practice, teaching, and administration. To articulate future directions and agendas for knowledge development in nursing, existing knowledge needs to be articulated and integrated.

Dr. Neuman, using her model as a guideline, provides us with an integrated and coherent whole with a depiction of the model and its use for practice, education, administration, and research. Models are developed in disciplines to enhance understanding of phenomena across fields of study. This model is no exception. It is used in diverse clinical settings and this volume enables those who use the model to understand the experiences of diverse populations in different clinical settings. The experiences of clinicians, educators, and researchers as described in the various sections of this book should support collaboration among members of the discipline. As the readers visit the different chapters, they are treated to a vast array of approaches to interpreting the model in their work.

The value of this book is in its demonstration of the utility of the Neuman Systems Model in the discipline of nursing. More importantly, it is essential reading for nurses and health care professionals who have shared goals, as well as those who have different goals. For users of the Neuman System Model, it provides a reference group who share the same framework, language, mission, and goals. It also provides them with exemplars in how to use the model, as well as forces and constraints in its implementation. In addition, it provides the state of the art and science that emanate from this model. For those who are interested in knowledge development, it provides strategies that are used in structuring findings related to the use of a model as an exemplar for other models. It supplies the knowledge base to compare and contrast progress in different theories and models in nursing. This is a challenging example of foundational bases of nursing knowledge.

The book demonstrates how the model is used in different practice settings: teaching, administration, and research; and demonstrates the diversity of use of the model. By consolidating existing findings, applications, and extensions, Dr. Neuman invites a critical appraisal of her model. She provides the reader with the opportunity to experience the whole as she sees it.

As we approach the turn of the century, we are faced with significant trends that profoundly influence the entire fabric of our society in general, and our discipline in particular. Globalization, collaboration, complexity, diversity, and home care are areas that require our attention. These goals and concepts resonate in nursing, and drive the need to experiment with models that facilitate these trends, as well as models that are trend setters for quality health care. This volume acknowledges and affirms the visibility of the Neuman System Model as it reflects these trends.

This book will serve as the basis for many dialogues in practice, research, teaching, and consultation. It celebrates progress related to the Neuman Systems Model, provides readers with consolidated findings, and invites collaboration in the further development of the model.

Progress in the development of knowledge requires commitment of the community of scholars in shared missions and common goals. Over the years, Dr. Neuman has demonstrated persistence in the development of a framework that reflects nursing and its mission, and a framework that nurses can use. This volume is a demonstration of Dr. Neuman's commitment to knowledge development in nursing and her vigilance in continuing to revisit the model. Her vision, commitment, vigilance, and persistence are hallmarks to be emulated if we want to witness dramatic progress in the development of nursing knowledge.

As nurses become more comfortable using different theories to uncover, understand, and explain nursing phenomena, the need for volumes such as this becomes imperative. Students schooled in nursing theory and colleagues committed to structuring foundational bases of nursing may be inspired to use this book to create other similar volumes.

Afaf Ibrahim Meleis, RN, PhD, DrPs (Hon)

Section I

Systems and Nursing: Conceptualization of the Neuman Systems Model

1

THE NEUMAN SYSTEMS MODEL

Betty Neuman

Chapter 1 is a revision of formerly published information (found in the 1982 and 1989 book editions) that presents the Neuman Systems Model and how it relates to nursing and systems theory.

The model components are specifically related to the four accepted subconcepts of nursing: client, environment, health, and nursing. The model spiritual variable is further described in Appendix B of this book edition. Although initially developed as protection, the created environment ultimately may have a negative system outcome because of the unavailability of bound energy. Health promotion is described as to how it relates to the primary prevention concept.

The use of a family case study briefly explains the process of determining a nursing diagnosis with the Neuman Systems Model. All former aspects of the Neuman Systems Model, and those currently developed by the author, are included in this chapter.

I. Nursing and the Systems Perspective

THE BEGINNINGS

A new direction for nursing has, indeed, become evident: that is, a comprehensive "systems approach," as is increasingly reflected in the nursing literature.

Systems theory has the potential for development of a totally new posture toward professionalism. The nursing system will benefit, as have other scientific disciplines, through use of a systemic structure for better organization, specificity, and cohesion of its increasingly complex components. Nursing is beginning to take notice of the growing use of systems theory as an important organizing structure by other disciplines, particularly the business field.

As early as 1971, Hazzard identified the significance of systems for nursing in her statement that "General Systems Theory is a theory of organized complexity, where all the elements are in interaction. Such a theory can be utilized well in nursing. Nursing is a system because it consists of elements in interaction." (p. 383) The systems concept is increasingly used as a unifying force for scholarly exploration in various scientific fields. The major question still exists: Will the nursing profession fully recognize and accept the exciting potential for and inevitable challenge to develop its scientific professional base within the breadth of a systems perspective as relevant to emerging trends? New frontiers are possible for the profession through research validation of systems use in rapidly evolving practice roles.

The growing complexity of the nursing field demands that an organizational system be able to change as required while preserving and even enhancing its inherent character. The systems approach has the potential for such organization, while allowing the assimilation of new demands through adjustive processes, which are requisite if new qualities are to emerge. The following statement of Myrtle Aydelotte in 1972 is still valid:

> Nursing leadership must reorient itself and restructure itself in such a way that nursing education and practice are inseparable, are symbolic, and are united in purpose. We must put aside inertia, apathy, competitiveness, personal animosities, and censorship. We must restructure a set of social relationships which will enable society to receive that which it has charged us to provide. If we do not do this, society will surely place the charge they have given us elsewhere. Portions of nursing leadership, in resisting change, have boldly overlooked the fact that nursing as an occupation is a social institution and social institutions, many of long standing, are crumbling and changing today as a result of the reordering of priorities and of values and services by current day society.
>
> There is a great need to accelerate these progressive movements now occurring in nursing: "striking changes in levels of nursing practice; greater development of clinical specialization; and significant alterations in the reciprocal roles held by nurses and other health personnel, particularly the physicians." There is increasing evidence that these movements are responsive to what society wants and are the directions that society will support. (p. 23)

Rapid societal changes, with concomitant new creative expectations, roles, functions, and conditions, create stress areas for nursing practice. A great challenge for nursing will continue as the profession attempts to remain stable yet flexible enough to meet the action and reaction effects of both internal and external environmental demands. As nursing functions become more diversified and complex, the traditional linkages or structures that hold all of nursing together are being severely challenged. Thus, nursing professional inconsistencies need closure to prevent others from making their decisions for them. The profession has become a complex system, if measured only by its diversity of role and function. A systems perspective adds to our appreciation of the system's complexity and to the valuing of its parts. Portions of the domain of nursing can be dealt with either as organized wholes within the larger superstructure or as parts or subparts of the defined whole system.

For example, a nurse manager is concerned with the broad, all-encompassing domain, while a clinical nurse specialist gives priority of function to a specific area as a part or subpart of the larger system. Using this example, the roles and functions of both the clinical specialist and the manager would contribute to the development of new alliances, providing truly wholistic client care. Other examples could be provided of new alliances that benefit the nursing profession and that enhance both education and practice. A reorientation to the functional domain of nursing, with subsystems clearly defined, is required; we must view structurally the logical overall system within which nursing education and practice take place. After the boundaries of the larger system are established, the parts and subparts inherent within it must be clearly defined. The use of systems can help nursing define itself in relation to new health mandates and care reform issues, such as major emphasis on wellness and disease prevention.

As nursing roles and functions expand, they become more complex and comprehensive, and a broader structure will be required to encompass them. Expansiveness as a result of assimilation of change is a characteristic of the systems concept. Complex nursing phenomena can be placed within a logical and empirically valid open systems perspective; as the number of parts or subparts increases, the whole expands. Regardless of the size of an identified system, its boundaries, as well as the characteristics of the interrelating parts, must be defined for analysis and utilization. Now is the time to consider the reorganization and application of systems science and systems thinking for the field of nursing. With an expansive systems perspective as a nursing base, we must overlook neither system implications for nursing education, practice innovations, and scientific exploration, nor the crossing of interdisciplinary boundaries where cooperation and collaboration are requisites.

Banathy (1973, 174) acknowledged that solutions to increasingly more complex technological and social problems cannot be found with the thinking and tools of single analytically oriented disciplines. We have had to evolve a new way of thinking and a new approach to disciplined inquiry: systems science. Systems science has demonstrated its effectiveness in attacking highly complex and large-scale problems. It evolves models—constructed of systems concepts— that are applicable to several traditional fields of knowledge. It also develops strategies that can be applied to the solution of problems. The integration of systems concepts into our thinking leads us to acquire the systems view. The systems view enables us to think of ourselves, our environment, and the entities that surround us (and that we are a part of) in a new way. This new way of thinking can be applied to analysis, design or development, and management of systems for the solution of complex problems. To adapt systems thinking to nursing demands a high degree of flexibility that allows for much creativity. A great risk for the nursing profession lies in failing to measure up to the flexibility required by rapid societal changes and demands and instead maintaining a tragic semblance of stability through defensive rigidity. Maintenance of a quasi-homeostatic or stability state through use of the systems approach must also be guarded against.

For nursing to mature as a profession and expand through systems methods, a wide variety of creative approaches to client care must be examined. A possible beginning point might well be to rethink the two major components of nursing: education and practice. In the systems approach, the two are interdependent and mutually affected by environmental changes. The forming of a cooperative, collaborative relationship between these two interdependent parts of the system creates favorable conditions for enhancement of the system. The ability to form meaningful relationships is requisite for the growth of any system.

Inherent within the systems concept are guidelines for system enhancement and expansion; this feature is particularly significant to nursing, which is becoming an increasingly complex system within the general health care system. Some advantages of the use of systems in nursing are (1) the integration of systems concepts with nursing phenomena, leading to new perspectives for nursing, and (2) the clarification and definition of nursing knowledge related to the social sciences. This is congruent with Fawcett and Downs's (1986) assertion that theory and research hold promise of advancing nursing knowledge. Orem (1971) also believes that a general concept of nursing is essential for knowledge production within the field since an adequate general concept of nursing makes explicit the proper object of the profession.

In the change process a stress-war is always being waged between the rigidity required to retain valued elements of the past and the uncertainty and flexibility required for new structures to emerge. Lazlo (1972) believes that without synthesis of the items of knowledge held valid in a society, neither individual nor long-term purposes can be identified or rationally pursued. Inherent in nursing, as within any other system, are factors for either maintenance or growth through change, as illustrated in the conceptualization below.

	Maintenance	**Growth**	
Rigidity and maintenance	⎧ Safety ⎪ Security ⎨ Certainty ⎪ Familiarity ⎩ Rigidity	Risk ⎫ Anxiety ⎪ Uncertainty ⎬ Difference ⎪ Flexibility ⎭	Flexibility and change

The more complex the nursing system becomes, the more difficult it is to maintain the status quo, and the greater is the need for a viable organizational structure that can maintain relative stability during the process of change. As the boundaries of nursing roles and functions continue to broaden or expand, paradoxically nursing is gaining freedom to assert itself, while simultaneously increasing its need for a valid organizational base or structure.

Implicit in the goal of attaining stability through use of systems is the risk of coordination and control to a degree that limits the flexibility necessary for adjusting the nursing system to the changing environment, thus producing a closed rather than the desired open system. An open system is one in which there is a continuous flow of input and process, output and feedback. Miller (1965) defines dimensions of the system as follows:

- Structure refers to the arrangement of parts and subparts of a system at any given point in time.
- Process and function refer to matter, energy, and information exchanges with interaction between the parts and subparts. . . . [L]iving systems are open systems and a steady state exists when the composition of a system is relatively constant despite continuous exchanges between the system and its environment.

THE DEVELOPMENT

Within the systems approach is the potential for self-determinative, creative, and adjustive effects in relation to internal and external environmental stressors imposed upon nursing, and a tangible structure within which change can safely take place. Although some alteration in the conception of and approaches to nursing is inherent in the use of the systems approach, the requisite structure allowing for flexibility exists for meeting the challenge of tomorrow's new nursing posture. In systems thinking, the "whole" is the structure; sharing is the function.

Discovering order is a major challenge of the systems approach. Florence Nightingale could well have been the first pioneer in systems thinking for nursing when she demanded that nursing laws be discovered and defined (Riehl and Roy, 1974). In determining these laws, we must carefully consider nursing as a rapidly evolving system. Ashby (1972) notes that we must treat systems as wholes composed of related parts between which interaction occurs. In analyzing the system, nursing could use general systems theory, defined by Klir (1972) as a collection of concepts, principles, tools, problems, methods, and techniques associated with systems.

The whole of nursing as a system must be clearly identified with boundaries defined before its parts can be properly analyzed. Then we can identify the interacting parts or subparts and their relationship to the whole system. The ways in which the combination of interacting system parts form the structure of the whole is significant.

The organization of nursing in relation to systems thinking may be classified as follows. The health care system is the larger system; it includes the field of nursing. The field of nursing includes two major components: nursing education and practice. Nursing education and practice contain many subparts, with specialized areas of concern.

By considering systemically specific interactions occurring within as well as among each of the parts and subparts, we can deal appropriately with the constraints the environment places on nursing, thus assuring that the profession meets its commitment both to the client and to the larger client system. Accelerated development and integration of nursing as a science can take place within the context of such an organized yet flexible structure. As a whole system, nursing must have a reciprocal relationship with the environment of the larger health care system and with the larger social system surrounding it, while sharing with the parts and subparts of its own smaller system. For example, nursing as a component of the health care system is related to other disciplines with the common goal of maintaining the integrity of the client/client system. The actions of nursing affect the health care system and in turn are affected by it. These sharing relationships of parts or subparts of the health care system represent a type of interdependency and accountability requisite for optimal system functioning and, in fact, for the evolutionary survival of the whole system.

The concept of "system"—something consisting of interacting components—is not limited and can apply to any defined whole. It is relevant to nursing in dealing with varied client system interrelationships, because the same terms and principles can be applied to facts in either system parts or the whole. Since the systems concept of organization or structure and process is of such major importance, it is surprising that the nursing profession has yet to subscribe to it without reservation. A clear conception of systems organization requires skill in viewing client situations abstractly. That is, client system boundaries and related variables may lose some clarity because they are dynamic and constantly changing, presenting different appearances according to time, place, and the significance of events. The uniqueness of the characteristic response of each system part implies that each must be studied and understood at its own level if we are to understand its significance in relationships and to the stability of the whole systems organization. Dunn (1961) describes the state of wellness as the integration of social, cultural, psychological, and biological functioning in a manner that is oriented to maximize the potential capabilities of the identified system. Components of a system, from a wholistic viewpoint, are not significantly connected except with reference to the whole. A system, then, can be defined as a pervasive order that holds together its parts. With this definition, nursing can readily be conceptualized as a complete whole with identifiable smaller wholes or parts. The whole structure is maintained by interrelationships of system components, through regulations that evolve out of the dynamics of the open system. As increasing organization becomes automatic in the course of development, regulations are ideally compensatory to system internal and external feedback.

The open systems concept increases understanding and has far-reaching implications for nursing; it provides an important working hypothesis for the development of new insights and statements for verification of new theoretical perspectives. The open systems concept, with possibilities inherent for stability, has been found to be increasingly relevant particularly to the sciences, contributing greatly to the expansion of scientific theory. The systems concept has significant potential for nursing, simultaneously representing both a great challenge and an opportunity as we move into the 21st century of evolving health care reform.

THE FULFILLMENT

For professional nursing to grow and expand, to become relevant to rapidly changing social demands, and to best articulate its future direction, it must subscribe to a broadly based organizing structure. The unifying effects of a systems approach should adequately provide the necessary structure for relatedness within the nursing field and point the way for discovery of commonalities and cooperative relationships with other health disciplines, while allowing nursing to declare emphatically its unique professional profile. Since systems terminology is understood by all health professions, important interdisciplinary sharing and communication should improve significantly.

In contrast to past mechanistic views in science is the newer concern with wholeness, dynamic interaction, and organization. Working terms derived from general systems usage such as *wholeness, order, differentiation, goal directedness, stressors, stability,* and *feedback* are homologous to nursing concepts. Principles and terminology can be readily transferred from one field to another, having a unifying effect on all the sciences. The trend toward cooperative interdisciplinary alliances is becoming increasingly clear.

New insights and principles for professional nursing are possible as new areas amenable to research and resolution are discovered. Valid, realistic, and operational systems principles can advance nursing toward becoming a scientific discipline bearing a new professional image. The systems perspective points the way for nursing to discover its own uniqueness, which lies in the way it organizes and uses knowledge rather than in its fund of knowledge per se. The use of systems should help clarify how the bridge is made between knowledge and nursing action; it should identify which nursing actions are beneficial to the client and should support research efforts toward the development of a science of nursing.

The staggering yet noble movement toward professionalism in nursing is at best arduous, prolonged, and often divisive; however, new tools are being acquired to meet this continuous and provocative challenge. Nurse theorists continue to expand their conceptual model components to include a more wholistic perspective. The rapid acceleration of model usage, a significant development for organizing nursing phenomena, is the precursor of the development of the profession into a recognized scientific discipline. The systems perspective offers new hope for those who seek professionalism in nursing and provides a basis for continued creativity in relatively unexplored arenas made possible by worldwide evolving health reform issues and opportunities.

For example, the relevancy of the Neuman Systems Model increases as the practice of nursing moves to the community. The client's environment is no longer controlled by nursing; thus, it becomes a necessity rather than an option to view the client as part of other systems, such as the family. The model's wide international acceptance and utility have much to do with its ease in crossing cultural boundaries as other countries increasingly program for wholistic client care.

The model will have future flexibility to incorporate the Neuman concept of caring—caregiving that includes empathy, acceptance, and continuity in cooperation with other scientific disciplines.

II. The Neuman Systems Model and the Systems Perspective

The basic task of nursing in using wholistic perspectives is the systemic study of the abstract characteristics of the client, the family, and the community, with the precise, comprehensive analysis of the relations in space and time on which they largely depend.

The Neuman Systems Model fits well with the wholistic concept of optimizing a dynamic yet stable interrelationship of spirit, mind, and body of the client in a constantly changing environment and society (Neuman and Young, 1972). It joins the World Health organization mandate for the year 2000, seeking unity in wellness states—wellness of spirit, mind, body, and environment. The Neuman Systems Model is also in accord with the views of the American Nursing Association, sharing its concern about potential stressors and its emphasis on primary prevention as well as world health care reform concern for preventing illness.

Wholism, implicit within the Neuman Systems Model, is both a philosophical and a biological concept, implying relationships and processes arising from wholeness, dynamic freedom, and creativity in adjusting to stressors in the internal and the external environments. Using a wholistic systems approach to both protect and promote client welfare, nursing action must be skillfully related to the meaningful and dynamic organization of the various parts and subparts of the whole affecting the client. The various interrelationships of the parts and subparts must be appropriately identified and analyzed before relevant nursing action can be taken. A system implies dynamic energy exchange, moving either toward or away from stability, which has a direct relationship to outcome predictability.

Basically, nursing functions within accepted, familiar, and often singular concepts. It is now imperative that the profession articulate its function within a comprehensive structure. That is, we must conceptualize nursing action in wellness–illness and organization–disorganization states more broadly. Consideration of a more broadly based organizing structure will help facilitate the professional goal of enabling clients to move toward optimal wellness in any setting.

The opposing systems concepts of entropy and negentropy, or evolution, describe the action of system energy flow. Energy moves either toward extinction (entropy), by gradual disorganization, increasing randomness, and energy dissipation, or toward evolution (negentropy), as a system absorbing energy to increase its organization, complexity, and development as it moves toward a steady or wellness state. A continuous dynamism and energy flow implicit within the systems concept adequately provide the most tangible structure within which the plethora of phenomena in nursing can meet its desired goal of protecting client/client system integrity.

The systems approach permits a reorientation to a scientific thinking approach to studying people. Ludwig von Bertalanffy (1968) finds that a different image of the person in society is needed. That is, the client must be considered an unlimited entity with an active personality system, whose evolution follows principles, symbolism, and systemic organizations, and it is not always possible to see the potential expansions of this entity and the ramifications of its actions.

The open systems approach begins by identifying and mapping repeated cycles of input, process, and output (which serves as feedback for further input); these cycles comprise the dynamic organizational pattern. Such a system is never at rest; rather, it tends to move cyclically toward differentiation and elaboration for further growth and survival of the organism. The Neuman Systems Model is an open systems model that views nursing as being primarily concerned with defining appropriate action in stress-related situations or in possible reactions of the client/client system; since environmental exchanges are reciprocal, both client and environment may be positively or negatively affected by each other.

I agree with Heslin (1986) that a revitalization occurs when an open system achieves stability in an equifinal process. She considers every restorative process and reconstitution following a reaction, interaction, and intervention to be the reestablishment of an equifinal steady state. She relates system output to the end product of the process and also sees it as input to further cycles, resulting in a redefined pattern of stability. Based on open systems theory, client variables are interrelated and organized in various patterns that serve as sources of system input and output alike. Her view, like mine (Neuman 1982, 8), that processed input provides output as feedback for further input, creating an organized pattern within the open system, supports the open systems theory of both Bertalanffy's (1968) and Lazarus' (1981) systemic views.

Arlene Putt (1978) identified that application of general systems theory is well suited to the assessment of client needs, the development of nursing care plans, and the determination of nursing actions. Believing the assessment of client needs for nursing to be the first step in providing professional nursing care, she found that, guided by systems models, one can more easily achieve a desired level or quality of nursing care.

According to the Neuman Systems Model and systemic perspective in general, health and wellness is defined as the condition or the degree of system stability, that is, the condition in which all parts and subparts (variables) are in balance or harmony with the whole of the client/client system. The client is an interacting open system in total interface with both internal and external environmental forces or stressors; the client is in constant change, with reciprocal environmental interaction, at all times moving either toward a dynamic state of stability or wellness or toward one of illness in varying degrees. Health is reflected in the level of wellness: when system needs are met, a state of optimal wellness exists. Conversely, unmet needs reduce the client wellness condition.

The consideration of environment is critical, since health and wellness vary as to the needs, predisposition, perception, and goals of all identifiable systems; environment is that viable arena that has relevance to the life space of the system, including a *created environment.* Environment has been generally conceptualized as all factors affecting and affected by the system. Putt (1972) considers variables inherent in the client's adaptation to the environment. She feels that as each system impinges upon another, it articulates with that system, and the relationship of both is changed.

A tendency exists within any system to maintain a steady state or balance among the various disruptive forces operating within or upon it. The Neuman Systems Model identifies these forces as stressors, which may have either a positive or negative outcome effect. Both possible reaction and actual reaction with identifiable symptoms may be mitigated through appropriate early interventions. The Neuman Model diagram identifies the *flexible line of defense* as determining whether or not a reaction might be likely to take place in an encounter with a stressor (Neuman, 1974). The ideal is to strengthen this protective mechanism, preventing or reducing a possible stressor reaction, or doing both. A dynamic stability state can exist within the system along the *internal lines of resistance,* following a reaction to a stressor. However, a violent energy flow occurs when a system is disrupted from its normal or stable state; that is, it expends energy to cope with disorganization. When more energy is used by the system in its state of disorganization than is built and stored, the outcome may be death. The degree of wellness is determined by the amount of energy required to return to and maintain system stability. When more energy is available than is being used, the system is stable. Putt (1972) believes that the two processes, entropy and evolution, can be assessed by the nurse in the clinical setting and that assessment can be utilized as a guide for determining appropriate intervention. Nursing intervention, then, is directed toward counteracting entropy with a form of evolutionary system adjustment in retaining, restoring, and/or maintaining a degree of stability between and among client system variables and environmental stressors, based on energy conservation.

Critical to system analysis is the identification of stressors as to type, time of encounter, and nature of a reaction or possible reaction to them. They may have a positive outcome, with the potential for beneficial temporary or even ultimate system change. For example, in an avoidance condition such as agoraphobia, anxiety may be clinically imposed as a stressor for the possible longer-term gain of mitigating the phobia, allowing for higher-level functioning. Various conditions and constraints accompany stressors. For example, a stressor may create a series of effects in more than one part or subpart of the client system and in response to these effects may itself in turn be affected. Stability implies a state of balance or harmony requiring energy exchange between the system and environment to cope adequately with imposing stressors, whether the goal is to retain, attain, or maintain system integrity. Primary, secondary, and tertiary prevention as intervention acts as a typology for nursing intervention to retain, attain, or maintain system balance.

Emery (1969) states that in adapting to its environment, an open system will attempt to cope with external environmental stressors by ingesting them or acquiring control over them for survival purposes. At the simplest level, a steady state, governed by a dynamic interaction of parts and subparts, is one of stability over time. This is analogous to the Neuman Systems Model concept of the normal line of defense; at more complex levels, a steady state preserves the character of the system through growth and expansion. As a system becomes progressively more organized, conditions of regulation or constraints become more complex. For example, as social organizations increase, their roles become more specialized in function. The process of development, evolution, and increasing order are beyond homeostasis or stability, just as the lack of development results in regression to lesser states and ultimately to extinction. Gray et al. (1969) find Menninger's notion of a continuum—that there is a circular motion in all living activity, regardless of limitation—highly useful. Examples may be the cycle of wellness to illness to wellness again or the balance process of homeostatic and heterostatic mechanisms.

Homeostasis (stability) preserves the character of the system. An adjustment in one direction is countered by a movement in the opposite direction, both movements being approximately rather than precisely compensatory. With opposing forces in effect, the process of stability is an example of the regulatory capacity of a system. Feedback of output into input makes the system self-regulated in relation to either maintenance of a desired health state or goal outcome. For example, much research is needed to determine client health status by identification of compensatory actions among one or more system variables. Interaction of parts can fuse the client/environment into a unit relationship as a system. Health, within a systemic perspective, is viewed as a continuum from wellness to illness. The end-states are opposites: wellness is a state of saturation or inertness, one free of disrupting needs; illness is a state of insufficiency with disrupting needs unsatisfied.

A system receives suitable satisfaction only by interacting with the available environment in order to take on its parts for fulfillment of survival needs. Energy flow is continuous between the client and the environment even when a relatively stable state is maintained. The Neuman Systems Model paradigm of wellness to illness on a continuum (Figure 1–1) reflects an open system; movement toward energy depletion (entropy) signals closure of the system as available energy fails to sustain life. This is in accord with the generally accepted definition of *entropy:* "increase in entropy with change signifies a reduced amount of available energy." Nursing acts to conserve energy to impede or arrest movement toward the entropic (illness) state and to facilitate movement toward the negentropic (wellness) state.

The whole system is bound by the available environment and constraints, whether they be nursing, the client, or other systems, as illustrated in Figure 1–2. A first constructive step in conceptualizing a system is to analyze processes occurring within the arbitrarily defined system. The next step is to relate wholes to their environment. A system is defined when its parts or subparts can be organized into an interrelating whole. Although organization is logical, structural differences may exist from system to system. The implied concept of wholistic organization is one of keeping parts intact or stable in their intimate relationships. The nature and number of parts and their relationships determine the complexity of the system. Both systems processes and nursing actions are purposeful and goal directed. That is, nursing vigorously attempts to control vari-

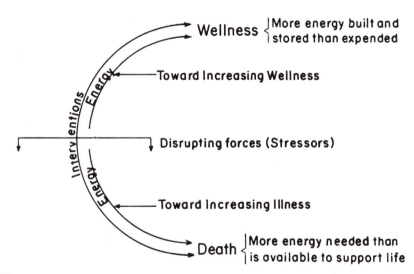

Figure 1–1. Neuman Systems Model paradigm of the wellness–illness continuum.

ables affecting client care, for example, toward the general improvement of client system capability or performance, better adjustment of behavior patterns, or perhaps better skill performance of a specific task. An inherent danger in the use of a systems model is oversimplification, especially when the phenomena and definition of entities under consideration are very complex. When used correctly, however, a systems model dramatically and convincingly demonstrates the nature of a process, which leads to better understanding and more accurate prediction.

Inherent in all systems are structure and dynamic organization, principles and laws, and terms affecting the constraints of their environments. Bertalanffy (1968) describes general systems theory as consisting of the scientific exploration of "wholes" and "wholeness." The interdisciplinary nature of concepts, models, and principles applying to systems provides a logical approach toward the unification of science. Beckstrand (1980) suggests furthering development of nursing knowledge by rigorous application of the methods of science, ethics, and philosophy to problems encountered in the professional experience of nurses. Since conceptual models represent reality, they are basic to any attempt at theory development. A model facilitates deductions from premises, explanations, and predictions, often with unexpected results. Oakes (1978) believes that general systems theory will prove to be the step toward the ultimate goal of improvement in the quality of client care. As nursing continues to use systems components knowledgeably over time, to the benefit of the client/client system, it should evolve into a logically defensible, wholistic, and scientific discipline.

The intent of the Neuman Systems Model or conceptual framework is to set forth a structure that depicts the parts and subparts and their interrelationship for the whole of the client as a complete system. The same fundamental idea or concept would apply equally well to a small group or community, a larger aggregate, or even the universe. The model provides the structure, organization,

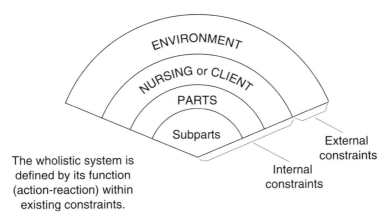

The wholistic system is defined by its function (action-reaction) within existing constraints.

Figure 1–2. Nursing or client, or both, in the wholistic system.

and direction for nursing action, and is flexible enough to deal adequately with the client's infinite complexity. Putt (1972) describes the concept of "living systems" as open to their environment, freely interchanging energy and information with surrounding matter, maintaining themselves, and seeking a steady state while existing in an interlocking hierarchy ranging in size from cosmic to microscopic.

III. The Neuman Systems Model for Nursing

The health care delivery system is becoming so complex that models are indispensable, providing needed structure and direction for information processing and goal-directed activities. Because of its broad, comprehensive wholistic and systemic approach to the client/client system, the utility of the Neuman Systems Model has been proven in a wide variety of nursing education and practice settings. Though the model as diagrammed in Figure 1–3 illustrates the client as an individual, it can be equally well applied to a group or larger community, or even to a social issue. The model was designed to be used in nursing, but it is appropriate for other health disciplines as well. The list of model definitions in Appendix A can be readily understood by caregivers in all health disciplines.

The Neuman Systems Model has the potential for unifying various health-related theories, clarifying the relationships of variables in nursing care and role definition. Use of the model can clarify role definition at various levels of nursing practice. Nursing practice goals should enable the client in creating and shaping reality in a desired direction, related to retention, attainment, or maintenance of optimal client system wellness, or a combination of these, through purposeful interventions. Nursing interventions should mitigate or reduce stress factors and adverse conditions that affect or could affect optimal client functioning at any given point in time. Specific "tools" for model implementation have been designed and tested (Tables 1–1 and 1–2). Both the Neuman Nursing Process and the Prevention as Intervention Formats were designed to implement the model by incorporating its terminology and satisfying the model's breadth of purpose.

A great need exists to clarify and make explicit not only the relationship of variables affecting a client during and following an illness, but also those variables related to ambulatory and evolving high-risk groups. Since health care focus is shifting increasingly toward primary prevention (including health promotion), an understanding of how these variables interface with those of secondary and tertiary prevention is important. These relationships are illustrated in

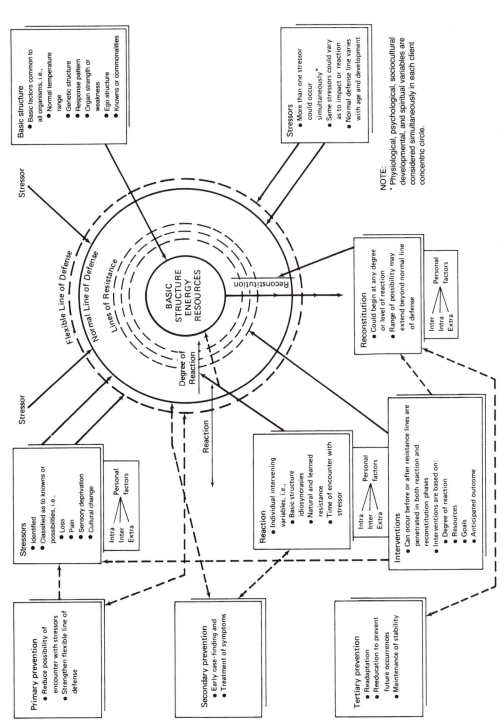

Figure 1–3. The Neuman Systems Model. *Original diagram copyright © 1970 by Betty Neuman.*

TABLE 1–1. THE NEUMAN NURSING PROCESS FORMAT

Nursing Diagnosis		

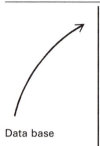
 	
Data base
	Variances from wellness are determined by correlations and constraints
	
	Hypothetical interventions are determined for prescriptive change
		I. Nursing diagnosis
		  A. Data base—determined by
		    1. Identification and evaluation of potential or actual stressors that pose a threat to the stability of the client/client systems.
		    2. Assessment of condition and strength of basic structure factors and energy resources.
		    3. Assessment of characteristics of the flexible and normal lines of defense, lines of resistance, degree of potential reaction, reaction, and/or potential for reconstitution following a reaction.
		    4. Identification, classification, and evaluation of potential and/or actual intra-, inter-, and extrapersonal interactions between the client and environment, considering all five variables.
		    5. Evaluation of influence of past, present, and possible future life process and coping patterns on client system stability.
		    6. Identification and evaluation of actual and potential internal and external resources for optimal state of wellness.
		    7. Identification and resolution of perceptual differences between caregivers and client/client system.
		    Note: In all of the above areas of consideration the caregiver simultaneously considers five variables (dynamic interactions in the client/client system)—physiological, psychological, sociocultural, developmental, and spiritual.
		  B. Variances from wellness—determined by
		    1. Synthesis of theory with client data to identify the condition from which a comprehensive diagnostic statement can be made. Goal prioritization is determined by client/client system wellness level, system stability needs, and total available resources to accomplish desired goal outcomes.
		    2. Hypothetical goals and interventions postulated to reach the desired client stability or wellness level, that is, to maintain the normal line of defense and retain the flexible line of defense, thus protecting the basic structure.

TABLE 1–1. (Continued)

Nursing Goals

Caregiver-client/client system negotiation for prescriptive change

Caregiver intervention strategies negotiated to retain, attain, and maintain client/client system stability

II. Nursing goals—determined by
  A. Negotiations with the client for desired prescriptive change or goal outcomes to correct variances from wellness, based on classified needs and resources identified in the nursing diagnosis.
  B. Appropriate prevention as intervention strategies are negotiated with the client for retention, attainment, and/or maintenance of client system stability as desired outcome goals. Theoretical perspectives used for assessment and client data synthesis are analogous to those used for intervention.

Nursing Outcomes

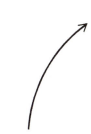

Nursing intervention using one or more prevention modes

Confirmation of prescriptive change or reformulation of nursing goals

Short-term goal outcomes influence intermediate and long-range goal determination

Client outcome validates nursing process and acts as feedback for further system input as required

III. Nursing outcomes—determined by
  A. Nursing intervention accomplished through use of one or more of three prevention modes:
    1. Primary prevention (action to retain system stability)
    2. Secondary prevention (action to attain system stability)
    3. Tertiary prevention (action to maintain system stability), usually following secondary prevention as intervention
  B. Evaluation of outcome goals following intervention either confirms them or serves as a basis for reformulation of subsequent goals based on systemic feedback principles.
  C. Intermediate and long-range goals for subsequent nursing action are structured in relation to short-term goal outcomes.
  D. Client goal outcome validates the nursing process.

the Neuman Systems Model diagram (Figure 1–3). The model is explained in relation to an individual client as a system, subject to the impact of environmental stressors, although as mentioned above, its concepts are equally applicable to groups of any size. The following former basic assumptions (Neuman, 1974, 101) inherent within the Neuman Systems Model may also be viewed as propositions:

TABLE 1–2. FORMAT FOR PREVENTION AS INTERVENTION

Nursing Action		
Primary Prevention	*Secondary Prevention*	*Tertiary Prevention*
1. Classify stressors that threaten stability of the client/client system. Prevent stressor invasion.	1. Following stressor invasion, protect basic structure.	1. During reconstitution, attain and maintain maximum level of wellness or stability following treatment.
2. Provide information to retain or strengthen existing client/client system strengths.	2. Mobilize and optimize internal/external resources to attain stability and energy conservation.	2. Educate, reeducate, and/or reorient as needed.
3. Support positive coping and functioning.	3. Facilitate purposeful manipulation of stressors and reactions to stressors.	3. Support client/client system toward appropriate goals.
4. Desensitize existing or possible noxious stressors.	4. Motivate, educate, and involve client/client system in health care goals.	4. Coordinate and integrate health service resources.
5. Motivate toward wellness.	5. Facilitate appropriate treatment and intervention measures.	5. Provide primary and/or secondary preventive intervention as required.
6. Coordinate and integrate interdisciplinary theories and epidemiological input.	6. Support positive factors toward wellness.	
7. Educate or reeducate.	7. Promote advocacy by coordination and integration.	
8. Use stress as a positive intervention strategy	8. Provide primary preventive intervention as required.	

Note: A first priority for nursing action in each of the areas of prevention as intervention is to determine the nature of stressors and their threat to the client/client system. Some general categorical functions for nursing action are initiation, planning, organization, monitoring, coordinating, implementing, integrating, advocating, supporting, and evaluating. An example of a limited classification system for stressors is illustrated by the following four categories: (1) deprivation, (2) excess, (3) change, and (4) intolerance.
Copyright © 1980 by Betty Neuman. Revised 1987 by Betty Neuman.

1. Although each individual client or group as a client system is unique, each system is a composite of common known factors or innate characteristics within a normal, given range of response contained within a basic structure.
2. Many known, unknown, and universal environmental stressors exist. Each differs in its potential for disturbing a client's usual stability level, or normal line of defense. The particular interrela-

tionships of client variables—physiological, psychological, socio-cultural, developmental, and spiritual—at any point in time can affect the degree to which a client is protected by the flexible line of defense against possible reaction to a single stressor or a combination of stressors.

3. Each individual client/client system has evolved a normal range of response to the environment that is referred to as a normal line of defense, or usual wellness/stability state. It represents change over time through coping with diverse stress encounters. The normal line of defense can be used as a standard from which to measure health deviation.

4. When the cushioning, accordion-like effect of the flexible line of defense is no longer capable of protecting the client/client system against an environmental stressor, the stressor breaks through the normal line of defense. The interrelationships of variables—physiological, psychological, sociocultural, developmental, and spiritual—determine the nature and degree of system reaction or possible reaction to the stressor.

5. The client, whether in a state of wellness or illness, is a dynamic composite of the interrelationships of variables—physiological, psychological, sociocultural, developmental, and spiritual. Wellness is on a continuum of available energy to support the system in an optimal state of system stability.

6. Implicit within each client system are internal resistance factors known as lines of resistance, which function to stabilize and return the client to the usual wellness state (normal line of defense) or possibly to a higher level of stability following an environmental stressor reaction.

7. Primary prevention relates to general knowledge that is applied in client assessment and intervention in identification and reduction or mitigation of possible or actual risk factors associated with environmental stressors to prevent possible reaction. The goal of health promotion is included in primary prevention.

8. Secondary prevention relates to symptomatology following a reaction to stressors, appropriate ranking of intervention priorities, and treatment to reduce their noxious effects.

9. Tertiary prevention relates to the adjustive processes taking place as reconstitution begins and maintenance factors move the client back in a circular manner toward primary prevention.

10. The client as a system is in dynamic, constant energy exchange with the environment.

Although recent trends reveal that nurse theorists have increasingly added systems components to their models, initially they predominantly viewed man collectively or the person singularly as a behavioral composite, a biological system, an organism at a particular stage of development, or part of an interactive process. The Neuman Systems Model, being wholistic, has always considered all these factors simultaneously and comprehensively within a systems perspective. That is, the client is viewed as a composite of interacting variables—physiological, psychological, developmental, sociocultural, and spiritual—that are, ideally, either functioning harmoniously or stable in relation to both internal and external environmental stressor influences. This approach to the client/client system prevents possible fragmentation and failure to interrelate various aspects of the client system as the nursing goal becomes that of facilitating optimal client system stability.

The Neuman Systems Model, a conceptual framework for nursing, is considered predominantly wellness-oriented or wholistically focused by its author; theoretically, the model is related to Gestalt, stress, and dynamically organized systems theories (deChardin, 1955; Cornu, 1957; Edelson, 1970; Selye, 1950). It is based on stress and reaction or possible reaction to stressors within the total environment of the defined client as a system. The client as a system represents an "individual," a "person," or "man." The client system may also represent more than one person in environmental interaction, for example, in groups of various sizes (i.e., family, community, or a social issue). The model components are equally applicable to narrowly defined systems and to those defined as broadly as situations dictate, that is, ranging from one client as a system to the global community as a system. What is defined or included within the boundary of the system must have relevance to nursing and represent the reality of its domain of concern.

The purpose of the model is to help nurses organize the nursing field within a broad systems perspective as a logical way of dealing with its growing complexity. Earlier, the model was criticized as being too broad; now this quality has become a major reason for increasing acceptance of the model and its proven utility.

The Neuman Systems Model is based on the two major components: stress and the reaction to stress. That is, the client is an open system in interaction and total interface with the environment. Using the model and systems terminology, the client is a system capable of both input and output related to intra-, inter-, and extrapersonal environmental influences, interacting with the environment by adjusting to it, or as a system, adjusting the environment to itself. The process of interaction and adjustment results in varying degrees of harmony, stability, or balance between the client and environment. Ideally, there is optimal client system stability.

Stressors are defined as tension-producing stimuli with the potential for causing system instability. For example, stressors may be present in situational or maturational crises, whether or not experienced as such by the client. As is implicit in the above interaction adjustment process, using the Neuman Model, variables contained within the flexible line of defense would ideally protect the client system from possible instability caused by stressors. Determining factors would include the client's physiologic condition, sociocultural influences, developmental state, cognitive skills, and spiritual considerations. It is important to view the whole client concept as dealing not with one or a few of these variables, but rather with all variables affecting the client at any given point in time. The whole-ness concept is based on appropriate consideration of the interrelationships of variables, which determine the amount of resistance an individual has to any environmental stressors, whether or not a reaction has occurred.

ENVIRONMENTAL STRESSORS

Stressors are tension-producing stimuli or forces occurring within both the internal and external environmental boundaries of the client/client system. More than one stressor may be imposed upon the client at any given time. According to Gestalt theory, any stressor to some degree influences the client's reaction to all other stressors.

Using the model terminology, environmental stressors are classified as intra-, inter-, and extrapersonal in nature. That is, they are present within as well as outside the client system in terms of the following environmental stressor typology:

- *Intrapersonal stressors:* Internal environmental forces occurring within the boundary of the client/client system (for example, conditioned response or autoimmune response).
- *Interpersonal stressors:* External environmental interaction forces occurring outside the boundaries of the client/client system at proximal range (for example, between one or more role expectations or communication patterns).
- *Extrapersonal stressors:* External environmental interaction forces occurring outside the boundaries of the client/client system at distal range (for example, between one or more social policies or financial concerns).
- Stressors have potential for reaction with the client or can cause a reaction with defined symptoms, and can influence reconstitution following treatment of symptoms. The time of stressor occurrence, past and present condition of the client, nature and intensity of the stressor, and the amount of energy required by the client to adjust are all important considerations. The caregiver may be able to predict possible client adjustment based on past coping behavior or patterns in a similar situation, all conditions being equal. Coping has a strong correlation to both client perception and cognition. Cognitive appraisal determines the degree of stress felt, while coping functions mediate (Lazarus, 1981). Although stressors are considered basically inert, client encounter will determine either a beneficial or noxious outcome.

The author presents the Neuman Systems Model for nursing as unique in that the profession is concerned with all variables affecting a client's possible or actual response to stressors. The purpose of the model is to provide a unifying focus for approaching a wide range of nursing concerns and for understanding basic nursing phenomena: the client and the environment. The model is dynamic because it is based on the client's continuous relationship to environmental stress factors, which have potential for causing a reaction, or obvious symptomatic reaction to stress, or could affect reconstitution following treatment of a stress reaction. Though it is designed to be used by nursing, it is readily applicable to other health professions. It is not in conflict with existing nursing models; rather, it has proven to be complementary and to encompass them because of its broad, comprehensive systemic wholistic perspective. It is easily implemented cross-culturally.

Theoretically, the Neuman Systems Model has some similarity to Gestalt theory, which implies that each client/client system is surrounded by a perceptual field that is in dynamic equilibrium. It also relates to field theories endorsing the molar view that all parts of the system are intimately interrelated and interdependent (Edelson, 1970). Emphasis is placed on the total organization of the field. In the wholistic Neuman Systems Model the organization of the field or system considers (1) the occurrence of stressors, (2) the reaction or possible reaction of the client to stressors, and (3) the particular client as a system, taking into consideration the simultaneous effects of the interacting variables—physiological, psychological, sociocultural, developmental, and spiritual. This is similar to Gestalt theorists' view of insight as the perception of relationships in a total situation.

Chardin (1955) and Cornu (1957) suggest that in all dynamically organized systems the properties of a part are determined to an extent by the wholes that contain it. This means that no part can be considered in isolation; each must be viewed as part of the whole. The single part influences our perception of the whole, and the patterns or features of the whole influence our awareness of each system part.

IV. The Neuman Systems Model

The Neuman Systems Model (see Figure 1–3) presents a comprehensive systems-based conceptual framework for nursing. It represents the client within the systems perspective wholistically and multidimensionally. It illustrates the composite of five interacting variables—physiological, psychological, sociocultural, developmental, and spiritual—ideally functioning harmoniously or stably in relation to internal and external environmental stressor influences upon the client, as a system, at a given point in time.

It is considered a wellness model by its author; wellness retention and optimal client/client system wellness attainment and maintenance are major considerations in its use.

The model is based on the concepts of stress and the reaction to stress. As defined, a system acts as a boundary for a single client, a group, and even a number of groups; it can also be defined for a social issue. The client system delineates the domain of nursing concern. The conceptual model, employing a systems-based perspective, explains how system stability is achieved in relation to stressors imposed upon it. The main nursing goal is to facilitate optimal wellness for the client through retention, attainment, or maintenance of client system stability. Optimal wellness represents the greatest possible degree of system stability at a given point in time. Thus, wellness is a matter of degree, a point on a continuum running from greatest negentropy (degree of wellness) to maximum entropy (see Figure 1–1).

Nursing action or intervention is based on a synthesis of comprehensive client data and relevant theory that is appropriate to the client's perception of need and is related to functional competence or possibility within the client's environmental context (see Table 1–1).

The outer boundary for the client as a system is designated by the protective flexible line of defense. The basic structure is similarly protected by lines of resistance. Moreover, a functionally interactive relationship exists jointly among all lines of defense and resistance, as each line individually contains the five system variables and protects the system components pertaining to it. Input, output, and feedback across these boundary lines (environmental exchanges) provide corrective action to change, enhance, and stabilize the system, with the goal of achieving the optimal wellness level.

The point of entry into the health care system for both the client and caregiver is either predominantly at the primary prevention level (before a reaction to stressors has occurred), at the secondary prevention level (after a stressor reaction has occurred), or at the tertiary prevention level (following treatment of a stressor reaction). The prevention-as-intervention format or modes (Table 1–2; also Figures 1–8, 1–9, and 1–10) act as a typology that not only identifies the entry point condition for the client into the health care system, but also indicates the general type of intervention or action required. This intervention modality allows for multilevel intervention, since more than one of the prevention-as-intervention modes can be used simultaneously, as the client condition warrants.

For further purposes of clarity, the Neuman Systems Model (see Figure 1–3) has been segmented into the four major nursing concepts or subcomponents accepted for the domain of nursing: man, environment, health, and nursing. Man is termed *client* or *client system* because of respect for newer client–caregiver collaborative relationships, and wellness perspectives of the model. For the purposes of reader clarity, the model will be explained in terms of the above four nursing concepts related to the complementary segmented portions of the Neuman Systems Model diagram as illustrated in Figures 1–4 to 1–7.

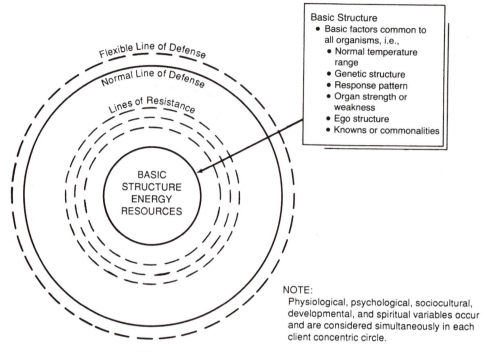

Figure 1–4. Client/client system.

THE CLIENT/CLIENT SYSTEM

The client/client system is illustrated in Figure 1–4. The client or client system is represented by a series of concentric rings or circles surrounding a basic structure. The central or core structure consists of basic survival factors common to the species, such as variables contained within it, innate or genetic features, and strengths and weaknesses of the system parts. Examples for the client as *man* or *person* are innate mechanisms for the maintenance of a normal temperature range, genetic response patterns, and the strength or weakness of body organs. In relation to the five variables, certain unique features or baseline characteristics also exist for each client or client system; an example is cognitive ability. The concentric circles function essentially as protective mechanisms for the basic structure, or client system, integrity.

The flexible line of defense protects the normal line of defense, which is the usual wellness state. The lines of resistance protect the basic structure. The flexible line of defense forms the outer boundary of the defined client system, whether a single client, a group, or a social issue. Each line of defense and resistance contains similar protective elements related to the five variables—physiological, psychological, developmental, sociocultural, and spiritual—while being distinguished by their specific protective functions.

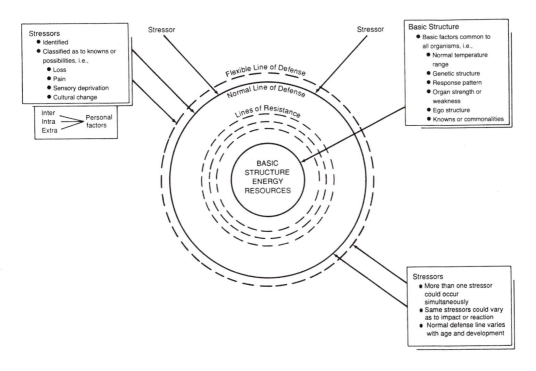

Figure 1–5. Environment.

Flexible Line of Defense

The flexible line of defense is shown by the outer, broken circle surrounding the normal (solid) line of defense. It acts as a protective buffer system for the client's normal or stable state. That is, it ideally prevents stressor invasions of the client system, keeping the system free from stressor reactions, or symptomatology. It is accordian-like in function. As it expands away from the normal defense line, greater protection is provided; as it draws closer, less protection is available. It is dynamic rather than stable and can be rapidly altered over a relatively short time period or in a situation like a state of emergency or a condition like under-nutrition, sleep loss, or dehydration. Single or multiple stressor impact has the potential for reducing the effectiveness of this buffer system. When the normal line of defense is rendered ineffective in relation to a particular *stressor* impact, a reaction will occur within the client system. That is, when the normal line of defense has been penetrated, the client presents with symptoms of instability or illness, caused by one or more impacting stressors. In all lines of defense and resistance are found elements that are similar, but specific functionally, related to the five client variables. Some examples are coping patterns, life-style factors, and developmental, sociocultural, and belief system influences.

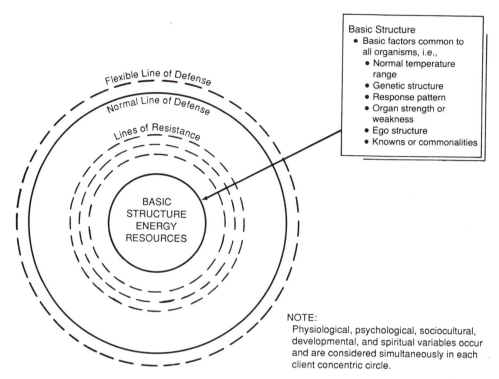

Figure 1–6. Health.

The Five Variables

The Neuman Systems Model considers the client, whether one or many, proximal or distal, as a system. Each system boundary must be identified or defined, along with the parts contained within it. In all client systems five variable areas are contained, with varying degrees of development and a wide range of interactive styles and potential. In the list below, the variables are defined broadly and generally; the first four are commonly understood by nursing. Since it was added to the model in the 1989 text, the spiritual variable continues to be described in some detail.

- Physiological—refers to bodily structure and function
- Psychological—refers to mental processes and relationships
- Sociocultural—refers to combined social and cultural functions
- Developmental—refers to life developmental processes
- Spiritual—refers to spiritual belief influence

The spiritual variable, now explicitly added to the Neuman Systems Model, has been successfully used with the model in several settings. This variable is viewed as innate, a component of the basic structure, whether or not it is ever acknowledged or developed by the client or client system. The author views it as being on a continuum of development that permeates all other client system variables. The client/client system can move from complete unawareness of this variable's presence and potential, or even denial of it, to a consciously and highly developed spiritual understanding that supports client optimal wellness; that is, the spirit controls the mind, and the mind consciously or unconsciously controls the body (see Appendix B). The spiritual variable positively or negatively affects or is affected by the condition and interactive effect of other variables, such as grief or loss (psychological states), which may arrest, decrease, initiate, or increase spirituality. The potential exists for movement in either direction on a continuum.

Through careful assessment of client needs in the spiritual area, followed by purposeful intervention such as fostering hope that affects the will to live, the relationship between the spiritual variable and wellness may be better understood and utilized as an energy source in achieving client change and optimal system stability. It is the author's belief that spiritual variable considerations are necessary for a truly wholistic perspective and truly caring concern for the client/client system.

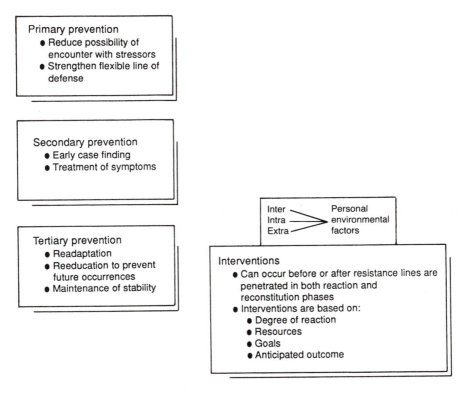

Figure 1–7. Nursing.

Lines of Resistance

The series of concentric broken circles surrounding the basic structure are identified as lines of resistance for the client; these are activated following invasion of the normal line of defense by environmental stressors. These resistance lines contain certain known and unknown internal and external resource factors that support the client's basic structure and normal defense line, thus protecting system integrity. An example is the body's mobilization of white blood cells or activation of immune system mechanisms. Effectiveness of the lines of resistance in reversing the reaction to stressors allows the system to reconstitute; ineffectiveness leads to energy depletion and death.

The Normal Line of Defense

The *normal line of defense* is the solid boundary line that encircles the broken internal lines of resistance. This line represents what the client has become, the state to which the client has evolved over time, or the usual wellness level. The adjustment of client system variables to environmental stressors determines client stability or usual wellness level. The normal defense line is a *standard* against which deviancy from the usual wellness state can be determined. It is the result of previous system behavior, defining the stability and integrity of the system and its ability to maintain them. Influencing factors are the system variables, coping patterns, life-style factors, developmental and spiritual influences, and cultural considerations. Any stressor can create a reaction within the client by invading the normal line of defense when it is insufficiently protected by the flexible line of defense. A client reaction may reduce the ability of the system to withstand additional stressor impact, especially if the effectiveness of the lines of resistance is reduced. The normal line of defense is considered dynamic in that it can expand or contract over time. For example, the usual wellness level or system stability may remain the same, become reduced, or expand following treatment of a stressor reaction. It is also dynamic in terms of its ability to become and remain stabilized to deal with life stresses over time, thus protecting the basic structure and system integrity.

ENVIRONMENT

The *environment* is broadly defined as all internal and external factors or influences surrounding the identified client or client system (Figure 1–5). The client may influence or be influenced by environmental forces either positively or negatively at any given point in time. A particular stressor with a negative outcome for a client at a particular point in time may not always be noxious. The adjustment of the system may alter the client response pattern. Input, output, and feedback between the client and the environment is of a circular nature; client and environment have a reciprocal relationship, the outcome of which is corrective or regulative for the system.

The internal environment consists of all forces or interactive influences internal to or contained solely within the boundaries of the defined client/client system. It correlates with the model intrapersonal factors or stressors. The external environment consists of all forces or interactive influences external to or existing outside the defined client/client system. It correlates with both the model's inter- and extrapersonal factors or stressors.

Environmental exchanges must be identified as to their nature and possible or actual outcome for the client or client system. Another important environment identified and presented by the author (Neuman, 1989, 1990), the *created environment*, represents an open system exchanging energy with both the internal and external environment. This environment, developed unconsciously by the client, is a symbolic expression of system wholeness. That is, it acts as an immediate or long-range safe reservoir for existence or the maintenance of system integrity expressed consciously, unconsciously, or both simultaneously.

The *created environment* is dynamic and represents the client's unconscious mobilization of all system variables (particularly the psycho-sociocultural), including the basic structure energy factors, toward system integration, stability, and integrity. It is inherently purposeful. Though unconsciously developed, its function is to offer a protective coping (Lazarus, 1981) shield or safe arena for system function as the client is usually cognitively unaware of the host of existing psychosocial and physiological influences. It pervades all systems, large and small, at least to some degree; it is spontaneously created, increased, or decreased, as warranted by a special condition of need. It supersedes or goes beyond the internal and external environments, encompassing both.

The insulating effect of the *created environment* changes the response or possible response of the client to environmental stressors, for example, the use of denial or envy (psychological), physical rigidity or muscular constraint (physiological), life-cycle continuation of survival patterns (developmental), required social space range (sociocultural), and sustaining hope (spiritual). Perception has a direct relationship to coping (Lazarus, 1981). All basic structure factors and system variables influence or are influenced by the *created environment*, which is developed and maintained through binding available energy in varying degrees of protectiveness; at any given place or point in time or over time, it may be necessary to change a situation or the self to cope with threat. The following environmental typology is now established for the Neuman Systems Model:

- Internal environment—intrapersonal in nature
- External environment—inter- and extrapersonal in nature
- Created environment—intra-, inter-, and extrapersonal in nature

The caregiver will need to determine through assessment (1) what has been created (nature of it), (2) the outcome of it (extent of its use and client value), and (3) the ideal that has yet to be created (the protection that is needed or possible, to a lesser or greater degree). These are all important areas for determination to best understand and support the client's created environment. After the nature and quality of the client's created environment is accurately assessed, further integration and synthesis of it may be desirable for optimal client wellness. The created environment is based on unseen, unconscious knowledge, as well as self-esteem, beliefs, energy exchanges, system variables, and predisposition; it is a process-based concept of perpetual adjustment within which a client may either increase or decrease available energy affecting the wellness state. The caregiver's goal is to guide the client in the conservation and use of energy as a force to move beyond the present condition, ideally preserving and enhancing the wellness level. What was originally created to safeguard the health of the system may have a negative outcome effect in the binding of available energy.

A major objective of the *created environment* is to stimulate the client's health. It has been well documented that a diseased condition is often created by cognitive distortions on the part of the client or the caregiver, although intervention traditionally focuses on physical and observable symptoms, overlooking causal factors like unexplored beliefs and fears. For example, a client's fear of job loss, with resultant lowered self-esteem and role conflict because of the inability to meet financial obligations, may lead to spinal problems. A client's ideas based on past experiences may also influence a current health state; for example, the belief in the length of time required to cure the common cold may have a positive or negative health outcome.

In wellness and illness states all causal factors must be evaluated as to internal, innate, and external factors (known as variables and stressors) affecting the client; known or potential interrelationships, interactions, and interdependencies that may have created a given health state must be identified and correlated. Optimal client wellness is dependent upon the evaluation of all causal factors, along with nursing action through relevant nursing intervention. Client awareness of the *created environment* and its relationship to health is a key concept that nursing may wish to pursue and further develop.

As the caregiver recognizes the value of the client *created-environment* and purposely intervenes, the interpersonal relationship can become one of important mutual exchange.

HEALTH

Figure 1–6 represents health or wellness, as viewed on a continuum; wellness and illness are on opposite ends of the continuum. Health for the client is equated with optimal system stability, that is, the best possible wellness state at any given time. The health of the client is envisioned as being at various, changing levels within a normal range, rising or falling throughout the life span because of basic structure factors and satisfactory or unsatisfactory adjustment by the client system to environmental stressors. The author views health as a manifestation of living energy available to preserve and enhance system integrity.

The wellness–illness continuum (Figure 1–1) implies that energy flow is continuous between the client system and the environment. To conceptualize wellness, then, is to determine the actual or possible effects of stressor invasion in terms of existing client system energy levels. Client movement is toward negentropy when more energy is being generated than used; when more energy is required than is being generated, movement is toward entropy, or illness—and possible death. Variances from wellness or varying degrees of system instability are caused by stressor invasion of the normal line of defense.

The author and a valued nursing colleague, Audrey Koertvelyessy (Neuman and Koertvelyessy, 1986), jointly identified the major theory for the model as being the theory of optimal client system stability; that is, stability represents health for the system. Several other theories inherent within the model could be identified and clarified with the goal of optimizing health for the client.

NURSING

The nursing component of the model (Figure 1–7) illustrates that the major concern for nursing is in keeping the client system stable through accuracy both in assessing the effects and possible effects of environmental stressors and in assisting client adjustments required for an optimal wellness level. *Optimal* means the best possible health state achievable at a given point in time. Nursing actions are initiated to best retain, attain, and maintain optimal client health or wellness, using the three preventions as interventions to keep the system stable. In keeping the system stable, the nurse creates a linkage among the client, the environment, health, and nursing.

Prevention as Intervention

The model format for prevention as intervention (Table 1–2) provides an intervention typology. First considered is *primary prevention as intervention*. This modality (Figure 1–8) is used for primary prevention as wellness retention, that is, to protect the client system normal line of defense or usual wellness state by strengthening the flexible line of defense. The goal is to promote client wellness by stress prevention and reduction of risk factors. This includes a variety of strategies for health promotion.

Intervention can begin at any point at which a stressor is either suspected or identified. Primary prevention as intervention is provided when the degree of risk or hazard is known but a reaction has not yet occurred. The caregiver may choose to reduce the possibility of stressor encounter or in some manner attempt to strengthen the client's flexible line of defense to decrease the possibility of a reaction. Ideally, primary prevention is also considered concomitant with secondary and tertiary preventions as interventions.

Assuming that either the above intervention was not provided or that it failed and a reaction occurred, intervention known as secondary prevention as

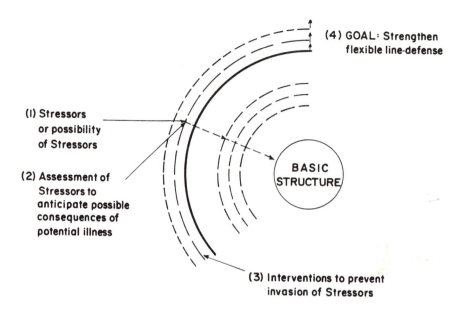

Figure 1–8. Format for primary prevention as intervention mode. *Copyright © 1980 by Betty Neuman.*

intervention or treatment would be provided in terms of existing symptoms. The *secondary prevention as intervention* modality (Figure 1–9) is used for secondary prevention as wellness attainment, that is, to protect the basic structure by strengthening the internal lines of resistance. The goal is to provide appropriate treatment of symptoms to attain optimal client system stability or wellness and energy conservation.

Treatment could begin at any point following the occurrence of symptoms. Maximum use of existing client internal and external resources would be considered in an attempt to stabilize the system by strengthening the internal lines of resistance, thus reducing the reaction. Relevant goals are established, based on use of the Neuman Nursing Process Format (Table 1–1), which has been designed to implement the model. Through its use the meaning of the experience to the client is discovered, as well as existing needs and resources for meeting them. Through the synthesis of comprehensive client data and relevant theory, an umbrella-like, or comprehensive, nursing diagnostic statement is made, from which nursing goals in collaboration with clients can be readily determined for nursing intervention.

If, following treatment, secondary prevention as intervention fails to reconstitute the client, death occurs as a result of failure of the basic structure to support the intervention. Reconstitution is identified as beginning at any point following treatment; it is the determined energy increase related to the degree

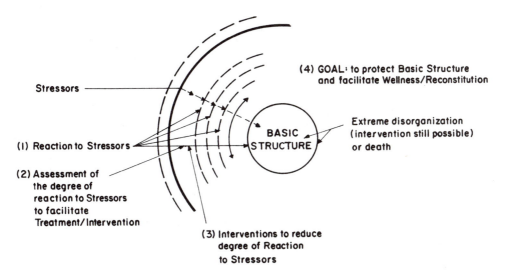

Figure 1–9. Format for secondary prevention as intervention mode. *Copyright © 1980 by Betty Neuman.*

of reaction. Complete reconstitution may progress well beyond the previously determined normal line of defense or usual wellness level, it may stabilize the system at a lower level, or it may return to the level prior to illness.

The *tertiary prevention as intervention* modality (Figure 1–10) is used for tertiary prevention as wellness maintenance, that is, to protect client system reconstitution or return to wellness following treatment. Reconstitution may be viewed as feedback from the input and output of secondary intervention. The goal is to maintain an optimal wellness level by supporting existing strengths and conserving client system energy.

Tertiary prevention as intervention can begin at any point in client reconstitution following treatment, that is, when some degree of system stability has occurred. Reconstitution at this stage is dependent upon the successful mobilization of client resources to prevent further stressor reaction or regression; it represents a dynamic state of adjustment to stressors and integration of all necessary factors toward optimal use of existing resources for client system stability or wellness maintenance.

This dynamic view of tertiary prevention tends to lead back, in circular fashion, toward primary prevention. An example of this circularity is either avoidance of specific known hazardous stressors or desensitization to them. In using this intervention typology, the client condition, in relation to environmental stressors, becomes readily apparent. One or all three prevention modalities give direction to, or may be simultaneously used for, nursing action, with possible synergistic benefits.

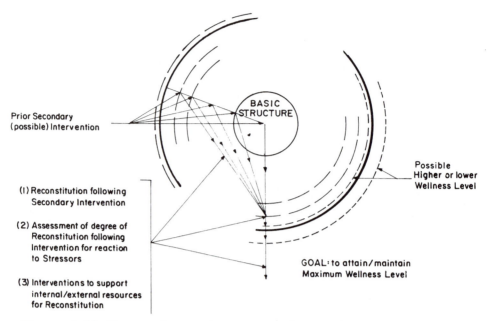

Figure 1–10. Format for tertiary prevention as intervention mode. *Copyright © 1980 by Betty Neuman.*

Koertvelyessy (personal communication, fall 1987) proposed the theory of prevention as intervention. She views the concept of prevention—whether primary, secondary, or tertiary—as prevalent and significant in the Neuman Systems Model, linked to each of the broad concepts of the model, that is, man (client), environment, health, and nursing. Since the prevention strategies are the modes instituted to retain, attain, or maintain stability of the client's health status, she considers the development of a theory statement linking these concepts a necessary next step.

Health promotion based on the Neuman Systems Model is a component of the primary prevention as intervention modality. This contradicts Pender's (1987) view that the two areas should be considered separate entities. In the Neuman Systems Model health promotion is subsumed within the area of primary prevention and becomes one of the specific goals within it for nursing action. For example, following need determination, intervention goals would include education and appropriate supportive actions toward achieving optimal client wellness, that is, augmenting existing strengths related to the flexible line of defense and thus decreasing the possibility of risk or threat of client reaction to potential or actual stressors. The major goal for nursing is to reduce stressor impact, whether actual or potential, and to increase client resistance. Ideally, health promotion goals should work in concert with both secondary and tertiary preventions as interventions to prevent recidivism and to promote optimal wellness, since the Neuman Systems Model is wellness oriented. Health promotion, in general, and within the primary prevention concept, relates to activities that optimize the client wellness potential or condition.

Since the Neuman Systems Model has always considered environmental stressors as impacting the client or client system on a continuous basis, health promotion is inherently a major area of concern for both client and caregiver, not only in retention, but also in attainment and maintenance of optimal client/client system wellness (Neuman, 1974, 104–106). Primary prevention as intervention with inherent health promotion is an expanding futuristic, proactive concept with which the nursing field must become increasingly concerned. It has unlimited potential for major role development that could shape the future image of nursing as world health care reform continues to evolve into the 21st century.

In summary, the multidimensionality and wholistic systemic perspective of the Neuman Systems Model is increasingly proving its relevance and reliability in a wide variety of clinical and educational settings throughout the world. Its comprehensive approach accommodates a variety of health-related theories. It also has the potential for generating important nursing theory through research into its components and by the unification of existing theories to serve world health care concerns well into the future.

THE NURSING PROCESS AND THE NEUMAN SYSTEMS MODEL

Insufficient methodology exists for truly scientific approaches to complex and rapidly changing nursing concerns. Nurses largely conceptualize and utilize their social science knowledge for nursing in their own unique way, thus contributing to general inadequacy in professional communication and often poorly defined client goals. The need is critical for meaningful definitions and conceptual frames of reference for nursing practice if the profession is to be established as a science. For example, though considerable progress has been made in the past few years, the profession is still without definitive criteria for establishing a nursing diagnosis within the nursing process. It is considered to be in an evolving state from its present NANDA guidelines. There is major concern that these criteria relate only in part to various nursing conceptual frameworks. Because of this concern, the author has recommended for Neuman model usage available and relevant diagnostic nomenclature, adding to it as required using Neuman concepts and terminology. Tables 1–1 and 1–2 illustrate the Neuman three-step nursing process and the preventions as interventions.

The nursing process for the Neuman Systems Model (Neuman, 1982) shown in Table 1–1 was designed specifically for nursing implementation of the Neuman Systems Model. The nursing process has been developed within the following three categories: nursing diagnosis, nursing goals, and nursing outcomes. These categories best fit the systemic perspective of the Neuman Systems Model. The utility of the format was first validated by doctoral students in 1982. Appendix C illustrates initial use of the Neuman Nursing Process Format; it has since proved its validity and social utility in a wide variety of nursing education and practice areas.

In using the Neuman Systems Model, the nurse is concerned with acquiring significant and comprehensive client data to determine the impact or the possible impact of environmental stressors upon the defined client system. Selected, prioritized client information is related to or is synthesized with relevant social science and nursing theories. This process fully explains the client condition, providing the logic or rationale for subsequent nursing action. That is, it provides the basis for a broad, comprehensive (umbrella-like) diagnostic statement concerning the entire client condition, from which logically defensible goals are easily and accurately derived. To complement the nursing process, a Prevention as Intervention Format (see Table 1–2 and Figures 1–8, 1–9, and 1–10) clearly sets forth a viable typology for nursing intervention. The intervention modalities of primary, secondary, and tertiary prevention as intervention have gained universal acceptance.

This format, presented as an organizing tool based on the prevention concept, provides a clear definition and refinement of strategies for meaningful nursing interventions. The prevention as intervention modalities facilitate integrative processes necessary to retain, attain, and maintain the stability and integrity of the client/client system.

Specifically unique to the Neuman Nursing Process Format is that both client and caregiver perceptions are determined for relevant goal setting. Another important feature is the mutual determination of client intervention goals. These characteristics follow current mandates within the health care system for client rights in health care issues.

Although many authors have set forth various characteristics as integral components of the nursing process as a whole and in each of its phases, Phaneuf (1976) points out that there is little to support assumptions concerning the outcomes of the nursing process unless they are made from an adequate data base. The Neuman Nursing Process Format attempts to offer some resolution to this awkward dilemma in the following manner. Sufficient client data are obtained to make a comprehensive diagnostic statement and objectively determine client variance from wellness. Relevant goal setting is then defensible in terms of the theoretical synthesis with client data. Through the use of this specially designed nursing format, analytical outcomes are possible since they are based on purposeful prevention as intervention modalities.

USE OF A FAMILY CASE STUDY ABSTRACT AND THE NEUMAN NURSING PROCESS FORMAT FOR DETERMINING A NURSING DIAGNOSIS

Because of often conflicting views on how to arrive at and state the nursing diagnosis, it is important to provide such information for use of the Neuman Systems

Model. Thus far, the author has received no satisfactory answer to her frequently asked question, "How do you use theory in making a nursing diagnosis based on the Neuman Model?"

In addition to the general problem of conflicting views on how the nursing diagnosis is arrived at and best stated, there are some specific factors that contribute to a confusing and faulty nursing diagnosis: (1) existing NANDA diagnostic nomenclature does not "fit" the entirety of nursing models; (2) interpretation of client data may be faulty, or information may be insufficient; (3) theory may not be explicitly used, or it may be improperly related to client data. It is more common for theory to be explicitly related to intervention than to assessment and the nursing diagnosis.

To best resolve the nursing diagnosis dilemma in using the Neuman Systems Model and the Neuman Nursing Process Format, a brief family case study abstract will be presented. It will be followed by an illustration of the way client data and theory are synthesized into what is known as "variance from wellness," that is, the difference from the normal or usual wellness condition. The areas of wellness variance, or those for major concern, provide the basis for a wholistic and comprehensive nursing diagnostic statement to include the entire client–family condition as a system. Since theory is related to client data, defensible and logical client goals are readily determined from the diagnostic statement for subsequent appropriate intervention, in order to retain, attain, and maintain system stability or wellness. Theory appropriate to the nursing diagnostic statement will also be found to be relevant for nursing intervention.

Family Abstract*

The B—— family moved from a metropolitan area, with Mr. B—— assuming the superintendency of a rural school district. Mrs. B—— had worked very hard at various jobs to help her husband acquire his doctoral degree and to advance his career goals. She had not wanted to make this move because of her mother's terminal condition with bone cancer, which would necessitate long trips every other weekend for family visits. They were both in their late thirties and had two teenage daughters aged 14 and 16. Mrs. B—— devoted all her time to family needs, keeping the home and environment immaculate. The family profile was one of happiness, togetherness, and religious centeredness, though there was little socialization in the home. Both daughters were obese and shy, with social contacts only while at school. The younger daughter was in competition with the older daughter, who was favored by the parents. There were frequent purchases of the newest styles in clothing for all family members. A public image of the ideal and proper family prevailed.

Then, to supplement the family income, Mrs. B—— assumed a position in a nearby dairy, rising early in the morning and riding to work with a close neigh-

*Based on information in J. P. Riehl-Sisca, *Conceptual Models for Nursing Practice,* 3d ed. (East Norwalk, Conn.: Appleton & Lange, 1989).

bor, Mrs. P——, who also worked there. During their one-and-one-half-year stay, the family had won the respect of all residents of the small village in which they lived. Mr. B—— had excelled in the school system. All family members kept a low social profile.

During the winter preceding the elder daughter's high school graduation and soon following her eighteenth birthday, she suddenly told the family that she was "in love" with the neighbor's wife with whom the mother rode to work. Following attempted violence toward Mrs. P——, the mother collapsed and was hospitalized for hypoglycemic shock; the elder daughter promptly moved into Mrs. P——'s home, with her husband present.

Two days following hospital discharge, Mrs. B—— attempted suicide with an overdose of sleeping medication. Mrs. B—— improved to some degree because of counseling while hospitalized. Neither the younger daughter nor Mr. B—— became involved, but rather continued with usual school activities. The older daughter completed high school while continuing to live across the street with Mrs. P——, whose husband finally moved out of their residence. She remained estranged from her family. Though the school system invited Mr. B—— to continue, he relinquished his position at the end of the school year, assuming a position near Mrs. B——'s mother, who died one week prior to their move. Mr. B——'s major concern was that he might lose his new position if the family crisis should become known. The younger daughter became more withdrawn and the crisis remained essentially unresolved for all family members. Since the family chose not to share their dilemma with distant family members, there was no support from relatives, neighbors were immobilized, and there was no appropriate follow-up therapeutic family intervention from the community agencies. The family moved away and failed to keep contact with the villagers.

Major Stressors for Each Family Member

- Mr. B—loss of status
- Mrs. B—questionable mothering role and loss
- Younger daughter—unmet developmental needs
- Older daughter—unmet developmental needs

Family Perception of Their Condition

Mrs. P—— had unjustly invaded the B—— family system, creating the major crises that occurred.

Caregiver Perception of Their Condition

The parents had failed to relate effectively to their daughters' developmental needs and to those of the family as a system.

Rigid family interaction patterns were considered a major causal factor in the crisis situation. Mr. B—— also failed to recognize and support the needs of his wife before and after the crisis. Community resources failed to provide appropriate family intervention, and unresolved family crises remained.

Determination of the Nursing Diagnosis

Variance from wellness is first determined by the following synthesis or integration of the data base, with various appropriate theories (placed in parentheses in relation to analyses of the data base) as follows:

> The family's past accumulated energy drain weakened the flexible line of defense, allowing stressors to penetrate the solid or normal defense line of the family, causing a series of near-fatal crises. A serious threat to the basic structure of the family existed for which there had been no previous coping mechanisms developed as internal lines of resistance. (Crisis, systems, communication, and nursing process theories)
>
> Social role and function as well as educational differences can influence family behavior. To integrate differing expectations, which can become internal and external stressors, into the intrafamily system is often difficult to accomplish while maintaining family stability. (Role and systems theories) Unless individual needs are identified and met, family integrity may be jeopardized, especially when new coping strategies are required. (Personality, developmental, change, and family theories)
>
> Excessive energy was required to maintain the public image of Mr. B——, while the growth and development needs of the two daughters and their mother were grossly compromised over the years. (Growth and development theory) The autocratic, rigid family interaction patterns failed to allow for free expression of emotions, differences, ideas, and individuation. The needs of one family part or member, Mr. B——, superseded the needs of the other three, creating a dysfunction of the family system. (Systems and family theories)

Variance from Wellness

1. Mother's suicide attempt
2. Father's public image
3. Younger daughter's immobilization
4. Older daughter's abandonment

From the specific areas of variance from wellness (theory and data base synthesis), the following wholistic and comprehensive nursing diagnostic statement was made:

> Erosion of the family system because of the continuous, unresolved stressor of rigid family rules to maintain Mr. B——'s public image resulted in bankruptcy of family emotions and energy, negating sustaining family communications during the crises.

Once a meaningful and comprehensive diagnostic statement of the overall situation can be made, major areas for goal setting and subsequent intervention can logically be determined and defended as required. The use of theory, then, is circular; that is, the same theories used in determining major wellness variance can also be used for purposeful outcome goals and intervention. Nurse professionalism is related to skill in synthesis of established scientific theory with client data to frame an accurate client diagnostic statement and present a logical, defensible justification for the decisions made.

The Neuman Nursing Process (Table 1–1) and Prevention as Intervention formats (Table 1–2 and Figures 1–8, 1–9, and 1–10) were designed as tools for model implementation to replace those earlier published in *Conceptual Models for Nursing Practice* (Neuman, 1974). A decision was made to place the earlier slightly revised assessment and intervention tool and explanation in Appendix D because of its past wide usage. This tool is considered by the author as a generic guide for assessment and intervention related to the Neuman Model. It has provided a base for further assessment tool refinement for use with specific client populations encountered in nursing specialty and clinical areas. Readers may choose to continue to use this earlier tool if it proves useful in conjunction with more recently developed tools or instead of them. This would also apply to the support data (slightly revised in 1989) in the assessment and intervention tool development guide, also included in Appendix D.

It is the author's hope that the Neuman Systems Model, with its comprehensive approach to clients, will not only further validate these model implementation tools in a wide variety of settings but also encourage creativity in their use and new development. The model should facilitate the socialization of nursing into the wellness perspective and the consideration of all aspects of client concern, replacing the limited and fragmented illness focus of the past. As nursing clearly articulates and presents scientific logic for its actions, other health professionals, as well as clients and consumers, will sanction a new image for the profession. The understanding and use of the Neuman Systems Model perspective is proving to be readily translatable to other cultures, facilitating important global sharing and resolution of universal nursing concerns.

The widespread and successful use of the model has largely discounted criticism set forth in earlier nursing literature. Nursing research and utilization in nursing education and practice areas are proving its value and social utility. Its comprehensive systems base and the reported relative ease of adaptation to other cultures are significant factors for its future increasing usage, relevance, and continued acceptance in nursing. The author is indeed proud of all the fine people who have pioneered the use of the model, both at home and abroad. Nursing education and practice area usage of the model can be found in Chapter 50; however, it is impossible to present a complete detailed account since new developments continue to emerge. Unfortunately, too, much existing research remains unavailable through lack of publication; for that reason, contributive research data, identified through a purposeful search, are set forth in abstract form in Chapter 33.

SUMMARY

The relationship of the Neuman Systems Model to nursing as a viable and relevant perspective for the nursing profession in the future has been presented. The model's future potential for research has been predicted, based on the past extent of its utilization in areas of nursing education, practice, administration, and research.

Philosophically, the model was set forth as a comprehensive guide for nursing practice open to creative implementation. However, the author does not sanction structural changes that could alter its meaning and purpose.

REFERENCES

Ashby, W. 1972. Systems and their informational measures. In *Trends in General Systems Theory,* edited by G. J. Klir. New York: Wiley.

Aydelotte, M. 1972. Nursing education and practice: Putting it all together. *Journal of Nursing Education* 2(4):23.

Banathy, B. 1973. Models of educational information systems. In *Systems in Society,* edited by M. D. Rubin. Washington, D.C.: Society for General Systems Research.

Beckstrand, J. 1980. A critique of several conceptions of practice theory in nursing. *Research in Nursing and Health* 3:69–70.

Bertalanffy, L. von. 1968. *General Systems Theory.* New York: Braziller.

Chardin, P. T. de. 1955. *The Phenomenon of Man.* London: Collins, 109–112.

Cornu, A. 1957. *The Origins of Marxist Thought.* Springfield, Ill.: Thomas, 12–17.

Dunn, H. 1961. *High-level Wellness.* Arlington, Va.: Beatty.

Edelson, M. 1970. *Sociotherapy and Psychotherapy.* Chicago: University of Chicago Press, 225–231.

Emery, F., ed. 1969. *Systems Thinking.* Baltimore: Penguin Books.

Fawcett, J., and Downs, F. 1986. *The Relationship of Theory and Research.* East Norwalk, Conn.: Appleton-Century-Crofts.

Gray, W., Rizzo, N. D., and Duhl, F. D., eds. 1969. *General Systems Theory and Psychiatry.* Boston: Little, Brown.

Hazzard, M. 1975. An overview of systems theory. *Nursing Clinics of North America* 6:383–384.

Heslin, K. 1986. A systems analysis of the Betty Neuman Model. Unpublished student paper, University of Western Ontario, London, Ontario, Canada.

Klir, G. J. 1972. Preview: The polyphonic general systems theory. In *Trends in General Systems Theory,* edited by G. J. Klir. New York: Wiley.

Lazarus, R. 1981. The stress and coping paradigm. In *Models for Clinical Psychopathology,* edited by C. Eisdorfer, D. Cohen, A. Kleinman, and P. Maxim, 177–214. New York: SP Medical and Scientific Books.

Lazlo, E. 1972. *The Systems View of the World: The Natural Philosophy of the New Development in the Sciences.* New York: Braziller.

Miller, J. 1965. Living systems: Structure and process. *Behavioral Science* 10:337–379.

Neuman, B., and Young, R. J. 1972. The Betty Neuman Model: A total person approach to viewing patient problems. *Nursing Research* 21:3.

Neuman, B. 1974. The Betty Neuman Health-Care Systems Model: A total person approach to patient problems. In *Conceptual Models for Nursing Practice,* edited by J. P. Riehl and C. Roy. New York: Appleton-Century-Crofts.

Neuman, B. 1980. The Betty Neuman Health-Care Systems Model: A total person approach to patient problems. In *Conceptual Models for Nursing Practice,* 2d ed., edited by J. P. Riehl and C. Roy. New York: Appleton-Century-Crofts.

Neuman, B. 1982. *The Neuman Systems Model: Application to Nursing Education and Practice.* East Norwalk, Conn.: Appleton-Century-Crofts.

Neuman, B., and Koertvelyessy, A. 1986. The Neuman Systems Model and Nursing Research. Paper presented at the meeting of the Nursing Theory Congress, Toronto, Canada, August.

Neuman, B. 1989. *The Neuman Systems Model.* East Norwalk, Conn.: Appleton & Lange.

Neuman, B. 1989. The Neuman Nursing Process Format: A family case study. In *Conceptual Models for Nursing Practice,* 3d ed., edited by J. P. Riehl. East Norwalk, Conn.: Appleton & Lange.

Neuman, B. 1990. Health on a continuum based on the Neuman Systems Model. *Nursing Science Quarterly* 3(3):129–135.

Oakes, D. L. 1978. A critique of general systems theory. In *General Systems Theory Applied to Nursing,* edited by A. Putt. Boston: Little, Brown.

Orem, D. E. 1971. *Nursing: Concepts and Practice.* New York: McGraw-Hill.

Pender, N. J. 1987. *Health Promotion in Nursing Practice,* 2d ed. East Norwalk, Conn.: Appleton & Lange.

Phaneuf, M. 1976. *The Nursing Audit: Self-Regulation in Nursing Practice,* 2d ed. New York: Appleton-Century-Crofts.

Putt, A. 1972. Entropy, evolution and equifinality in nursing. In *Five Years of Cooperation to Improve Curricula in Western Schools of Nursing,* edited by J. Smith. Boulder, Colo.: Western Interstate Commission for Higher Education.

Riehl, J. P., and Roy, C. 1974. *Conceptual Models for Nursing Practice.* East Norwalk, Conn.: Appleton-Century-Crofts.

Selye, H. 1950. The physiology and pathology of exposure to stress. Montreal, Quebec, Canada: ACTA, 12–13.

APPENDIX A ─────────────────

The Neuman Systems Model Definitions

BASIC STRUCTURE: The basic structure consists of common client survival factors, as well as unique individual characteristics. It represents the basic system energy resources.

BOUNDARY LINES: The flexible line of defense is the outer boundary of the client system. All relevant variables must be taken into account, as the whole is greater than the sum of the parts; a change in one part affects all other system parts.

CLIENT/CLIENT SYSTEM: A composite of variables (physiological, psychological, sociocultural, developmental, and spiritual), each of which is a subpart of all parts, forms the whole of the client. The client as a system is composed of a core or basic structure of survival factors and surrounding protective concentric rings. The concentric rings are composed of similar factors, yet serve varied and different purposes in either retention, attainment, or maintenance of system stability and integrity or a combination of these. The client is considered an open system in total interface with the environment. The client is viewed as a system, and the term can be used interchangeably with the client/client system.

CONTENT: The variables of person in interaction with the internal and external environment comprise the whole client system.

DEGREE OF REACTION: The degree of reaction is the amount of system instability resulting from stressor invasion of the normal line of defense.

ENTROPY: A process of energy depletion and disorganization moving the system toward illness or possible death.

ENVIRONMENT: The environment consists of both internal and external forces surrounding the client, influencing and being influenced by the client, at any point in time, as an open system. The created environment is an unconsciously developed protective environment that binds system energy and encompasses both the internal and external client environments.

FEEDBACK: The process within which matter, energy, and information, as system output, provide feedback for corrective action to change, enhance, or stabilize the system.

FLEXIBLE LINE OF DEFENSE: The flexible line of defense is a protective, accordion-like mechanism that surrounds and protects the normal line of defense from invasion by stressors. The greater the expansiveness of this line from the normal line of defense, the greater the degree of protectiveness. Examples are situational, such as recently altered sleep patterns or immune functions.

GOAL: The system goal is stability for the purpose of client survival and optimal wellness.

HEALTH: A continuum of wellness to illness, dynamic in nature, that is constantly subject to change. Optimal wellness or stability indicates that total system needs are being met. A reduced state of wellness is the result of unmet systemic needs. The client is in a dynamic state of either wellness or illness, in varying degrees, at any given point in time.

INPUT/OUTPUT: The matter, energy, and information exchanged between client and environment that is entering or leaving the system at any point in time.

LINES OF RESISTANCE: Protection factors activated when stressors have penetrated the normal line of defense, causing a reaction symptomatology. The resistance lines ideally protect the basic structure and facilitate reconstitution toward wellness during and following treatment, as stressor reaction is decreased and client resistance is increased.

NEGENTROPY: A process of energy conservation that increases organization and complexity, moving the system toward stability or a higher degree of wellness. Stability and degree of wellness have a direct relationship.

NORMAL LINE OF DEFENSE: An adaptational level of health developed over time and considered normal for a particular individual client or system; it becomes a standard for wellness-deviance determination.

NURSING: A unique profession concerned with all variables affecting clients in their environment.

OPEN SYSTEM: A system in which there is a continuous flow of input and process, output and feedback. It is a system of organized complexity, where all elements are in interaction. Stress and reaction to stress are basic components.

PREVENTION AS INTERVENTION: Intervention typology or modes for nursing action and determinants for entry of both client and nurse into the health care system. Primary prevention: before a reaction to stressors occurs. Secondary prevention: treatment of symptoms following a reaction to stressors. Tertiary prevention: maintenance of optimal wellness following treatment.

PROCESS/FUNCTION: The function or process of the system is the exchange of matter, energy, and information with the environment and the interaction of the parts and subparts of the client system. A living system tends to move toward wholeness, stability, wellness, and negentropy.

RECONSTITUTION: Represents the return and maintenance of system stability, following treatment of stressor reaction, which may result in a higher or lower level of wellness than previously.

STABILITY: A state of balance or harmony requiring energy exchanges as the client adequately copes with stressors to retain, attain, or maintain an optimal level of health, thus preserving system integrity.

STRESSORS: Environmental factors, intra-, inter-, and extrapersonal in nature, that have potential for disrupting system stability. A stressor is any phenomenon that might penetrate both the flexible and normal lines of defense, resulting in either a positive or negative outcome.

WELLNESS/ILLNESS: Wellness is the condition in which all system parts and subparts are in harmony with the whole system of the client. Wholeness is based on interrelationships of variables, which determine the amount of resistance an individual has to any stressor. Illness indicates disharmony among the parts and subparts of the client system.

WHOLISTIC: A system is considered wholistic when any parts or subparts can be organized into an interrelating whole. Wholistic organization is one of keeping parts whole or stable in their intimate relationships; individuals are viewed as wholes whose component parts are in dynamic interdependent interaction.

APPENDIX B

The Spiritual Variable

An analogy of the "seed" will be used to further qualify and clarify the statement made in the 1989 Neuman text that "the spirit controls the mind and the mind controls the body" as it relates to the Neuman Systems Model Spiritual Variable.

It is assumed by the author that each person is born with a spiritual energy force, or "seed," within the spiritual variable as identified in the Basic Structure of the Neuman Systems Model. The seed or human spirit with its enormous energy potential lies on a continuum of dormant, unacceptable or undeveloped to recognition, development, and positive system influence. Traditionally, a seed must have environmental catalysts such as timing, warmth, moisture, and nutrients to burst forth with energy that transforms it into a living form that then in turn, as it becomes further nourished and developed, offers itself as sustenance, generating power as long as its own source of nurture exists.

The human spirit combines with the power of the Holy Spirit as a gift from God when the innate human force, or "seed," becomes catalyzed by some life event such as humility, joy, or crisis; this energy begins to magnify and become recognizable within the thought patterns as something whose truths must become known and tested in life situations. Ideally in the testing, mental and physical expressions of, for example, understanding, compassion, and love become manifested.

As thought patterns are positively affected, the body becomes increasingly nourished and sustained through positive use of spiritual energy empowerment. For example, it has been proved that a joyous thought enhances the immune system; the opposite is also true, with a negative outcome for the body.

Thus, it is assumed that spiritual development in varying degrees empowers the client system toward well-being by positively directing spiritual energy for use first by the mind and then by the body.

The beginning of spiritual awareness and development can take place at any stage of the life cycle. The supply of spiritual energy, when understood and positively used by the system, is inexhaustible except for the death of the living system as we know it.

However, the author believes that the human spirit or soul returns to the God source to live on into eternity when death occurs and it is no longer needed to empower the living mind and body.

APPENDIX C

A Case Study Analysis Using the Neuman Nursing Process Format: An Abstract

Patricia Prophet Lillis
Virginia Lee Cora

Use of a theoretical framework as a foundation for client systems increases nurse professionalism. The Neuman Systems Model has proved its utility as a most effective framework for unique and comprehensive approaches to the individual, family, or community as client. The authors wish to share their experiences to confirm that the case study method both complements and facilitates progressive understanding of the Neuman systems approach, by using the nursing process designed for model implementation. This learning method has major implications for staff development, continuing education, classroom teaching, and practice situations. It could be particularly valuable for nursing case management, primary care, clinic treatment, and home visiting.

The case study method of learning, using the B——— family case study presented in brief in Chapter 1, was utilized by four graduate students as they studied the Neuman Systems Model during a series of five consecutive daily doctoral seminars in the summer of 1982.* The content, process, and impact of the seminars using the case study method of learning is presented, based on the progressive nature of the Neuman Nursing Process Format.

*The four graduate students—Patty Lillis, Virginia Lee Cora, Jean Braun, and Lucille Pulliam—attended the 1982 Summer Doctoral Seminar presented by Dr. Neuman at the University of Alabama at Birmingham School of Nursing.

NURSING DIAGNOSIS DETERMINATION

Following oral presentation of the B——— family case study by Neuman (see pp. 39–43), general impressions were formulated for the entire family and each of the members. Students were unfamiliar with the model, and many questions followed concerning the family, as well as the intent and purpose of the model. Because of initial uncertainty, some noncompliance was noted; it soon dissipated as students worked together in small groups to dissect the case material to gain an overall perspective of the family.

During the consecutive five-day seminars, in-depth questioning of the instructor provided increasingly detailed client information. The relationship of family or client data to the format of the Neuman Nursing Process became increasingly obvious as to the format's purpose for implementing the model. Though it was laborious to secure a detailed and comprehensive data base, following the steps of the process proved the viability and utility of such a structure for both organizing and placing into perspective family system information.

First, students identified major actual stressors, as well as the potential ones that either were impacting or might impact the family as a system. Some examples of identified stressors were the lack of individuation of family members, family energy directed toward sustaining Mr. B———'s image, and rigidity of the entire family system. Family strengths related to basic structure and energy resources were identified by students as family religious beliefs, their close intergenerational linkages, and continuing attempts at family cohesiveness. The rigidity with which rules were imposed upon family members severely limited effectiveness of both normal and flexible lines of defense. Similarly, following reaction to stressors, the lines of resistance failed to provide adequate protection in relation to current and continuing major stressors impacting the life process of the B——— family. Genograms of both the B——— and P——— families, along with other interacting systems, graphically confirmed the complexity of their total situation or condition.

The Neuman Nursing Process Format and the case study method of learning allowed for a progressively increasing depth of assessment, which led to the making of a defensible, comprehensive, and wholistically based nursing diagnostic statement. They also structured a systematic perspective for ordering massive amounts of information that otherwise might not have been processed sufficiently for relevant nursing goals to be developed. For example, following in-depth analysis of available data, four major theories best correlated with family assessment data for synthesis and determination of wellness variance. They were as follows: communication theory based on interaction patterns repetitive within and between the B——— and P——— families, crisis theory based on several developmental and situational crises, family theory based on unmet developmental needs of mother and daughters, and role theory based on unrecognized family needs and expectations. All of these reduced the family system's stability and ability to cope with impacting stressors.

To complement the above theories being used for further system analysis, a time line of major events and impacting stressors was developed to organize the data longitudinally. Using the Neuman classification system of intra-, inter-, and extrapersonal interactions between the client and environment was most helpful in clarification of the dynamics operating within the B—— family system. Through information processing, identification and prioritization of various aspects of the family condition, and relating selected theories and relevant themes from client data, a synthesis to formulate a wholistic, defensible, and comprehensive family diagnosis was possible, with help from the instructor, as follows:

> Erosion of the family system related to the rigidity required to maintain Gregory's (father's) public image. Bankruptcy of family emotions negated sustaining effective family communications.

From the above family diagnosis the following major areas of concern for individual members have been identified.

- Marie (mother)—loss associated with sibling abandonment and mothering image
- Angela (younger daughter)—self-concept deficit associated with stuttering and obesity
- Rose (older daughter)—unmet developmental needs acted out
- Gregory (father)—status maintenance based on fear and competition

NURSING GOALS

Hypothetical intervention goals and perceptual differences were identified for ideal use with the family prior to establishment of short-, intermediate-, and long-range goal plans for nursing intervention.

NURSING OUTCOMES

Based on identified family strengths, needs, and available resources, intervention strategies for management and problem resolution were planned, based on the three levels of prevention as intervention designed by Neuman to implement nursing actions based on the Neuman Systems Model. Immediate, intermediate, and long-range goals for the family and each of its members were developed.

The major family goal was to stabilize the family system, conserving available energy by meeting its individual member needs. Examples of individual goals included:

- Marie—settle unresolved grief over loss of daughter.
- Angela—develop self-assertive skills.
- Gregory—reexamine career goals and family needs.
- Rose—contact and accept family when possible.

For this simulated family situation, students wrote a prescription of practical interventions for both resolution and management of family and individual needs and concerns as presented in the family simulation. Examples of these prescriptions included relating to the type of goal and intervention strategy most appropriate, as follows:

1. Family (immediate/secondary): Establish ways for openly communicating with Rose, such as using telephone conferences.
2. Rose (intermediate/secondary): Write regular reassuring letters of acceptance and concern.
3. Marie (long-range/tertiary): Pursue development of latent artistic talent with a view toward future employment and compensation.
4. Angela (intermediate/tertiary): Develop plans for fitness to control weight and increase self-confidence.
5. Family (long-range/primary): Attend nutritional classes and family counseling, if possible, to support existing strengths and energy level.
6. Gregory/family (long-range/primary): Focus on family socialization to improve member interaction patterns.

OUTCOME FOR STUDENTS

A high level of excitement with feelings of both personal and professional satisfaction resulted from learning to use the Neuman Systems Model and its implementation tools, the Neuman Nursing Process Format's step-by-step analysis of family system data and intervention strategy development. Through use of the case study method of learning and the above structure for organizing client system data, the model became fully and clearly operational as an important organizing framework for nursing.

To provide closure for the teaching and learning process, the four students and Neuman examined the relevance of the B—— family situation to their own personal and professional lives. Each student identified one aspect from the family case study and problem-solving learning process that could be used with other client systems. Their successful experience validated the Neuman Nursing Process Format designed to implement the model prior to its publication in Neuman (1982).

SUMMARY

The case study method proved to be an effective strategy for increasing both the depth and scope of understanding in relating the Neuman Systems Model to a simulated family situation.

The use of five consecutive daily seminars for detailed analysis of case study material and discovery of appropriate relationships in the data, facilitated in-depth learning of how a nursing model relates to relevant nursing actions. Also, it clarified the process of operationalizing a nursing model, with the potential for improving nursing practice.

The case study method/process may be used as a teaching strategy for any practice or educational setting that seeks a wholistic perspective of the client/client system in order to develop nurse skill in critical thinking and high-level problem solving. This method originated with Hippocrates and has been successfully used by many disciplines, including law, business, and medicine. It may be timely for a revisitation by nursing. By altering the complexity of the case situation, the case study as a learning method is also applicable to all levels of education and purposes within practice settings. Increasingly, case study methodology is being used in qualitative research designs. The doctoral seminar students were the first to validate use of the Neuman Nursing Process Format and to demonstrate the relevance of the case study method for student learning to operationalize the Neuman Systems Model.

REFERENCES

Heidergerkin, L. E. 1965. *Teaching and Learning in Schools: Principles and Methods,* 3d ed., 487–502. Philadelphia: Lippincott.

Neuman, B. 1974. The Betty Neuman Health-Care Systems Model: A total person approach to patient problems. In *Conceptual Models for Nursing Practice,* edited by J. P. Riehl and C. Roy, 99–114. New York: Appleton-Century-Crofts.

Neuman, B. 1980. The Betty Neuman Health-Care Systems Model: A total person approach to patient problems. In *Conceptual Models for Nursing Practice,* 2d ed., edited by J. P. Riehl and C. Roy, 119–134. New York: Appleton-Century-Crofts.

Neuman, B. 1982. *The Neuman Systems Model: Application to Nursing Education and Practice.* New York: Appleton-Century-Crofts.

Schweer, J. E. 1976. *Creative Teaching in Clinical Nursing.* St. Louis: Mosby, 128–130.

APPENDIX D

Nursing Assessment and Intervention Based on the Neuman Systems Model

Nurses who wish to develop their own specific assessment and intervention tools for use with the Neuman Systems Model should consider the following:

1. Proper assessment would include all knowledge of factors influencing the client's perceptual field.
2. The meaning of a stressor should be validated by both the client and caregiver, should highlight discrepancies for resolution, and should lead to relevant nursing action.

Table 1–3, An Assessment and Intervention Tool Development Guide, is a revision of the former table, Intermediate Step in the Neuman Model, which appeared in Riehl and Roy (1974, 1980). Because of its wide usage, the guide is included for those who may continue to benefit from it in developing their own tools. The guide should facilitate the linkage of Neuman Systems Model concepts to an operational assessment and intervention tool by identifying some facts and conditions from which client goals are established and modified. Its utility for care continuity and clarification of caregiver role relationships needs exploration.

THE ASSESSMENT AND INTERVENTION TOOL

The following assessment and intervention tool is designed to include the various aspects of the Neuman Systems Model while allowing for inclusion of other

TABLE 1–3. AN ASSESSMENT AND INTERVENTION TOOL DEVELOPMENT GUIDE

Primary Prevention	Secondary Prevention	Tertiary Prevention

Stressors[a]
  Covert or potential
	Stressors[a]
	  Overt, actual or known
		Stressors[a]
		  Overt, or residual-possible covert

Reaction
  Hypothetical or possible, based on available knowledge
	Reaction
	  Identified symptoms or known stress factors
		Reaction
		  Hypothetical or known residual symptoms or known stress factors

Assessment
  Based on client assessment, experience, and theory
  Risk or possible hazard based on client and nurse perceptions
  Meaning of experience to client
  Life-style factors
  Coping patterns (past, present, possible)
  Individual differences identified
	Assessment
	  Determined by nature and degree of reaction
	  Determine internal and external available resources to resist the reaction
	  Rationale for goals–collaborative goal setting with client
		Assessment
		  Determined by degree of stability following treatment and further potential reconstitution for possible regression factors

Intervention as prevention
 	
  Strengthen client flexible line of defense
  Client education and desensitization to stressors
  Stressor avoidance
  Strengthen individual resistance factors
	Intervention as treatment
	
	  Wellness variance—overt symptoms—nursing diagnosis
	  Need priority and related goals
	  Client strengths and weaknesses related to the five client variables
	  Shift of need priorities as client responds to treatment (primary prevention needs and tertiary prevention may occur simultaneously with treatment or secondary prevention)
	  Intervention in maladaptive processes
	  Optimal use of internal and external resources, such as energy conservation, noise reduction, and financial aid
		Intervention as reconstitution following treatment
		  Motivation
		  Education and reeducation
		  Behavior modification
		  Reality orientation
		  Progressive goal setting
		  Optimal use of available internal and external resources
		  Maintenance of client's optimal functional level

Assessment should include information concerning the relationship of the four variables—physiologic, psychologic, sociocultural, and developmental. (Since 1989 a fifth variable has been added—spiritual.)
Appendix D is reproduced, with revision (1987), from B. Neuman, "The Betty Neuman Health Care Systems Model: A Total Approach to Patient Problems," in Conceptual Models for Nursing Practice, *edited by J. P. Riehl and C. Roy (New York: Appleton-Century-Crofts, 1974).*

areas of information, such as individual specific client or larger client system needs—age, situational differences, special requirements, and so on.

The assessment and intervention tool is readily adaptable for use by nursing to determine limited needs of individual clients, as well as broadly based concerns of a client system like an entire community or a social issue. A unique feature is that the kind of data obtained from the client's own perception of his, her, or its condition influences the overall goals for nursing action. Hence, the form itself is not to be submitted to the client but should be used as a question guide for obtaining comprehensive data. It may be used also as a guide for development of specific tools for select client homogeneous groups.

The following format should offer a progressive total view of facts and conditions from which client goals are developed and modified as needed. Since all caregivers can relate to this assessment and intervention format, continuity of care should be facilitated through its use, and role relationships clarified.

An Explanation of the Assessment/Intervention Tool

CATEGORY A—Biographical data

- A–1. This section includes general biographical data. However, certain agencies may require additional data in this area.
- A–2. Referral source and related information are important. They provide a background history about the client and make possible any contacts with those who interviewed the client earlier. Requests from agencies for reciprocal relationships might be recorded in this area.

CATEGORY B—Stressors as perceived by client

- B–1. It is important to find out from the client how he or she perceives or experiences the particular situation or condition. By clarifying the client's perception, data are obtained for optimal care planning.
- B–2. The client should be encouraged to discuss how present life-style is related to past, or usual, life-style patterns. A marked change may be significantly related to the course of an illness or possible illness.
- B–3. This area relates to coping patterns. It is important to learn what similar conditions may have existed in the past and how the client has dealt with them. Such data provide insight about the type of resources available that were mobilized to deal with the situation. Past coping patterns may be significantly related to the present situation, making possible certain predictions as to what a client may or may not be able to accomplish. For example, symptoms of present loss might be exaggerated following unresolved past losses.
- B–4. The area of client expectations is important in planning health care interventions. Goals for care could be inappropriate if not based on clarification of how the client perceives his or her situation or con-

dition. For example, a client might erroneously think the situation is terminal while the caregiver attempts to prepare the client for living.

- B–5. If the extent of client motivation to help him- or herself can be known, available internal and external resources can be more wisely used in the client's behalf.
- B–6. The health care cost factor can often be a source of stress for the client. Sufficient data should be obtained from the client about the health care services the client feels are needed. However, the practitioner should bear in mind that the client frequently requires help in determining what services are realistic.

CATEGORY C—Stressors as perceived by caregiver

The fact that caregivers have a perspective different from that of the client is considered a positive factor. Education, past experiences, values, personal biases, and unresolved personal conflicts can, however, distort the caregiver's clear conception of the client's actual condition. Category C was included to reduce this possibility. Questions 1 through 6 are essentially the same as those in Category B so that the client's perception can be compared with the caregiver's perception. The interviewer should know the basis for his or her own perceptions, as well as the client's, so that the reality of the client's situation or condition can be fairly accurately described in a summary of impressions.

CATEGORIES D, E, and F—As perceived by both caregiver and client

These categories deal with the intra-, inter-, and extrapersonal factors illustrated on the model diagram. In order to assess an individual's total situation or condition at any point, it is necessary to know the relationships among internal environmental factors, factors occurring between the individual and the environment, as well as external environmental factors that affect or could affect the individual. This set of questions attempts to clarify these relationships so that goal priorities can be established.

CATEGORY G—Nursing diagnosis

A clear, comprehensive statement of the client condition requires the reconciliation of perceptual differences between client and caregiver. All pertinent aspects of client data must be ordered according to need priority before appropriate client goals can be determined.

CHART 1–1–Summary of goals with rationale

Once the major problem has been defined in relation to all factors affecting the client situation or condition, further classification is needed. A decision must be made as to what form of intervention should take priority. For example, if a reaction has not yet occurred and the client has been assessed as being in a high-risk category, intervention should begin at the primary prevention-as-intervention level. Moreover, one should be able to state the logic or rationale

CHART 1–1. SUMMARY OF GOALS WITH RATIONALE

Primary Prevention (Prevention of treatment)	Secondary Prevention (Treatment)	Tertiary Prevention (Follow-up after treatment)
Immediate Goals: 1. 2. 3. Rationale:		
Intermediate Goals: 1. 2. 3. Rationale:		
Future Goals: 1. 2. 3. Rationale		

for the intervention. If a reaction is noted on assessment (that is, symptoms are obvious), intervention should begin at the secondary prevention level (treatment). When assessment is made following treatment, intervention should begin at the tertiary prevention level (follow-up after treatment).

By relating all factors affecting the client, it is possible to determine fairly accurately what type of intervention is needed (primary, secondary, or tertiary), as well as the rationale to support the stated goals. At whatever point interventions are begun, it is important to attempt to project possible future health care requirements. These data may not be readily available on initial assessment but should be noted when possible to provide a comprehensive and progressive view of the client's total condition. It is important to relate this section of the assessment and intervention tool to the intervention (worksheet) plan (Chart 1–2).

CHART 1–2—Intervention plan to support stated goals

This portion of the assessment and intervention tool is a form of worksheet that provides progressive data as to the type of intervention given, by goal, as listed and ranked by priority. The type of interventions, and their outcomes, are noted. The comment section might include data useful for future planning, such as new goal priorities based on changes in the client's condition or responses and success or failure of past or present interventions, or both. This format classifies each intervention in a consistent, progressive, and comprehensive manner to

CHART 1–2. INTERVENTION PLAN TO SUPPORT STATED GOALS

Primary Prevention	Secondary Prevention	Tertiary Prevention
Date		
Goals[a]	Goals[a]	Goals[a]
1.	1.	1.
2.	2.	2.
3.	3.	3.
Intervention:	Intervention:	Intervention:
Outcome:	Outcome:	Outcome:
Comments:	Comments:	Comments:

[a]Goals are stated in order of priority.

which any caregiver can meaningfully relate. This system of classifying data over time allows one to see the relationship of the part to the whole, that is, to view the client in total perspective, thereby reducing the possibility of fragmentation of care and possibly reducing cost factors.

An Assessment and Intervention Tool Based on the Neuman Health Care Systems Model

Client

A. *Intake Summary*
   1. Name _____
      Age _____
      Sex _____
      Marital status _____
   2. Referral source and related information.
B. *Stressors as Perceived by Client* (If client is incapacitated, secure data from family or other resources.)
   1. What do you consider your major stress area, or areas of health concern? (Identify three areas.)
   2. How do present circumstances differ from your usual pattern of living? (Identify life-style patterns.)
   3. Have you ever experienced a similar problem? If so, what was that problem and how did you handle it? Were you successful? (Identify past coping patterns.)
   4. What do you anticipate for yourself in the future as a consequence of your present situation? (Identify perceptual factors, that is, reality versus distortions—expectations, present and possible future coping patterns.)
   5. What are you doing and what can you do to help yourself? (Identify perceptual factors, that is, reality versus distortions–expectations, present and possible future coping patterns.)
   6. What do you expect caregivers, family, friends, or others to do for you?

(Identify perceptual factors, that is, reality versus distortions–expectations, present and possible future coping patterns.)

C. *Stressors as Perceived by Caregiver*

1. What do you consider to be the major stress area, or areas of health concern? (Identify these areas.)
2. How do present circumstances seem to differ from the client's usual pattern of living? (Identify life-style patterns.)
3. Has the client ever experienced a similar situation? If so, how would you evaluate what the client did? How successful do you think it was? (Identify past coping patterns.)
4. What do you anticipate for the future as a consequence of the client's present situation? (Identify perceptual factors, that is, reality versus distortions–expectations, present and possible future coping patterns.)
5. What can the client do to help him- or herself? (Identify perceptual factors, that is, reality versus distortions–expectations, present and possible future coping patterns.)
6. What do you think the client expects from caregivers, family, friends, or other resources? (Identify perceptual factors, that is, reality versus distortions–expectations, present and possible future coping patterns.)

Summary of Impressions

Note any discrepancies or distortions between the client perception and that of the caregiver related to the situation.

D. *Intrapersonal Factors*

1. Physical (examples: degree of mobility, range of body function)
2. Psycho-sociocultural (examples: attitudes, values, expectations, behavior patterns, and nature of coping patterns)
3. Developmental (examples: age, degree of normalcy, factors related to present situation)
4. Spiritual belief system (examples: hope and sustaining factors)

E. *Interpersonal Factors*

Examples are resources and relationship of family, friends, or caregivers that either influence or could influence Area D.

F. *Extrapersonal Factors*

Examples are resources and relationship of community facilities, finances, employment, or other areas that either influence or could influence Areas D and E.

G. *Formulation of a Comprehensive Nursing Diagnosis*

This is accomplished by identifying and ranking the priority of needs based on total data obtained from the client's perception, the caregiver's perception, or other resources, such as laboratory reports, other caregivers, or agencies. Appropriate theory is related to the above data.

With this format, reassessment is a continuous process and is related to the effectiveness of intervention based on the prior stated goals. Effective reassessment would include the following as they relate to the total client situation:

1. Changes in nature of stressors and priority assignments
2. Changes in intrapersonal factors
3. Changes in interpersonal factors
4. Changes in extrapersonal factors

In reassessment it is important to note the change of priority of goals in relation to the primary, secondary, and tertiary prevention as intervention categories. An assessment tool of this nature should offer a current, progressive, and comprehensive analysis of the client's total circumstances and relationship of the five client variables (physiological, psychological, sociocultural, developmental, and spiritual) to environmental influences.

2

THROUGH THE LOOKING GLASS
Back to the Future

Lois W. Lowry
Patricia Hinton Walker
Rosalie Mirenda

This chapter represents a looking back, by three long-standing, dedicated trustees, in order to best view the future of the Neuman Systems Model. Predictions are then made as to relevancy for 21st-century use of the model in helping structure and shape the future of nursing.

The '90s are indeed a critical decade. Solutions to rapidly increasing economic, social, and health problems will require a radical shift in societal thinking, perceptions, values, problem-solving, and even life-styles. With a current paradigm shift from an illness-focused health care system to an illness prevention health promotion system, will the nursing models and theories, constructed twenty years ago to guide the profession, remain relevant to the challenge facing the nursing community of tomorrow?

The answer to this rhetorical question is that some models will continue to be useful well into the 21st century, while others will not. What will make the difference? One must search the literature to rediscover why models are developed. All disciplines use models to replicate, reproduce, or represent something in the world. Models can be classified according to their level of abstraction, with physical models, such as automobile replicas, at one end of the continuum and abstract mental models, such as mathematical symbols, at the other. All models focus on the details of reality that are perceived to have the greatest relevance to the situation at hand (Lancaster and Lancaster, 1981).

Nursing models were developed to provide a clearer definition of nursing. Faced with complex human problems, nurses have always used a problem-solving process to interpret the realities confronting them. Nursing models allow part of reality to be represented by organizing and structuring complex events while limiting extraneous factors and only portraying essential components of the situation (Lancaster and Lancaster, 1981). Each nursing model provides a particular view or perspective of nursing as interpreted by the author of the model. Model assumptions and values must be congruent within the arena it represents, with clear definitions of concepts and relational statements. Since models have no truth in and of themselves, their usefulness lies in how well they describe the reality they represent.

What was the reality within the discipline of nursing in the 1960s and 1970s when nursing theories began to emerge? Nursing leaders of the day resisted the implication that nursing was merely a chapter of medicine (Meleis, 1991), and patients a collection of biological systems needing medical attention (Rogers, 1973). In fact, Johnson's (1959) analysis of the nature of science in nursing was a milestone in drawing attention to the potential of nursing as a scientific discipline. Johnson conceptualized patients as behavioral systems as opposed to biological systems, thus setting the stage for development of nursing models that placed ideas and concepts relevant to nursing into comprehensive constructs that could guide nursing practice and education (Rogers, 1973).

Dr. Neuman developed her systems model in 1970 (first published in 1972) in response to expressed needs of graduate students for an overview course containing content relevant to the breadth of nursing prior to selection of a specific area for clinical specialization (Neuman and Young, 1972). Although Neuman, Roy, and Johnson were faculty colleagues at UCLA during this time period, Dr. Neuman developed her wholistic model from her philosophic views and insights gained through experiences while originating and teaching in a postmaster's community mental health program. The major concepts in the Neuman Model (client, environment, health, and nursing) are those presented by Yura and Torres (1975) as the paradigm for nursing that was readily accepted by nurse scientists.

HISTORICAL PERSPECTIVE

During the early years, the Neuman Systems Model was used primarily to guide education and practice and as a conceptual framework for some master and doctoral level research. Its 23-year history is phenomenal in terms of its escalating growth, utility, and future potential. The model, never in an embryonic stage, has remained relevant and unchanged since Neuman first developed and utilized it in 1970 at UCLA as a wholistic nursing concepts course integrative tool for graduate students. It was not until the early to mid-1970s that educational programs began to initiate curricular development based on nursing models. In

1975 Neumann College, Division of Nursing began its work on developing a curricular design based on the Neuman Systems Model. However, the first Neuman-based programs implemented were at the University of Pittsburgh undergraduate program and Texas Woman University graduate program in the late 1970s. During the 1980s exploration and utilization of the Neuman Systems Model greatly accelerated in education at all levels of practice in varied settings throughout the United States, Canada, Europe, Australia, and Far Eastern areas within the Republic of China, Japan, and Korea.

Through the years from 1970 to the present (late 1994), the relevance and utility of the Neuman Systems Model can be organized under the following four major categories:

1. The model provides a full representation of nursing, that is, a world view of the profession of nursing and the full scope of responsibility of the professional nurse (Neuman, 1989).
2. The model serves as a curriculum guide, or blueprint, for curriculum development (Fawcett, 1989).
3. The model guides clinical nursing practice in a variety of health care settings and for individuals, families, and communities (Whall, 1983).
4. The model, through its major concepts and propositions, provides guidelines for nursing research (Fawcett, 1989).

REPRESENTATION OF NURSING

The model represents a way of viewing clients wholistically and multidimensionally, within a systemic perspective. It considers all variables affecting a client's potential or actual response to environmental stressors. The model illustrates the dynamic nature of "client" as being a composite of five interacting variables—physiological, psychological, sociocultural, developmental, and spiritual—ideally functioning harmoniously for system stability.

The model is considered dynamic because of continuous client system interactive relationships with environmental stress factors during both wellness and illness. The model presents nursing as a unique profession in its consideration of all client system variables requiring a wholistic, comprehensive care approach to client situations. The dynamic wholistic nature of client system functioning requires multidimensional thinking, acting, and coordinating. The systemic approach provides a unifying effect for nursing through organization and structure of its component parts relevant to the profession and to the health care system in general. The increased emphasis on primary prevention (wellness retention) is a rapidly expanding futuristic concept with which nursing as a profession must be concerned. The Neuman Systems Model holds unlimited potential for major role development that could shape the future of nursing within the overall health care system. It will remain relevant to and incorporate outcomes of worldwide health care reform issues.

CURRICULUM GUIDE

Fawcett (1989) stated that the utility of the Neuman Systems Model for nursing education is well documented. The use of the Neuman Systems conceptual model as a curriculum guide has been described in a number of publications and presentations (Bourbonnais and Ross, 1985; Kilchenstein and Yakulis, 1984; Lowry, 1985; Mirenda, 1986).

Bower (1982) developed a curricular blueprint consistent with the Neuman Systems Model. The blueprint provides direction for curricular development to include terminal and level outcomes, course content, sequence, and course descriptions. Knox, Kilchenstein, and Yakulis (1982) have described the University of Pittsburgh integrated baccalaureate program based on their adaptation of the Neuman Model. The model provides a logical conceptual base for broadly focused and flexible programming in nursing education for those wishing to design a wholistic curriculum focused on total quality care of individuals, families, and communities within multiple and diverse systems. The second book edition of the Neuman Systems Model (1989) included an entire section describing application of the Neuman Systems Model to nursing education. Examples of model application included: baccalaureate and graduate nursing programs at California State University, Fresno; a cooperative baccalaureate program in Minnesota; an associate degree program in transition to a baccalaureate program; a baccalaureate program undergoing curriculum revision at the University of Saskatchewan; and the utilization of the Neuman Model in multilevel nurse education programs at the University of Nevada, Las Vegas. More recently, communication with the Neuman trustees reveals that the University of Guam, Indiana University–Purdue University, and State University of New York at Brockport are in various stages of curriculum development based on the Neuman Systems Model.

Use of the Neuman Systems Model as a curriculum guide for the future will assist in making the necessary paradigm shift for health care reform by providing (1) a collaborative, cooperative model for approaching clients; (2) a client-centered focus; (3) emphasis on primary prevention; and (4) a coordinated, managed care model.

NURSING PRACTICE

The utility of the Neuman Systems Model from the mid-1970s through the early 1990s is also well documented. The first edition of the Neuman text (1982) includes examples of model use in various clinical situations within community and public health settings, nursing centers, family therapy, acute medical and surgical situations, and rehabilitation centers. Neuman (1990) provided an overview of model usage for nursing clinical practice around the world. Her examples included worldwide use of the model for psychiatric nursing, critical care, primary care, public health, community mental health, various clinics, long-term care facilities, and family health nursing.

Critical to evolution of the Neuman Systems Model in practice are three dimensions that link the model to the future. The first of these is its consideration of caring caregiving. Central to the concept of systems is stability and/or balance and harmony in the face of continuous change, a major goal when utilizing the Neuman Model. Neuman (1990) stated that caring caregiving implies that nurses act to protect clients' own preferences, privileges, wants and desires, health, and needs rather than their own. Caring caregiving is best seen in one's ability and willingness to seek ways to protect the rights of clients, which implies acceptance of responsibility to administer, coordinate care, and establish health policies that reflect social justice. The second dimension that links Neuman Model relevance to the future is its potential for use by other health care disciplines because of its common terminology, concepts, and comprehensive nature. The current trend is toward increased interdisciplinary sharing and cooperation. For example, currently (1994), the model is used for physical therapy (University of Michigan at Flint) and occupational therapy (Sheffield, England) as a model from nursing that assists development of interdisciplinary curricula and practice evaluation formats from a wholistic client system perspective. A third dimension is the model's proven utility as a comprehensive base for both nursing education and practice in a variety of cultures. The model is being successfully used in many cultures worldwide, for example, the Far East, the United Kingdom, Australia, and others. The model's breadth, flexibility, and comprehensive nature will foster its relevancy for structuring and organizing nursing phenomena well into the 21st century.

GUIDELINES FOR NURSING RESEARCH

While the primary model contribution has largely been pragmatic, Neuman-based research activity is becoming increasingly well documented (for example, Ziegler [1982], Ziemer [1983], Capers [1987], Hanson and Berkey [1991], and Fulton [1992]). Louis and Koertvelyessy (in Neuman, 1989) report the results of their 1987 international survey, which identified Neuman as one of the three most frequently used models for nursing research. At the spring 1993 International Symposium meeting, the Neuman Systems Model Trustee Group, Inc., identified major research areas for the model as being the further explication of the five system variables, the levels of prevention as intervention modes, and the basic energy structure when the client system is identified as family or community. Dr. Jacqueline Fawcett shares her views on future Neuman research protocols in the research section of this text.

Therefore, as we look forward to the 21st century and to health care reform, with implications for a strong emphasis on primary health care services, it is imperative that the social utility of nursing models be evaluated. For example, will the assumptions on which the Neuman Systems Model was based in 1970, though relevant today, continue to be so for tomorrow's sociopolitical environment? Further, can a "mature" model (20 or more years in use) be flexible enough to meet the demands of a changing society?

To explore these questions, it is important to revisit the former Neuman Model assumptions.

> Though each individual is viewed as unique, he is also considered to be a composite of common "knowns" or characteristics within a normal, given range of responses. There are many known stressors. Each stressor is different in its potential to disturb an individual's equilibrium or normal line of defense. Moreover, particular relationships of the variables—physiological, psychological, socio-cultural, and developmental—at any point can affect the degree to which an individual is able to use his flexible line of defense against possible reaction to a single stressor or combination of stressors. Each individual, over time, has evolved a normal range of responses which is referred to as a normal line of defense. When the cushioning, accordion-like effect of the flexible line of defense is no longer capable of protecting the individual against a stressor, the stressor breaks through the normal line of defense. The interrelationship of variables determines the nature and degree of the organism's reaction to the stressor. Each person has an internal set of resistance factors (lines of resistance), which attempt to stabilize and return to his normal line of defense should a stressor break through it. Man is in a state of wellness or illness in varying degrees in relation to the dynamic composite of interrelationships of the four variables . . . that are always present. Primary prevention relates to general knowledge that is applied to individual client assessment in an attempt to identify and allay the possible risk factors associated with stressors. Secondary prevention relates to symptomatology, appropriate ranking of intervention priorities, and treatment. Tertiary prevention relates to the adaptive process as reconstitution begins, and moves back in a circular manner toward primary prevention. (Neuman, 1974, 101)

These assumptions reflect similar truths in today's world. It is important to note, however, that in 1989 Dr. Neuman added the spiritual variable to the initial four making a total of five client system variables. The original model was derived from a synthesis of broad concepts and philosophic beliefs from other disciplines, supporting continued model relevancy for today. Health care disciplines currently are being challenged to listen closely to one another and to develop collaborative liaisons to deliver high-quality health care. The consumer, viewed by Neuman as client (individual, family, or group), is considered to be the center of the health care system of tomorrow. Consumers (or clients) are customers who will choose what is best for them. Nurses forming partnerships with consumers can assist in influencing them to be active participants in their care. Models broad enough to encompass multiple health care disciplines can provide a language understandable and usable by nurses and other health care providers. With increased focus on care outcome criteria that benefit the client, comprehensive models will be sought as health care reform evolves.

The Neuman Systems Model (earlier titled the *Neuman health-care systems model*), developed in 1970, may have been "before its time" when many models were nursing discipline specific. As we look to the future, however, the Neuman Model meets the criteria for health care outcomes reached through an evolving interdisciplinary approach. Thus, it is concluded that the Neuman assumptions (now considered propositions) are as relevant today as 20 years ago.

A second question addresses the attributes of a mature model vis-à-vis a young model. Youth implies flexibility, vigor, creativity, and developing habits. Maturity, on the other hand, is viewed as a process of reducing initial flexibility and adaptiveness to a more predictable, less chaotic habit pattern. Is it possible for a model to advance toward maturity without moving toward rigidity and decreasing vitality? If the process of maturity encompasses change as a positive value, the result is a dynamic model. "In an ever-renewing society that matures is a system or framework within which continuous innovation, renewal and rebirth can occur" (Gardner, 1965, 5). Ideally, continuity and change must be interwoven. Continuity provides the long-term values, purposes, and direction for change; change is the innovation within the continuity (Gardner, 1965). A system ideally provides for its own continuous renewal, through input, output, and process. In its dynamism a system can remain stable while in the process of change. The Neuman Systems Model meets this criterion.

Dr. Neuman designed a comprehensive framework to guide students in selecting and synthesizing knowledge critical to their practice. Further, the model, as an open systems structure, permits creativity in its use. Dr. Neuman encourages innovative use of her work so long as the basic intent and purposes are retained. This view is congruent with Smith's (1992) perception that models are "works in process." Each new contribution to or innovation with the model should contribute to its vitality and longevity. Thus, we can predict that since the Neuman Systems Model has continued to be flexible with a high degree of social utility throughout its past years of use in the United States and internationally, it will continue to be relevant in the future. As use of the model accelerates, its vitality will increase.

TOWARD NEW CHALLENGES

Past Neuman Systems Model disputes have centered around an interpreted incompatibility of world views. For example, the mechanistic theory of stress and adaptation and client reaction to stressors appears to be in conflict with statements concerning wholistic persons and interrelationships of the variables (Fawcett, 1989). Within the model, however, the organismic world view, stemming from Gestalt and field theories, is predominant. From a pedagogical point of view, it is often necessary to "break down the whole" into its constituent parts in order to study the parts and relationships among them. This dispute has occurred primarily within nursing education programs.

Furthermore, whereas Neuman statements concerning stress and reaction to stress are explicit (which is consistent with Selye's [1950] biological view of stress), other perceptions are implied related to psychological stress and coping. For example, the Neuman construct of the created environment as a dynamic interface with the internal and external environments, protecting the client system, implies the integration of all five variables in perceiving and coping with stress. Dr. Neuman writes:

> The insulating effect of the created-environment changes the response or possible response of the client to environmental stressors, for example, the use of denial or envy (psychological), physical rigidity or muscular constraint (physiological), life cycle continuation of survival patterns (developmental), required social space range (sociocultural), and sustaining hope (spiritual). (Neuman, 1989, 32)

These examples illustrate that the model clearly reflects continuous interaction occurring between clients and their environment, dynamic and reciprocal in nature, leading to growth and congruence with an organismic world view.

An important attribute of the model has been its breadth in defining nursing interventions within three prevention modalities. Throughout the past 20 years of its use, emphasis was primarily on secondary and tertiary nursing care, particularly in associate and baccalaureate degree programs that prepared graduates for more generalist roles within acute and chronic care settings. However, today, as health care becomes more broadly based, health promotion and primary prevention will receive the educational priority long deserved in nursing education. The relationship among the three preventions is specific enough to provide the link necessary for nurse graduates to incorporate health promotion as a strategy in discharge planning and reeducation by supporting client strengths.

A second significant model attribute is the strong emphasis on consideration of both client and nurse perceptions of stressors and client coping strategies. Both will receive considerable emphasis in the future consumer-driven health care system. Consumers are increasingly becoming recognized as the nurse's best ally. Consumers, as individuals and families, are being encouraged to assume primary responsibility for their own health care decisions. Nurses are in a pioneering position to facilitate this process as they provide wholistic client care. Outcome potential for increasing client wellness is markedly enhanced through wholistic nursing practice.

A third attribute of the Neuman Systems Model is its common language. The terminology of the model is clearly "user friendly" (Walker, 1992). Since its terms are not "unique," the model is easily adaptable in international settings, in workings with other health care professionals, and in the community with clients.

International use of the model is growing significantly, and regardless of the language, stressors, wholism, lines of resistance, and categorization of interventions provide helpful guidelines in the health care arena. Health-conscious clients recognize the impact of stressors and are increasingly interested in participating in and accepting responsibility for their own primary prevention strategies when risk is identified. In addition, many individuals and families who must cope with chronic illness understand and practice tertiary prevention strategies for self-care. Also, as mentioned previously, the client is becoming increasingly concerned about participating in decisions regarding secondary interventions or treatment. Decisions regarding cost, quality of life, and longer-term impact of use of technology in treatment are rapidly becoming issues that consumers of health care want to participate in. The language of the Neuman Systems Model is "user friendly" and invites participation in decision making through the premise that requires development and implementation of mutual goals and decisions for care.

The fourth attribute of the Neuman Systems Model is that the client as a system can be an individual, family, group, or community. With the focus of care and evaluation shifting from the individual to aggregate and community levels, the Neuman Systems Model is well positioned for the future. Applications of the model in administration will continue to develop as nursing and other professions search for ways to categorize interventions across settings and across disciplines. Our current health care delivery system's focus has been primarily on acute care in institutional settings (secondary prevention). Primary and tertiary prevention interventions, such as prevention of specific diseases and health promotion, and tertiary prevention, including rehabilitation, health maintenance, and reconstitution for the chronically ill and elderly, will emerge as a framework to guide the definitions and outcomes of care. The increase of community-based organizations providing care, such as community nursing centers, will redefine health care. Health along the continuum will finally challenge the health care systems previously focused only on the illness paradigm. The Neuman Systems Model, originally developed with the "community as client" in mind, has an advantage in that it has always been prepared for the future.

VISION FOR THE FUTURE

Nursing's vision for a quality, equitable, and cost-effective health care delivery system is within reach. Health care reform in the 1990s provides hope for consumers to have access to affordable care and for nurses to be finally recognized as key providers of health care. Although much of the emphasis on the nursing role and nursing models of care is new to many legislators and the general public, for nurses it is "back to the future."

Lillian Wald, responding to societal needs of her time, developed the Henry

Street Settlement House in 1893. As we listen back to the future, we remember that "Ms. Wald further stated that nurses not only serve the individual but promote the interest of a collective society" (Kippenbrock, 1991, 209). Does this sound familiar? Nursing has historically been positioned for and providing care at the front-end and back-end of the health care delivery system. Schorr writes that medical care is only a part of health care, yet nurses provide 90 percent of what the patient needs before and after the diagnosis is made (Schorr, 1993, 294). She identifies nursing as "first class health care" and describes numerous examples where nurses provide primary care and preventive services to satisfied populations in the community. These include community nursing centers, school-based family health centers, nurse midwifery outreach projects, gerontologic care in nursing homes, and home health, and in occupational settings where occupational health nurses serve as care managers and caregivers for workers and families (Schorr, 1993, 295).

According to de Tornyay, "the future will be more oriented to health, stressing disease and injury prevention, health promotion, elimination of environmental hazards, and individual responsibility for health-related behaviors. . . . In addition, the systems will be more population-based with more attention paid to risk factors in the physical and social environments—many of which must be addressed at the community rather than the individual patient level" (de Tornyay, 1993, 303). Management of care across settings and systems will require coordination of care across disciplines. This "coordination requires the ability to use language others can readily understand" (de Tornyay, 1993, 304). The impetus for increased individual responsibility and interdisciplinary care will require use of language and terminology that emphasizes the collaborative role between practitioner and client and among nurses and other disciplines.

Three significant societal changes and forces contribute to a changing role for the nursing profession as health care reform evolves. These changes include (1) feminism and the women's movement, (2) the American health care crisis influenced by increased specialization and high-tech care crisis, and (3) a growing internationalism or "global" community with an emphasis on primary care and health for all by the year 2000. According to Fagin, "interdependence—of nations, of economies, and of people—is at the heart of the new internationalism. Interdependence is also the heart of nursing models of care" (Fagin, 1992, 208–209).

Where does the Neuman Systems Model fit into this picture? Neuman's clients have and will continue to be at the center of the health care system. The client according to Neuman can be the individual, family, or community. With increasing emphasis on care of aggregate populations and communities, the Neuman Systems Model and instruments that have been developed to assess the client as individual, family, and community will provide direction and guidance. The perception and goals of the client (now often referred to as the consumer) have also been and will continue to be at the center of the Neuman Systems Model. Bringing the client in as a full participant in health care decisions is not new to Neuman Model users; consequently, the Neuman Systems Model is congruent with the evolving priority of the consumer as participant in health care.

Neuman's clients (individual, family, or community) interact reciprocally with the external and internal environment. As we look to the future, external and internal environments will increasingly influence health states of clients. The relationship and influence of the external environment to the client have taken on new meaning during this last decade of the 20th century, and there will be an even greater emphasis on the influence of the external environment in the next century. These influences include but are not limited to the impact of violence in the home and community; sexual messages and information in the media; environmental contaminants in air, food, and water; and increasing global disasters and wars. Such factors will force health care providers to increasingly focus analysis of the impact of the external environment on care of the client (for example, see Chapter 6). The internal environment and its reciprocal relationship to the client system is also becoming much more complex, with societal issues such as crack babies, alcohol-dependent newborns, genetic engineering as treatment, and altered mind states from addiction to drugs. Patient care studies and research are already emphasizing an expanding role for prevention as intervention for those at risk because of stressors in the environment. Because of environmental dangers, secondary and tertiary prevention is critical for those who have already experienced changes in one of the five variables areas: physiological, psychological, sociocultural, developmental, and spiritual, as identified by Neuman.

The wholistic approach to assessment of the client system variables is a hallmark of the Neuman Model. The addition of the spiritual variable in the 1989 second book edition particularly positions the Neuman Systems Model for the future. Naisbitt and Aburdene write that "at the dawn of the third millennium is a worldwide multidenominational religious revival . . . that religious belief is intensifying worldwide under the gravitational pull of the year 2000, the millennium" (Naisbitt and Aburdene, 1990, 270–271). They state, however, that it is spirituality, not organized religion, that is on the rise. One conclusion is that the return to faith is a sign of "the refusal to define life only in terms of science and technology" (Naisbitt and Aburdene, 1990, 297). For these reasons, the new impetus and interest in the spiritual variable in the Neuman Systems Model will continue to flourish. Donley emphasizes the importance of the spiritual dimension of care at a time when the health care system promotes material and technical values (Donley, 1991, 179). She believes that the "crisis in health care is one of meaning and values" (Donley, 1991, 178). New chapters in this third edition highlight evolving issues and discussions regarding the spiritual variable. Exploring the spiritual dimension in practice and research and the potential for understanding spiritual implications on a global perspective are included in Chapters 3 and 41. It is clear that this variable will continue to be a critical contribution of the Neuman Systems Model to the future.

International health, health of communities of clients, impact on health policy, and interdisciplinary practice will characterize the future development of the Neuman Systems Model. Categorizing care and determining the cost-benefit and utility of primary, secondary, and tertiary preventions as interventions are logical next steps for the Neuman Systems Model. Applications for managed care and interdisciplinary practice will flourish as the emphasis on primary care, prevention, health promotion, and health maintenance worldwide provides a ready climate for Neuman Model advocates.

Nurses functioning as primary care providers will further emphasize primary and tertiary interventions, forming partnerships with clients who are active participants in their own care. An increased focus in the health care system on prevention as intervention will bring the historical value of the Neuman Model to the forefront of health care delivery. According to Hillary Rodham Clinton, "The nurses in the ambulatory and community clinics, health departments, school based health clinics and perinatal units will make preventive health care a priority. In addition, collaborating with others in health settings can eliminate barriers to access" (Clinton, 1993, 288).

Collaboration as a part of secondary preventions will require new and different arrangements within the interdisciplinary team to provide linkages into the acute care or "medical" system. Community nursing centers and other community-based care environments will offer opportunities for new collaborative and consultative models of practice with physicians. Case management will also move more to the forefront as providers struggle with coordination of care across settings. This will stimulate new interest in data and information; consequently, information systems will be developed using nursing models of care. There will also be renewed interest in "tertiary prevention" as Neuman describes it in order to deal with health maintenance compounded by the increased high-tech care provided by our current delivery system. Many Americans are living longer, and more individuals and families are experiencing some form of chronic illness. Concepts of prevention, maintenance of function, and client participation are critical to successful management of individual clients and families with chronic illness. The Neuman Systems Model provides a framework for care of this often neglected population in the current health care delivery system.

FUTURE IMPLICATIONS FOR USE OF THE NEUMAN SYSTEMS MODEL

The Neuman Systems Model is clearly poised and ready for the challenges of the future. Sometimes characterized in the past as too broad, complex, and comprehensive, the model is coming into its own with the challenges of the 21st century. The complexities of the global society, of crises in health care delivery, and of changing patterns and dangers from the environment provide stimulus for new applications of the Neuman Systems Model. The model is not only broad and comprehensive enough to provide structure for nursing interventions, but also for other disciplines interested in focusing on wellness and wholistic care for patients and clients. Meleis writes that "time and sociocultural conditions are right for the development of theoretical nursing, which in turn is significant for patient care and nurses are "going for it' " (Meleis, 1991, 67). The ongoing use and scholarly development of the Neuman Systems Model in practice, education, administration, and research in domestic and international settings is evidence of this.

REFERENCES

Bourbonnais, F. F., and Ross, M. R. 1985. The Neuman Systems Model in nursing education: Course development and implementation. *Journal of Advanced Nursing* 10: 117–123.

Bower, F. L. 1982. Curriculum development and the Neuman Model. In *The Neuman Systems Model: Application to Nursing Education and Practice,* by B. Neuman, 94–99. Norwalk, Conn.: Appleton-Century-Crofts.

Capers, C. F., and Kelly, R. 1987. Neuman Nursing Process: A model of holistic care. *Holistic Nursing Practice* 1(3):19–26.

Clinton, H. R. 1993. Nurses in the front lines. *Nursing and Health Care* 14(6):288.

de Tornyay, R. 1993. Nursing education staying on track. *Nursing and Health Care* 14(6):303–304.

Donley, R. 1991. Spiritual dimensions of health care. *Nursing and Health Care* 12(4):178–179.

Fagin, C. 1992. President's message. *Nursing and Health Care* 13(4):208–209.

Fawcett, J. 1989. *Analysis and Evaluation of Conceptual Models of Nursing,* 2d ed. Philadelphia: F. A. Davis.

Fulton, B. 1992. Curriculum integration using the Neuman Systems Model. Unpublished doctoral dissertation.

Gardner, John W. 1965. *Self Renewal.* New York: Harper & Row.

Hansen, S., and Berkey, K. 1991. Development of a family health stressor/strength assessment-intervention guide. Research in progress.

Johnson, D. E. 1959. The nature of a science of nursing. *Nursing Outlook* 7(5):291–294.

Kilchenstein, L., and Yakulis, I. 1984. The birth of a curriculum: Utilization of the Betty Neuman Health Care Systems Model in an integrated baccalaureate program. *Journal of Nursing Education* 23:126–127.

Kippenbrock, T. A. 1991. Wish I'd been there. *Nursing and Health Care* 12(4):209.

Knox, J. E., Kilchenstein, L., and Yakulis, I. M. 1982. Utilization of the Neuman Model in an integrated baccalaureate program: University of Pittsburgh. In B. Neuman, *The Neuman Systems Model: Application to Nursing Education and Practice,* 117–123. Norwalk, Conn.: Appleton-Century-Crofts.

Lancaster, J., and Lancaster, W. 1981. Models and model building in nursing. *Advances in Nursing Science* 3(3):31–42.

Lowry, L. W. 1985. Application of Betty Neuman's framework. Paper presented at Nursing Theory in Action Conference, Edmonton, Alberta, Canada, August.

Meleis, A. 1991. *Theoretical Nursing: Development Progress,* 2d ed. Philadelphia: J. B. Lippincott.

Mirenda, R. M. 1986. The Neuman Systems Model: Description and application. In *Case Studies in Nursing Theory,* edited by P. Winstead-Fry, 127–166. New York: National League for Nursing.

Neuman, B. 1989. *The Neuman Systems Model,* 2d ed. New York: Appleton & Lange.

Neuman, B. 1982. *The Neuman Systems Model: Application to Nursing Education and Practice.* Norwalk, Conn.: Appleton-Century-Crofts.

Neuman, B. 1974. The Neuman Health Care Systems Model: A total person approach to patient problems. In *Conceptual Models for Nursing Practice,* edited by J. P. Riehl and C. Roy. New York: Appleton-Century-Crofts.

Neuman, B. 1990. The Neuman Systems Model chronology. Paper presented at the Ohio Nurses Association Nursing Theory Conference, Ohio, June.

Neuman, B. 1990. Reflections on caring and future of the model. Paper presented at the Third Biennium of the Neuman Systems Model Conference, Dayton, Ohio, November.

Rogers, C. G. 1973. Conceptual models as guides to clinical nursing specialization. *The Journal of Nursing Education* 12(4):2–6.

Schorr, T. M. 1993. The term is "health care." *Nursing and Health Care* 14(6):294–295.

Selye, H. 1950. The physiology and pathology of exposure to stress. Montreal: ACTA.

Smith, M. C. 1992. Distinctiveness of nursing knowledge. *Nursing Science Quarterly* 5(4):148–149.

Whall, A. L. 1983. The Betty Neuman Health Care Systems Model. In *Conceptual Models of Nursing: Analysis and Application,* by J. J. Fitzpatrick and A. L. Whall. Bowie, Md.: Brady.

Yura, H., and Torres, G. 1975. Today's conceptual frameworks within baccalaureate nursing programs. In *Faculty-Curriculum Development Part III: Conceptual Framework—Its Meaning and Function,* 17–25. New York: National League for Nursing.

Ziegler, S. M. 1982. Taxonomy for nursing diagnosis derived from the Neuman Systems Model. In *The Neuman Systems Model: Application to Nursing Education and Practice,* by B. Neuman, 55–68. Norwalk, Conn.: Appleton-Century-Crofts.

Ziemer, S. M. 1986. Effects of information on postsurgical coping. Paper presented at the First Neuman Systems Model Symposium, Aston, Pa., October.

3

THE SPIRITUAL VARIABLE
Essential to the Client System

Ruth Ann B. Fulton
Introduction by Verna Carson

Spirituality, a concept both difficult to define and to operationalize, is nonetheless an integral part of our humanity. Our spirituality allows us to strive for coherent meaning in the most trying of life's circumstances, including the most painful losses of our own health and the death of those closest to us; it allows us to relate to the Ultimate Being or Reality as we define that reality; it allows us to seek and offer forgiveness, experience joy, and enter into relationships that are loving, committed, and steadfast; it allows us to see the best in the other and to see potentials for goodness in those who display the worst of human behavior; it allows us to maintain a dynamic hope and to believe in the possibility of a reality that at present does not exist.

Certainly, a concept as important as spirituality must also be an important focus of the profession of nursing, which has always claimed a wholistic domain when it comes to caring for the needs of others. This importance is being acknowledged by nurse practitioners, educators, and researchers. However, much of the current research and expository writing on spirituality relegates the concept as an "add-on" to nursing theory. The writings of nonnursing theorists are frequently used to explain the essence of spirituality and the crucial role that spirituality and spiritual concerns play in the lives of people. There has been no coherent model or theory that integrates the spiritual variable into the domain of nursing's concern. The Neuman Systems Model is unique in making the spiritual variable an explicit aspect of nursing theory.

Reviewed by Verna Carson and Lois W. Lowry.

In this chapter Dr. Fulton provides the reader with an excellent and comprehensive review of the "state of the art" of the spiritual variable as a focus of nursing's concern. The multiple approaches to the spiritual variable, including spiritual dimension, spiritual well-being, spiritual needs, spiritual care, and spiritual distress, are presented and integrated into the Neuman Systems Model in a manner that provides linkage among the many approaches and a sense of continuity lacking in much of the literature she cites.

In a succinct fashion, Dr. Fulton examines the research presently available regarding the multiple aspects of the spiritual variable. From this review she suggests that these studies facilitate decision making and future direction for research using the Neuman Systems Model. She posits that the most important priority for quantitative research is the development of valid and reliable instrumentation; for the qualitative researcher the most important priority is to identify relationships among spiritual constructs and categories relevant to the spiritual variable. Further, she identifies the paucity of studies that examine the spiritual variable in children and recommends this as an appropriate area for research inquiry using the Neuman Systems Model.

Dr. Fulton proceeds to examine the "fit" of the Neuman Systems Model with nursing education and practice. Her review of the literature concludes that (1) nursing education is not providing enough instruction regarding spirituality; and (2) content that focuses on the spiritual variable makes a positive difference to students of nursing in terms of their own spirituality and their ability to meet the spiritual needs of clients. She suggests two remedies for the apparent lack of spiritually related content and practice within nursing curricula. The first approach involves developing an increasing awareness of the spiritual self in faculty and students. The second approach, which actually operationalizes the first approach, is for nursing educational programs to adopt the Neuman Systems Model as the organizing framework for choosing, organizing, sequencing, and delivering relevant nursing content. In addition, the Neuman Systems Model offers a framework for evaluating the outcomes of educational interventions and developing educationally focused research agendas. Dr. Fulton directs the reader to the many resources already available to educators interested in incorporating the spiritual variable in both secular and Christian nursing programs.

The chapter next highlights nursing practice, focusing on spiritual care, and the use of the Neuman Systems Model. The model identifies the role of spiritual care as a primary, secondary, and tertiary mode of prevention as intervention. The focus on spiritual care as a primary prevention represents a quantum leap in nursing's understanding of the place of spiritual care. Frequently, spiritual care is identified with endings and losses—and spiritual care becomes not a primary intervention but usually a secondary or tertiary one. Dr. Fulton informs the reader regarding available studies and resources that guide the practitioner in assessing the spiritual variable. She reviews the literature for identified spiritual interventions and describes how these resources are easily integrated into the Neuman Systems Model.

Dr. Fulton concludes this excellent overview of spirituality and the Neuman Systems Model with an examination of the future implications in the areas of nursing research, education, and practice using the Neuman Systems Model as an organizing and explanatory conceptual framework. She extends an implicit invitation to the reader to consider both the importance of the spiritual variable and the usefulness of the Neuman Systems Model for understanding, clarifying, and putting into practice this most important dimension of nursing practice.

THE SPIRITUAL VARIABLE

The spiritual variable of the client/client system of the Neuman Systems Model is "innate, a component of the basic structure, whether or not it is ever acknowledged or developed by the client or client system" (Neuman, 1989). It is integrated among the physiological, psychological, sociocultural, and developmental variables of the client. Neuman (1989) considers the spiritual variable to be on a developmental continuum that may range from denial to full understanding and that, ultimately, influences the illness and wellness outcomes of the client. This description of the spiritual variable is congruent with the broad and general definitions noted in the literature (Burkhardt, 1989; Emblen, 1992; Fulton, 1991; Haase et al., 1992). The spiritual variable is often overlooked or ignored by nurses as a resource to move clients toward wellness.

The purposes of this chapter are to present knowledge about and resources for aspects of the spiritual variable in nursing research, nursing education, and nursing practice; and to consider the spiritual variable and nursing in the 21st century.

ASPECTS OF THE SPIRITUAL VARIABLE

Spiritual dimension, spiritual well-being, spiritual needs, spiritual care, and *spiritual distress* are terms in the health professionals' literature that are similar to "aspects of spirituality" (Fawcett, 1989). After a review of the literature and analysis of these terms (Fulton, 1991), each was superimposed onto the Neuman Systems Model, which provides organization, congruence, and consistency to the ordering (Figure 3–1).

An explanation of this adapted model is based on the assumption that the spiritual variable and spiritual needs exist in the client. If these needs are being met, the client experiences spiritual wellness (well-being); however, spiritual care involving primary prevention as intervention can strengthen the flexible line of defense to retain optimal wellness. If the needs are not being met, stressors can result in spiritual illness (distress); penetration of the flexible line of defense, normal line of defense, and lines of resistance; and, possibly, death. Spiritual care at the secondary and tertiary prevention as intervention levels should result

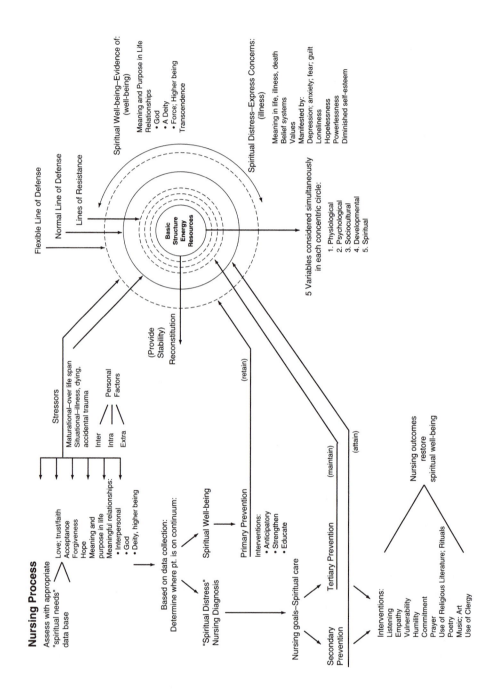

Figure 3–1 Adaptation of selected components of Neuman Systems Model for Spirituality-based on literature review. © 1994 Ruth Ann B. Fulton, RN, DNSc.

in the desired outcomes of stabilization and reconstitution, for example, when the client demonstrates behaviors of optimal spiritual wellness, or well-being.

NURSING RESEARCH

Direction for qualitative and quantitative nursing research is provided by using the Neuman Systems Model as a framework to operationalize the aspects of spirituality (Figure 3–1). Available instrumentation and research findings about each aspect are presented to guide scientific inquiry. An extensive reference list is provided to make available instrumentation and research findings for each aspect of spirituality presented in this diagram.

Spiritual Well-Being

There are three measures of spiritual well-being. The Spiritual Well-Being (SWB) Scale (Paloutzian and Ellison, 1982a) is the most widely used measure despite its Judeo-Christian bias. It has established reliability and validity, although Kirschling and Pitman (1989) contend the SWB lacked construct validity after administration to a group of older hospice caregivers. Moberg (1984) developed an 82-item Subjective Spiritual Well-Being instrument that has seven indexes. It requires further testing to develop validity and reliability. Nurses developed the JAREL Spiritual Well-Being Scale (JAREL) from indicators of spiritual well-being described by 65- to 85-year-old adults (N=31), including "Christians, . . . non-Christians, . . . atheists" (Hungelmann et al., 1985) to minimize a religious bias. Twenty indicators on a 6-point Likert-type scale were administered to 286 adults whose ages were 65 years old and older (Hungelmann et al., 1989). DeCrans (1990) found a high correlation (r=.82, p=.000) between the JAREL and Paloutzian and Ellison's (1982a) Spiritual Well-Being Scale. Fulton (1992) found the Chronbach's alpha to be .81 for 260 adults between the ages of 19 and 64 years, which is similar to .85 and .91 reported by Hunglemann et al. (1989) and DeCrans (1990), respectively.

Research reports suggest a relationship between spiritual well-being and health, and spiritual well-being is, indeed, a factor of wholistic health (Bauwens and Johnson, 1984). Meaning in life, inner peace, and relationships with self, other persons, God, or a higher being are described as characteristics of spiritual well-being (DeYoung, 1984; Fulton, 1992). Persons with illness use spiritual strategies to restore spiritual well-being (Granstrom, 1985; Miller, 1985; Reed, 1986, 1987). Other studies suggest spiritual well-being is a mediator in response to life change (Fehring, Brennan, and Keller, 1987) and that it correlates highly with hope among persons with AIDS (Carson, Soeken, Shanty, and Terry, 1990), women with breast cancer (Mickley, Soeken, and Belcher, 1992), and healthy persons (Carson, Soeken, and Grimm, 1988). Spiritual well-being was a predictor of hardiness for persons with AIDS (Carson and Green, 1992).

Four studies suggest spiritual well-being does not necessarily have a positive effect on persons. Buchanan (1987) found length of illness and hospital stay reduced spiritual well-being among oncology patients when they were compared to cardiovascular patients. Kaczorowski (1989) reported lower spiritual well-being scores and higher anxiety scores among women with breast cancer in comparison to women with other kinds of cancers. Two studies showed a negative correlation between loneliness and spiritual well-being (Miller, 1985; Paloutzian and Ellison, 1982).

Spiritual Needs

Spiritual needs are meaning and purpose in life; the need to receive love and to give love; the need for hope and creativity (Highfield and Cason, 1983); and the need for forgiving, trusting relationships with self, others, and God or a deity, or a guiding philosophy (Stoll, 1989a). Available instruments should be considered in terms of validity and reliability. Measures include a scale developed by Martin, Burrows, and Pomilio (1976), a questionnaire developed by Highfield and Cason (1983), and Boutell's Inventory for Identifying Nurses' Awareness of Spiritual Needs (Boutell and Bozett, 1990). Five scales that pertain to spiritual needs include Crumbaugh's (1968) Purpose in Life Test, Trainor's (1980) forgiveness scale, the Patient Spiritual Coping Interview (McCorkle and Benoliel, 1981), the Religious Perspective Scale (Reed, 1986), and the Intrinsic/Extrinsic Religiousness Scale (Feagin, 1964).

Hope, as a spiritual need, sustains persons through periods of suffering and may be rooted in religious beliefs or in a humanistic philosophy. Nurses have developed hope scales (Herth, 1989; Miller and Powers, 1988; Nowotny, 1989), and psychiatrists (Beck et al., 1974) have developed a hopelessness scale.

Research findings suggest that women express their spiritual needs more often than men (Martin, Burrows, and Pomilio, 1976); that a high priority need is support from others (Bean, 1987; Martin, Burrows, and Pomilio, 1976); and that other needs include God's love, a hopeful future, and meaning in life (Slaughter, 1979). Additionally, illness and hospitalization increase patients' perceptions of reliance on spiritual needs (Francis, 1986; Hoskins, 1986; Schomus, 1980); nurses identify spiritual needs to be in the psychosocial domain (Dettmore, 1986; Highfield and Cason, 1983; Piles, 1990); older nurses acknowledge the spiritual domain and use listening and observing skills to do so (Boutell and Bozett, 1990); and nurses are perceived as helpful to support spiritual beliefs (Richter, 1987).

Spiritual Distress

The nursing literature describes characteristics of spiritual distress (Carpenito, 1992; Carson, 1989; Fehring and McClane, 1989; Labun, 1987; McFarland and McFarlane, 1989; Stoll, 1989). Flesner (1982) initiated a measure of spiritual distress, which requires refinement. Soeken (1989) suggests "loneliness, powerlessness, . . . anxiety, trust, guilt, anger, grief, . . . religious immaturity" are existent tools in psychiatric literature to measure characteristics of spiritual distress. The Abbreviated Loneliness Scale (Paloutzian and Ellison, 1982b) is one example.

Weatherall and Creason (1987) performed a qualitative study to initiate validation of the defining characteristics of spiritual distress developed by the North American Nursing Diagnosis Association (NANDA). Five characteristics that emerged were concerns about the meaning of suffering, statements concerning relationship with deity, expressions of inner conflict about beliefs, a sense of hopefulness, and concerns about relationships with others.

Spiritual Care

Anecdotal nursing literature about spiritual care includes care across the life span; care specific to cultures, religions, and disease entities; and care provided in specialty areas of practice. Instrumentation is limited to questionnaires.

Research findings suggest nurses provide spiritual care by being concerned, cheerful, and kind, and through listening and touching (DeYoung, 1984; Fulton, 1992; Hoskins, 1986; Martin, Burrows, and Pomilio, 1976); however, nurses state they are uncomfortable about spiritual matters (Sodestrom and Martinson, 1987). Other studies suggest religion is an important aspect of spiritual care for the elderly (Nelson, 1989) and is integral to life satisfaction of persons with life-threatening and chronic illnesses (Stoll, 1983). A qualitative study reported themes of the hospice nurse–family spiritual relationship were nurses' ways of being, of knowing, of doing, of giving and receiving, and of welcoming a stranger (Stiles, 1990).

Clark, Cross, Deane, and Lowry (1991) state that nursing care must include a "spirit-to-spirit encounter between caregiver and patient." An interdisciplinary team used the Neuman Systems Model as a framework to explore how health care professions address spiritual needs and spiritual care. Responses from interviews of hospitalized persons suggest that nurses promote hope and well-being, and create negative feelings if they lack sensitivity or competence, and that support systems contribute to well-being. This study provides direction for nursing research about aspects of the spiritual variable of the Neuman Model. The authors encourage operationalization of the terms *spiritual needs* and *spiritual care.*

Summary

Studies about spirituality are evident in the nursing literature, but, unfortunately, a large number of masters' theses, doctoral dissertations, and conference presentations have not been published. It is possible to synthesize and accept what is known about each aspect of the spiritual variable within the context of the Neuman Systems Model to facilitate decision making and direction for further research. The greatest needs are to develop instrumentation; to use phenomenology, ethnography, and grounded theory to construct "categories and relationships . . . from direct interaction" between researcher and phenomenon (Walker and Avant, 1988); to explore development of the spiritual variable across the life span; and to describe relevance among nursing, spiritual care, and optimum wellness of clients.

NURSING EDUCATION

A synthesis of studies suggests that practicing nurses and nursing students do not receive adequate education about spirituality (Dettmore, 1986; Piles, 1980, 1990); educational interventions about spirituality improve students' perceptions of spiritual care (Hitchens, 1988) and religious beliefs (Carson, Winkelstein, Soeken, and Brunins, 1986); spiritual well-being of nursing students is positively correlated with hope (Carson, Soeken, and Grimm, 1988) and perceptions of the health professional's role to provide spiritual care (Soeken and Carson, 1986); spiritual well-being mean scores of nursing students and faculty are high (Fulton, 1992); and nursing students and faculty intuitively and spontaneously describe spiritual well-being and spiritual care of persons (Fulton, 1992).

Nursing students and faculty have, at a minimum, an awareness about spirituality and state the desire for education about this topic. Lack of educational preparation may result in not meeting spiritual needs of patients (Highfield and Cason, 1983; Piles, 1990) with subsequent spiritual disequilibrium and, possibly, death. Disregard of the spiritual variable of clients is antithetic to the premise that nurses care for clients wholistically. Two approaches may remedy this dilemma. One approach is to initiate an awareness of a spiritual self before nursing faculty and students are expected to recognize and care for the spiritual needs of clients. Strategies that promote a personal spirituality are evident in the literature (Arnold, 1989; Burnard, 1988; Clifford and Gruca, 1987; Dugan, 1987/88; Hately, 1984; Hover-Kramer, 1989; Lane, 1987; Nagai-Jacobsen and Burkhardt, 1989; Rew, 1989; Richardson and Nolan, 1984; Shelly and Fish, 1988; Smythe, 1985; Taylor and Ferszt, 1990).

A second approach is through continued adoption of the Neuman Systems Model to guide nursing curricula. Organization of course content may be facilitated by Figure 3–1. Resources are available for educators to address spirituality in both secular and Christian nursing programs (Shelly, 1993); in life-span coursework (Carson, 1989; Clutter, 1991; Feiser and Rogers-Seidl, 1991; Hall, 1985; Hill and Smith, 1985); and in use of the nursing process to attain, retain, and maintain spiritual wellness (Beck, Rawlins, and Williams, 1988; Carpenito, 1992; Carson, 1989; Craven and Hirnle, 1992; Dossey et al., 1988; Johanson, Dungca, and Hoffmeister, 1988; Kozier, Erb, and Olivieri, 1991; Stoll, 1989b; Swinford and Webster, 1989). Research related to outcomes of these two approaches can be beneficial to education and practice.

NURSING PRACTICE

Aspects of spirituality and the Neuman Systems Model (Figure 3–1) guide the nursing process. Neuman (1989) states that the "major concern for nursing is in keeping the client/client system stable" through accurate assessment of stressors in order to move the client toward spiritual wellness. Available resources are adaptable to assess the spiritual variable, depending on specific situational and maturational stressors of the client (Carpenito, 1992; Carson, 1989; Colliton, 1981; Dossey et al., 1988; Hill and Smith, 1985; O'Brien, 1982; Shelly and Fish, 1988; Stoll, 1979; Swinford and Webster, 1989).

Assessment between client and nurse may result in concluding that the spiritual needs aspect of the spiritual variable is intact and that spiritual wellness, or well-being, prevails. Thus, primary prevention as intervention minimizes stressors and strengthens the flexible line of defense to retain and optimize the wellness level. Primary prevention spiritual care involves, basically, identification of client/client system coping strengths and support of health-facilitating activities of education, role-play strategies, and anticipatory guidance.

When a variance from wellness exists, the degree of spiritual illness, or distress, is described in a diagnostic statement. Spiritual care at the secondary prevention as intervention level involves collaboration between the client and the nurse to set goals that alleviate symptoms of the maturational or situational stressor(s) and avoid penetration of the flexible line of defense, normal line of defense, and lines of resistance. Protection of the basic structure and restoration of spiritual wellness are desired goals. Their achievement may result from interventions of listening, being empathetic, touching, personal sharing, and other therapeutic nurse's use of self. Additional interventions are use of music, art, and bibliotherapy. Religious interventions include offering prayer, reading religious literature, and assisting with rituals. The nurse provides spiritual care in order to attain the normal line of defense and promote stabilization and reconstitution. The outcome of spiritual wellness results when the client expresses meaning and purpose in life, re-establishes relationships, and resumes practices of a belief system.

Tertiary prevention is described by Neuman (1989) as "wellness maintenance," which begins when treatment of the stressor(s) is underway and stability results. Spiritual care interventions that support "existing strengths" and conserve "client system energy" include facilitating adaptation to and education about spiritual resources in order to maintain the client's lines of resistance and lines of defense during stabilization and reconstitution. These interventions are directed toward the goal of maintaining optimal wellness.

Spiritual care interventions are individualized to protect the basic structure, alleviate stressors, and begin reconstitution. The ultimate goal is to have the client recognize and mobilize personal spiritual resources that maintain stability and strengthen other interacting variables of the client system. In the event that spiritual care interventions are not employed, the effectiveness of the lines of resistance may be reduced with energy depletion, or death, occurring.

FUTURE IMPLICATIONS FOR USE OF THE NEUMAN SYSTEMS MODEL

Aspects of the spiritual variable are supported in the literature by research reports and concept analyses that are congruent with the organization and terminology of the model (Figure 3–1). For example, the terms *spiritual dimension* and *spiritual domain* tend to include the developmental, perceptual, and integral language of Neuman (1989). It is from this perspective that the Neuman Systems Model is poised to meet the needs of nursing research, practice, and education in the 21st century.

Research will need to focus on the spiritual care of markedly increased high-risk groups and conditions of cultural concerns, homelessness, aging, and AIDS that are anticipated in the 21st century. To keep pace with the resultant rapid societal changes, research is imperative to describe, explain, and predict the meaning of the spiritual variable for clients who will be recipients of nursing care. Nurses can provide a leadership role in promotion of the Neuman Model to guide interdisciplinary research. This research initiative has begun, as evidenced by the increasing use of the model to organize aspects of the spiritual variable and scholarly presentations at the Third and Fourth Biennial Neuman International Symposia.

The model provides direction to develop nursing practice that is wholistic and wellness oriented. This paradigm shift from the medical model requires nurses to explain what they do and to develop new, exciting roles. Future nursing will take place in new environments with new problems inherent in promoting wellness. The roles of parish nursing, block nursing, and nurse-managed centers are examples. The creation of nursing roles will also be necessary during exploration for human habitation in outer space and in the sea. Spiritual wellness is an important goal for clients in these and other rapidly evolving new practice areas.

An increasing number of nursing schools have adopted the Neuman Systems Model at all education levels. The spiritual variable as described in *The Neuman Systems Model,* 2d and 3d book editions, assures a wholistic approach to the client as a system. The model provides important direction for developing relevant nursing curricula as health care is reformed, redefined, and reshaped. As the practice of nursing and new nursing roles develop, the Neuman Model has the potential to adequately prepare nursing students for wholistic practice in the 21st century. With wellness as the focus of care, the Neuman model provides the appropriate structure for organizing teaching protocols for primary prevention as intervention and integrating the important spiritual variable into a wholistic client care profile.

SUMMARY

The Neuman Systems Model has major implications for nursing research, practice, and education in the future. The focus of wellness, the spiritual variable, and the systematic, wholistic, individualized nursing care approach enable the nursing profession to define its uniqueness in a world order of major social and scientific changes. Understanding and appropriate use of spiritual concepts are imperative for future nurse professionalism.

REFERENCES

Arnold, E. 1989. Burnout as a spiritual issue: Rediscovering meaning in nursing. In *Spiritual Dimensions in Nursing Practice,* edited by V. B. Carson, 320–353. Philadelphia: Saunders.

Bauwens, E. E., and Johnson, R. 1984. Perceived health status, life satisfaction and spiritual well-being. In *Proceedings of the Conference on Spirituality: A New Perspective on Health,* edited by R. J. Fehring, J. Hungelmann, and R. Stollenwerk, 9–1 to 9–21. Milwaukee: Marquette University.

Bean, C. A. 1987. Needs and stimuli influencing needs of adult cancer patients. Unpublished doctoral dissertation. University of Alabama, Birmingham.

Beck, A. T., Weissman, A., Lester, D., and Trexler, L. 1974. The measurement of pessimism: The hopelessness scale. *Journal of Consulting and Clinical Psychiatry* 42:861–865.

Beck, C. K., Rawlins, R. P., and Williams, S. R., eds. 1988. *Mental Health-Psychiatric Nursing: A Holistic Life-Cycle Approach,* 2d ed. St. Louis: Mosby.

Boutell, K. A., and Bozett, F. W. 1990. Nurses' assessment of patients' spirituality: Continuing education implications. *Journal of Continuing Education in Nursing* 21:172–176.

Buchanan, D. 1987. Loneliness and spiritual well-being of hospitalized and healthy adults: A quality of life study. Unpublished doctoral dissertation, University of Alabama, Birmingham.

Burkhardt, M. A. 1989. Spirituality: An analysis of the concept. *Holistic Nursing Practice* 3:69–77.

Burnard, P. 1988. Discussing spiritual issues with clients. *Health Visitor* 61:371–372.

Carpenito, L. J. 1992. *Nursing Diagnosis: Application to Clinical Practice,* 4th ed. Philadelphia: Lippincott.

Carson, V. B. 1989. *Spiritual Dimension in Nursing Practice.* Philadelphia: Saunders.

Carson, V. B., and Green, H. 1992. Spiritual well-being: A predictor of hardiness in patients with Acquired Immunodeficiency Syndrome. *Journal of Professional Nursing* 8:209–220.

Carson, V. B., Soeken, K. L., and Grimm, P. M. 1988. Hope and its relationship to spiritual well-being. *Journal of Psychology and Theology* 16:159–167.

Carson, V. B., Soeken, K. L., Shanty, J., and Terry, L. 1990. Hope and spiritual well-being: Essential for living with AIDS. *Perspectives in Psychiatric Care* 26:28–34.

Carson, V. B., Winkelstein, M., Soeken, K., and Brunins, M. 1986. The effect of didactic teaching on spiritual attitudes. *Image* 18:161–164.

Clark, C. C., Cross, J. R., Deane, D. M., and Lowry, L. W. 1991. Spirituality: Integral to quality care. *Journal of Holistic Nursing Practice* 5:67–76.

Clifford, M., and Gruca, J. A. 1987. Facilitating spiritual care in the rehabilitation setting. Rehabilitation Nursing 12:331–333.

Clutter, L. B. 1991. Fostering spiritual care for the child and family. In *Comprehensive Child and Family Nursing Skills,* edited by D. P. Smith, 263–272. St. Louis: Mosby.

Colliton, M. A. 1981. The spiritual dimension of nursing. In *Clinical Nursing,* 4th ed., edited by I. Beland and J. Y. Passos, 492–501. New York: Macmillan.

Craven, R. E., and Hirnle, C. J. 1992. *Fundamentals of Nursing: Human Health and Functioning.* Philadelphia: Lippincott.

Crumbaugh, J. C. 1968. Cross validation of the purpose in life test based on Frankl's concepts. *Journal of Individual Psychology* 24:74–81.

DeCrans, M. 1990. Spiritual well-being of the elderly. Unpublished master's thesis, Marquette University, Milwaukee, Wisc.

Dettmore, D. 1986. Nurses' conceptions of and practices in the spiritual dimension of nursing. Unpublished doctoral dissertation, Columbia University Teachers' College, New York, N.Y.

DeYoung, S. 1984. Perceptions of the institutionalized elderly regarding the nurse's role in supporting spiritual well-being. In *Proceedings of the Conference on Spirituality: A New Perspective on Health,* edited by R. J. Fehring, J. Hungelmann, and R. Stollenwerk, 10–1 to 10–11. Milwaukee: Marquette University.

Dossey, B. M., Keegan, L., Guzzetta, C. E., et al. 1988. *Holistic Nursing: A Handbook for Practice.* Rockville, Md.: Aspen.

Dugan, D. O. 1987. Death and dying: Emotional, spiritual and ethical support for patients and families. *Journal of Psychosocial Nursing* 25:21–29.

Emblen, J. D. 1992. Religion and spirituality defined according to current use in nursing literature. *Journal of Professional Nursing* 8:41–47.

Fawcett, J. 1989. Analysis and evaluation of the Neuman Systems Model. In *The Neuman Systems Model,* 2d ed., edited by B. Neuman, 65–92. Norwalk, Conn.: Appleton & Lange.

Feagin, J. R. 1964. Prejudice and religious types: A focused study of Southern fundamentalists. *Journal for the Scientific Study of Religion* 4:3–13.

Fehring, R. J., Brennan, P. F., and Keller, M. L. 1987. Psychological and spiritual well-being in college students. *Research in Nursing and Health* 10:391–398.

Fehring, R. J., and McClane, A. N. 1989. Value belief. In *Mosby's Manual of Clinical Nursing,* 2d ed., edited by J. M. Thompson, G. K. McFarland, J. E. Hirsch, et al., 1821–1825. St. Louis: Mosby.

Feiser, K. O., and Rogers-Seidl, F. F. 1991. Spiritual distress. In *Geriatric Nursing Care Plans,* edited by F. F. Rogers-Seidl. St. Louis: Mosby.

Flesner, R. S. 1982. Development of a measure to assess spiritual distress in the responsive adult. Unpublished master's essay, Marquette University.

Francis, M. R. 1986. Concerns of terminally ill adult Hindu cancer patients. *Cancer Nursing* 9:164–171.

Fulton, R. A. 1991. Dimensions of spirituality: A concept analysis. Paper presented at the Third Biennial Neuman Systems Model International Symposium, Dayton, Ohio, November.

Fulton, R. A. 1992. Spiritual well-being of baccalaureate nursing students and faculty and their responses about spiritual well-being of persons. Unpublished doctoral dissertation, Widener University, Chester, Pa.

Granstrom, S. L. 1987. A comparative study of loneliness, Buberian religiosity and spiritual well-being in cancer patients. Unpublished doctoral dissertation, Rush University, Chicago.

Haase, J. E., Britt, T., Coward, D. D., et al. 1992. Simultaneous concept analysis of spiritual perspective, hope, acceptance and self-transcendence. *Image* 24:141–147.

Hall, E. G. 1985. Spirituality during aging. *Pastoral Psychology* 34:112–117.

Hateley, B. J. 1984. Spiritual well-being through life histories. *Journal of Religion and Aging* 1:63–71.

Herth, K. A. 1989. The relationship between level of hope and level of coping response and other variables in patients with cancer. *Oncology Nursing Forum* 16:67–72.

Highfield, M. F., and Cason, C. 1983. Spiritual needs of patients: Are they recognized? *Cancer Nursing* 6:187–192.

Hill, S., and Smith, N. 1985. *Self-Care Nursing: Promotion of Health*. Englewood Cliffs, N.J.: Prentice-Hall.

Hoskins, N. A. 1986. Patients' perceptions of spiritual needs. Unpublished master's thesis, Vanderbilt University, Nashville, Tenn.

Hover-Kramer, D. 1989. Creating a context for self-healing: The transpersonal perspective. *Holistic Nursing Practice* 3:27–34.

Hungelmann, J., Kenkel-Rossi, E., Klassen, L., et al. 1985. Spiritual well-being in older adults: Harmonious interconnectedness. *Journal of Religion and Health* 24:147–152.

Hungelmann, J., Kenkel-Rossi, E., Klassen, L., et al. 1989. Development of the JAREL Spiritual Well-Being Scale. In *Classification of Nursing Diagnoses: Proceedings of the Eighth Conference*, edited by R. M. Carroll-Johnson, 393–398. Philadelphia: Lippincott.

Johanson, B. C., Dungca, C. U., Wells, S. J., et al. 1988. Emotional and spiritual care of the critically ill. In *Standards for Critical Care*, 3d ed., 324–332. St. Louis: Mosby.

Kaczorowski, J. M. 1989. Spiritual well-being and anxiety in adults diagnosed with cancer. *The Hospice Journal* 5:105–115.

Kirschling, J. M., and Pittman, J. F. 1989. Measurement of spiritual well-being: A hospice caregiving sample. *The Hospice Journal* 5:1–11.

Kozier, B., Erb, G. L., and Olivieri, R. 1991. *Fundamentals of Nursing Practice: Concepts and Procedures*, 2d ed. Menlo Park, Calif.: Addison-Wesley.

Labun, E. 1988. Spiritual care: An element in nursing. *Journal of Advanced Nursing* 13:314–320.

Lane, J. A. 1987. The care of the human spirit. *Journal of Professional Nursing* 3:332–337.

Martin, C., Burrows, C., and Pomilico, J. 1988. Spiritual needs of patients study. In *Spiritual Care: The Nurse's Role*, 3d ed., edited by J. A. Shelley and S. Fish, 160–176. Downers Grove, Ill.: InterVarsity.

McCorkle, R., and Benoliel, J. Q. 1981. *A Manual of Data Collection Instruments*. Unpublished manual, University of Washington.

McFarland, G. K., and McFarlane, E. A. 1989. *Nursing: Diagnosis and Intervention*. St. Louis: Mosby.

Mickley, J. R., Soeken, K., and Belcher, A. 1992. Spiritual well-being, religiousness and hope among women with breast cancer. *Image* 24:267–272.

Miller, J. F. 1985. Assessment of loneliness and spiritual well-being in chronically ill and healthy adults. *Journal of Professional Nursing* 1:79–85.

Miller, J. F., and Powers, M. J. 1988. Development of an instrument to measure hope. *Nursing Research* 37:6–10.

Moberg, D. O. 1984. Subjective measures of spiritual well-being. *Review of Religious Research* 24:351–364.

Nagai-Jacobsen, M. G., and Burkhardt, M. A. 1989. Spirituality: Cornerstone of holistic nursing practice. *Journal of Holistic Nursing Practice* 3:18–26.

Nelson, P. B. 1989. Ethnic differences in intrinsic/extrinsic religious orientation and depression in the elderly. *Archives of Psychiatric Nursing* 3:199–204.

Neuman, B. 1989. *The Neuman Systems Model,* 2d ed. Norwalk, Conn.: Appleton & Lange.

Nowotny, M. L. 1986. Measurement of hope as exhibited by a general adult population after a stressful event. *Dissertation Abstracts International* 47(08), 3296-B. (University Microfilms No. 8626494).

O'Brien, M. E. 1982. The need for spiritual integrity. In *Human Needs 2 and the Nursing Process,* edited by H. Yura and M. B. Walsh, 85–114. Norwalk, Conn.: Appleton-Century-Crofts.

Paloutzian, R. F., and Ellison, C. W. 1982a. Loneliness, spiritual well-being and the quality of life. In *Loneliness: A Sourcebook of Current Theory, Research and Therapy,* edited by L. A. Peplau and D. Perlman, 224–237. New York: Wiley.

Paloutzian, R. F., and Ellison, C. W. 1982b. Loneliness, spiritual well-being and quality of life. In *Loneliness: A Sourcebook of Current Theory, Research and Therapy,* edited by L. A. Peplau and D. Perlman. New York: Wiley.

Piles, C. L. 1980. Spiritual care as part of the nursing curriculum: A descriptive study. Unpublished master's thesis, St. Louis University, St. Louis.

Piles, C. L. 1990. Providing spiritual care. *Nurse Educator* 15:36–41.

Reed, P. G. 1986. Religiousness among terminally ill and healthy adults. *Research in Nursing and Health* 9:35–41.

Reed, P. G. 1987. Spirituality and well-being in terminally ill hospitalized adults. *Research in Nursing and Health* 10:335–344.

Rew, L. 1989. Intuition: Nursing knowledge and the spiritual dimension of persons. *Holistic Nursing Practice* 3:56–68.

Richardson, G. E., and Nolan, M. P. 1984. Treating the spiritual dimension through imagery. *Health Values* 8:25–30.

Richter, J. M. 1987. Support: A resource during crisis of mate loss. *Journal of Geriatric Nursing* 13:18–22.

Schomus, I. G. 1980. Hospital stress and the patient's perception of the importance of spiritual needs. Unpublished master's thesis, Arizona State University, Tempe.

Shelly, J. A. 1993. *Teaching Spiritual Care: A Resource Book for Nursing Faculty,* 2d ed. Madison, Wisc.: Nurses Christian Fellowship.

Shelly, J. A., and Fish, S. 1988. *Spiritual Care: The Nurse's Role,* 3d ed. Downers Grove, Ill.: InterVarsity.

Slaughter, T. A. 1979. Identifying the spiritual needs of the oncology patient. Unpublished master's thesis, University of Arizona, Tucson.

Smythe, E. E. M. 1985. *Surviving Nursing.* Menlo Park, Calif.: Addison-Wesley.

Sodestrom, K. E., and Martinson, I. M. 1987. Patients' spiritual coping strategies: A study of nurse and patient perspectives. *Oncology Nursing Forum* 14:41–46.

Soeken, K. L. 1989. Perspectives on research in the spiritual dimension of nursing care. In *Spiritual Dimensions of Nursing Practice,* edited by V. B. Carson, 354–378. Philadelphia: Saunders.

Soeken, K. L., and Carson, V. B. 1986. Study measures nurses' attitudes about providing spiritual care. *Health Progress* 67:52–55.

Stiles, M. K. 1990. The shining stranger: Nurse–family spiritual relationship. *Cancer Nursing* 13:235–245.

Stoll, R. I. 1979. Guidelines for spiritual assessment. *American Journal of Nursing* 79: 1374–1377.

Stoll, R. I. 1983. Indicators of life satisfaction in persons with life threatening diagnosis and those with non-threatening diagnosis. Unpublished doctoral dissertation, Catholic University of America, Washington, D.C.

Stoll, R. I. 1989a. The essence of spirituality. In *Spiritual Dimensions of Nursing Practice,* edited by V. B. Carson, 4–23. Philadelphia: Saunders.

Stoll, R. I. 1989b. Spirituality and chronic illness. In *Spiritual Dimensions of Nursing Practice,* edited by V. B. Carson, 180–216. Philadelphia: Saunders.

Swinford, P. A., and Webster, J. A. 1989. *Promoting Wellness.* Rockville, Md.: Aspen.

Taylor, P. B., and Ferszt, G. G. 1990. Spiritual healing. *Holistic Nursing Practice* 4:32–38.

Trainor, M. F. 1980. Forgiveness: Intrinsic, role-expected, expedient in the context of divorce. Unpublished doctoral dissertation, Boston University.

Walker, L. O., and Avant, K. C. 1988. *Strategies for Theory Construction in Nursing.* Norwalk, Conn.: Appleton & Lange.

Weatherall, J., and Creason, N. S. 1987. Validation of the nursing diagnosis; Spiritual distress. In *Classification of Nursing Diagnosis: Proceedings of the Seventh Conference,* edited by A. M. McLane, 182–185. St. Louis: Mosby.

4

THE NEUMAN SYSTEMS MODEL REVISITED

Glenn Curran

The aim of this chapter is to revisit the Neuman Systems Model and examine its basic premise as a visionary wholistic model for nursing. The Neuman Systems Model represents an important shift in nursing towards wholism, systems theory, and spirituality. This chapter explores the meaning of these ideas to nursing and their potential contribution to health care in the 21st century.

WHOLISM: A KEY TO UNDERSTANDING SYSTEMS THEORY

The Neuman Systems Model (1989) describes a system as ". . . any defined whole" (p. 8). Therefore, a system may be an individual, an issue, a society, or the earth. It is assumed that as a system expands and becomes more complex, the principles governing the relationships within the system remain the same.

Neuman (1989) opens the conceptual doors to wholistic thinking. There is a beautiful simplicity within the idea of wholism as Neuman (1989) claims:

> Wholism, implicit in the Neuman Systems Model, is both a philosophical and a biological concept implying relationships and processes arising from wellness, dynamic freedom and creativity in adjusting to stress in the internal and external environment. (p. 10)

Wholism is a major assumption of the Neuman Systems Model which has functional and conceptual definitions. Wholism refers to the complex interdependent, interactive processes occurring within a system. Nurses draw on this

Reviewed by Rosalie Mirenda, Diane Breckenridge, and Patricia Hinton Walker.

multidimensional perspective (personal, social, and environmental) as a way to focus on client well-being. Wholism supports the idea of implementing ongoing assessments of the client before, during, and after nursing interventions. In this way wholism influences nursing practice.

Furthermore, wholism as a conceptual framework encourages an expanding philosophy in nursing. The abstract concept of wholism requires a broad description and understanding of the phenomena that surround health care. The Neuman Systems Model may be used to provide a wholistic framework for health care in general. Pearson and Vaughan (1988) suggest that the strength in the Neuman Systems Model is the ability to support an interdisciplinary team approach.

Another assumption in the Neuman Systems Model (1989) is that the components of a system ". . . are not significantly connected except with reference to the whole" (p. 8). This idea suggests that every element of every concept has a relationship but only with reference to the whole. There is always the danger in oversimplifying systems when considering nursing interventions. It takes studied and skillful assessment to recognize and piece together the relationships that influence the system. The potential weakness of systems thinking also lies in this idea. One only has to uncover an inconsistency in the model at any point and the whole idea is flawed.

It is proposed that the indigenous peoples of America and Australia understand the idea of wholism and systems far better than their dominating Western societies. The reason for this knowledge belongs to an understanding of the sacred relationships, and respect for the balance and diversity of life in the land they inhabit. Nursing can learn and understand ideas about wholism by listening to these indigenous peoples.

Wholism as an idea is not difficult to grasp, although it requires abstract thinking. Neuman (1989) suggests that:

> A clear conception of systems organization requires skill in viewing client situations abstractly. That is, client system boundaries and related variables may lose some clarity because they are dynamic and constantly changing, presenting different appearances according to time, place, and the significance of events. (p. 8)

The metaphorical ideas of a tree and forest are used to describe the link between wholism, systems theory, the individual, and the community. It takes training to see the tree and forest, or the person and community as a system within a system. Systems thinking makes sense when there is a focus on oneness and unity. The ability to see the tree–forest and person–community as one can be extrapolated to the global system where all life is interconnected.

The stability of system earth is dependent on simple relationships (tree, flora, fauna) and complex ecosystems (forest). One tree cut down may not seem important. The removal of one million trees alters local ecology. One billion trees taken out of the system affects the earth's respiration and disrupts the carbon cycle; watersheds are destroyed; biodiversity is reduced; entropy as wasted nonrenewable energy increases; and all living systems are threatened.

There is a balanced wholistic order to system earth, and humanity belongs to this system. Currently, our global system is under threat as the earth's lines of defense and resistance are weakened. The inhabitants of system earth are approaching the possibility of dealing with a positive feedback scenario in climate change that may cause irreparable damage. It appears that the recent failure of affluent countries to come to terms with the issue of biodiversity is a foreboding sign (Rio de Janeiro Earth Summit, 1992).

The threat of an unstable global system impacts heavily on the basic needs of people, such as water, food, and shelter. These health-related issues cannot be seen in isolation but as a connection with the whole. The Neuman Systems Model offers a conceptual framework to understand this connection because it acknowledges and seeks to identify the implicit relationships and processes involved.

The challenge is to view these relationships with other defined systems, be they individuals, issues, communities, or global systems. It is a pleasant surprise to discover the scope of the Neuman Systems Model where the complexity of any given system is governed by wholism.

THE NEUMAN SYSTEMS MODEL: A CONTRIBUTION TO NURSING

Betty Neuman draws on personal insight and experience, and scientific and social disciplines to create a unique and visionary nursing model. Nursing is considered a system; therefore it follows that the Neuman Systems Model offers an organized way of thinking and practicing as a nurse.

Nursing is experiencing a paradigm shift away from the empirical biomedical paradigm toward the qualitative human sciences. A paradigm shift may well take several generations before the new ideas eventually become the model of everyday practice. The Neuman Systems Model is an example of a nursing shift away from the biomedical paradigm. The characteristics that define this shift in the Neuman Systems Model include the following:

- The client is seen as a unique individual.
- Decision making is shared between the nurse and client.
- Knowledge developed is essentially qualitative and noncompetitive.
- The system is open, and diversity is valued and respected.
- Wholism is the philosophical base of the model.
- Spirituality is innate to every system.
- Order, unity, and wellness are the primary nursing goals of the model.

It is at the practice level where the Neuman Systems Model excels and therefore is of most interest to nursing. Neuman (1982, 1989) provides a comprehensive explanation of nursing and the individual client system. The important aspect when considering a client system is that the nurse unravels those distinct lines of defense and variables, as they interact with environment, to provide individualized nursing interventions.

Neuman (1989) focuses on the nurse–client relationship as a mutual sharing that assures the participation of the client in prevention as intervention. The client is valued as a unique, dynamic, open system where a reciprocal role can develop between the nurse and client. Reciprocity is a complementary exchange between two people, where the nurse understands and acts on what the client is saying and doing. The ideal represented in the Neuman Systems Model is that respect, trust, and sharing can develop as the nursing process is determined by the client and nurse.

The community is another client system. By thinking about the community as a client system, the nurse has a rationale for understanding and exploring how a community interacts and relates to prevention as intervention. It is necessary to see the community as a system when considering health promotion and community development initiatives (Anderson, McFarland, and Helton, 1986; Beddome, 1989). Therefore, nursing interventions are promoted as an important component of a community health care plan.

Neuman (1989) suggests that every system is in unity, strengthened and supported by the diversity of its subsystems. Styles (1987) commented that ". . . nursing's maximum contribution for social good is dependent upon . . . the ability of the profession to maintain unity in diversity" (p. 8). Nurses by professional interest and education have a diversity of roles where practitioners are involved at all levels (primary, secondary, and tertiary) of health care. The cultural diversity of clients is another factor that is assessed by the nurse's attention to the five variables (Sohier, 1989). In presenting nursing as a system, the Neuman Systems Model encourages and respects diversity of roles and culture as necessary to system wellness and vitality.

Unfortunately, the health system does not always support such ideals. The health sector is a combination of private interests, intransigent organizations, hierarchical bureaucratic control, and biomedical domination that tend to impinge on personal liberty. When an individual client or community surrenders or lose its rights to participate in health care, primary, secondary, and tertiary interventions are limited. The ideas of inequitable and unequal power relationships in health care are not new to nursing. Bevis (1982) makes a pertinent comment about this:

> Individual or group power is remarkable in that it cannot be taken away by another person, or group. Power is never taken, it is surrendered. Nurses often surrendered to others their power, their self identity, and the direction of their own affairs. (p. 42)

It is necessary for nurses to understand and modify these power relationships so that the will of the client (individual and community) is valued and respected. This may sound easy but is often a most difficult decision for a nurse to carry out. It is suggested that the value of nursing intervention may be measured by the way the client perceives and participates in the health care process.

From a global perspective nursing is affected by and can affect the institutions that govern health care delivery. The decisions made at the international, national, and state levels have the potential to develop or constrain the nursing interventions provided or available at the community level.

In an increasingly complex health environment, nursing has to order its affairs and work with other health professionals to influence decision making. The wave of economic rationalism is an example where the nursing profession has to compete with pragmatists and entrenched vested interests to maintain a role in health care reform. The nursing role in health care reform will continue to expand through ongoing education, research, and a vision of future practice.

Nursing faces the challenge of crisis and opportunity. The crisis arises from an inability to respond to and manage a fast-changing health care climate. The opportunity is to create a vision of the future and be clear about where nursing is headed. This requires organization, flexibility, skill, and a conceptual and philosophical base that is consistent with nursing ideals and practice.

It is suggested that there is a need in the nursing world for a model capable of incorporating nursing with other systems. A first step for nursing in managing the complex ideas of wholism and systems theory involves a workable guide to nursing practice. The philosophical underpinnings of this model must be consistent with the meaning, aims, and goals of nursing. Lastly, this model needs to have the capacity to explain and develop a scope of nursing practice as it becomes more diverse and complex.

The Neuman Systems Model offers such a model for nursing as it has the dynamic expansiveness of systems thinking. The ability to expand and adapt to multiple systems while maintaining a cohesive integrity in practice is a quality necessary for present and future nursing.

In summary, the philosophy and practice of the Neuman Systems Model offers a consistent change in direction toward wellness in health care, respect for clients' rights in decision making, and the promotion of nursing as a rich, diverse system. The Neuman Systems Model reaffirms the ideals of equity and client participation in health care interventions. The Neuman Systems Model has the capacity to bring together the complexities of other systems into a workable health care framework.

SPIRITUALITY AND NURSING

Spirituality is the most important evolutionary concept in the Neuman Systems Model (1989). The Neuman Systems Model has the scope to create an image of nursing that can claim to be wholistic. Neuman (1989) harmonizes the complex interrelationships in systems with a description of the spiritual variable.

> This variable is viewed as innate . . . whether or not it is ever acknowledged or developed by the client . . . as being on a continuum of development that permeates all other client system variables. The client/client system can move from complete unawareness of this variable's presence and potential, or even denial of it, to a consciously and highly developed spiritual understanding that supports client optimal wellness; that is, the spirit controls the mind and the mind consciously or unconsciously controls the body. . . . The spiritual variable positively or negatively affects of is affected by the condition and interactive effect of other variables, such as grief or loss (psychological states), which may arrest, decrease, initiate, or increase spirituality. The potential exists for movement in either direction on a continuum. (pp. 29–30)

This bold statement by Neuman is considered as a leap of certainty into the unknown. In simple terms, the spiritual variable describes the essence of any defined system. Neuman (1992) acknowledges the spiritual variable as the "major and dominant variable" within her model, as spirituality implies the existence of a creative transcendent spiritual force.

The Neuman Systems Model representation of the spiritual variable is not viewed as a pseudoreligious statement but offers a unique gift wrapped in reason and knowledgeable experience. There is no attempt to change or deny a person's belief or value system, nor is there an esoteric or ritualistic structure to follow.

Neuman (1989) has the courage and conviction to explicitly state the relationship of the spiritual variable to the client and nursing. Neuman (1992) maintains that the spiritual variable was always present in her model. She explains the spiritual variable developed from

> my own observation and experience in life and nursing as seen acted out in human situations. . . . [N]urses have not investigated these phenomena nor called it by a spiritual name. . . . I find that a little strange in that nursing is a caring profession. . . . We need to set forth our beliefs. (personal communication)

Spirituality, most notably likened to the caring act of one person for another, is considered rich in nursing (Dobbie, 1991; Samarel, 1992; Trice, 1990). Neuman (1989) also claims this motive for the development of the Neuman Systems Model, which ". . . was facilitated by my own basic philosophy of helping each other live" (p. 458).

In summary, Neuman (1989) makes a clear, unequivocal statement about the dominant spiritual nature of any defined system. The explanation of the spiritual variable opens up new meaning for the client system and is integral to an understanding of the Neuman Systems Model.

A NURSING MODEL FOR THE 21ST CENTURY

The Neuman Systems Model's wholistic perspective views the client as a dynamic and unique system. Neuman (1989) provides a conceptual framework with wellness as a primary focus. The application of nursing interventions based on systems thinking presents a practical and visionary approach to nursing.

In conclusion, the Neuman Systems Model (1989) has the capacity to project nursing into the 21st century. The opportunity for the nursing profession is to understand wholism and demonstrate, by research and practice, the value of systems thinking.

REFERENCES

Anderson, E., McFarland, J., and Helton, A. 1986. Community-as-client: A model for practice, *Nursing Outlook* 34(5):220–224.

Beddome, G. 1989. Application of the Neuman Systems Model to the assessment of community as client. In *The Neuman Systems Model,* by B. Neuman, 363–373. Norwalk, Conn.: Appleton & Lange.

Bevis, E. O. 1982. *Curriculum Building in Nursing: A Process,* 3d ed. St Louis: C. V. Mosby.

Dobbie, B. J. 1991. Women's mid life experiences: An evolving consciousness of self and children. *Journal of Advanced Nursing* 16:825–831.

Neuman, B. 1989. *The Neuman Systems Model,* 2d ed. East Norwalk, Conn.: Appleton & Lange.

Neuman, B. 1992. The spiritual variable. Personal communication, June 13.

Pearson, A., and Vaughan, B. 1988. *Nursing Models for Practice,* 105–123. Heinemann Nursing.

Rio de Janeiro Earth Summit. 1992. Conference on Environment and Development, United Nations, June.

Samarel, N. 1992. The experience of receiving therapeutic touch. *Journal of Advanced Nursing* 17:651–657.

Sohier, R. 1989. Nursing care for the people of a small planet; Culture and the Neuman Systems Model. In *The Neuman Systems Model,* by B. Neuman, 139–154. Norwalk, Conn.: Appleton & Lange.

Styles, M. 1987. Professionalism—What is it? In *Proceedings of the College of Nursing Australia Conference.* 9th National Conference, Hobart, May 14.

Trice, L. B. 1990. Meaningful life experience to the elderly. *Image: Journal of Nursing Scholarship* 22(4):248–251.

5

NURSING CARE FOR THE PEOPLE OF A SMALL PLANET
Culture and the Neuman Systems Model

Raphella Sohier

As we approach the year 2000, national and geographic boundaries continue to exist but no longer contain all the members of each individual nation or define the cultural mix to be encountered within the boundaries. The rapidity and availability of international and intercontinental travel and the burgeoning technology of the information age combine to diffuse cultures across boundaries. The people of the planet earth have become earth-citizens rather than citizens of the place or nation of their origin. This population diffusion has created, and presents, an increasing challenge to health care providers in terms of the appropriateness and quality of care for people of diverse cultures.

Highly developed and affluent societies lure poorer citizens from all over the world seeking their share of the world's resources. Third World or New Wave immigration has created a situation in which increasing numbers of health professionals do not speak the languages or understand the life-styles of the consumers of health care with whom they interact on a day-to-day basis. Entry into a new society—even when it is deeply desired, and the new life-styles are endorsed—does not presuppose immediate or functional levels of adaptation on the part of the newcomer. Culture change in individuals (acculturation) takes time. Greeley (1981) has demonstrated that cultural beliefs influence health care decisions for as long as four generations after immigration. Recent work by Kosko and Flaskerud (1987) supports this observation.

Plurality of origin, culture, and purpose and multilingual expression are part and parcel of American life. Together, these multicultural, multiethnic influences form a rich tapestry or setting for the American heritage. Nevertheless, comparatively little consideration has been given to these deeply cherished, rich perspectives of individual life or the influences they exert on health belief systems and health behaviors. Few nurse–client or health care provider–client interactions in the U.S. occur within a common culture context. In the majority of cases provider and recipient belong to distinctly different cultural backgrounds. They approach problem solving using different languages, and a consequent primary variation in symbolic and semantic structural systems. It is difficult to know if the person addressed understands what one has said in the way one has meant it to be understood. These variations often inhibit and frequently prohibit common comprehension between caregiver and the recipient of care. Even when the two appear to belong to one culture group, subtle or not so subtle variations, based on religion, ideology, or social and educational class, can intervene. They inhibit the flow of interaction, impede the process, and hinder the achievement of health goals.

The flexibility and dynamism of the Neuman Systems Model provide a conceptual approach capable of circumventing the problems detailed above. The wholistic nature of the model requires assessment data to be collected on physical, psychological, sociocultural, developmental, and spiritual variables. The model can be applied successfully in a cross-cultural context and accommodates the culture-centered approaches indispensable to every thorough assessment. The visual image provided by the model facilitates organization and reorganization of the elements in such a way that it simplifies understanding of the "client" focus. Subjective elements of client problems or perceptions of stress are brought to the forefront. Neuman (1982) describes this as a "unique feature" of the model, stating, ". . . the kinds of data obtained from the client's own perception of his/her condition influence the overall goals of care" (p. 16). Neuman's model is clearly client-centered rather than professionally driven, a characteristic that is consistent with the emic perspectives emphasized in anthropological inquiry and incorporated in the nursing process.

Writing on the subject of individual and family, Neuman (1983, 1989) describes the core structure of person, group, and human community as a composite of characteristics that originate as "culturally determined or transmitted values." She further cautions that the integrity of this basic structure must be preserved at all costs because ". . . all transactions take place against the backdrop of the basic structure" (p. 242). Implicit in her position is the imperative to understand culture in the application of the Neuman Systems Model or at least comprehend the implications presented by cultural variation.

This chapter will explain the basic elements of culture, the influence of culture on human and health care decision making, and the implications of culture for applying the Neuman Systems Model in multicultural populations.

BASIC ELEMENTS OF CULTURE

Basic human needs can be typified from an anthropological perspective in two categories.

1. Existential: those needs related to daily survival, such as environmental temperature within certain limits of variation and the availability of food and shelter. Human beings cannot survive without these needs being met.
2. Persistential: human groups cannot persist unless a second set of needs are met, those that enable the transmission of human seed (sex) and those that provide for the care and early education of the helpless human infants born to members of our species.

In the animal kingdom many offspring gain independence within hours, days, or weeks of their birth. In the case of human infants, achieving independence from adult caretakers is a longer, slower process. It is this set of "persistential" needs that produces a demand for acceptable ways to frame the transmission of seed (sex) and the care and early education phases of development for human infants (family).

Whether we speak of existential (minute-to-minute, day-to-day) needs for survival or persistential needs (the set of social, interpersonal interactions that sustain family lines, groups, or cultural communities), we are referring to the common and shared needs of all members of the human species—"commonalities" across cultures. In every cultural group the nurse encounters modes of provision for basic needs and also social structures that support mating, marriage, and early family education. The ways in which these needs are met and the form of the structure that ensures their continuance varies from culture to culture. Fundamental details that influence this "variability" are geography, demography, time in space, history, availability of resources, level of technological development, and an esoteric characteristic of human life called ethos.

ETHOS AND VALUES

Ethos is the root of ethics, morality, and values. Understanding the functional value of ethos provides the nurse with a tool of immeasurable importance in working with persons from a multiplicity of cultures. Webster (1975) defines ethos as "distinguishing characteristics, sentiment, or guiding beliefs" (p. 393). Anthropologists, however, accord ethos a more mysterious character, visualizing the concept as some innate, not learned, somewhat intuitive apprehension of what is right. According to anthropologists, ethos is not a learned moral sense, but an elusive quality attributed to infused, intuitive group perspective. Sociobiological theory might be applied in explicating this elusive quality of human life. Despite its mystery, ethos remains a major defining characteristic of values.

According to Geertz (1973) values are composed of three elements—ethos, world view, and religion or moral definition. Ethos is the human understanding of "how things should be" (idealism). World view comprises human awareness of "how things are" (reality). Religion, ritual, and group or community moral perspectives serve as "an organizing framework" (stabilizer) between the other two elements. Ethos is of the dream world; world view expresses sometimes harsh reality or sober realism; and religious or philosophical perspectives serve to make sense of the discrepancy between the two, establishing balance or equilibrium. Religion and ritual have also been characterized as a "bridge" supporting communication between ethos and world view. An illustration of values that my students enjoy is contained in the words of a Negro spiritual:

> Nobody knows the trouble I've seen (world view)
> Nobody knows but Jesus (religion)
> Nobody knows the trouble I've seen (world view)
> Glory, Alleluia! (ethos—dream of how the perfect life is)

Out of these three elements there emerges a group sense of value. The values held and expressed by each cultural group are passed on from generation to generation in the early childhood learning process that anthropologists call "enculturation." Early education is tenacious. It is probably justified to suggest that all of us carry some elements of early values training with us throughout our entire life and leave this life only after we have made our children or students the repository of some of them. Value elements are sometimes modified or changed in a conscious process called "acculturation."

ACCULTURATION

Acculturation takes two forms—developmental or situational. Erikson (1968) theorizes that each of us experiences changes in early adulthood associated with the establishment of adult identity. This author interprets early adult adaptation in terms of conscious values change, or a "developmental" form of acculturation. In this phase of human development we consider and evaluate the usefulness of early education, particularly the moral teaching received from early childhood caretakers. We set it into a frame that includes the world as we understand it, the world as we were taught to view it by our parents, and the moral or philosophical perceptions that are ours at that time. We compare and contrast one element with the others, evaluating the usefulness of what we were taught in the past in relation to present needs. From this composite evaluation there emerges an autonomous or personal vision of the world and its demands.

We consciously choose to accept all of the value elements prescribed by our family and group or adapt and modify them to fit the contemporary world as we understand it. It is usual for young adults to view their world and times as quite different from the world that confronted their parents in their youth. Thus a different world view, even when related to a previously held ethos, may demand adaptation. The basis of philosophical and religious views may remain consistent with those of parents or be changed in this process that describes developmental acculturation.

In its second and more clearly recognized form, "situational" acculturation occurs when persons move from one culture to another, experience some major traumatic event, or experience a charismatic change as religious conversion. The critical attributes in both forms of acculturation are *change* and *consciousness*. One must choose to change values. Tenacious as they are, values do not undergo spontaneous, unintended change. Religious conversion does account for a more spontaneous version of change. The importance of understanding values, and the process of change related to values, is imperative for an accurate interpretation of the Neuman Systems Model when applied to persons, families, or groups of cultures different from that of the care provider. Understanding both the tenacity with which people cling to values and the essential nature of the attributes represented by values supports nurses in their interventions for change.

Nursing is directed at interpretation of and intervention in human behavioral responses to health and illness situations. Human behavior is influenced by values. Customary patterns, culturally acceptable or appropriate reactions, and responses to nursing interactions and interventions must be understood by the nurse in order to assess, diagnose, and treat successfully, wherever the nursing situation presents cultural barriers.

CULTURAL CONCEPTS AND THE NEUMAN MODEL

Neuman's conceptual model of nursing has been described as a comprehensive, dynamic view of individuals, groups, and communities subject to environmental stressors (1974). The individual is described by Neuman as a unique (variable) composite also presenting characteristics that reside within a normal range (commonalities). Paraphrasing Neuman, Mirenda (1986) states, "The Neuman systems model has as its central focus a holistic view of person or client, from both a philosophic and biologic perspective, which implies relationships, dynamic freedom and creativity in adjusting to stress situations occurring in the internal and external environments" (p. 130). This description of the individual can also be adapted to families and groups and related to the anthropological concepts of individual, family, and group described on the previous pages. Neither the anthropological assumptions nor Neuman's assumptions are violated by relating the two.

The model focuses on the stressors that impinge on individuals, families, groups, and communities, and their reactions to stress as well as those factors that influence reconstitution. The term "client" was chosen by Neuman because it can be applied equally to the individual, family, or group, as well as community or population at risk. Whoever or whatever is identified as the focal system for nursing interaction is termed "the client."

Stressors according to Neuman have the power to disturb equilibrium in the client. This holds true for an individual or aggregate. "By a process of interaction and adjustment the individual maintains varying degrees of harmony or balance between his/her internal and external environments" (Neuman, 1982, 14). The measure of disequilibrium that occurs as a reaction to stress is variable. The actual state of the client at the moment of impact and the developmental level of the client in terms of physiology, psychology, sociocultural evolution, and spirituality together define the potency of the stressors and their range of effect on the client. Further, the nature and vitality of the stressor must also be considered. All human beings are capable of reactions within a normal range. When moderate stress occurs, the cushioning or accordion-like reaction of the flexible line of defense protects the core structure by supporting adaptations within the range normal for this client. As long as the flexible line of defense is not breached, and stressors are accommodated within the normal range of variation on all variables, equilibrium is maintained. When the stressor is extreme, and/or the client is functioning at the extreme end of the range of variation, the flexible line of defense will no longer be capable of maintaining equilibrium, and the stressor will break through to the normal line of defense, threatening the client's inner lines of resistance. The lines of resistance in their turn—by reacting—attempt to stabilize and return the client system to a normal state (within the normal line of defense). In the presence of extreme stressors, all lines of resistance may be destroyed, and the core structure of the client system compromised.

Neuman's representation of the client as a system capable of extensive adaptation in response to internal and external environments is consistent with anthropological concepts of human adaptation and environment (Dubos, 1965; Hockett, 1973; Pelto and Pelto, 1976).

THE NURSING PROCESS, CULTURE, AND THE NEUMAN MODEL ASSESSMENT

Utilization of the Neuman Model in practice requires the application of the nursing process. An extensive and thorough assessment of the client system forms the basis for nurse–client interaction. Neuman (1974, 1982, 1989) delineates the following principles to support quality assessment.

1. Knowledge of all the factors influencing a client's perceptual field.
2. Understanding the subjective (emic) meaning a stressor presents to the client as well as the objective (etic) meaning of the caregiver.

3. Perceptual elements that influence the caregiver's understanding of the client situation.

The caregiver in cross-cultural situations is presented with magnificent dilemmas. It is unlikely that a person whose perspectives are those of the dominant culture group will be able to understand and evaluate all the factors influencing the perceptual field of a client belonging to the Laotian Hmong. Nevertheless, an attempt at comprehending is demanded if quality of client–nurse interaction is to be achieved and maintained. In a complex pluralistic society such as the United States, health providers cannot afford the luxury of ethnocentrism. The unusual amount of literature on noncompliance gives rise to the thought that a lack of cultural understanding and its importance for interpreting client perspectives and defining needs is an important variable in care planning. Labeling a client noncompliant is more comfortable for many care providers than acknowledging his or her failure to assist the client in structuring and achieving health goals that can be understood by the client. Mirenda (1986) implicitly supports this position; ". . . as persons are unique composites of variables so are their environments." Neuman characterizes human beings as open systems in interaction with the environment. Mirenda writes further, "The degree of stability or harmony attained and/or maintained by the client system as it relates to the environment becomes that client's level of wellness at any specific point in time" (p. 133). If as Mirenda indicates harmony with the environment "becomes that client's level of wellness," it behooves the health care provider to understand the environmental context in which the client functions by considering the client's culture during the assessment phase and in planning for care.

CULTURAL DEFINITIONS AND CARE

How does the caregiver proceed? Understanding that cultural values shape the perceptions of each one of us is a beginning. In all cultures there exist emphases (values) regarding the ideal person, ideal health, ideal behavior, and the role of the caregiver (Leininger, 1988). The normal line of defense as identified by Neuman represents this ideal. It is this composite view of the world and personal equilibrium in relation to it that symbolizes health in all cultural contexts. For example, in the course of research with Mormons (Latter Day Saints), the author discovered that there exists an "Ideal Profile of the Saint." The Ideal Saint is perceived as an individual whose physical person is healthy, clean, and trim; a fitting temple for the Holy Spirit; and constantly available to meet the demands of church, community, and country. Procreation is central to the beliefs of Mormonism, and therefore the Ideal Saint also has healthy attitudes toward sexuality, marriage, children, and the responsibilities inherent in marriage and family. Responsible management of home, family, and finances are all attributes that are valued, and commitment to spiritual development of self and family is considered supreme. Further, extended family, church family, and community and civic interaction create the framework within which the Ideal Saint strives to achieve and maintain wholeness. It is this "total concept" of the Ideal that constitutes "health" in the mind of the Saint.

Most nursing assessment tools would produce basic information about the Mormon client, either individual or aggregate. However, only sensitive understanding of the value placed on motherhood, procreation, and child rearing could present to the caregiver a true measure of the disequilibrium experienced by a young Mormon wife who has been informed that she is unable to bear children. The value system that supports her life and in this case her spiritual survival are threatened. This scenario would be a painful one for any young woman hoping for a family, but for women of this subculture the discovery is a tragedy of great magnitude. For a young woman it could constitute a threat in psychological and sociocultural terms that could convert to a somatic physiological state or become life-threatening from a psychological perspective. In light of personal and professional goals, motherhood could conceivably seem undesirable to a modern caregiver. As a consequence the nurse might fail to understand the impact of the pronouncement on the client or the stress evoked by the diagnosis unless he or she had a good understanding of the subculture in question.

ASKING THE RIGHT QUESTIONS

Assessing clients in ways that produce culture-specific information is essential. Getting the right answers demands appropriate questions. If a nurse in the course of an obstetric or gynecological examination asks a Navajo woman "How many children do you have?" he or she may receive a baffling response such as "36." Traditional kinship lines in the Navajo culture are extended via the maternal blood lines, and traditional Navajo women regard the children born to their sisters, as well as those to whom they have given birth, as their own children. Therefore the appropriate question would take this form: "To how many children have you given birth?"

Inviting an Asian immigrant or a Mexican American immigrant to describe "the immediate family" may not provide an accurate picture of the living situation. Knowing that the couple being assessed has two children and lives at such-and-such an address does not necessarily provide an accurate family assessment or home assessment profile. Only a visit to the home will make it clear how many persons are perceived as part of that family. It may turn out that they are living in a space that is judged to be too small for the size of the extended family when evaluated in terms of hygiene, ventilation, and so on. Without a clear comprehension of the concept "family" in that particular culture, the nurse will fail to comprehend the responses of the client and will deliver erroneous information to the agency. By including inaccurate details in care plans, he or she will unknowingly program the interaction for failure.

NURSING DIAGNOSIS

Neuman (1982) describes stressors as occurring in three modes—intrapersonal, interpersonal, and extrapersonal. Determining the nature of stressors and their potential effect on the client in a way that supports the development of a valid nursing diagnosis requires an understanding of the nature of the client system. The value placed by the client system on self–family–extended family–group–community and national character is also necessary to this phase of the nursing process. It is difficult to determine the subjective importance of a stressor without a measure of understanding regarding the value placed by the client system on the threatened aspect or life attribute.

Wellness and illness are culturally defined. Related to the definition of wellness or illness there is a value system that colors interpretation of the nature of the stressor and the impact it exerts on the client. In cultures where intellectualism and learning are valued more than physical prowess, small stature and lack of brawn go relatively unnoticed. But the wrestler who is diagnosed with a cardiac neuropathy and told he may not work, much less wrestle in the future, is faced with tragedy unless intervention is tailored in such a way that it supports reconstitution and stabilization or the development of a new sense of equilibrium based on adapted values.

Average caregivers cannot arm themselves with all the information required to explain values in every segment of a multicultural population. A raised consciousness regarding the importance of cultural values will assist caregivers in probing for the necessary assessment data. Further, they will ask themselves whether culture is an intervening variable in situations where the diagnosis has led to interventions that prove unsuccessful in assisting reconstitution or facilitating the adaptations necessary following acute illness states.

NURSING INTERVENTIONS

Nursing interventions are formulated in three modes according to Neuman (1974, 1982, 1989). These are primary prevention, secondary prevention, and tertiary prevention. In each case the interventions are directed at maintaining or restoring equilibrium to the system. Primary modalities are directed at reducing the possibility of encounters with stressors and strengthening the flexible and normal lines of defense. Educational interventions are the common ones used by nurses to prevent disequilibrium and reduce stress while strengthening the flexible lines of defense. Therapeutic touch is another example of primary nursing intervention. Immunization, prenatal care, and nursing physical evaluations all serve to prevent stressors from breaching the flexible line of defense. Client education in cross-cultural situations demands extraordinary ingenuity. Teaching approaches must be tailored to the cultural comprehension and language of each group. Values must be given careful consideration in plans for intervention.

In Spanish-speaking groups of low socioeconomic status (for example, illegal Mexican immigrants), children are greatly valued. In situations where there is a shortage of food, there is a temptation to urge women to limit the size of their families. An undisguised confronting approach is unlikely to convince and may destroy trust in such a manner that future teaching is disregarded. However, many poor women will listen to the same information if it is tailored in appropriate ways or provided by indigenous caregivers. For example, it is possible to teach cultural aids who are members of the target community and allow them to teach the women in their group. San Diego State University College of Nursing developed an interactive video in Spanish to teach pregnant women about breast and bottle feeding. The subjects in the film are Spanish-speaking Americans from the target community, and the video is enjoying success.

Strengthening the normal line of defense in cross-cultural situations requires a nonjudgmental acceptance of variation in self-perception, the nature of interpersonal relations, and the ramifications of family and social structures that often appear very strange to the care provider. The level of acculturation of the client must be assessed. Language comprehension ability and number of years in the new country are important variables that provide the caregiver with clues when assessing acculturation levels. Desire to change, to Americanize, is a useful variable to assess also. The client who desires to become more American is more amenable to Western medicine. It is also important to know whether new immigrants are constantly infused into the family, group, or community. In groups where new immigrants are infused with regularity, cultural modes, customs, and traditions remain vital and attachment to culture-based perceptions more deeply entrenched. Two groups in urban settings that reflect this trend are Greeks and Mexican Americans.

Attempts to strengthen the flexible lines of defense in acculturating populations must reflect acceptance of variation, and tolerance for practices and perceptions that are appropriate in and for that culture. The care provider who is capable of approaching clients with an open mind will intervene successfully in many instances and serve as a catalyst for change. Most immigrants want to adapt to their new home and its culture; it is simply a slow and often confusing process. Sometimes it is necessary to support a combination of traditional and scientific interventions in order to maintain trust and provide effective care.

SECONDARY PREVENTION

Interventions of a secondary preventive nature are directed toward reconstitution or strengthening of the internal lines of resistance. They are called for whenever the flexible lines of defense have been breached and some deviation from health has been experienced by the client. A good example of the importance of understanding culture in order to intervene appropriately surfaced in contact with Hmong families in the area. A religious sister who conducted a preschool for Hmong children and a day school for their mothers explained that she could not get the mothers to push fluid intake for their small children suffering from a common cold with accompanying fever. No matter how she tried to explain the need for fluids, the children arrived at preschool seriously dehydrated, and occasionally children had to be hospitalized as a result. The graduate student working with the preschool group brought this problem to my attention. We called the sister and asked her what she advised the mothers to give the children to drink. She responded, "Well, fruit juice, Kool-Aid, and ice water." Asked further if all the recommended drinks were cold drinks, she said "Yes." I suggested that she advise the mothers to feed the children lots of warm chicken soup instead of cold drinks and report what happened. The sister was amazed; the problem resolved itself. Persons who have a background in Eastern religions often believe that warm remedies are the only ones appropriate to treat certain ailments and cold remedies for others. In the same way, they advise certain vegetables (for example, green vegetables) for some problems, and certain health deviations demand avoidance of certain foods.

A failure to understand the differences in value and belief systems expressed in health beliefs and practices could result in harmful advice. The small child who has fever and does not receive enough fluid is in jeopardy. Infants and small children quickly become dehydrated, and the nurse who does not understand the cultural approaches necessary to reach the client risks further breakdown of the normal lines of defense, a threat to the lines of resistance, and potential compromise of the core structure. The Hmong are very shy, and they are also very desirous of becoming American. Accepting American ways is part of being American. However, traditional health beliefs are such that the Hmong women will not give cold liquids to a child with a fever. We suspected that as a result of the sister's instructions, the mothers ended up giving less rather than more liquid to their children who had fevers. They did not want to appear un-American, nor did they want to violate their own health beliefs. In an attempt to instill order in the dissonant situation, they did neither. Warm chicken soup proved to be the right solution.

Thus it is necessary at each intervention step to inquire whether or not the proposed advice can be accepted by the client, or whether it constitutes a violation of traditional health beliefs. As people acculturate or change, they adjust automatically. But culture change is a slow, arduous process. In time parents see that other children survive who are fed cold liquids and cold foods even when they have fevers. To assume that our customs and approaches are the only ones, or worse, the only valuable ones, is ethnocentric and destroys trust. Most members of less-developed cultures, and many of well-developed cultures, apply mixed traditional and scientific methods in self-care. For example, many of us also combine the traditional chicken soup with aspirin when we have a cold. Some of us are fairly firm in the belief that one will not work without the other.

TERTIARY PREVENTION

An example of culture-centered prevention at the tertiary level is demonstrated in this narrative about a Navajo child. A 10-year-old Navajo child was admitted to a regional university medical center suffering from end stage renal failure. After a general work-up he was placed on dialysis and responded well to treatment. It was decided that the boy was a good candidate for renal transplant. Some effort was made on the part of the doctors to convey this to the mother. While the woman seemed to understand all that the doctor told her, she was very unresponsive when asked if members of her family would be willing to be tested as potential donors for the boy.

For a long time she failed to visit her son. Meanwhile it was decided to put the boy on a waiting list for a cadaver kidney. When the mother came to visit the child accompanied by her brother, the medical team met with her and shared the information that they were searching for a suitable cadaver kidney for her son. They also explained that they needed the necessary permission to proceed should the kidney become available. The mother asked for time to consider the plan and request and refused to sign the forms at that moment. The medical team was puzzled, feeling that the mother ought to be very grateful.

When the nurse in charge made rounds at midnight the same night, the child was missing. After 12 hours of frantic effort it was discovered that he was at home on the reservation with his extended family. Without dialysis for any extended period of time, his life was in jeopardy. The medical center sent out the life-flight in an attempt to bring the boy back to the hospital or at least to set up a dialysis unit in the local hospital. While this was being accomplished, a social worker, accompanied by a local medicine man, talked with the boy's mother and her brothers. They explained to the social worker that it was not acceptable in Navajo culture to take an organ from one person and insert it in another. Because Navajos believe that each person is complete and must remain inviolate, it could not be countenanced that the boy receive another person's kidney. The only acceptable tertiary intervention at that time was to maintain the child on dialysis. Eventually, in a triumph of cooperation between the medicine man and Western medicine, the boy received a kidney transplant. After the surgery the medicine man provided a "sing" directed at restoring equilibrium between the child and creation and ridding him of the influences of the intervention. Only a creative culture-centered intervention could succeed in this situation.

WHOLISTIC VISION

The prior attempts to separate out primary, secondary, and tertiary interventions in cross-cultural or transcultural situations in no way negate the importance of wholistic care. In many situations tertiary interventions will fail over time unless additional interventions have been structured at secondary and primary levels.

Space considerations make it impossible to explain this in this chapter, but a forthcoming chapter in Breckenridge (1994) will address this phenomenon in detail.

WHOLISTIC CARE

Neuman visualized human beings as wholistically organized systems, a composite of variables, with a core or basic structure surrounded by concentric protective rings. The individual's wholeness is dependent on maintaining stability physiologically, developmentally, psychologically, socioculturally, and spiritually. It is culture that proposes what wholeness comprises in any group. A very ancient grandmother or grandfather is perceived as whole and evolved in many Asian culture groups, while the American ideal of wholeness is that of strong, beautiful, unblemished youth. The concentric, protective circles are defined by culture also. Some people are less than whole when they are alone without family ties, whereas others reach wholeness only when they are totally self-supporting. In the first interpretation it is desirable to include extended family and community in care planning. In the other, the important factor is the client's personal wishes and directives. Thus the concentric circles may be defined as extended family, community structures, and/or religious community.

A shrewd caregiver understands that while cultural diversity in the population produces dilemmas on one hand, it offers care modalities in some situations that are unavailable in others. The community health nurse knows that structuring round-the-clock supervision for a patient with an extended family is simple compared to meeting the same need in a single elderly person with no relatives. Further, where strong bonds of community and culture exist, it is possible to obtain support from structures beyond the family. These organizational systems that reflect cultural values can be involved in the provision of educational units for primary prevention. Their persuasive influence (appropriately defined) can be incorporated in plans for change in groups or in the entire community.

RELIGION, RITUAL, AND SPIRITUALITY

In this chapter a value scheme has been presented that identifies religion or ritual as the organizing element between a person's perception of how things should be and his or her awareness of how they actually are. Formal religion and ritual (organized expression of religious or metaphysical beliefs) are to groups what spirituality is to persons or individuals. Without some element of spirituality or philosophy, human beings exhibit little hope.

Undermining or attacking the spiritual underpinnings of persons or groups is ill-advised since it is this element that creates order and infuses meaning into everyday situations. As Geertz (1973) states, "The religious perspective differs from the common sensical in that . . . it moves beyond the realities of everyday life to wider ones which correct and complete them, and its defining concern is not action upon those wider realities but acceptance of them, faith in them." And, ". . . it deepens the concern with 'fact' and seeks to create an aura of utter actuality" (p. 112). No matter how strange beliefs may appear to be, they sustain the person or family.

Leaving aside for the moment the occasional beliefs that appear destructive to health, consider those that sustain. Even sustaining religious ideas may seem nonproductive in situations where we imagine the need to be one for modern scientific intervention. Nevertheless, creative adaptations that allow the person to express beliefs or use alternative treatments to supplement those prescribed are more likely to support reconstitution and assist in restoring equilibrium than scientific and prescribed methods divorced from traditional methods.

Any aspect of the whole person can destroy or disturb equilibrium when it is overemphasized. The spiritual variable of humanness cannot sustain the total organism in this world if the other aspects of human dynamics are totally ignored. Even Teresa of Avila, the great mystic, drank water as well as ingesting the communion host daily, though it is documented that she ate nothing. Some words of T. S. Eliot are germane to this subject. He said that religious poetry is a minor form of poetry, and that the religious poet is not a poet who is treating the whole of poetry from a religious perspective but rather one who deals with a confined part of the subject matter of poetry. Thus, in applying the Neuman Model, it is important to evaluate the total or integral subject with emphasis on restoring or maintaining the equilibrium of the interacting whole. Neuman describes the human organism as one with physiological, psychological, developmental, sociocultural, and spiritual aspects. While spiritual dystony may be the basis for a diagnosis, one must continue to assess the integral effect of the spiritual element on the other variables and them on it.

A conscious awareness of wholeness is seldom encountered in individuals who deny a spiritual component in their lives. This spiritual element may be elusive, inexplicable, or merely philosophical, but because it creates order out of chaos, sense out of madness, or harmony out of disharmony, it is indispensable in nursing care. Care providers must take their cues from the client, family, or group. Spirituality is variously defined, and the presence of spiritual strength is very valuable for healthy living as well as in assisting reconstitution. Even when the client faces threats to core stability, the presence of spiritual health and strength may support a kind of equilibrium expressed as hope, or at the end of life, expressed as peace and acceptance.

CULTURE AND EVALUATION OF THE PROCESS

Evaluation, which is described as the final phase of the nursing process, actually provides the basis for reassessment and continued process. In cross-cultural situations each evaluative outcome must be validated by the client. Since the care provider's perspective is different, the nurse must elicit the client's perspective in order to establish the success or failure of interventions. This aspect of the Neuman Model calls once again for awareness of the client perspective. Those who are conscious of the importance of culture in forming values, and the fact that human responses are based on values, are able to approach clients from an emic perspective, or the perspective of the client and that of his or her culture. An objective or external perspective (the caregivers' own) is called etic. Evaluation is an ongoing process. Eliciting the client's perspective at each phase of the nurse–client interaction helps reduce the likelihood of failure in terms of interventions. This is true of all nurse–client interactions, but it is of particular importance in cross-cultural situations. Asking clients what they have understood, urging return demonstration of techniques taught, or recitation of information regarding prescribed behaviors, medical regimes, and diets is very important.

HARMONY AND THE NEUMAN SYSTEMS MODEL

Neuman describes health as equilibrium, balance, or harmony. The perception of harmony or equilibrium that each individual expresses in his or her life relies heavily on culture for its definition. Interaction, adjustment, and wholeness are all terms employed by Neuman to express her conception of nursing in our world. The definitions of an acceptable adjustment, appropriate forms of interaction, and the persons with whom it is appropriate to interact, as well as the concept of wholeness are formulated by each of us in living the life of the culture group into which we were born and enculturated or the culture we have consciously chosen (acculturation). Without some understanding of cultural ways, beliefs, and values, the health care professional can offer very little help toward restoration of the ". . . varying degrees of harmony and balance" between internal and external environments that Neuman characterizes as the process of reconstitution of health (1982, 14). However, a health care provider who does understand this need can apply the Neuman Systems Model in assessing, planning, and evaluating care in any cross-cultural interaction.

CONCLUSIONS

The primary conclusion that has emerged from application of the model in teaching and practice settings is its universality. The model can be applied successfully across the subfields of nursing and across situations. It also lends itself as an explicatory tool for planning care with interdisciplinary teams. The systems foundations of the model are familiar to most health professionals and facilitate their comprehension of the plan of care. This is particularly true for the community or public health team.

The Neuman assessment guide outlined by Mirenda (1986) provides a thorough approach to data collection on the client, which facilitates interdisciplinary care. Quality data support the nursing care process through the phases of diagnosis, care planning, and intervention and provide the basis for meaningful objective–subjective evaluation sessions. The universality of the model increases its value for nursing and for other health care providers interacting with nurses. This is of exceptional value in the primary care team. Because it is flexible and dynamic in nature, the model tolerates and incorporates culture specifics without distortion of the model or violation of its conceptual foundations.

A model capable of these applications has an increased value for planning care in multicultural populations. America has been described as "a conglomerate of 200 million people with little in common" (Moore, Van Arsdale, Glittenberg, and Aldrich, 1986), and while multiculturalism is a hallmark of American society, many other democratic countries are also confronted with increasing numbers of immigrants whose care presents an extraordinary problem for ordinary people.

It is for these reasons—to assist health care professionals in general, and nursing care professionals in particular—that the discussion of cultural variables and their implication for extending the use of the Neuman Systems Model is included in this volume. The chapter constitutes an attempt to assist contemporaries concerned with the task of providing quality nursing care to the citizens of this small planet earth.

REFERENCES

Dubos, R. 1965. *Man Adapting*. New Haven, Conn.: Yale University Press.

Erikson, E. 1968. *Identity: Youth and Crisis*. New York: Basic Books.

Geertz, C. 1973. *The Interpretation of Cultures*. New York: Basic Books.

Greeley, J. E. 1981. An interagency exploration of domestic violence in the Potomac Highlands: A rural study. *Journal of Rural Community Psychology* 2:46–50.

Hockett, C. F. 1973. *Man's Place in Nature*. New York: McGraw-Hill.

Kosko, D. A., and Flaskerud, J. H. 1987. Mexican American nursing practitioner and lay control group beliefs about cause and treatment of chest pain. *Nursing Research* 36(4):226–230.

Mirenda, R. M. 1986. The Neuman Systems Model: Description and application. In *Case Studies in Nursing Theory,* edited by P. Winstead-Fry, 127–166. New York: National League for Nursing.

Moore, L., Van Arsdale, P., Glittenberg, J., and Aldrich, B. 1987. *The Biocultural Basis of Health,* 2d ed. Prospect Heights, Ill.: Waveland Press.

Neuman, B. 1974. The Betty Neuman health-care systems model: A total person approach to patient problems. In *Conceptual Models for Nursing Practice,* edited by J. P. Riehl and C. Roy, 119–178. New York: Appleton-Century-Crofts.

Neuman, B., ed. 1982. *The Neuman Systems Model: Application to Nursing Education and Practice*. East Norwalk, Conn.: Appleton-Century-Crofts.

Neuman, B. 1983. Family interventions using the Betty Neuman Systems Model. In *Family Health: A Theoretical Approach to Nursing Care,* edited by I. W. Clements and F. B. Roberts. New York: Wiley.

Neuman, B. 1989. *The Neuman Systems Model,* 2d ed. East Norwalk, Conn.: Appleton & Lange.

Pelto, G. H., and Pelto, P. J. 1976. *The Human Adventure.* New York: Macmillan.

6

NURSES' ROLE IN WORLD CATASTROPHIC EVENTS
War Dislocation Effects on Serbian Australians

Nicholas G. Procter
Julianne Cheek

This chapter reports on an Australian study that demonstrates the use of the Neuman Systems Model to understand the experiences of Serbian Australians at a time of civil war in the former Yugoslavia with implications for the role of nursing in world catastrophic events.

CIVIL WAR IN THE FORMER YUGOSLAVIA AND THE NEUMAN SYSTEMS MODEL

Since June 1991 a tragic war has raged in the states of the former Yugoslavia—a civil war that can be described as a complex collision of emotional, social, cultural, and spiritual intensities involving both the togetherness and cohesion of individual ethnic groups and mass destruction and dislocation of people and property. It links historical, religious, and cultural events of the recent and distant past to ethnic rivalry and tensions of the present. Representatives from the European Community and warring factions have on numerous occasions sat down and attempted to negotiate a peaceful settlement to this war, as the destruction of cities and lives in the former Yugoslavia continues. As television

Reviewed by Raphella Sohier and Patricia Hinton Walker.

and newspaper images of destruction, human misery, and loss of life send shock waves throughout the world, what of the lives and experiences of people who originate and now feel displaced from this country, In particular, those whom the United Nations and European Community see as the main perpetrator of this war—Serbians? Whether or not Serbia is "at fault" is not the authors' concern. Instead, within a framework provided by the Neuman Systems Model, the authors will closely examine the meaning and experiences that individuals from the Australian Serbian community ascribe to this war, its impact on their health and well-being, and how nursing can become more fully involved in future worldwide catastrophic events.

Despite their existence thousands of kilometers away, many Serbians who live outside Serbia have experienced major stress over what they believe to be bias by the mainstream media in reporting of this war (Horsburgh, 1993; Stone, 1992) and concern for the safety of friends and family who remain in the former Yugoslavia (Totaro, 1991). In Australia stressors such as these have forced many of Serbian origin into a dynamic and complicated interplay between their sense of belonging, pride, nationalism, and intimacy with the people and places of their original homeland and Australia. The authors have chosen the Neuman Systems Model as the framework to examine the Australian Serbian experience since it is a model capable of embracing not only phenomena of complex personal, social, or technical dimensions but also small-scale problems in our environments and within our very selves.

Given that the Neuman Systems Model views the "client" as either an "individual, group, community, or social issue" (Neuman, 1989, 28), the clients discussed in this chapter will be both Australian Serbs and the Australian Serbian community itself. The Neuman Systems Model is suited to analysis of this kind because it allows for significant factors inherent in the nursing profession's concern for individual and community well-being (i.e., the ability for change, growth, and reconstitution, and the interplay between personal and environmental variables across the life-span) to be examined. At the clinical interface both nurse and client are in a collaborative process of mutual inquiry and discovery that allows for creativity and flexibility of both personal and global problem-solving. The goal of nursing using Neuman is to identify and prevent or reduce the impact of stressors on the client system—either noxious or beneficial "depending on their nature, timing, degree, and potential for ultimate change" (Neuman, 1982, 9). All parts and subparts of each are related and interrelated and can only be examined separately if removed temporarily and later placed back into the scheme of things or system-defined boundaries. For scholars of nursing the model offers "an important working hypothesis for the development of new insights and statements for verification of new theoretical perspectives" (Neuman, 1989, 9). That is, new ways of exploring breadth and depth in clinical and scholarly nursing inquiry.

Clearly, with breadth and depth in its analysis and interpretation of phenomena in and around the client system, the Neuman Systems Model provides a unifying focus for understanding clients and their environment. For the clients reported on in this chapter the Neuman Systems Model promotes consideration of ongoing interactions with stressors in their culture, spirituality, psychosocial functioning, and physical well-being across intra-, inter-, and extrapersonal dimensions.

METHOD

This study draws upon biographical research techniques that aim to present

> the experiences and definitions held by one person, one group, or one organisation as this person, group, or organisation interprets those experiences. (Denzin, 1989, 183)

As such it has a qualitative interpretative focus in that the way individuals understand and perceive events is central to the research being undertaken. Of particular interest is the *meaning* that individuals ascribe to certain central or critical events being studied.

The analysis is based on the case histories of two individuals from the Australian Serbian Community. These two individuals were chosen from a convenience sample (see Nieswiadomy, 1993, 179) of Serbian Australians derived from their location and the previous contact that one of the researchers had with the community from which they came. As with all case-based studies, which are in-depth examinations of people or groups, the generalizability of this study is limited. However, what this study does generate are theoretical analyses that can be tested in further research. As Younger (1985) points out, case studies are not used to test hypotheses, but rather hypotheses, or in this case theory, may be generalized from case studies.

A case history is a "full story of some temporal span or interlude in social life" (Glaser and Strauss, 1968, 182). In this instance the temporal span or interlude is the conflict in the former Yugoslavia. The attempt to gain the "full story" is an attempt to develop thick description and hence thick interpretation (Denzin, 1989). Thick description goes beyond the "mere or bare reporting of an act (that is; individual A did B). This is their description" (Ryle, 1968, 8–9). Moreover, a thick description "describes and probes the intentions, motives, meanings, context, situations and circumstances of action" (Denzin, 1989, 39). The notion of thick description is allied to the notion of theory as critique of the social world that is derived from the interpretations of those being studied. As Geertz (1973) contends, "the essential task of theory building is not to codify abstract regularities but to make thick description possible" (p. 24).

The purpose of such a study and approach is theory generation rather than theory testing. Once theory has been developed, it is possible to test it empirically or otherwise. In that way the thick description produced in the case study provides an ideal vehicle for the analysis and testing of the applicability of the Neuman Systems Model to understanding the effects of civil war and disturbance on the health of Serbian Australians. At all times the aim is to try to understand the conflict from the perspective of the individuals in the study. Of great interest and import is the definition of reality that these individuals have with respect to the conflict. It is this definition that provides insights into the stressors involved for these people and the resultant impact that such stressors have on their health or system stability and well-being. It is important to acknowledge that such perceptions and meanings cannot be seen in isolation since they relate to, and are influenced by, the structural units in which individuals function, such as the Australian Serbian community as a system isolated from Australian society.

Case histories were obtained by means of exploratory, unstructured interviews. Denzin (1989) points out that

> A careful transcription of an interview, provided it does not intermix the interviewer's own interpretations, is as much a form of life history data as a personal diary. (p. 183)

Each interview was recorded, with the consent of the individual concerned, on microcassette and later transcribed. The confidentiality of the transcript and the anonymity of the participants were maintained at all times. Transcripts of the interview were then coded and analyzed in order to reveal the themes and issues implicit in them pertaining to the health effects of the crisis on these individuals. The themes and issues identified were then explored using the theoretical framework and orientation provided by the Neuman Systems Model. From the data obtained at this "micro" level of analysis, it is possible to move the discussion into a more "macro" level. The themes and issues involved can be used to illustrate the effects of catastrophic world events on individuals and communities. This level of analysis also serves as a means to explicate the contribution nurses can make in dealing with similar events and influencing health policy regarding service provision for these individuals.

PRIMARY, SECONDARY, AND TERTIARY PREVENTIONS AS NURSING INTERVENTIONS FOR BOTH INDIVIDUAL AND COMMUNITY AS CLIENT

Appendix A and Appendix B summarize data pertaining to the meaning and experiences that both Serbian individuals and the Serbian community ascribe to this war and its impact on their cultural, spiritual, psychosocial, and physical well-being across intra-, inter-, and extrapersonal domains.

Appendix A reveals that the spiritual and emotional wholism for these clients has been shattered despite desperate attempts by the Serbian community to repair and reconstitute this domain. This has been further complicated by intra- and extrapersonal stressors characterized by adverse media, a breakdown in long-term friendships and social relationships, and feelings of deception by, and mistrust toward, the Australian government.

Appendix B demonstrates that the Australian Serbian community is an open system interacting environmentally with the media, Australian politicians, each other, and the wider Australian community that is not directly involved in the conflict. The inner core of the Australian Serbian community is characterized by a unique blend of basic survival factors such as nationalism, history, religion, gender, and a sense of geographical belongingness with names and places of the former Yugoslavia. For the Australian Serbian community, these factors include mechanisms for maintenance of normal communication of events both overseas and at a national level.

Usual prewar stressor coping patterns with the goal of facilitating wellness and adaptation for both the individual and community have included "shying away" from militant political activities and spending time away from the public gaze and mainstream media. Small-scale religious and cultural events tended to dominate the Serbian community's calendar rather than large-scale street rallies. Prewar, Australian Serbians would tend to communicate anger, disappointment, and/or frustration, in relation to a particular issue or concern, to their own print and electronic media operations within Australia rather than to mainstream media, always conforming to language, cultural, religious, and gender norms in concert with both community and social expectations. Today, however, many members of the Australian Serbian community have made significant steps toward a new profile in the mainstream electronic and print media and local, state, and federal government bodies as well.

Based on Neuman's model, the lines of resistance represent the internal factors that help the Serbians as clients defend against stressors. An example of this type of defense is the community's highly organized media watch campaign and monitoring of events (more precisely their corrective reporting) outside the mainstream media (see Appendix B).

The central and overriding themes that emerge from Appendix A and B are an estranged "sense of belonging" and loss of identity within the context of Australian society. Sense of belonging is a powerful emotional quality with significant personal and community health implications as a vital mental health concept (see Hagerty et al., 1992). Yet exploration and discussion of sense of belonging as a significant factor in the provision of care has been largely ignored by the international nursing community.

NURSING ROLE

It is against this background that the following Neuman-derived (Neuman, 1989, 57) primary, secondary, and tertiary nursing preventions as interventions for both individual and community are proposed to help ease the risk of deep cultural penetration by stressors and Serbian community system breakdown.

Primary Prevention as Intervention

This form of intervention is characterized by the client counteracting harmful circumstances or events *before* the production of stress reaction and system instability. Primary interventions occur when a stressor is suspected or identified and serve to strengthen the client's flexible lines of defense by decreasing the possibility of a reaction. Primary preventions as interventions should be concerned with the evolution and nature of events in the client's past, as well as the "here and now." In the case of civil war, it is necessary to closely examine the client's inner thoughts, motivations, and ideas, that is, the "self" and the influences of civil war upon it. Although a reaction may have not yet occurred, the degree of stressor risk is known. It is the knowing of potential stressor outcomes that should be a catalyst for the client to seek out creative ways of preventing system instability by promotion of system strengths. This is where the nurse as a sociopolitically knowledgeable caregiver can be most helpful in facilitating education and client coping development to offset potential stressor reactions.

For the Australian Serbian individual and community, civil war has caused a regeneration of spiritual intensities that have brought reunification, solidarity, and greatly increased nationalistic spirit. Primary prevention has acted as a client/client system buffer for intra-, inter-, and extrapersonal stressors such as distressing media reports often with images of a shattered homeland, feelings of betrayal by the Australian government, and loss of a "voice" and identity in mainstream Australian society. Both individual and community experience a catastrophic and powerful mix of emotion charged by the homeland civil war and subsequent change in lifeways. Serbian culture, spirituality, and psychosocial functioning all continue to suffer as events in the former Yugoslavia unfold and influence life in Australia. As life in former Yugoslavia becomes more distressing, so too does life for the Australian Serbian individual and community.

Secondary Prevention as Intervention

Evidence is clear from the data found in Appendix A that client-driven attempts to reduce levels of distress or disturbance in their system stability and well-being caused by this war are being moderately successful. For example, anger, frustration, and powerlessness experienced by clients in response to the loss of contact with their homeland has been reduced because of intervention activities that seek to legitimate the integrity of individual cultural mores and beliefs. Analysis of this critical dimension would not be complete without acknowledgement of stressor penetration that has increased the momentum of the client's self-direction away from the Australian community. Where the clients seek to re-establish their new place in the midst of a changing world, old friendships and relationships from the former Yugoslavia must be sacrificed. This painful resetting of boundaries is not unique to Australian Yugoslavs. For example, in the United Kingdom live approximately 60,000 people from the former Yugoslavia. This United Kingdom Yugoslav community was until recently "a 'close-knit' family embracing all its ethnic nationalities" (Cohen, 1991, 22). Many have been life-long friends and live only a few streets from each other. But since the recent civil war began, the walls have gone up between the communities, making such close ethnic friendships a thing of the past.

Only when the client feels safe to venture out into mainstream activities do they feel able to confirm through a voice their cultural identity. Feelings of safety come from sharing a common belief and purpose to sustain difficult circumstances. A great need exists for the Australian Serbian individual and community to establish a new sense of belonging and identity against implicit and explicit stressors that encourage isolation and rejection by the larger social order.

In the light of the preceding analysis, the goal of secondary preventions as interventions for these clients should be to protect their basic internal and external structures and facilitate wellness through participation and sense of belonging in the context of their immediate environment. The Neuman Model concentric circles surrounding and protecting system integrity and vitality of "the self" and basic structure should be nourished. That is, there must be appropriate and effective monitoring and interventions in stressor situations that could compromise the emotional integrity and inner peace of the client. One goal in these interventions is to change harmful thought patterns and beliefs that instigate and/or perpetuate feelings of "not belonging" and social isolation. When both the nurse and client collaborate in working toward protection of the client's basic structure in this manner, the possible outcome of the journey goes beyond optimum wellness. A broad sociocultural nursing approach of this kind should enhance stability of both individual client functioning and the larger community system as client through identification and specific ownership of positive system strengths to facilitate securing their "place in the world." In so doing, the individual and larger client system continue to enhance each other.

Tertiary Prevention as Intervention

Here the nurse attempts to reduce the client impact of residual effects caused by stressor penetration. Tertiary interventions focus on readaptation and reconstitution of the client system stability by maximizing their strength and closely monitoring areas of weakness or potential reactions from stressors. Tertiary interventions require the coordinated, often multidisciplinary strengthening of resistance to current and potential stressors by evaluating what has enhanced the healing process to date and what resources remain viable for future use. It is essential that nursing carefully monitor client progress and remain knowledgeable of intra-, inter-, and extrapersonal environmental factors that could increase client risk of regression in any of the five Neuman variable areas. To best accomplish this goal, considerable reflection and understanding of past events by both client and nurse are essential. This reflection should also support new coping strategies and enhance full appreciation of the circumstances in both their respective worlds that have contributed to optimal wellness and that define their subsequent relationship. Whether the client is defined as an individual or larger community, it is the responsibility of nursing to facilitate client extraction of important components of their journey together in order to create positive future evolvement and secure change in the everyday life of the client system.

The nature of the need for tertiary interventions for these clients is evident in both Appendix A and B and includes the re-establishment of connectedness with all that is intrinsic to being Serbian, that is, establishment of new and supportive structures for, and with, people that promote autonomy and a sense of belonging to the community's spiritual, social, psychological, and physically defined client system. Nursing should further seek to reward and complement whatever client system progress is being made to attain internal and external environmental mastery and optimal wellness. To achieve this end, realities of greatest concern and priority to the client (i.e., political and cultural beliefs) must be seen as features central to the therapeutic process.

The Neuman Systems Model accommodates this broad issue approach to catastrophic world events. It serves as a framework for care by negotiation, that is, on the basis of what definitions and beliefs are most idiosyncratic to the client and all that exists in the client's world.

IMPLICATIONS FOR NURSING IN THE CARE AND COMFORT OF PEOPLE FOLLOWING GLOBAL CATASTROPHIC EVENTS

For over two decades the Neuman Systems Model has established itself as a theoretical and practical framework for comprehensive analysis and understanding of phenomena in and around the client system in worldwide nursing education and practice arenas. As we enter the 21st century, it is indeed time to chart a new course in breadth in use of the model that goes beyond existing experience. In relating its use to worldwide catastrophic events through active coordination and facilitation of health care services that help clients better understand and cope with environmental stressors such events bring, nursing is continuing its worldwide commitment toward support of professionalism in fostering global unity, peace, and wholism for the client as a system.

This study has brought the researchers into direct dialogue with the internal and external environments of the client system. Each has been seen to have a unique response pattern, level of intensity, and existing interrelationships. It is with these factors that comprise the inner and outer world of the client that nursing should be most concerned. At times of catastrophic dislocation and distress it is the responsibility of nursing to learn how to reach out and find a connectedness with the breadth and depth of all factors impacting on the client's stability as a system. Evaluation of the need for primary, secondary, and tertiary preventative interventions is critical to system strength, stability, and maintenance. A major goal of client–nurse interventions in catastrophic world events should be to help restore and nourish existing strengths to offset a feeling of life's fragmented emptiness in a world that no longer makes sense—a world where (as in the former Yugoslavia),

> ...a new generation of European families is learning what it means to flee from a home, to lose a father killed or fighting on some unknown front, to travel the roads with bags and bundles and hungry children, to be the prey of armed bands who beat, steal, rape and sometimes kill, to be at best refugees in a foreign land without possessions or hopes. For this generation, like that of its grandparents in the 1940s, the world reveals itself as incomprehensible, unmanageable, and meaningless. (Ascherson, 1992, 25)

The goal of nursing in worldwide catastrophic events should be to retain maximum wellness and system stability for individuals and communities as clients as they strive for a sense of inner peace and contentment against impossible odds, a journey that encompasses changing and often hostile internal and external world environments. For nursing to properly fulfill its commitment to caring for the human impact of catastrophic world events such as this chapter illustrates, it must also be prepared to work closely with appropriate resources and place great emphasis on the use of strategies that enhance the self, family (immediate and extended), and community. It must also facilitate national identity and character of the client's larger world with the overall purpose of protecting its core survival and wellness potential.

FUTURE IMPLICATIONS FOR USE OF THE NEUMAN SYSTEMS MODEL

This chapter has highlighted the plight of one cultural group that is enduring a unique struggle against violence and destruction in their own homeland, and the destabilization of individual and community life in Australia. This chapter has also articulated the way in which the Neuman Model can be used to explore and explicate aspects of the current conflict in former Yugoslavia at personal, community, national, and international levels of analysis. The Neuman Model has the flexibility and capacity inherent within it to be used at all or any one of these levels, depending on the specific focus of a particular study. Such flexibility highlights the potential value of the Neuman Systems Model as a theoretical framework for research. It will continue to expand its contribution to debate and scholarly activity in the world health arena. The applicability of the Neuman Model to an analysis of the conflict in former Yugoslavia demonstrates model congruence for the development of in-depth understandings of global issues of great importance and concern.

Concomitant with highlighting the increased potential for use of the Neuman Systems Model within the global context is a plea for broadening the focus of nursing practice to incorporate global catastrophic care perspectives. Hopefully, nursing will be challenged to heighten its vision and abandon constraints on its future role and function. This chapter is intended to urge nurses to embrace a more active and critical role in contributing to the understanding of the nursing and health implications inherent in major social crises such as the civil war in former Yugoslavia. Clearer understanding, facilitated by organizing structures such as the Neuman Systems Model, will inevitably lead to quality humane nursing practice worldwide.

The Neuman Systems Model, by the analysis it allows and by the debate that such analysis promotes, will continue to contribute to better health care outcomes at local, community, national, and/or global levels.

REFERENCES

Ascherson, N. 1992. To be healthy and happy is sometimes to be mad. *Independent,* September 20, p. 25.

Cohen, D. 1991. Real Life: My wife, my friend, my enemies. *Independent,* October 13, p. 22.

Denzin, N. K. 1989. *The Research Act.* Englewood Cliffs, N.J.: Prentice Hall.

Geertz, C. 1973. *The Interpretation of Cultures.* New York: Basic Books.

Glaser, B. G., and Strauss, A. L. 1968. *The Discovery of Grounded Theory.* London: Weidernfeld Nicholson.

Hagerty, M. K., et al. 1992. Sense of belonging: A vital mental health concept. *Archives of Psychiatric Nursing* 6(3):172–177.

Horsburgh, S. 1993. Centre opens window on the Balkans. *The Australian,* January 20, p. 19.

Neuman, B. 1989. *The Neuman Systems Model.* East Norwalk, Conn.: Appleton-Century-Crofts.

Neuman, B. 1982. *The Neuman Systems Model: Application to Nursing Education and Practice.* East Norwalk, Conn.: Appleton-Century-Crofts.

Nieswiadomy, R. M. 1993. *Foundations of Nursing Research,* 2d ed. Norwalk, Conn.: Appleton & Lange.

Ryle, G. 1968. "The thinking of thoughts." University of Saskatchewan University Lectures, No. 18, University of Saskatchewan, Regina.

Stone, A. 1992. Yugoslavia's war tears at U. S. communities. *USA Today,* June 16, p. 8.

Totaro, P. 1991. Our local Balkan war. *The Bulletin,* December 10, pp. 30–34.

APPENDIX A
PERSON AS A CLIENT

	Intrapersonal Stressors	Interpersonal Stressors	Extrapersonal Stressors
PHYSICAL	Physiological functioning is compromised by stressful episodes of interaction between internal and external environments, resulting in poor diet, tachycardia, poor sleep, poor concentration, poor information processing, and information overload.	Circadian rhythm interrupted by poor sleep and generalized sleep disturbance. This follows "worry and concern" for family at "home" and offensive media reports. Poor family diet due to reduced enthusiasm for preparation of food.	Fatigue caused by sleeplessness, depression, anxiety, and preoccupation with catastrophic events. Loss of answers to why the war has happened. Tachycardia and other symptoms reflective of a sympathetic nervous system response.
PSYCHOLOGICAL	Sense of self, well-being, belonging, and companionship with family and individual's place within it are fabricated by family. When compromised, depression, emotional pain, loss of self, brooding, aggressive thoughts, and isolation from others occur.	Bond between relatives and friend in former Yugoslavia is lost or prohibited by sanctions, damage, and dislocation following war. Depression and emotional pain of loss of relationships; decreased will or desire to make contact with others.	Loss of the dream that one day individual may return to homeland (motherland). Loss of bond between country and culture, the self, and what might have been for the remaining life span. Loss of credibility as an Australian citizen, "no one is listening to me." Depression and loss of "new country" as well as feeling of being displaced and alone, not belonging anywhere at all.
SOCIOCULTURAL	Cultural beliefs influence parenting and gender styles (sex role stereotypes). Loving friendships since birth now changed due to differences made explicit. Several hundred years of history and nationalism are internalized; "self" is defined by belonging to this cultural group.	The sociocultural norms among self, former Yugoslavia, Australia, and Australian government are marked by feelings of anger, disappointment, betrayal, and disbelief. Loss of intimacy with Croatian girlfriend and sharing of symbols of childhood evolution together. Feelings of guilt and of being an outcast and victim of a conspiracy.	Loss of cultural connection as shared with Australian society leading to alienation complicated by loss of "motherland." Loss of identity with homeland has caused decreased cultural identity. Feels betrayed by Australian government and Australian media. Loss of intimacy with Australian sociopolitical system, yet struggling to maintain some form of identity within it.
DEVELOPMENTAL	Early childhood messages of cultural and gender role behavior. Dance and music grow within the person. When under stress, more lumbar and upper back pain—discomfort due to stoop in posture. Feelings of sadness and isolation.	Companionship with friends of same age and sex has been fragmented and dislocated by war. Depths of meaningful relationships made more shallow with non-Serbian members of former Yugoslavian community.	Loss of self and self-development after leaving homeland at an early age and forced separation caused by current conflict. Loss of a "dream" that has maintained and life span significance.
SPIRITUAL	Spiritual belonging influences weekend and other social activities, parenting styles. Notion of "self" intertwined with spiritual beliefs.	Resurgence of spiritual beliefs associated with Serbian Orthodox religion and significant events on the religious calendar. Reunited with blend of nationalism and religiousness—a spirit of all that is Serbian, and all that is me.	Loss of spiritual and religious symbols such as churches and icons in former Yugoslavia have been revealed by images of mass destruction on TV media. Loss of solidarity with other Orthodox and socialist countries in Eastern Europe (e.g., Soviet Union).

D O M A I N S

APPENDIX B
COMMUNITY AS A CLIENT

	Intrapersonal Stressors	Interpersonal Stressors	Extrapersonal Stressors
PHYSICAL	Maintenance of "heart and soul" of being a Serbian community—representing community interests at local and national levels in key areas such as health, education, aged care. Identification of Serbian "community" is internal yet collective—maintained by activities both cultural and religious. Intracommunity activity is fueled by birth of new members into community.	Rights of passage vis-à-vis immigration to Australia seems blocked by Australian government. This makes the community angry and unable to fairly represent itself in key areas of decision making.	Heart and soul" of Australian Serbs is compromised by constant attack by media and members of Australian society. It has become difficult for Australian Serbians to undertake preventative activities such as ongoing relationships with communities and groups within former Yugoslavia to avert fragmentation of "heart and soul" of current community identity.
PSYCHOLOGICAL	Sense of belonging is inextricably related to historical, familial, and spiritual events of the past, engendered by family tradition resulting in a sense of well-being and completeness. It is compromised by competing demands set by contemporary Australian society and isolation by outside community action and beliefs.	Anger, frustration, and resentment against Australian immigration departments that lack of understanding for refugees and asylum seekers from former Yugoslavia. Activities of community are not endorsed by existing sociopolitical structures in Australia. Younger members of Serbian community seek out ways to best express their anger and frustration against loss of homeland and symbols of identity. Need to psychologically legitimate and appease disequilibrium in the system to restore homeostasis.	Isolation, anger, and frustration by the community with Australian media and government structures do not allow for community development and participation free of stress and distress. The constant battle by the Australian Serbian community for credibility and identity in the Australian landscape is a distraction from the community's identification of risk factors that may place the community at risk of distress, dysfunction, "depression," or stagnation.
SOCIOCULTURAL	Cross-cultural and intracultural marriages, christenings, and funeral services all occur within the context of intra-Serbian norms. However, these are challenged by nationalism and withdrawal from mainstream Australian society and lead to a fragmentation of families. Serb-Croat (i.e., mixed) marriages, for example, are put under extreme risk due to conflict of allegiance to either group.	Loyalties to Australian society and citizenship expectations are placed under pressure by negative stereotypes of Serbian Australians set by the popular media and government bodies. Intercommunity (two Serbian community groups) solidarity emerges and is mobilized by well-orchestrated activities (street rallies, etc.) into the wider Australian sociopolitical and community landscape.	Conflict between Australian norms and values and Serbian cultural norms, values, expectations, and beliefs at a time of dislocation, feeling an outcast, personal losses, and traumas. Since postwar immigration to Australia 1947–50s, Australians have slowly accepted migrants from Eastern Europe as part of its ethnocultural landscape. Now, civil war has cast a dark cloud over the positive identity and intention of people with Serbian background, making them reluctant to openly identify themselves to this community unless in large numbers.

D O M A I N S

DEVELOPMENTAL	Prior to conflict two district Serbian churches and communities existed. This involved separate senior religious and community figures and spokespeople. The pressure of civil war and all it brings to the Australian Serbian community has forced the two groups to come together with common purposes and goals; a moving forward in collaborative strength has been achieved. Intracommunity "heart and soul" has meant a strengthening of community systems (church; recreation, newspapers, and other media activities).	Negative stereotypes of Serbians both by media and the dominant culture adversely affect a majority of the population already at risk, i.e., persons from the Australian Serbian community who before the conflict felt unsupported or isolated with limited ability to solve personal problems. Here, the developmental issue is personal enhancement of coping behaviors across the life span.	Children's education and socialization are disadvantaged by victimization at school by children of differing ethnic and social backgrounds. These conditions adversely affect the social and emotional development of children from Serbian backgrounds at a time of visible distress and hardship experienced in both home and community life. Distinct changes and stressors bring major developmental differences to the evolution of Australian Serbian community identity.
SPIRITUAL	Intracommunity consciousness has been penetrated and made to coexist with a strong blend of nationalism and theology that strengthens the collective resolve of community action and determination.	Stressors between Orthodox and Roman calendar events such as Christmas and New Year further emphasize the "difference" between Serbian Australians and mainstream society. Spiritual beliefs of community are also challenged by the notion of a Christian religion being associated with atrocities and serious acts of violence.	Spiritual and religious norms have evolved over hundreds of years and in contrast to mainstream Australian society.

7

FAMILY HEALTH AND THE NEUMAN SYSTEMS MODEL

Patricia Short Tomlinson
Kathryn Hoehn Anderson

This chapter examines a perspective of family health and relates that perspective to nursing mandates. A family health systems nursing paradigm is defined and related to the Neuman Systems Model.

The influence of the family in health promotion is of long-standing interest in the practice of nursing (Whall, 1986b). However, theories for practice have varied in their perspective about the centrality of the family in health care, and few, if any, have identified the family system as the primary client. One of the contributions of the Neuman Systems Model (Neuman, 1989) is the articulation of a system of nursing practice that has a pervasive order that unifies assessment and intervention and fosters understanding of the reciprocal relationships between client and caregiving systems. Rooted in general systems theory, the Neuman Systems Model is philosophically consistent with the perspectives of a family system approach and can be expanded to include the family as client.

Neuman was one of the first to acknowledge the need for a systems approach for organizing nursing care. Her concern that the profession fully accept the challenge to develop within a systems basis has been important to subsequent theory development. With respect to a family health perspective, the long-standing emphasis in most theories is on the family as the context in which caregiving is done. This is being supplanted by growing recognition of the whole family as client in the health promotion enterprise. However, despite the increasing focus on the family system as a health entity, there is not a universally accepted definition of family health as a systems phenomenon. The family health system paradigm proposed by Anderson and Tomlinson (1992) explicitly defines family health as a wholistic function of the family system and its health promotion capability. Integrating this concept of the family system with the Neuman Systems Model is a step toward a synthesis of a full family systems perspective in health care.

The merging of a family health systems nursing theory with a conceptual framework for practice is extremely timely. There has been a burst of interest from both the political and health care sectors regarding the importance of the family in promoting health, in providing sustained care for the chronically ill, and in adapting to the stressors of their expanded role in caretaking. These forces compel us not only to think of health as the wholistic system Neuman describes in her model, but also to incorporate the family explicitly in an integrative paradigm.

The purpose of this chapter is to examine the development of the concept of family health, propose a perspective of family health based on a family health system paradigm (Anderson and Tomlinson, 1992), and relate that to the Neuman Systems Model.

FAMILY HEALTH

The centrality of the family in health care is emphasized in the ANA futuristic policy statement of 1985 (Cabinet on Nursing Research, 1985), as well as in the legal definitions of nursing in many states, thus mandating nursing to provide family care (American Nurses' Association [ANA], 1980; Donaldson and Crowley, 1978). However, the literature (King, 1983; Neuman, 1983; Newman, 1983; Rogers, 1983; Roy, 1983; Whall, 1986a) clearly shows there are alternate views of the family in health care: as individual persons who comprise the family unit; as the environment for family members, particularly for caretaking of the acutely or chronically ill; and more recently as a unit of health care and analysis. These views are generally concerned with the health of the family and its members, and the nursing intervention designed to improve family health (Gilliss, Highley, Roberts, et al., 1989). The discipline has thus expanded its metaparadigmatic view of health, shifting the unit of care and analysis from person to include the family system (Anderson and Tomlinson, 1992; Fawcett and Whall, 1988; Gilliss, 1991; Murphy, 1986; Wright and Leahey, 1984), challenging the more traditional focus of individual health care and redefining "person" in the nursing metaparadigm to include the "family as the unit of care or family as a context of care" (Feetham, 1984, 1990; Wright and Leahey, 1988). This redefined focus also represents a paradigm shift requiring greater consistency in the approach to practice.

However, the concept of health itself, a central goal for nursing practice, reflects differing degrees of specificity, reductionism, and centrality (Meleis, 1985), as well as differing paradigmatic influences (Newman, 1986; Newman, Sime, and Corcoran-Perry, 1992). Consideration of these factors leads to alternate definitions of health: (1) health as a dichotomous variable, (2) health as a continuum, and (3) health as a more inclusive, wholistic state (Tripp-Reimer, 1984).

Within the wholistic view there are two perspectives. The first, a eudaemonistic view (Smith, 1983), defines health as a dynamic state or a process of obtaining physical, psychological, social, and spiritual well-being (Smith, 1983; Woods, Laffrey, Duffy, Lentz, Mitchell, Taylor, and Cowan, 1988; World Health Organization, 1973). The Neuman Systems Model falls within this perspective.

A second wholistic view, expressed in the Man-Environment Simultaneity paradigm (Parse, 1987), sees humans as more than and different from the sum of their parts in continuous multiple interrelationships with the environment. Health is viewed as an expression of the process of living or becoming. Nurse theorists consistent with this paradigmatic focus include Newman (1986), Parse (1987), Paterson and Zderad (1976), Rogers (1983), and Watson (1985). Despite the continuing development of these paradigms, all were originally structured on assumptions of an individualistic perspective where health is a state or process of the whole person in interaction with the environment and/or where the family represents a significant factor of the environmental matrix.

Outside of nursing, the concept of family health may "denote the health (absence of disease) of family members, or it may denote the condition of the family itself" (McEwan, 1974, 487). McEwan concluded that "family health" refers to the comparative health status of the individuals within the family and that "familial health" refers to evaluative descriptions of the functions and structure of the family, with dual focus on both the health of individual members and the health of the family as a whole (McEwan, 1974).

Using a more integrative wholistic view, Pratt (1976) described "family health" as the "general level of health in a family so inextricably intertwined with the pattern of family relations that health itself becomes a vital aspect of the fabric of family life" (p. 139). From a sociological perspective, Pratt views the family as a personal care system within which health is molded and health care is mobilized, organized, and carried out within a societal context. She introduces the idea of "energized family" as one whose structure encourages and supports persons to develop their capacities for full functioning and independent action, thus contributing to family members' health. Clearly Neuman's perspective of health is synchronous with this view. Like Neuman, Pratt argues that the energized family structure includes the family's ability not only to be responsive to individual members' needs and interests and to actively cope with life's problems and issues, but also to demonstrate an energized pattern of family health care. This includes both positive personal health practices and the composite health practices of the family group.

In other disciplines the meaning of family health has generally been synonomous with family functioning (deChasney, 1986), using systems concepts developed by family scientists (Burr, 1979; Hill, 1958; McCubbin and Patterson, 1983; and Olson et al., 1983) or concepts developed by family therapists (Bowen, 1978; Minuchin, 1974; Satir, 1972). In addition to the focus on family functioning, some of these family health definitions incorporate limited biopsychosocial factors, aspects of wellness, and the environmental interaction affecting both family members and the family unit.

However, there is relatively little empirical support for this perspective. This has led to growing interest in the interface of health and the family, particularly among family scientists and family physicians (Doherty and Campbell, 1988). Olson (1989) in particular has urged more research to increase understanding of the changes in family processes related to physical and emotional illness, especially in determining the difference in families that have a quick recovery and families that have a difficult recovery from significant health events (Tomlinson, Kirschbaum, Harbaugh, and Anderson, in press).

Within the nursing discipline, several theorists use a partial family health system in their theoretical framework. Neuman's (1989) systemic model itself implies a potential for inclusion of the family system perspective, but explicitly indicates a role for the family more as context for the individual, with a system interface. She suggests that the same systemic principles apply in consideration of an individual, group, community, or issue defined as a system. Johnson's (1984) definition of the family relationship to health includes the interactive relationship of the family with the community, and the role of the family unit as developer of members' concept of health and health habits. Mauksch's (1974) concept of the "family health estate" focuses on the interdependence of the health of the family and the health of the individual family members, health-related roles, and task allocations.

While these frameworks do not include a family health system construct in the definition of health, they could be expanded to do so. Family frameworks for practice in nursing are distinguished from those of other disciplines in a number of ways. For one thing, family health must be considered a dialectic. That is, health must include simultaneously both health and illness (Moch, 1990), and the individual and the collective in defining the family as a unit of care. Nursing frameworks also must incorporate nursing actions on behalf of or in conjunction with the family and its members (Fawcett and Whall, 1988), and must have a specific view of the family and health promotion, health maintenance, and health restoration. As a result of nursing's expanding family health care function, it has been suggested that the discipline also needs to consider family culture in relation to health of individual family members and the family as a whole in determining symptom/illness interpretation, health priorities, and health care practices (Friedman, 1987). Moreover, the definition of family health also needs to link to a theoretical framework for professional clinical practice (Loveland-Cherry, 1988).

Because family health incorporates both wellness and illness within a variety of health experiences and contexts, the scope of family nursing practice means that knowledge generation in family health for nursing must be broad.

This view of family health, which links nursing practice in wellness and illness, is important to the process of developing prescriptive family health theory. Thus, the developing definitions of family health in nursing are clearly more complex than those used in other disciplines.

THE FAMILY HEALTH SYSTEM

From the above review there is evidence that nursing is concerned with a central family health system and that the analysis of family health from the nursing perspective must include explicit assumptions regarding both health and the family unit as a system. If health is a wholistic concept, then its definition must incorporate at least those realms that evidence has shown are related to health and those phenomena that are part of nursing practice.

We have argued that the nursing perspective of family health should link family structure, function, and health variables (including both wellness and illness); incorporate the biopsychosocial and contextual system aspects of nursing; specify the paradigm view; and address the levels of family interaction with the nurse (Anderson and Tomlinson, 1992). This definition suggests a paradigm shift where family health embraces more than the health of individuals as a part of a family and recognizes the family health system as a central phenomenon of nursing practice.

This definition of family health fits into the wholistic family health view and incorporates wellness and illness in interaction with the environment. The proposed family health systems paradigm prescribes inclusive use of five realms of family experience that influence nursing practice and provide a structure for both practice and systematic knowledge development—the interactive processes, the developmental processes, the coping processes, the integrity processes, and the health processes of the family—all systems level phenomena.

The *interactive processes* include such concepts as family relationships, communication, nurturance, intimacy, and social structure maintenance as they relate to health and illness. The *developmental processes* include family transitions and the dynamic interaction between family development and individual developmental experience in both health and illness. The *coping processes* involve decision making, problem solving, and adaptation to stressors that are part of health promotion and maintenance. The *integrity processes* include such concepts as shared meaning of experiences, family identity and commitment, family history, family values, boundary maintenance, and family rituals that relate to health experiences. Finally, *health processes* embrace family health beliefs, family health status, family health responses and life-style practices, and family-centered health care provision during illness and wellness.

This paradigm of family health (1) is systemic and processural, (2) includes an interaction of biopsychosocial and contextual phenomena, (3) incorporates the health of the collective and the interaction of health of the individual with the collective, and (4) embraces the assumption that the health system of the family can only be apprehended through an inclusive appraisal of the above processes.

RELATIONSHIP OF A FAMILY HEALTH SYSTEMS PARADIGM TO THE NEUMAN SYSTEMS MODEL

The Neuman Systems Model has proved to be a very useful guide to assess families in health care (Herrick and Goodykoontz, 1989; Berkey and Hanson 1991) by utilizing the flexible comprehensive systemic structure of the model and concepts such as stressors and lines of defense. Others have used an explicit family systems perspective to extend theory based on the Neuman Model. By combining the Neuman Model with a general family systems perspective and substituting the family for the individual in the Neuman original model, Herrick and Goodykoontz (1989) identify stressors related to developmental transitions as part of the primary level of prevention and identify the threat to family integrity that chronic long-term health problems can create.

The proposed view of a family health system described above extends the Neuman Systems Model in different ways. The promotion of the processes of interactions in the family unit, enhancement of family/individual development and interaction, support of active coping with stressful experiences, promotion of family identity and integrity, and promotion of the life-style and health practices that enhance family life in wellness and illness are all system-related goals in a family health systems practice.

Several areas of interface between the Family Health System paradigm (Anderson and Tomlinson, 1992) and the Neuman Systems Model (Neuman, 1989) show their complementary and supplementary relationship with respect to these goals. Five major areas were selected for this discussion: (1) the complexity of the system, (2) the conceptualization of the core of the family, (3) the goal of family health, (4) the entry point in caring for families, and (5) the nursing interaction.

Complexity of the System

The authors show their views on substituting the family system for the individual system in the Neuman Model. Neuman (1989) acknowledges that as a system becomes more organized, the regulations and constraints become more complex. She warns of the dangers of oversimplification in the use of a systems model. Conceptualization of the family as a system using her model requires the addition of unique features of that client system related to the basic structure of its resources. For example, transitions are of great interest in understanding the energy of the family and source of stressors and, according to Neuman, may be strongly related to clients' ability to effectively use their lines of defense and resistance. The level of complexity would need to shift when using the family health systems perspective to consider not only the individual stressor response in relation to the family but also the family's response relative to lines of defense and resistance. Thus at the individual level we may be interested in an individual's developmental status, while at the family systems level we are interested in the multiple developmental transitions in the system at any one given time.

The Neuman Systems Model related to family health, like individual health, has the goal of optimal client system stability or wellness. However, the concept of health in families must include the collective family system's definition of health to reflect the complexity of the construct. Perception of health thus rests within the family's construction of the meaning of health and illness. As Mu (1993) argues, the way in which families construct these meanings influences how they will use their energy. This inclusion of the family health system as defined above relates to client perception found in the Neuman Model Nursing process format.

The Core of the Family

According to Neuman, the core of the family is composed of its individual members, and assessment of the family is done in relation to the dynamics of individual member contributions to the whole within their environmental interactive context. Reed (1989) elaborates on the family approach in the Neuman Systems Model to suggest that "the family is viewed as a composite having individual member identity" (p. 386). The family health systems paradigm goes beyond looking at the collective in that sense and postulates that consideration for individual family members should be viewed from the perspective of the collective tension between the individual, dyadic, and family systems in meeting their unique goals in relation to the environment. Thus the core of the family system is viewed as the interface of its members in interaction with the environment.

The Goal of Family Health

Neuman's primary health goal is "to facilitate optimal level wellness for the client by retaining, attaining, and maintaining client system stability" (Neuman, 1989, 24). Stressors from the internal or external environment can penetrate the flexible and normal lines of defense, causing a systemic reaction of varying degrees or deviation from wellness. Neuman views her work as a wellness-oriented model with strengths or resources utilized by the nurse to keep the system stable while adjusting to stressor reactions toward ultimate optimal wellness and desired change. In relation to family health Neuman incorporates the following five important interacting factors: coping patterns, life-style, development, spiritual influences, and cultural concerns. These factors, although more general, are related to the overall family health goals within the realm of the family health system: interaction, development, coping integrity, and health.

A primary difference in the two views is the goal for nursing action in relation to family health. Neuman's (1989) central concern is to facilitate optimal client system stability or wellness in the face of change. However, since change is inevitable in a family system as a result of life events, the optimal system goal is viewed by the authors as system flexibility to respond to the dynamics of family life while maintaining connectedness (Boss, 1988; Olson, 1989). A certain mutability is thus established that facilitates family adaptation to stress. Thus, from a family health system perspective, it is most desirable to facilitate client system wellness using strengths to reduce stressor effects and enhance family growth toward positive transformation of its central structure as a result of a significant illness experience. (Anderson, 1993; Orton and Tomlinson, 1993; Kirschbaum, 1993).

For the concept of stability and change, the Neuman Systems Model focuses on the nurse's collaboration with the family and other resources to best deal with stressors threatening the lines of defense and resistance that could result in system instability or even "demise of the family as a system" (Neuman, 1989, 392). Using the family health systems paradigm, illness stress is known to have a significant influence on family functioning. The salutogenic effects of strengths or family resources that interact with the stressors families encounter in health and illness are considered to be equally important. While illness or stressor reactions may adversely impair family functioning and health, the family may successfully utilize both its form and function to meet the challenge of illness. For example, in families with early chronic illness, Anderson (1993) found that the families' view of the world as comprehensible, manageable, and meaningful was much more important to family quality of life than was the effect of illness stress. This perspective is consistent with the Neuman view that family strengths are important determinants in the core energy of the family system.

Nurse Entry Point in Caring for Families

The Neuman Model directs the pivotal role of nurse involvement with the family in identifying the entry point into the family and determining the appropriate type of intervention (Neuman, 1984). Perceptual difference resolution between both nurse and client system for cooperative and relevant subsequent nursing action in collaboration with the family is important. The family is thus empowered in making decisions about their own family health issues; ideally, they become partners in health care. The nurse utilizes both acquired knowledge and family assessment data, considering family needs, desires, dynamics, and response to stressor reactions to plan collaboratively with the family for relevant preventive/interventive care. Consistent with Neuman's philosophical focus, family strengths are used as resources to combat stressors. According to Neuman, nursing functions to conserve system energy, thus impeding movement of the system toward illness and enhancing the wellness condition toward an optimal level of client health.

Nursing Interaction

The Family Health Systems paradigm operationalizes the Neuman Systems boundary concept. While the Neuman Model levels of prevention as intervention, or nursing actions, relate to retaining, attaining, and maintaining client system stability or wellness, the nurse role creates an explicit cooperative alliance with the client. As with the individual client, a family systems approach by the caregiver becomes a "shared caregiver role" to help conserve family system energy as it moves toward optimal stability or wellness. Ideally, when the professional caregiver is guided by a systemic model, a portion of the family system's responsibility for nurturance, caregiving, and protection, complex transactions move the caregiver into the family system in a circumscribed manner, as well as out of the family when the need is finished. Based on a family systems perspective, the boundary between the individual client system and caregiver is viewed by the authors as semipermeable; that is, in the family caregiving situation there may be considerable boundary ambiguity (Boss, 1988) as to when the nurse is either inside or outside the system boundary. Differing perceptions between caregivers and family members as to each other's rights and obligations in their shared caregiver role may create role uncertainty. The greater the primacy of the caregiving role, the greater the potential for ambiguity in that transaction (Tomlinson and Mitchell, 1993; Mu, 1993).

CONCLUSION

In summary, it is important for the dialogue to continue between theorists who have by and large used an individualistic perspective of health and those who are using a family systems approach in order to synthesize these perspectives. One of the major contributions of Dr. Neuman's work is her insistence on use of the systems perspective to define nursing as interactions in reciprocal relationship with the client, the family, and larger health care system and her recognition that the same principles apply to a defined system of any size. The Neuman Systems Model will serve well in providing major constructs toward full evolvement of family health within a systems perspective. It is critical that nursing develop consensus of approach to families since nurses essentially determine the client system entry point and appropriate type of intervention. In the future, both an individual and family system focus will become necessary, as nursing intervention with families is now mandated.

As we approach the 21st century, it is anticipated that nursing will increasingly develop practice autonomy within comprehensive community-based health systems for client health promotion and health maintenance. Families will require increased support in maintaining their system integrity and health. The nurse who can function using the broad concepts of the Neuman Model, enhanced by the shared family health system perspective, will be well prepared to meet future nursing challenges.

REFERENCES

American Nurses' Association. 1980. *Nursing: A Social Policy Statement.* Kansas City, Mo.: The American Nurses' Association.

Anderson, K. H. 1993. The relative contributions of illness stress and family system variables to family quality of life during early chronic illness. Unpublished dissertation, University of Minnesota, Minneapolis, Minn.

, Anderson, K. H., and Tomlinson, P. S. 1992. The family health system as an emerging paradigmatic view for nursing. *Image: A Journal of Nursing Scholarship* 23(1):57–63.

Berkey, K., and Hanson, S. M. 1991. *Pocket Guide to Family and Intervention*. St. Louis, Mo.: Mosby Year Book.

Boss, P. 1988. *Family Stress Management*. Newbury Park, Calif.: Sage.

Bowen, M. 1978. *Family Therapy in Clinical Practice*. New York: Jason Aaronson.

Burr, W., Hill, R., Nye, F. I., and Press, I., eds. 1979. *Contemporary Theories about the Family*. Vol. 2. New York: Free Press.

Cabinet in Nursing Research. 1985. Directions for nursing research: Toward the 21st century. Kansas City, Mo.: American Nurses' Association.

de Chasney, M. 1986. Promoting healthy family functioning in acute care units. *Journal of Pediatric Nursing* 1:96–101.

Doherty, W. J., and Campbell, T. 1988. *Families and Health*. Newbury Park, Calif.: Sage Publication.

Donaldson, S. K., and Crowley, D. M. 1978. The discipline of nursing. *Nursing Outlook* 26:113–120.

Fawcett, J., and Whall, A. 1988. Family theory development. Paper presented at the International Family Nursing Conference, Calgary, Alberta, Canada, May 27.

Feetham, S. L. 1984. Family research: Issues and direction for nursing. *Annual Review of Nursing Research* 3:3–25.

Feetham, S. L. 1990. Conceptual and methodological issues in research of families. In *The Cutting Edge of Family Nursing,* edited by J. Bell, W. Watson, and L. Wright. Calgary, Alberta, Canada: Family Nursing Unit Publications.

Friedman, M. M. 1988. *Family Nursing: Theory and Assessment*. Norwalk, Conn.: Appleton-Century-Crofts.

Gilliss, C. L. 1983. The family as a unit of analysis: Strategies for the nurse researcher. *Advances in Nursing Science* 5(3):59–67.

Gilliss, C. L. 1991. Family nursing research, theory and practice. *Image: Journal of Nursing Scholarship* 22:19–22.

Gilliss, C. L., Highly, B. L., Roberts, B. M., and Martinson, I. M. 1989. *Toward a Science of Family Nursing*. Menlo Park, Calif.: Addison-Wesley.

Herrick, C. and Goodykootnz, L. 1989. Neuman's systems model for nursing practice on a conceptual framework for a family assessment. In *The Neuman Systems Model,* 2d ed., edited by B. Neuman, 98–108. Norwalk, Conn.: Appleton & Lange.

Hill, R. 1988. Social stresses on the family: Generic features of families under stress. *Social Casework* 39:139–158.

Johnson, R. 1984. Promoting the health of families in the community. In *Community Health Nursing: Process and Practice for Promoting Health,* 1st ed., edited by M. Stanhope and J. Lancaster, 330–360. St. Louis: C. V. Mosby.

King, I. M. 1983. King's theory of nursing. In *Family Health: A Theoretical Approach to Nursing Care,* edited by J. W. Clements and F. B. Roberts, 177–188. New York: Wiley & Sons.

Kirschbaum, M. 1993. Deciding to authorize, forego, or withdraw life support: The meaning for parents. Unpublished dissertation, University of Minnesota, Minneapolis, Minn.

Loveland-Cherry, C. 1989. Family health promotion and health protection. In *Nurses and*

Family Health Promotion: Concepts, Assessments and Interventions, edited by P. Bomar, 13–25. Baltimore: Williams & Wilkins.

Mauksch, H. 1974. A social science basis for conceptualizing family health. *Social Science and Medicine* 8:521.

McCubbin, H. I., and Patterson, J. M. 1983. The family stress process: The double ABCX model of adjustment and adaptation. *Marriage and Family Review* 6:7–37.

McEwan, P. J. M. 1974. The social approach to family health studies. *Social Science and Medicine* 8:487–493.

Meleis, A. I. 1985. *Theoretical Nursing: Development and Progress.* Philadelphia: J. B. Lippincott.

Minuchin, S. 1974. *Families and Family.* Cambridge: Howard University Press.

Moch, S. D. 1990. Health within illness: Conceptual evolution and practice possibilities. *Advances in Nursing Science* 11(4):23–31.

Mu, P. F. 1993. Parental perception of family stress in pediatric health crisis: A phenomenological study. Unpublished dissertation, University of Minnesota.

Murphy, S. 1986. Family study and family science. *IMAGE: Journal of Nursing Scholarship* 80:170–174.

Neuman, B. 1983. Family intervention using the Betty Neuman health-care system model. In *Family Health: A Theoretical Approach to Nursing Care,* edited by I. W. Clements and F. B. Roberts, 239–254. New York: Wiley & Sons.

Neuman, B. 1989. The Neuman Systems Model. In *The Neuman Systems Model,* 2d ed., edited by B. Neuman. Norwalk, Conn.: Appleton & Lange.

Newman, M. A. 1983. *Newman's health theory.* In *Family Health: A Theoretical Approach to Nursing Care,* edited by I. W. Clements and F. B. Roberts, 239–254. New York: Wiley & Sons.

Newman, M. A. 1986. *Health as Expanding Consciousness.* St. Louis: C. V. Mosby.

Newman, M. A., Sime, A. M., and Corcoran-Perry, S. 1992. The focus of the discipline of nursing. *Advances in Nursing Science* 14(1):1–6.

Olson, D. H. 1989. Circumplex model and family health. In *The Science of Family Medicine,* edited by C. N. Ramsey, Jr., 75–94. New York: Guilford Press.

Olson, D. H., McCubbin, H. I., Barnes, H. L., Larsen, A. S., Muren, M. J., and Wilson, M. A. 1983. *Families: What Makes Them Work.* Beverly Hills, Calif.: Sage Publishers.

Orton, M., and Tomlinson, P. In process. *Shock, Recovery, and Transformation: Stages of Parental Reaction to Pediatric Critical Illness.*

Parse, R. 1987. *Nursing Science: Major Paradigms, Theories, and Critiques.* New York: W. B. Saunders.

Paterson, J., Zderad, L. 1976. *Humanistic Nursing.* New York: Wiley & Sons.

Pratt, L. 1976. *Family Structure and Effective Health Behavior: The Energized Family.* Boston: Houghton Mifflin Company.

Reed, K. 1989. Family theory related to the Neuman Systems Model. In *The Neuman Systems Model,* 2d ed., edited by B. Neuman. Norwalk, Conn.: Appleton & Lange.

Rogers, M. 1983. Science of unitary human beings: A paradigm for nursing. In *Family Health: A Theoretical Approach to Nursing Care,* edited by J. W. Clements and F. B. Roberts, 219–228. New York: Wiley & Sons.

Roy, C., Sr. 1983. Roy adaptation model. In *Family Health: A Theoretical Approach to Nursing Care,* edited by J. W. Clements and F. B. Roberts, 255–278. New York: Wiley & Sons.

Satir, V. 1972. *Peoplemaking.* Palo Alto, Calif.: Science and Behavior Books.

Smith, J. A. 1983. *The Idea of Health: Implications for the Nursing Profession*. New York: Teachers College Press.

Tomlinson, P. S., Kirschbaum, M., Harbaugh, B., and Anderson, K. In press. The relationship of family resources, severity, and maternal uncertainty during critical pediatric hospitalization. *American Journal of Critical Care*.

Tomlinson, P. S., and Mitchell, K. 1992. On the nature of social support for families of critically ill children. *Maternal Child Nursing Journal* 19(1):45–62.

Tripp-Reimer, T. 1984. Reconceptualizing the construct of health: Integrating emic and etic perspectives. *Research in Nursing and Health* 7:101–109.

Watson, J. 1985. *Nursing: Human Science and Human Care*. Norwalk, Conn.: Appleton-Century-Crofts.

Whall, A. L. 1986a. *Family Therapy Theory for Nursing*. Norwalk, Conn.: Appleton-Century-Crofts.

Whall, A. L. 1986b. The family as the unit of care in nursing: A historical review. *Public Health Nursing* 3:240–249.

Woods, N. F., Laffrey, S., Duffy, M., Lentz, M., Mitchell, E., Taylor, D., and Cowan, K. 1988. Being healthy: Women's images. *Advances in Nursing Science* 11(1):36–46.

World Health Organization. 1973. *Pharmacogenetics Technical Report Series—524*. Geneva: World Health Organization.

Wright, L. M., and Leahey, M. 1988. Family nursing trends in academic and clinical settings. Plenary paper presented at the International Family Nursing Conference, Calgary, Alberta, Canada, May.

Section II

Application of the Neuman Systems Model to Nursing Education

8

CULTURAL CONSIDERATIONS IN A NEUMAN-BASED CURRICULUM

Eleanor M. Stittich
Filomena C. Flores
Patricia Nuttall

The role of an educator in a multicultural classroom is both exciting and challenging. The rich kaleidoscope of learning experiences at California State University, Fresno (CSUF), are likewise rewarding to both the educator and the students. Different ethnic groups of students analyze, interpret, and communicate their comprehension of concepts taught in the nursing programs in interesting patterns. The inductive and deductive reasoning processes of these groups have definite cultural implications and need to be considered by all nursing educators. These considerations will be the focus of this chapter.

Change, an expected constant in everyone's life, has meaningful implications for the nurse educator. Continuous objective evaluation and revisions of the curriculum ensure currency of content in keeping with societal health care demands. Population migration has accelerated this process for some groups (Robbins, 1991), the result of political and economic chaos and crises. This increased migration of refugees has magnified the demand for a deliberate focus on the cultural variable within the Neuman Systems Model (Neuman, 1989). How the concept is introduced, developed, nurtured, and implemented throughout the curriculum needs to be a major concern for all faculty in this changing society.

TABLE 8-1. 1980–1992 ETHNIC POPULATION GROWTH IN FRESNO

Year	Euro-Americans	African Americans	Mexican Americans	Asian Americans
1992	174,893	27,653	105,757	45,869
1990	180,765	30,292	100,186	21,696
1980	136,800	20,106	51,489	9,807

Demographically, the San Joaquin Valley in California is home to over 70 distinct ethnic and cultural groups. The largest populations are the Mexican Americans and the Asian Americans, especially the recent Asian refugees. Fresno County has the highest number of Hmong, Laotian, and Vietnamese immigrants in the United States. Table 8–1 compares the 1980–1992 statistics of the ethnic composition of the city of Fresno (Fresno 1992 Statistical Abstract). Enrollment of ethnic minority students at the CSUF Department of Nursing increased from 10 percent in 1980 to 17 percent in the spring of 1988. In the fall of 1988, enrollment of minority nursing students showed a dramatic rise to 44 percent. This enrollment pattern has continued over a five-year period ranging from 21 percent to 47 percent (Table 8–2).

Understanding the concept of culture is essential for nurses when assessing and evaluating behavioral responses regarding health practices, illness, and care. Culture is defined in many ways. It is generally described as a pattern of social interaction, traits, attitudes, beliefs, norms, life-style, folklore, and behavioral responses. Culture is not a pure concept. Many environmental factors influence cultural characteristics. Multicultural and subcultural traits germinate into a unique blend of culture for groups and particularly for individuals. Culture implies an established way of life, or a social heritage, that includes religious beliefs, customs, and values that culminate in the development of a unique individual. Cultural diversity indicates differences, and this, indeed, is a basic characteristic of all human beings. In the process of enculturation, the cultural traits of all groups may be altered. Nurses need to be sensitive to cultural diversity and the

TABLE 8-2. ETHNIC MINORITY NURSING STUDENT ENROLLMENT IN THE FIRST SEMESTER

Term		Percent
Fall	1988	44%
Spring	1989	47%
Fall	1989	45%
Spring	1990	42%
Fall	1990	20%
Spring	1991	33%
Fall	1991	37%
Spring	1992	21%
Fall	1992	34%
Spring	1993	28%

dynamic nature of culture. Changing demographics require changing attitudes. Ethnocentricity, the belief that one's own culture is the only "right" culture (Leininger, 1984), results in a biased attitude and may have detrimental regressive outcomes.

Support for cultural beliefs begins with cultural awareness, identification, and sensitivity. This leads to the development of a nonjudgmental understanding about health culture and an appreciation for the client's belief and values regarding health care practices. Relativism and repatterning are also important in supporting cultural diversity (Watson, 1982). While emphasis is placed on determining the client's perception of health, illness, and care, each nurse must begin with an introspective view of his or her own values, beliefs, and traits. To know and understand one's own biases enhances objectivity and respect for diverse viewpoints and customs. Demonstration of an honest and sincere interest in determining what is significant to the client encourages establishment of rapport and discussion of folk health practices. It is through this exchange of viewpoints that trust is established between the client and the provider of care. It is also through this process that the ultimate therapeutic benefits for the client are achieved.

Although the concept of culture is a thread in all courses, the focus of this chapter is on the actualization of this concept in the undergraduate courses of Basic Concepts of Nursing, Nursing of the Child-Rearing Family, and Concepts of Complex Clinical Nursing. At the graduate level, the discussion is related to the Nurse Practitioner program.

Culture is studied within the realm of the five variables of the Neuman Systems Model—physiological, psychological, sociocultural, developmental, and spiritual (Neuman, 1989)—and what it signifies and how it influences and interrelates with other variables. The model assists the student to identify, organize, and analyze cultural concepts. It also enables the student to consider controversial issues related to transcultural nursing. The main thrust is to recognize and reduce cultural stressors and enhance positive client responses. By instituting interventions to strengthen the flexible and normal lines of defense and the lines of resistance, client response resources are increased. Data collection becomes more feasible and meaningful when the nurse is cognizant of cultural verbal and nonverbal cues. The Asian student/client may reply "yes," indicating an acceptable response that demonstrates respect and the desire to foster harmonious relationships rather than agreement. Thus explorative feedback is essential to determine specific and accurate meanings of responses.

Recognizing that cultural diversity is a basic necessity for quality nursing care, the CSUF nursing faculty (Department of Nursing NLN Self Study, 1993) identified culture as one of the concepts to be integrated throughout the curriculum. Concurrent clinical experience with culturally diverse clientele is provided when feasible. Teaching approaches vary with the cultural structure of each group of students. In multicultural classes, exchange of cultural ideas and experiences is encouraged and used to nurture understanding of the importance of cultural traits to the individual (Felix, 1992). This sharing of cultural knowledge among students provides an authentic resource of information and an appreciation of variables in beliefs and values. Projects are used in monocultural classes to increase understanding of cultural stressors and responses.

The importance of culture is reflected in the university mission statement, and departmental philosophy, terminal objectives, conceptual framework, and course objectives (Department of Nursing NLN Self Study, 1993). The Department of Nursing has a faculty support program to assist culturally diverse students who are educationally disadvantaged and at risk for failures because of language and other cultural differences. Memmer and Worth (1991) cite that a rapidly growing number of California's ethnic minority nursing students are individuals whose primary language is not English and that English-as-a-second-language (ESL) students have a high attrition rate in nursing.

The faculty support program at CSUF, for cultural minority students, encompasses orientation classes that emphasize effective study and classroom skills: note- and test-taking skills, time management, postclass review sessions, conceptual learning, cognitive mapping, graphic organization of concepts through models, diagrams, or paradigms, and networking through a minority peer group. To trace the patterns of test-taking errors, the director of this support program conducts an item-analysis of test responses. Test errors related to ethnic differences are identified and appropriate teaching and learning strategies are instituted to assist the student.

BACCALAUREATE PROGRAM IN NURSING

The Neuman Systems Model facilitates integration of cultural components throughout the curriculum and serves as a framework for the selection of course sequence and content in a systematic and logical manner. The model enhances the application of the nursing process in meeting cultural needs and implementing quality care. The initial focus is on the individual student and cultural diversity within the group of students in the first nursing course. As the learner progresses in the nursing program, the emphasis is on the cultural needs of the client, family, and community.

This section discusses cultural components in the following courses: Basic Concepts in Nursing Practice offered in Level I, Care of the Child-Rearing Family in Level II, and Concepts of Complex Nursing in Level III.

Level I: Basic Concepts of Nursing Practice

Neuman describes client care in terms of four constructs: person, environment, health, and nursing.

Neuman (1982, 1989) describes man as a *person*—a composite of physiological, psychological, sociocultural, developmental, and spiritual variables. This wholeness characterizes all participants in the health care delivery system: client/client system and health care provider.

In the first nursing course, Basic Concepts of Nursing, students are introduced to the Neuman Systems Model and to the concept of cultural diversity. General systems theory provides the basic introduction to the model with the discussion of what a system is and how it operates. Initial introduction also embodies clarification of the following: open and closed systems; entropy and negentropy; micro-, mezzo-, and macrosystems; environmental stressors; and the system's responses to maintain, regain, or restore client stability. The person is viewed within three types of systems: as a microsystem (individual with subsystems); as a mezzosystem (an individual within the boundaries of a small group such as family, work, study, or church); and as a macrosystem (an individual within the matrix of large-scale relationships as society).

Communication is an essential process in the achievement of equilibrium or client stability. Different ethnic groups have unique communication patterns. To focus on these variances, specific cultural traits are identified. For example, behaviors such as eye contact or direct questioning have different meanings in some cultures. An Asian child often is taught to converse with adults with eyes cast downward because direct eye contact is interpreted as a sign of defiance or disrespect for elders. Another cultural difference occurs when Euro-American women are interviewed. They tend to answer questions directly, while Hmong women defer questions to the husband or other male family member.

Neuman describes the *environment* as forces within or outside the person surrounding the client or client system (Neuman, 1989). The stressors experienced by the individual are forces that affect not only persons coming from the dominant culture but also the ethnic clientele whose beliefs and practices may not be fully understood by the caregivers. Some of the stressors may be life-threatening. Students are taught that health care encompasses both scientific and indigenous health care delivery systems. This wholistic belief is gaining universal acceptance and support (Leininger, 1988). Thus students develop an understanding of folk medicine and the use of indigenous plants, many of which are also basic ingredients of contemporary pharmacotherapeutics.

Classroom discussions stress the diversity of the sociocultural variables that influence human behavior related to the microsystem (individual), mezzosystem (family), and macrosystem (society) (Neuman, 1989). The variables impinging on the family mezzosystem of the African American may be dissimilar to those of a Hispanic. For example, in the area of language, while the African American may experience stress from discrimination problems, the Mexican migrant worker may have language difficulties in addition to discrimination. Among migrant families, these issues may be accelerated. The external stressors of the Southeast Asians are compounded by language, discrimination, and relocation. The voyage across the seas has resulted in many changes and challenges for individuals and their families.

Actual clinical cases reflect Neuman's concept of *health* as balance and harmony between and among the systems. Scenarios depict multifarious health problems of the various ethnic client populations. Students are encouraged to share personal experiences and observations to vitalize an objective discussion of unique needs. Thus biases and prejudices are minimized as beginning students increase their understanding of culturally diverse individuals/groups.

The impact of the intra-, inter-, and extrapersonal stressors occurring within both the internal and external boundaries of the client systems also have cultural considerations. Students are taught that responses to these stressors are individualistic, not clone-like, with unique characteristics reflective of different cultures. For example, in discussions related to pain, students analyze client responses and consider the variety of treatment modalities that could be used to overcome the discomfort. The Asian patient, being stoic in nature, may delay complaints of pain, making minimal dosages of pain medications ineffective (Nguyen, 1985). The utilization of cultural assessment enhances interventions and therapeutic results.

In teaching the construct of *nursing* in the basic course, the Neuman Systems Model is interwoven with Gordon's 11 Functional Health Patterns and the assessment of the individual across the life span. Discussions of each health pattern reflect ethnic differences in client responses to stressors. The nature of entropy and negentropy is emphasized. The South Asian family's belief in the efficacy of home remedies such as herbs, oils, animal parts, and prayers illustrates indigenous measures that promote negentropy (McKenzie, 1977).

First-semester nursing students perform the primary prevention mode of care for elderly clients in nursing homes. The focus of each nursing care plan is to strengthen the normal and flexible lines of defense through assessment of the client's learning needs. Client education based on empathy and consideration of folk beliefs and practice facilitates the adaptation process needed to strengthen normal lines of defense over time. The *machismo* (Spanish for masculine) image dictates the need to deny pain until it becomes unbearable and threatens the core. In this situation, cultural traits are competitive forces to the innate lines of resistance.

To highlight the impact of imposing one's own values and beliefs on another person, newspaper articles of cultural issues underlying client care in the hospital are used. An example of this was an article regarding a Hmong child with a clubfoot. Southeast Asian students led the discussion about the family's refusal of surgical correction of the abnormality. Students clarified the cultural reasons for the family's decision. This type of class discussion enhances class learning through real problem analyses.

Emphasis on professional assertiveness may be in conflict with cultural traits. The Asian nurse may outwardly demonstrate acceptance of an unorthodox or undesirable assignment simply to maintain harmonious relationships. In reality, there may be no intention of performing the assignment because it is incongruent with personal and professional standards.

People who have been taught from birth to be assertive find it difficult to understand why other persons are not. In cultures where respect for the elders or for authority is the primary value, expression of assertiveness is difficult. In discussing role relationships, students develop strategies for assertiveness. These are useful in caring for patients and in establishing meaningful working relationships.

Particular attention is directed toward the selection of clinical nursing experiences. Cultural conflicts may occur in the patient assignment process from clients who have unpleasant memories related to specific ethnic groups. This was demonstrated by a Vietnam War veteran who refused care from a Vietnamese nursing student. Thus nursing educators need to be cognizant of the cultural implications of all nursing activities and assignments.

Level II: Care of the Child-Rearing Family

In the child-rearing course, the focus is on the introduction of current theories and concepts in the care of the pediatric client/family with emphasis on wellness and illness. Knowledge and understanding of the Neuman based core concepts, in addition to clinical skills, are needed to enhance quality nursing interventions. All Neuman Model variables are considered with particular emphasis on developmental and sociocultural variables. Appreciation of cultural implications helps to decrease noncompliance and alienation of the family, and their lack of trust in health care providers. It is usual for the nursing student to feel insecure in the care of infants and children, and this problem can be intensified if the student is unable to relate to parents and children of different cultural groups. The pediatric client currently enters the health care system from a variety of cultural settings, and many of these children have serious health care problems such as malnutrition, fetal alcohol/drug syndrome, and child abuse.

Many pediatric health care problems are the result of impoverished living conditions, lack of accesss to primary care, and lack of parental understanding of infant and child care. The cultural life-style at home influences behavior of the pediatric client in both the primary care and hospital setting. With an understanding of the cultural variables, the nurse can assist the child and family in this new and unfamiliar environment. Cultural differences of clients are evident in dress, food, behavior, language, and health care beliefs. Emphasis is placed on assessing and appreciating the child's natural life-style and family health care practices. This promotes the establishment of mutual respect between the family and health care providers, as the nurse assists the family to develop competence in the care of their child. Encouragement of the use of safe traditional foods, home remedies, and health practices can help the family achieve the ultimate goal of health care while maintaining important cultural traditions. Acceptance of client's life-styles also promotes self-care and self-reliance.

Both child and family stability are threatened when hospitalization occurs. This experience also challenges the flexible and normal lines of defense as well as the lines of resistance for all persons and may contribute to disorientation and increased anxiety. Unfamiliar caregivers and the hospital environment are frightening to both the child and parents. Thus multiple stressors impinge upon the child and family. The child's behavior in this altered environment will be dependent on age, culture, and developmental level. Behaviors that are universally understood by children such as a smile, touch, kindness, music, picture books, and play help the child adapt to the health care environment, foster growth and development, and diminish fear.

As in all cultures, the establishment of rapport is essential between health care providers and the mother or primary caregiver. Effective working relationships promote the child's/family's confidence and willingness to assist in the planning and implementation of care. Encouraging the parent or relative to participate in the child's care enhances security and family life stability. Whether the child is seen in a primary, acute, or chronic setting, respect of culture is a critical variable affecting the totality of the therapeutic intervention. The pediatric nursing student needs to develop an appreciation about other cultures to be able to provide meaningful interventions for all children, including the homeless, the migrant, and those from single-parent families.

A goal of the child-rearing course is to provide learning experiences in the care of children from various cultural backgrounds and to learn more about the characteristic health care practices of major cultural groups. Well care and hospital/agency settings are used to provide concurrent clinical experiences with children from different cultures. Learning includes use of case studies that address family kinship bonds, religious beliefs, health practices, and communication patterns. Students learn to assess and understand barriers to health care. The focus of primary care includes a well child and the family during which students assess child development and behavior related to the child's age and culture.

Erikson's (1963) and Piaget's (1969) theories of child development are used to describe developmental parameters and to determine variance in height, weight, body structure, and behavioral patterns in children. Some cultural groups are smaller due to malnutrition, illnesses, or constitutional factors. Inherent in each plan of nursing care are measures to promote growth and development, nutritional health, safety, exercise, and the development of self-concept within Neuman parameters of primary prevention as intervention modality for health retention. Learning includes content on primary interventions, such as immunizations, anticipatory guidance, and health-promoting behaviors. When the child becomes ill, secondary interventions are instituted.

The child and the family may experience cultural shock as they enter the unfamiliar setting of the hospital, and this may be expressed by confusion, anxiety, and fear. The student learns to care for these families as a system and to develop cultural sensitivity. Often care includes the use of an interpreter. Entertainment, education, and play programs are provided as part of the child life activities in the hospital setting. Students participate in these programs and engage children of all cultures in the universal activity of play. In addition, to enhance cultural sensitivity, customs and traditions are emphasized during the various holidays.

Using the Neuman Systems Model (1989), the student performs a cultural assessment that identifies family structure, health beliefs, healing practices, cultural practices, and child-rearing approaches. Opportunities are provided to study health resources and to assist families with community referrals. Students develop the nursing care plan focusing on primary, secondary, and tertiary prevention as intervention modes of care needed to retain wellness, promote recovery, and facilitate appropriate growth and development.

Level III: Concepts of Complex Clinical Nursing

In the critical care nursing course, Concepts of Complex Clinical Nursing, the primary focus is on the theory and concepts relative to care of clients with complex health problems during crises. Emphasis is on the synthesis of concepts and principles derived from nursing and other disciplines in the implementation of primary, secondary, and tertiary prevention as intervention for clients of all ages. All of the concepts relative to cultural diversity introduced in the previous courses are elaborated upon and used in the critical care setting. The life-saving measures, utilization of monitors, and other complex technology may, as the result of urgency of care, supersede consideration of cultural components. However, in using the wholistic framework of the Neuman Systems Model (1989), recognition and care must be given within the context of the unique cultural needs of the client. While the urgency of implementation of life-support measures is important, effectiveness may ultimately be dependent upon the degree of compatibility with the client's culture. In this class, emphasis is placed on recognition of cultural differences or "mind set" of critically ill clients and families and how this influences behaviors and responses to interventions.

Focus is on environmental stressors and the need to reduce or eliminate them. Sensory deprivation, sensory overload, and sleep deprivation are a few examples of experiences that clients encounter in the high-tech environment of intensive care units. Stressors experienced by all critically ill clients are magnified for those with culturally diverse backgrounds. The client's expression of pain, for example, reflects culturally learned and expressed behaviors. Culture will also influence whether resuscitative measures and organ donation are permitted. Some cultures may hesitate to participate in the organ donation program. At times, the essence of critical care mandates rapid utilization and application of the Neuman Systems Modoel with more detailed data collection postponed until feasible.

Admission to a critical care unit is an overwhelming experience with multiple stressors for both the client and family. The separateness of single rooms provides privacy but also contributes to development of feelings of aloneness, bewilderment, isolation, and loss of support. Each stressor is intensified when combined with specific parameters of individual sociocultural heritage. Thus it is essential that the nursing student in critical care learns to customize care based on the unique needs of each client and family. Cultural assessments are vital for identification of the client's perception of current illness, hospitalization, and care as well as priority intra-, inter-, and extrapersonal stressors. Hence, the psychosocial stressors associated with critical illness must be viewed within the context of culture and potential determinants for subsequent prognosis and recovery.

In the critical care setting, the nurse not only anticipates the usual stressors common to all clients but must also seek to identify the changes in perspectives of these stressors specifically related to cultural influences. The ultimate goal of all nursing interventions is to meet wholistic needs of each client as a system and facilitate re-establishment of a homeodynamic status—one of system stability free from entropy.

An example of the application of the Neuman Systems Model is depicted in this course through the discussion of the stress response experienced by the client and family and the inherent mechanisms that serve to protect the client system core structure from insult and injury during crisis. Exposure to stress results in increased anxiety, apprehension, instability, uncertainty, potential injury, and destruction. The protective processes of the flexible and normal lines of defense and the lines of resistance are all severely challenged during critical illness.

The flexible line of defense, the outermost protective measure, is the individual's dynamic buffering system in constant motion in direct response to situational changes. When encountering stress and stressful situations, this line expands and protects the normal line of defense and client core structure by facilitating avoidance, protection, or system adjustment to environmental stressors. This line represents adaptors that need to be strengthened through education regarding risk factors, needed changes in life-styles, and perceptual sets. Prehospitalization visits, teaching, and preparation for elective care in critical care units are used to establish positive understandings of what to expect in care and support. Thus anticipatory preparation is used to avoid stress that occurs with unfamiliar experiences. Nursing interventions need to be directed toward changing coping patterns, decreasing stress, promoting relaxation, and increasing confidence in staff and care.

The normal line of defense represents coping behaviors developed by each individual client as a system over time and is influenced by cultural background factors that culminate in unique reactions and responses to environmentally stressful situations. This line also represents and identifies determinants of the nature and the degree of reaction or potential reaction to stressors. Here, the goal for nursing is secondary prevention as intervention, to support effective coping abilities, prevent entropy, and regain system stability. Cultural coping measures need to be identified, accepted, and used to full advantage for the client. Beliefs, values, and customs, especially when assumed to be in conflict with the "usual practices," may have underlying adverse effects on client care and progress. Effective coping mechanisms redirect the client's energy toward re-establishment of a state of system balance, halting further invasion of stressors that threaten the client's core or basic structure. Data relevant to past coping behaviors need to be elicited from the client or family. Behavioral responses to stress need to be identified in the assessment process as indicators of energy expended in the acceleration of the tension state versus adaptation and re-establishment of stability.

When the normal line of defense succumbs to a stressor, the lines of resistance are activated through the stress/adaptation response. This involves the stimulation of the autonomic nervous and neuroendocrine systems, which prepare the individual for "fight or flight" in stressful situations. This activation of the adrenal-adaptive process is the body's autoregulatory mechanism to achieve negentropy. These physiological responses attempt to stabilize and return the client to the wellness state. Although the physiological responses to stress are well defined, the psychosocial responses are individualistic and socioculturally related, making them more difficult to determine. Thus cultural implications also have an impact on the internal protective process. For example, external complacency seen in some cultures or by stoic clients may indeed obliterate the degree of internal expenditure of energy being used to overcome the stressor and the extent of resultant damage to the core. Nursing interventions are directed toward maintaining open communication with clients, promoting establishment of effective coping abilities, and enhancing both internal and external environmental defensive processes or system resources.

Cultural distinctiveness and diversity are important facets of this critical care course. Emphasis is placed on the need for critical care nurses to maintain objectivity, recognize cultural needs, and strive to adapt nursing care to meet the unique and wholistic needs of the client and family during a critical illness.

THE PEDIATRIC AND FAMILY NURSE PRACTITIONER PROGRAMS

The Neuman Systems Model (1989) is the organizing framework for the nurse practitioner programs that embody primary, secondary, and tertiary care. Within this framework, core concepts of systematic inquiry, advanced practice, and social organization are taught in relation to Neuman's concepts. Students learn to elicit health beliefs from culturally diverse clients and to mutually negotiate treatment plans for effective and satisfactory care toward client optimal wellness.

The goal of the nurse practitioner programs is to prepare the graduate nursing student to provide wholistic health care to children, adults, and families. The focus of each program is on health assessment, health maintenance, and health promotion. A cross-cultural perspective is reflected at all three levels of prevention as intervention with clinical practicum in a variety of community settings serving most cultural groups. Some examples of these include Indian and refugee health centers, migrant and school-based clinics, health departments, medical health centers, and private medical practices.

An increasing number of culturally diverse students in the program have previous varied nursing experiences and expertise in caring for clients from different cultural groups. Because of the large Hispanic population in the San Joaquin Valley, many nurse practitioner students study Spanish to facilitate interaction with and understanding of the needs of Latino clients.

Courses are organized within the Neuman three modes of care: primary, secondary, and tertiary prevention as intervention. In the first course, emphasis is placed on primary prevention across the life span with a focus on health promotion, health maintenance, and illness prevention. Guest speakers representing different ethnic groups discuss culturally related practices. Students care for clients of all ages and cultures. Student journals describing cultural learning and experiences are shared with peers.

A major focus is on health teaching related to the establishment and maintenance of wellness behaviors, including nutrition, exercise, stress reduction, and recognition of healthy life-styles. Students discuss the wellness practices of various cultures, including cultural beliefs, home remedies, use of alternate health healers, and health care. Nurse practitioner students learn to identify, incorporate, and encourage health remedies practiced by clients that are congruent with safe health care. This facilitates understanding and preserves cultural heritage. Thus clients maintain control and more readily assume responsibility for self-care. Additional activities center on studying dominant cultures, cultural sensitivity, and the advocacy role of the nurse practitioner. Students also prepare position papers on current and significant transcultural trends and role transitions of men and women.

Consideration of the cultural attributes of all individuals and families promotes nurse–client rapport. It also provides comfort and enhances mutual respect between clients and providers. The wholistic approach to client and family includes prevention and early screening activities to identify potential or early health problems and improve the quality of life for clients. In this way, students develop an understanding of the cultural barriers and their role in the provision of health care for all clients. Students develop an appreciation for differences as to history, traditions, values, customs, and folkways that are important components of clients' lives needing to be preserved and incorporated into contemporary health care practices. A major objectivee is to provide quality nursing interventions within appropriate cultural parameters. Health care teaching focusing on wellness and self-care is an integral part of each intervention.

Many medically underserved groups present health conditions that have been aggravated by lack of care and require secondary and tertiary preventions as interventions. Some of these problems prevail because clients are often unaware of available health care resources and preventive services within their locale. The nurse practitioner's role includes assessing health needs and assisting the client to access appropriate health care facilities. Throughout the program, students learn about health care practices of various cultures and specific health care beliefs. This includes the hot/cold theory of food, alternate health care practitioners (i.e., faith healers, *curandarism,* and spiritual healers), the healing power of herbs and other medicinals, and alternate world views such as the concept of harmony that relates to opposing forces of *yin* and *yang* (Wadd, 1983; Jackson, 1993; Lenart et al., 1991).

Health is believed to be a balance of many factors, and an imbalance may cause illness. Some cultures believe that evil spirits (evil wind, evil eye, and evil tongue) cause disease that enters the body during illness (Flores, 1968). In some cases, human excrement has been placed on open wounds and on intravenous sites by well-intentioned family members to ward off these evil spirits. Likewise, objects such as amulets, talismans, and red bracelets believed to have preventive and supernatural powers have been used to prevent or treat illness (McKenzie and Chrisman, 1977). Other specific cultural practices include acupuncture, suction over body areas, coining (rubbing a coin over the body), and massage (Muecke, 1983; Robbins, 1991). Within this realm, students are also taught to formulate plans of care congruent with cultural needs and available health information and resources.

Many cultures have strong family structures and kinship groups with members expressing an interest in participating in the care of the ill person. In some cultures, the father is the primary caregiver, and a senior male or elder must be consulted regarding family health care decisions (Nguyen, 1985). The nurse practitioner needs to use this knowledge to encourage family participation and enhance nurturing behaviors and wholistic care.

IMPLICATIONS

The implications of cultural considerations in a Neuman-based curriculum are threefold: (1) for nursing education in terms of curriculum development and teaching, (2) for nursing practice, and (3) for the future of the Neuman Systems Model.

Nursing Education

It is important that nurse educators be sensitive to the challenges of a multiculturally diverse student group. Humanism is considered a vital component of professional nursing. Cultural components should enrich the nursing curriculum without sacrificing scientificity. Ideally, application of theories and concepts includes diversity of the client population that students will eventually serve, with students being recruited from these ethnic groups. When nurses with varied cultural heritages share their personal experiential background with other students, all benefit by broadening their perspectives of client care needs and processes unbounded by parameters of race, color, or creed.

Students learn to be culturally sensitive and aware and to appreciate meeting clients with unique needs. Changed beliefs and values for both students and faculty result from increased cultural sensitivity to changing national demographics. For example, self-disclosure, self-assessment, and self-actualization are "techniques" used by wholistic practitioners to be most effective in planning and implementing cultural care considerations.

Teaching strategies should continue to include the five client variables and all client system components of the Neuman Systems Model in presentation of specific classroom content. Shared examples of cultural differences in client responses to a variety of stressors will maximize learning of important cultural variations with care plan focus on client differences to improve nurse–client relationships. Clinical conferences that discuss appropriate interpretation of cultural cues provide reality-based teaching. Student/faculty discussion of cultural differences, use of modular programs, role playing of ethnic variance in client response to stressors or illness, and videotaping of student presentations for subsequent classes where specific cultures are not represented have all proved to be effective strategies in promoting cultural sensitivity.

The implications for future curricular development include the need for continued faculty review, and evaluation and revision of courses and programs in keeping with culturally sensitive curricular goals and objectives. Other considerations are to view health care practices and alternate methods of care in terms of validity or benefit to clients; to determine the value of separate versus integrated courses in priority focus on culture; and to evaluate student, faculty, and clinical staff outcome feedback in education and practice settings.

Nursing Practice

Philosophically, emphasis is on developing and maintaining an attitude of enthusiasm, openness, interest, equality, and respect for the unique individuality of each person. Ideally, both client and nurse are involved in decision making. Client response to stressors of illness may influence members of the mezzosystem in acceptance and utilization of all modes of care: primary, secondary, or tertiary preventions as interventions. All client system variables—physiological, psychological, sociocultural, developmental, and spiritual—may become vulnerable during illness.

The nurse is viewed as a promoter/facilitator of a collaborative relationship that elicits what the client perceives as best for self, while the nurse develops the plan of care with the client and implements care based on assessed needs. Emphasis should be given to the nature of cultural diversity leading to increased sensitivity and effective nursing intervention outcomes. Specific cultural assessment tools enhance data collection. That is, they are deliberate and purposeful in both identification and goal setting to meet cultural needs. Mobilizing and maximizing family cultural customs, traditions, and support will enhance the healing process and ultimate wellness outcome. Mutual client and family involvement in care planning and implementation are encouraged. They are recognized as critical resources in meeting present early discharge care mandates.

The current trend is toward increased home care services for tertiary mode of care within the home setting. Many nurses need additional knowledge and skill in providing optimal care for culturally diverse clients/families. For example, there is a need to understand beliefs, behavioral and perceptual differences, and cultural cues and to motivate family/client involvement in mutual goal setting for achievement of wholistic care and optimal wellness outcomes.

Neuman Systems Model

The Neuman Systems Model has been used for six years as the curricular base for the CSUF nursing program. Student evaluations support the gradual introduction of concepts basic to the Neuman Systems Model, as described previously in the undergraduate Level I, Basic Concepts of Nursing course. This approach has resulted in a strong theoretical foundation and increased student ability to use the model in clinical practice.

An increasing number of health care agencies now endorse the trend for use of nursing models to enhance theory-based nursing practice. The benefits of using the Neuman Systems Model in clinical practice include the following:

- Nurse–client relationships have improved with increased understanding of client stressors.
- Quality care has improved with specific focus on the client as a system interacting with the environment (internal and external).
- The length of hospitalization has decreased with the focus on primary, secondary, and tertiary modes of care.

These benefits also have the potential for decreasing the cost of hospital care. The Neuman Systems Model provides a logical framework for viewing the client in a humanistic manner, that is, as a whole person with physiological needs for survival, psychological needs to be loved and esteemed, and sociocultural and spiritual needs to be valued and respected.

In summary, the implications for the use of the Neuman Systems Model at CSUF are to continue to provide continuing education programs for staff and faculty on cultural diversity and use of the Neuman Systems Model throughout the nursing program; to assist student affiliating community agencies and other agency nursing staff in use of the model toward a scientific theory-based practice; and to encourage research in use of the model to help in meeting cultural needs of clients and families.

CONCLUSION

Provision of quality nursing care is highly dependent upon the quality of cultural awareness expressed between clients and nursing caregivers. Skill in nurse flexibility, openness to new ideas, and receptivity in learning clients' perceptions and health beliefs are all critical to client optimal wellness. The caring process of offering respect and sincere concern are key components to enhance understanding and cooperation from culturally diverse client populations. With increasing demands for professional competence in meeting the needs of a multicultural society, the authors of this chapter advocate that respect for cultural diversity begin with the professional nurse.

REFERENCES

CSUF, Department of Nursing. 1993. *NLN Self Study Report. 1993.* Fresno, Calif.: California State University, Fresno.

Erikson, E. 1963. *Childhood and Society.* New York: Norton.

Felix, N. 1992. Multicultural education in the college classroom. *Delta Kappa Gamma Bulletin* 59(1): 31–35.

Flores, F. 1968. Superstitious beliefs and practices of Cebuano parents in pregnancy and childbirth. Unpublished master's thesis, University of San Carlos, Cebu City, Philippines.

Fresno. 1992. *Fresno Statistical Abstract.* Fresno, Calif.: Development Department Annexation & Research Division.

Jackson, L. E. 1993. Understanding, eliciting and negotiating clients' multicultural health beliefs. *Nursing Practitioner* 18(4): 30–43.

Leininger, M. 1984. Transcultural nursing: An essential knowledge and practice field for today. *Canadian Nurse* December:41–45.

Leininger, M. 1988. Leininger's theory of nursing: Cultural care diversity and universality. *Nursing Science* 1(4):152–160.

Lenart, J., St. Clair, P., and Ball, M. 1991. Childbearing knowledge, beliefs and practices of Cambodian refugees. *Journal of Pediatric Health Care* 5(6): 299–305.

McKenzie, J., and Chrisman, N. 1977. Health herbs, Gods and magic: Folk health beliefs among Filipino Americans. *Nursing Outlook* 25(5): 326–329.

Memmer, M., and Worth, D. 1991. Retention of English-as-a-second language students: Approaches used by California's 21 generic BSN programs. Unpublished doctoral dissertation abstract, California State University, Chico, Calif.

Muecke, M. 1983. In search of healers—Southeast Asian refugees in the American health care system. *Western Journal of Medicine* 139(3): 835–840.

Neuman, B. 1982. *The Neuman Systems Model: Application to Nursing Education and Practice.* East Norwalk, Conn.: Appleton-Century-Crofts.

Neuman, B. 1989. *The Neuman Systems Model.* East Norwalk, Conn.: Appleton & Lange.

Nguyen, D. 1985. Culture shock: A review of Vietnamese culture and its concepts of health and disease. *Western Journal of Medicine* 142(3). 409–412.

Piaget, J., and Inhelder, B. 1969. *The Psychology of the Child.* New York: Basic Books.

Robbins, R., and Blackburn, M. 1991. Study pinpoints college student population shifts. *Higher Education Advocate* IX(1):1.

Wadd, L. 1983. Vietnamese postpartum practices. *Journal of Obstetrical & Gynecological Nursing* (July/Aug.:252–258.

Watson, W. 1983. *Aging and Social Behaviors.* Monterey, Calif.: Wadsworth Health Sciences.

9

CURRICULUM TRANSITION BASED ON THE NEUMAN SYSTEMS MODEL
Los Angeles County Medical Center School of Nursing

Sharon A. Hilton
Marilyn D. Grafton

Sensitive to the changing needs in the health care delivery system and the demand for well-prepared nurses within the community, the faculty and administration of Los Angeles County Medical Center School of Nursing studied ways that the school could best prepare nurses for the future. The faculty recognized that nursing educational patterns of the future must be different than educational patterns of the past.

Today's applicants, more concerned about educational mobility, have frequently requested information about academic degrees. Employers have expressed a need to hire nurses prepared in a broader range of competencies than in the past. Increasing numbers of nurses with baccalaureate and advanced degrees in nursing are needed in the delivery of care. The number of diploma programs closing or transitioning to a single-purpose degree-granting college of nursing has continued to grow. These developments and others have provided the impetus for the faculty and administration of the school to plan for ways that the educational program can best serve students and the community.

In determining a new direction for the educational program, the purpose, mission, and resources of the sponsoring institution provided a focus and a reality that were crucial. Graduates of the future would need to be prepared to practice in different settings, with different populations, and in different roles than those currently emphasized in academic settings. It was predicted that a high demand for well-prepared nurses within the county would continue into the 21st century.

The educational program has enjoyed a rich learning environment within the country's health care system. The campus, shared by students from the School of Medicine and School of Pharmacology, has offered a stimulating and exciting practice setting. There has been a consistent focus on learning, and opportunities have been available for collaboration with other disciplines.

Although the campus has a wealth of learning opportunities, cost remained a major issue in determining a new educational pattern. Tuition has remained a major consideration for students in determining the type of nursing program in which to enroll. The majority of students have worked while attending school and have needed to complete the curriculum within a relatively short time period. Therefore it was determined that most students would find it necessary to follow an educational ladder in order to complete a baccalaureate degree.

A thorough needs assessment resulted in a proposed model to offer an associate degree nursing program. The current agreements with a Los Angeles community college for the provision of general education components would be maintained. The curriculum would be designed so that articulation could continue with baccalaureate degree nursing programs within the community.

PLANNING FOR CURRICULUM CHANGE

The need to update the curriculum was discussed at several faculty meetings. This discussion was in response to the California State Board of Registered Nursing's recommendation that the curriculum framework be strengthened. Students gave evaluative input expressing a need for more consistency in teaching the nursing process, in the use of nursing assessment tools, and in the organizational approach to content. The appointment of Dr. Betty Neuman to the School of Nursing Faculty in 1989 had a major effect in determining the developmental direction of the new curriculum. Her commitment to a conceptual framework greatly influenced the faculty decision to consider a model that would support their philosophical beliefs and provide organizational structure from which the curriculum could be developed.

The faculty's concerns and need for information led the school's curriculum committee to develop and present a two-day workshop demonstrating ways in which frameworks could provide curriculum structure. Two conceptual models were chosen to be explored in depth. Faculty workshop presenters provided examples of curriculum components based on each conceptual framework. The components included a written statement describing the conceptual framework and identification and descriptions of concepts, subconcepts, theoretical formulations, and curriculum threads.

Following the workshop a faculty decision was made to accept the Neuman Systems Model as the basis for curriculum development. The selection was influenced by the fact that the model was congruent with the philosophical beliefs of the faculty and would provide a conceptual base upon which the graduate could draw well into future. Another factor influencing the selection was the ability of faculty to easily understand the model. The large minority student population served by the school would benefit from a model that utilized clear terminology and concepts. The faculty also realized that the expert knowledge and leadership required to operationalize the model existed within the group. This expertise lessened to some degree the anxiety that accompanied change.

A steering committee of faculty with knowledge of the Neuman Systems Model and the program's director and associate director participated in planning and coordinating curriculum development activities. The steering committee designed an action plan with completion dates for each step of the process. The steps included the development of philosophy, purpose, program objectives, conceptual framework, curriculum plan, level objectives, course descriptions, and course objectives. The committee involved all faculty members through the use of workshops, questionnaires, and small group activities. Committee members encouraged the exchange of thoughts and ideas, while providing support and assistance to faculty during the process.

Vital in planning for the transition to an associate degree nursing program was for the faculty to develop the curriculum within the accreditation guidelines of the California State Board of Registered Nursing, the National League for Nursing, and the Western Association of Schools and Colleges. After reviewing the work completed in each step, the curriculum committee made recommendations to the faculty organization for acceptance.

As the curriculum developed, each faculty member grew in knowledge of and commitment to using the Neuman Systems Model. The process of adapting the model as a basis for organizing the curriculum has been a unifying experience. The faculty has been encouraged by a growing understanding of the curriculum process, a sharing of values and perspectives, and an increasing level of agreement.

CURRICULUM FRAMEWORK

The first step toward the development of the curriculum framework occurred when the faculty reached agreement on its beliefs (philosophy) about the specific concepts of man, health, and nursing. When completed, the philosophical statements of faculty described their beliefs about man, health, environment, and nursing, the elements of the Neuman Systems Model. Beliefs about education and learning were stated as well.

The philosophical statements served as the basis for the development of the curriculum framework (organizational structure). The faculty formulated a conceptual framework that demonstrated the relationship of and provided definitions for man, health, environment, and nursing. The curriculum framework shown in Table 9–1 provides a schematic overview of the discussion relating to

TABLE 9–1. CURRICULUM FRAMEWORK

Concepts (Vertical Threads)	Major Subconcepts	Defining Subconcepts	Theoretical Formulations	Organizing Principles
Man	Wholism	**5 Variables:** Physiological Psychological Sociocultural Developmental Spiritual	**Stress and coping** (Lazarus and Selye) **General systems** (Lazlo) **Change theory** (Lewin) **Developmental** (Erikson, Maslow, Piaget)	**Life span** ("The individual moves through the life span as a composite of five variables. . . .")[a]
Environment	Stressors	Intrapersonal Interpersonal Extrapersonal	**Stress and coping** (Lazarus and Selye) **General systems** (Lazlo)	**Client/client systems** ("Dynamic adjustment to stressors must consistently be made for system stability. . . .")[a]
Health	Wellness continuum	Retain, attain and maintain system stability	**General systems** (Lazlo) **Stress and coping** (Lazarus and Selye) **Wellness** (Dunn and Ardell) **System model** (Neuman)	**Wellness/illness** ("Health is viewed as being on a continuum from wellness to illness. . . .")[a]
Nursing	Role	Provider Manager Member of a discipline	**General systems** (Lazlo) **Systems model** (Neuman) **Role theory** (Mead)	**Prevention as intervention** ("Nurses . . . utilize interventions to assist the patient to retain, attain, and maintain optimal system stability. . . .")[a]

[a] From conceptual framework.

concepts, major subconcepts, defining subconcepts, theoretical formulations, and organizing principles developed by the faculty.

Concepts (Vertical Threads)

The concepts of man, health, environment, and nursing were selected to be the vertical threads of the curriculum framework. The four concepts as vertical threads provided for the overall organization and sequencing of content within the curriculum and further assured integration of the philosophy and conceptual framework into the curriculum.

Major Subconcepts

The faculty identified a major subconcept for each vertical thread. The major subconcepts served to operationalize the threads for curriculum development. The major subconcepts identified in the conceptual framework were wholism under the concept of man; stressors under the concept of environment; and wellness continuum under the concept of health. Role was identified as the major subconcept under the concept of nursing.

A review of the Neuman Systems Model was made. The identified major subconcepts were clearly components of the model. The subconcept of role is implicit in the concept of nursing as described by Neuman in her model.

Definition Subconcepts

The delineation of the defining subconcepts as part of the curriculum framework further integrated the philosophy and the conceptual framework into the curriculum. These served as a vehicle to more specifically identify, organize, and sequence curriculum content. The defining subconcepts, integral parts of the vertical threads, flowed directly from the concepts and major subconcepts. The major subconcept of wholism was expanded by the defining subconcept of the five variables of the client/client system. The types of stressors were specifically identified as intrapersonal, interpersonal, and extrapersonal. To retain, attain, and maintain system stability was the defining subconcept of the wellness continuum. The defining subconcepts for role are provider of care, manager of care, and member of a discipline. These related directly to the roles basic to associate degree nursing practice (NLN, 1990).

Theoretical Formulations

The faculty discussed and agreed upon the major theories to be utilized as the basis for curriculum and content building. The theories, called theoretical formulations, assisted in the operationalization of the vertical threads, major subconcepts, and the defining subconcepts. The selection of the theoretical formulations was based on theorists utilized by Neuman and those favored by the faculty.

Organizing Principles

The curriculum development process then moved from the philosophical and conceptual into the more concrete task of placement of content within the curriculum. Organizing principles were identified to provide for a clear mapping of sequencing of content throughout the curriculum. The organizing principles selected were life span under the concept of man; client/client systems under the concept of environment; wellness/illness under the concept of health; and prevention as intervention under the concept of nursing.

Scientific Foundations

The scientific foundations utilized as part of the curriculum framework flowed from the philosophy and conceptual framework. The philosophy stated,

> Nursing education is a continuous process that builds upon a theoretical base from related disciplines. Nursing education provides conceptualizations that influence the perspective of nursing practice. It is essential for nursing education to maintain a strong theory-practice relationship.

The conceptual framework stated,

> Foundation content provides a scientific base for understanding human functioning, communication, social behaviors and growth development. (LAC, School of Nursing, 1991)

The scientific foundations are operationalized by selected required courses from the biological and social sciences. Table 9–2 shows the specific courses selected.

Horizontal Thread (Unifying Theme)

A process thread (horizontal thread) was identified. The process thread, a constant, served as the unifying theme for the curriculum framework.

Nursing Process.   A study of the conceptual framework revealed that the nursing process was the unifying theme for the curriculum framework.

> The nursing process is used as an organized, systematic method of analyzing the wellness status, and is directed toward maximizing system adjustment. (LAC, School of Nursing, 1991)

The nursing process format designed specifically for the Neuman Model has three categories: nursing diagnosis, nursing goals, and nursing outcomes

TABLE 9–2. SCIENTIFIC FOUNDATION COURSES

Understanding Human Functioning	Social Behavior	Communication
• Anatomy and physiology	• Psychology	• English composition
• Microbiology	• Sociology	• Speech

(Neuman, 1989). The faculty agreed to operationalize the nursing process in five steps: assessment, diagnosis, planning, implementation, and evaluation.

Functional Health Patterns.   A consistency in the structural methodology used in facilitating the students' learning of the nursing process and its application was needed. A departure from a body-systems or a medical model was desired. The Functional Health Patterns, as developed by Gordon, were chosen and were perceived to be directly applicable to the Neuman Systems Model. Gordon (1991) states,

> Functional Health Patterns of clients, whether individuals, families, or communities, evolve from the client-environmental interaction. . . . Functional patterns are influenced by biological, developmental, cultural, social and spiritual factors. (p. 2)

Gordon (1991) grouped the NANDA taxonomy under related Functional Health Patterns. Assessment and diagnosis of the client's response to actual or potential stressors became operationalized by the use of the Functional Health Patterns and the corresponding nursing diagnosis.

CURRICULUM DESIGN

The curriculum was designed with four courses in nursing for each of the four academic semesters (levels): three theory courses and one clinical applications course. Each course developed one or more of the concepts, and its related major subconcept, defining subconcepts, and organizing principle. Table 9–3 provides an overview of major components of the curriculum design.

Man

Courses in this series were designed to have a growth and development emphasis for the age group that is the focus for the level. Material related to the normal functional patterns upon which to base assessment for the focal age group was included.

Human Response Patterns and Nursing Care (Environment and Health)

The concepts of environment and health were integrated into this group of courses. The content was directed toward the effect of impact of environmental stressors on the wellness/illness of the client/client systems focused on for the level.

The Functional Health Patterns and related nursing diagnosis were the basis for the presentation of the content. Each course presents appropriate primary, secondary, and tertiary prevention as intervention. Nursing knowledge

TABLE 9-3. CURRICULUM DESIGN

Courses	Level (Semester)	Course Number	Focus
Man[a]	I	N10	Open system
	II	N20	Conception to young adulthood
	III	N30	Middle adult years
	IV	N40	Late adult years
Human Response Patterns and Nursing Care[a]	I	N11	Individual: secondary prevention
			Common/noncritical human response patterns that require strengthening of: 1. Flexible lines of defense 2. Normal lines of defense
	II	N21	Individual and family: primary and secondary prevention
			Common human response patterns that require strengthening of: 1. Flexible lines of defense 2. Normal lines of defense 3. Lines of resistance
	III	N31	Individual, family, groups: primary and secondary prevention
			Human response patterns that require strengthening of: 1. Flexible lines of defense 2. Normal lines of defense 3. Lines of resistance
	IV	N41	Individual, family, community: primary, secondary, and tertiary prevention 1. Flexible lines of defense 2. Normal lines of defense 3. Lines of resistance (Acute, chronic, rehabilitative)
Professional Role[a]	I	N12	Standards of practice, provider of care
	II	N22	Client advocacy, provider of and manager of care
	III	N32	Health care system, provider of and manager of care
	IV	N42	Accountable practice, provider and manager of care, and member of discipline
Prevention as Intervention[b]	I	N14	
	II	N24	Application of the theory courses via the use of the nursing process
	III	N34	
	IV	N44	

[a] Theory courses
[b] Clinical courses

related to pharmacology, client education, and nutritional aspects of care were included.

Professional Role (Nursing)

The legal-ethical responsibilities and the behaviors required for functioning safely and effectively in the provider and manager of care roles were developed. Legal accountabilities and common ethical issues were included as appropriate for the age group focused on in the level.

The rights and responsibilities as a member of a discipline as well as leadership styles are incorporated in the fourth level.

Prevention as Intervention (Nursing)

This series of clinical courses further operationalized the concept of nursing and its relationships with man, health, and environment. The use of the nursing process focused on the provision of nursing care of patients within the age group covered in the level based upon assessments of the patient's Functional Health Patterns. Opportunities were given to the students to implement various methods and strategies and evaluate their effectiveness in the promotion and maintenance of the system stability of the client.

IMPLEMENTATION

Dr. Neuman in discussion with the authors suggested that psychiatric nursing, her own specialty field, be utilized to demonstrate the implementation of the model in the curriculum. The limitations of the parameters of the chapter prevents a detailed discussion.

Table 9–4 demonstrates the focused psychiatric content of each of the four courses within the level provided for the student in Level III (third semester) of the educational program. The companion content in Level III is focused in medical-surgical nursing. Table 9–5 demonstrates the operationalization of one response to stressors, mood disorders, in a lesson plan. The authors, with the willing agreement of the psychiatric nursing faculty, presented this information.

FUTURE IMPLICATIONS FOR USE OF THE NEUMAN SYSTEMS MODEL

As nursing education prepares to meet the demands of the 21st century, it will be necessary to redesign curricula that are cost-effective and accountable to the public. It is expected that over time work described in this chapter will continue to evolve. In the redirected health care system the Neuman Systems Model will continue to provide an effective organizing framework in which to establish economical nursing educational delivery patterns and nursing practice systems.

TABLE 9–4. LOS ANGELES COUNTY MEDICAL CENTER SCHOOL OF NURSING LEVEL III: PSYCHIATRIC NURSING CONTENT[a]

Nursing 30:   Development and Assessment of Man: Middle Adult Years

The theories of growth and development introduced in Level I and II are built upon. Allen's Cognitive Assessment Theory is introduced. The focus is on the assessment of man in the middle years.

Development and assessment basis for psychiatric nursing
- Health management for coping/stress tolerance and sexuality/reproduction
  Erickson's stage of ego development
  Crisis theory
- Psychosocial assessment
  Concept of self
  Concept of role
  Life-threatening illness phases
  Psychosocial assessment
  Allen's cognitive level assessment

Nursing 31:   Human Response Patterns and Nursing Care III

The focus of the course is on the environmental stressors that may result in acute, single-system health problems. The nursing process will be utilized as the basis for presentation of the content. Therapeutic communication is introduced in Level I and built upon in this course. Nursing interventions include the pharmacological, nutritional, and teaching aspects:

Response to stressors: psychiatric focus
- Chronically mentally ill
- Substance abuse and dependence
- HIV/AIDS
- Thought disorders
- Mood disorders
- Anxiety disorders
- Manipulative behavior

Nursing 32:   Professional Role Development III

This course focuses on the role of the nurse and the nursing profession as part of the societal-political system. Emphasis is placed on patient rights and protection and the influence of regulatory agencies.

Legal issues: psychiatric focus
- Rights of individuals in legal-ethical situations
- Criteria for holds, hearings, and conservatorships

Nursing 34:   Prevention as Intervention III

This clinical course focuses on the use of the nursing process in the provision of nursing care for patients with acute medical-surgical and psychiatric illnesses. The five variables are utilized in formulating, implementing, and evaluating a plan of care. Maintenance of system stability in the care of acute and chronic medical-surgical and psychiatric illnesses is implemented.

Clinical criteria: psychiatric focus
- Apply the concepts of wholism (6 weeks) in the psychosocial assessment.
- Apply the nursing process in the care of a patient or groups of patients with acute and chronic mental illness to promote optimal system stability.
- Utilize therapeutic communication techniques.
- Perform nursing care according to established standards.

[a] Excerpted from course syllibi prepared by Level III (third semester) faculty.

TABLE 9-5. LESSON PLAN

LOS ANGELES COUNTY MEDICAL CENTER SCHOOL OF NURSING

Nursing 31:   Human Response Patterns
                                                                  and Nursing Care III

Section A: Psychiatric Nursing   Date:
                                                                  Instructor:
                                                                  Hours: 3.0

Course Objectives:
   Upon satisfactory completion of this course, the student:
   1. Identifies human response patterns to actual or potential stressors resulting from acute
       health problems common to the middle years.
   2. Describes the implementation of the nursing process in the promotion of optimal system
       stability for the individual and groups of adult patients with acute illness.
   3. Describes therapeutic communications utilized to accomplish patient and nursing goals
       for the individual and groups of patients.

Unit Objectives:
   Upon satisfactory completion of this course, the student:
   1. Describes the nursing process in the care of patients with mood disorders in relation
       to stressors.

Topic: Mood Disorders
Instructional Objectives:
   At the completion of the lesson, the student will describe the nursing process in the care of
   patients with mood disorders in relations to stressors by:
   1. Identifying the specific related intra-, inter-, and/or extrapersonal stressors and how they
       related to the five variables.
   2. Identifying the characteristics of an individual's lines of resistance.
   3. Describing clinical manifestations that occur in the lines of resistance of individuals with
       severe mood disturbances.
   4. Examining the assessment data to formulate a nursing diagnosis for individuals with
       severe mood disturbances.
   5. Discussing a plan of care that will assist the individual to attain/maintain his/her
       maximum level of wellness.
   6. Identifying actions that will decreases the individual's stressor response.
   7. Describing criteria to evaluate the effectiveness of medical and nursing interventions.

Significant future curriculum modifications that this program expects the Neuman Systems Model to provide direction for include:

1. A community health care focus.

2. A seamless associate degree–baccalaureate degree articulation approach that utilizes differentiated competencies.

3. Increased educational opportunities for faculty and students to provide health care services.

4. Increased curriculum emphasis on processes, as content (i.e., adaptations to sociocultural changes, shared decision making, and collaborative relationships).

Thus the Neuman Systems Model can be relied upon to continue to provide a sound foundation for associate degree education to address the future—a future that promises continuous change.

REFERENCES

Gordon, M. 1991. *Manual of Nursing Diagnosis, 1991–1992*. St. Louis, Mo.: Mosby-Year Book, Inc.

National League for Nursing, Council of Associate Degree Programs. 1990. *Educational Outcomes of Associate Nursing Programs: Roles and Competencies*. New York: National League For Nursing.

Neuman, B., ed. 1989. *The Neuman Systems Model*. East Norwalk, Conn.: Appleton & Lange.

10

TEACHING CONTENT AND PROCESS OF THE NEUMAN SYSTEMS MODEL

Carol Bloch
Carolyn Bloch

This two-part chapter first presents the highly successful process and content, used by the author Carol Bloch, for an introductory course on teaching the Neuman Systems Model to beginning level nursing students.

The second part presents the sociocultural variable format in collaboration with her twin sister Carolyn. Both authored the second portion of the chapter. This teaching process is congruent with the Los Angeles County Medical Center, School of Nursing, their Neuman-based curriculum, school philosophy, and glossary of definitions.

This school is uniquely and highly multicultural in terms of its large student body, faculty, and client population community where learning takes place. The authors have pioneered a teaching format that gives beginning students a firm foundation in the parameters of wholistic nursing and early socialization into the importance of multicultural sensitivity. The authors welcome further inquiry from readers. They both feel that these teaching formats can be used for higher level learning.

Reviewed by Barbara Freese and Lois Lowry.

THE TEACHING PROCESS AND CONTENT FORMAT

It is both exciting and a great challenge to introduce theories used by nursing as content linked to a conceptual framework. The clear terminology and systems perspective of the Neuman Systems Model facilitate linking theory as content with the model. Based on Neuman, the curriculum concepts of man, environment, health, and nursing are used as a framework for a four-part six-hour component of a course on Man as a System: A Nursing Perspective (Nursing Course 10). The content is sequenced into four major categories:

- Part 1: The Client as a System—Comprehensive View of the Neuman Model to Structure Nursing
- Part 2: Environment—Systems Perspective and Nursing
- Part 3: Health—Health and Illness Continuum
- Part 4: Nursing—Wholistic Nursing Process

INSTRUCTIONAL FORMAT

Part 1: The Client as a System (1.5-hour lecture/discussion)

Content	Process
Conceptual frameworks and nursing. Definitions and use of conceptual frameworks to structure nursing activities. Role definition and trends related to model usage. Explanation and history of the Neuman systems perspective and how it provides a wholistic approach to nursing. Relationships explored between the model and the school's philosophy and curriculum, the Nurse Practice Act, and ANA definition of nursing.	Lecture with interactive dialogue. Dynamic relationships made with specific examples provided. Media and handouts used to illustrate. Students relate to self as a system and use same process to view family and community as systems. School glossary of Neuman-based definitions explained.

Frames of Reference
Interdisciplinary use and importance of models, theories, and other resources are explained by: 1. Wholism—social trends; individual, family, community as a system. 2. Nursing trends. 3. Human response to stressors; optimal wellness—systems related to Neuman Model. 4. Common stressors, e.g., pain. 5. Developmental change. 6. Loss/grief; self-care issues. 7. Future perspective, e.g., sociocultural, political.

Summary Statement. Nursing conceptual frameworks provide a structure for organizing a multitude of phenomena into a meaningful whole. They facilitate communication among nurses by establishing a common vocabulary and enable nurses to identify and address client problems more effectively because nurses are sharing the same interpretation of client problems. Conceptual frameworks support nursing practice by defining the goals and focus of nursing and providing structure to direct assessment and information processing to meet client needs.

The Neuman Systems Model provides a set of concepts that unify thinking and provide common purpose, direction, and language. It gives direction for identifying and forming relationships and illustrates how the five variables (as subconcepts) interrelate within the concept of client (whether person, family, or community).

Nursing is the only health care provider concerned with the whole person, with helping clients meet unmet needs from a wholistic perspective. As caregivers, nurses maintain a lateral, collaborative relationship with clients as nurse and client confront the phenomenon of illness together. Nursing interventions become significant as client responses are influenced through the caring process. A vital aspect of the nurse's role is resolving perceptual differences as to how clients view their own health problems versus the perception held by nurses and other health care professionals. As the nurse clarifies and demystifies faulty perceptions, clients are empowered to confront their health conditions. The outcome of this intervention is relevant client care.

Part 2: Environment (1.5-hour lecture/discussion)

Content	Process
Systems theory—terminology. Systems base and wellness perspective of the Neuman Systems Model. Systems: individual, group, or community. System characteristics; i.e., boundaries, input and output, adjustment to stressors, stability, types of environmental stressors (intra-, inter-, and extrapersonal), internal and external. Perception of stressors. Goal-directed/client-negotiated activities of a system. How a system remains viable. Client as a systems concept. Variables of the client system as illustrated by Neuman and environmental interaction.	Media and teaching aids. Definitions and analyses of individual, family, and community as a system. Dynamism of a system illustrated as interrelated, interactive, and interdependent parts of whole in constant change. Interactive student exchange. Student and instructor as environmental influence.

Frames of Reference:

Systems theorist: Lazlo
Stress theorists: Selye, Lazarus, Gestalt
Growth and development
Learned behavioral response or patterning
Cultural considerations

Summary Statement. The combination of teaching content and process socializes students into an understanding of systems as entities that consist of interrelated and interacting parts with arbitrarily established boundaries as well as inherent goal-directed activities. For example, as the concept of health versus illness is considered from this perspective, health is viewed on a continuum by Neuman as negentropy, while illness is entropy; the goal of the system is maintenance of stability or health.

Nursing deals primarily with client system response to stressors. The focus of nursing is to prevent, detect, promote, and maintain a desired wellness level and to treat illness and disability to conserve energy and enhance client wellness. Nurse and client ideally negotiate the goals of the caring system. In representing reality, the Neuman Systems Model provides a broad perspective within which to view nursing phenomena and organize nursing activities based on theoretical knowledge.

The Neuman Systems Model as a framework is an open system consisting of two components: stress and reaction to it (Neuman, 1982). A client as an open system interacts with the environment by adjusting to it or by adjusting it to the client. Ideally, the client system is in a stable, harmonious condition; nursing both strengthens wellness factors and corrects imbalances and illness. At all times, the environment, internal and external to the client system, contains a variety of stressors. The nurse identifies high-risk stressors as well as those that have caused a reaction or system instability and prioritizes them for nursing action. Nurses will increasingly be held accountable for interdisciplinary collaboration to benefit the client as a system.

Part 3: Health (1.5-hour lecture/discussion)

Content	Process
Significance of wholistic health trends with interdisciplinary cooperation and the Neuman Systems Model. Health viewed on the Neuman wellness–illness continuum. Wellness defined in systems terms of available energy and energy conservation. Role of the nurse. System strengths and weaknesses systematically and culturally defined. Deviations from normal health status using Neuman Model. Wellness	Case studies. Vignettes. Normal line of defense explained as wellness standard. Wellness relationships explored in relation to stability vs. instability.

Content	Process
orientation. Illness as reaction of varying degrees caused by stressors. Wholism related to all client system variables in interaction with environment. Optimal wellness. System stability related to health retention, attainment, and maintenance. Sociocultural factors, life-style, and coping effects on health.	Coping strategies.

Frames of Reference
Developmental
Psychological
Physiological
Sociocultural
Spiritual
Life-style
Role
Health beliefs
Values/mores
Dunn's High Level Wellness

Summary Statement. The teaching of both content and process adds dynamism to student learning. Through this format students learn first what wholistic wellness is by asssessing client system stability as the model's normal line of defense. To learn about wellness variance, students progress through assessment of degrees of client system instability (i.e., illness). Students can then plan logically for use of the three prevention as intervention modes to retain, attain, and/or maintain an optimal level of wellness or health for the client as a system.

Part 4: Nursing (1.5-hour lecture/discussion)

Content	Process
The model's major concern for nursing is in keeping the system stable through accuracy in assessment of the effects (actual and potential) of environmental stressors and in assisting client adjustments required for optimal wellness. Nursing actions are initiated to retain, attain, and maintain optimal client health or wellness, using the three prevention modes as interventions to keep the system stable. Thus the nurse creates a linkage between the client and	Nurse role and responsibilities explained. Values inherent within the model discussed. Comparison/contrast of Neuman three-step vs. traditional five-step nursing process. Case study assessment and goal planning based on Neuman terminology, nursing process, and model components. Case study based on Johnson (see references).

(cont.)

Content	Process
environment, health, and nursing. Operationalizing the Neuman Systems Model components into the nursing process, using five steps. Nursing diagnosis. New health mandates and nurse's role in client assessment. Goal negotiation/decision making. Prevention as intervention modality. The Neuman three-step nursing process format.	

Frames of Reference
Thibodeau Ziegler PES format (NANDA)

Summary Statement. Both content and process teaching provide model concept linkage and direction for students to apply the traditional five-step nursing process within each of the three prevention as intervention modes. Through this instructional format, the model's relevancy is actualized within the nurse–client interaction and care processes.

Course Evaluation Process

Student evaluations of the instructional format have been positive. As one student stated, "This is how nursing should be." Another said, "This is how nursing of the future will be."

Longitudinal evaluation will continue to include student course comments and program success rates on the National Council Licensure Examination for Registered Nurses (NCLEX-RN). Ongoing evaluation will take place to acquire data for curriculum refinement and evolvement in meeting the changing and challenging health priorities for the 21st century.

THE SOCIOCULTURAL VARIABLE

As the United States approaches the 21st century, diversity within our society is creating a multicultural client population that requires nurses to acquire new knowledge and skills to provide care that is culturally appropriate. In a multicultural environment such as Los Angeles county, students quickly learn that increasing cultural diversity is having a significant impact on nurse role/function and that this diversity requires specific knowledge and skill development to serve these multicultural populations effectively.

Transcultural concepts must be taught to increase student awareness, appreciation, and understanding of culture-specific client system similarities and differences. To help meet this need, the Los Angeles County Medical Center School of Nursing has included in the existing assessment tool a specific cultural component for determining client needs and planning specific goal-relevant care for all clients. This focus socializes students, moving then from an ethnocentric care approach to one of tolerance, appreciation, and understanding of differing client values within a multicultural population. Within Nursing Course 10, a faculty lecture with interactive student dialogue is used to present the following sequenced content:

- A video is presented on "Transcultural Nursing" to provide a general overview of transcultural concerns.
- A recent news article is used to illustrate the contemporary impact of cultural issues on health care delivery.
- The Neuman Systems Model sociocultural variable is explained as it relates wholistically to other client system variables and is defined as "includ[ing] social and cultural functions" (Neuman, 1982). Sociocultural variable congruence to school philosophy and Neuman-based definitions is clarified.
- Learned behavioral patterning of cultural values, priorities, and culture-specific characteristics commonly shared within a particular cultural group (Leininger, 1978) is discussed.
- Students identify features of the cultural group to which they belong.
- Components of a cultural system are identified using the cultural ethnic views of Orque et al. (1983) on religion, diet, family life processes, healing beliefs and practices, language and communication processes, social group interactive patterns, value orientation, art, and history.
- Cultural specifics related to the school client population are examined in terms of the culture of poverty, its myths and realities, and health practices such as natural folk medicine (plants, herbs, minerals, and other substances) used to prevent and treat illness. Magico-religious folk medicine (often considered occult), such as ritual use of charms, crystals, and holy actions as believed to prevent and cure illness (Spector, 1991), is discussed. Acquiring knowledge of specific aspects of a select culture helps the nurse assess client system needs and plan care within the context of that particular culture using Neuman-based concepts and intervention modalities.
- Particular emphasis is placed on assessment of ethnic affiliation, family system stability and patterns of interaction (intra-, inter-, and extrapersonal environmental influences), food patterns and preferences, health belief system, and ethnic health care patterns.
- Students are asked to share what they would like the caregiver to know about their cultural differences for best professional care.

The ideal outcome of a culturally congruent assessment is to decrease misunderstandings and frustrations and increase client satisfaction and compliance.

Processes used can be validated in terms of desired health care outcome data.

Nurse behaviors that express acceptance of cultural differences have been stated (Sheppard, 1990). The following may be used as indicators to evaluate sociocultural variable content mastery by students:

1. Paying attention to cultural belief cues that may contribute to illness or promote wellness.
2. Recognizing and facilitating family wishes for involvement in client care.
3. Considering that treatment priorities may differ from the traditional.
4. Combining folk and Western medicine as possible.

The content provided in this lecture contributes to effective consideration of the sociocultural component of the client system toward relevant wholistic caregiving.

> By knowing the language of a culture,
>   you know its voice.
> By knowing its values,
>   you know its heart.
>
> —Anonymous

REFERENCES

American Nurses Association. 1980. *Nursing: A Social Policy Statement.* Kansas City, Mo: American Nurses Association.

Johnson, S. E. 1989. A picture is worth a thousand words: Helping students visualize a conceptual model. *Nurse Educator* 13(3):21–24.

Lazlo, E. 1972. *The Systems View of the World: The Natural Philosophy of the New Developments in the Sciences.* New York: Braziller.

Leininger, M. M. 1978. *Transcultural Nursing—Concepts, Theories, and Practices.* New York: John Wiley and Son.

Monat, A., and Lazarus, R. S. 1977. *Stress and Coping—An Anthology.* New York: Columbia University Press.

Neuman, B., ed. 1982. *The Neuman Systems Model,* 1st ed. Norwalk, Conn.: Appleton & Lange.

Neuman, B., ed. 1989. *The Neuman Systems Model,* 2nd ed. Norwalk, Conn.: Appleton & Lange.

Orque, M., Bloch, B., and Monrroy, L. 1983. *Ethnic Nursing Care.* St. Louis, Mo.: C. V. Mosby Co.

Spector, R. E. 1991. *Cultural Diversity in Health and Illness,* 3d ed. Norwalk, Conn.: Appleton & Lange.

Sheppard, H. 1990. How Hispanic cultural patterns affect caregivers. *Nurseweek* 3(3):15–16.

Thibodeau, J. A. (1983). *Nursing Models: Analysis and Evaluation.* Belmont, Calif.: Wadsworth Health Sciences Division.

Ziegler, S. M., et al. 1986. *Nursing Process, Nursing Diagnosis, Nursing Knowledge—Avenues to Autonomy.* Norwalk, Conn.: Appleton & Lange.

11

INTEGRATION OF THE NEUMAN SYSTEMS MODEL INTO THE BSN CURRICULUM AT THE UNIVERSITY OF TEXAS AT TYLER

Linda Campbell Klotz

THE NEUMAN-BASED BACCALAUREATE PROGRAM

The University of Texas at Tyler, an upper-level and graduate educational institution, has as its purpose achievement of a variety of goals to satisfy the needs of its many constituencies. As a component of the university community, the Division of Nursing provides baccalaureate and master's nursing education programs. The BSN program is designed to include generic, registered nurse, and licensed vocational nurse students, with a Mobility in Nursing Education (MINE) track for the licensed students. Courses in the generic program span four semesters (Appendix A). The first-semester content addresses concepts and theories, health assessment, pharmacology, nursing competencies, and community health. Medical-surgical and psychiatric nursing content is explored in the second

Reviewed and edited by Virginia Strickland.
Reviewed by Rae Jean Memmott.

semester, while obstetrical and pediatric content provides the focus for the third semester. The program concludes with leadership, research, an advanced nursing process seminar, and advanced medical-surgical nursing.

As an alternative progression plan for the BSN curriculum, the MINE curriculum recognizes the prior learning and professional experience of registered nurses and licensed vocational nurses. This plan incorporates planned classroom activities, independent learning experiences, and individualized clinical assignments to achieve undergraduate program objectives. The MINE track includes two specially developed courses, Clinical Applications I and II. The first course incorporates a nursing perspective while examining in detail client physiological processes and responses; the second course uses a modular approach to broaden and update student knowledge in pharmacology, competencies, and medical-surgical, psychiatric, obstetrical, and pediatric nursing content. MINE students take concepts and theories, community health, and health assessment along with the generic students. Clinical Applications I is also taken in the first semester, Clinical Applications II in the second. MINE students join with generic students again in the leadership, research, and advanced nursing process seminar courses during the final semester. The program requires LVN students to take the advanced medical-surgical nursing course, while RNs may choose to take an elective course instead.

The Division of Nursing's philosophy is based on human-centered caring that supports the intrinsic value of persons, the wholeness of their being, the richness of human interaction, and the enhancement and preservation of hu-man dignity. Humanistic caring supports the individual's growing awareness and acceptance of self, freedom of choice, social responsibility, and accountability. The Neuman Systems Model (NSM) fully supports existing faculty beliefs regarding wholistic beings as open systems interacting as individuals, families, groups, and communities with internal, external, and created environments. The model provides a framework of structure and direction for information processing and goal-directed activities within an increasingly complex health care delivery system.

IMPLEMENTATION INTO THE CURRICULUM

Introduction and Application

Utilization of the Neuman Systems Model (NSM) begins in the first semester and continues throughout the curriculum. The model provides a unifying construct from which to view clients and nursing, integrating primary, secondary, and tertiary levels of prevention. Primary prevention receives greatest emphasis in Nursing Process I and II (Health Assessment and Community Health) but is incorporated throughout the entire curriculum. Students focus on secondary prevention in Nursing Process III, IV, V, and VI (Medical-Surgical, Psychiatric, Obstetrical, Pediatric, and Advanced Medical-Surgical Nursing). Learning experiences related to tertiary prevention appear in all nursing courses.

In Concepts and Theories I, a general discussion of nursing theories and the metaparadigm concepts progresses to an in-depth discussion of the NSM, utilizing the systems diagram first developed by Neuman in 1970 and later refined (1982, 1989). Nursing process is presented as a systematic mechanism for providing nursing care at any level for individuals, families, and groups. The Neuman Systems Model and interpersonal caring are viewed as adjunctive elements upon which to build a nursing knowledge base. Students are expected to utilize the model as part of their efforts as providers of health care in assisting clients to retain, attain, and maintain a maximum level of wellness through purposeful interventions. These interventions are to be aimed at reduction of stress factors and adverse conditions that either affect or could affect optimal functioning in a given client situation. Primary, secondary, and tertiary levels of intervention are discussed within a multicultural practice arena. Health Assessment students first examine the course content in the context of the major concepts of the NSM and advance through group work to organize and document case study client data into the Neuman framework using an assessment tool based on the model in order to develop a nursing care plan based upon the NSM. In Community Health, students are exposed to a variety of community resources that focus on primary prevention, and they apply the NSM in analyzing the health care of individuals, families, groups, and communities. In Competencies, students provide care for chronically ill clients utilizing the Summary of Assessment Data Tool based on the NSM to guide their application of the nursing process. MINE students in the first clinical applications course explore physiological processes of humans, emphasizing health promotion and maintenance.

The second semester medical-surgical and psychiatric nursing courses and clinical rotations blend didactic content with clinical experiences in an effort to encourage students to be aware of the "person beneath all the tubes" and to approach care planning with a wholistic view of the client and his or her internal, external, and created environments. Application of the NSM in the care planning tool broadens to incorporate the psychological, sociocultural, and spiritual variables as well as the physiological dimensions of human needs. Faculty encourage beginning recognition of developmental variables at this level. MINE students take the second clinical applications course during this semester. Course content enables the RN and LVN students to apply the NSM in care planning through the five specialty modules. Students use faculty-developed case studies in each module to facilitate application of the NSM into practice. Assessment includes all five variables with incorporation of rehabilitation, health promotion, and health maintenance.

Third-semester generic students in obstetrical and pediatric nursing courses apply the NSM assessment strategies to planning care for families. Developmental variables receive strong emphasis during this semester.

By combining the generic and MINE tracks for the leadership, research, advanced nursing process seminar, and advanced medical-surgical nursing courses in the final semester, students gain the opportunity to share experiences and enthusiasm during classroom and clinical rotations. Students synthesize previous knowledge in each selected clinical area and collaborate with other disciplines in problem solving, goal development, and selection of implementation strategies. Written work reflects incorporation of the NSM with current research to guide clinical management experiences.

Tool Development and Modifications

Faculty modified the NSM health history and assessment tool (Neuman, 1982, 26–27) when the BSN program began in 1982. Original adaptations reflected first-semester content emphasis on assessment of clients in the healthy state with only slight deviations from normal. Application of the model focused on identifying elements of the basic structure, lines of resistance, normal and flexible lines of defense, and stressors prior to organizing this data into a plan of care that incorporated nursing inverventions in the realm of primary, secondary, or tertiary prevention, as appropriate for the identified goals.

Difficulties in differentiating assessment data into the elements of basic structure, lines of resistance, and occasionally the normal line of defense, as well as student complaints regarding faculty inconsistencies in utilization of these three concepts, prompted faculty workshops to address the problem. Discussions identified some assessment data that could be placed in multiple categories. Examples included the following:

1. A client with an intact immune system (basic structure) experiences a situation that activates the immune system (line of resistance or line of defense).
2. A client who has smoked three packs of cigarettes a day for 25 years (normal line of defense) contracts bronchitis and quits smoking entirely (flexible line of defense or line of resistance).

To alleviate the intra-, inter, and extrapersonal stressors for faculty and students, faculty collapsed the assessment categories and combined elements of the basic structure, lines of resistance, normal line of defense, and flexible line of defense into a category labeled system strengths (see Summary of Assessment Findings, Appendix B). This system works well, allowing students to gain comfort with other concepts of the NSM while incorporating this framework into the care planning process during each nursing course. As students expand their knowledge of the model and its application, they become more flexible and develop the ability to think critically, making distinctions between the assessment concepts that may be defended through critical thinking. An example of nursing care planning using the Summary of Assessment Findings is provided in Appendix B.

EVALUATION

Utilization in a Variety of Settings

Among the many advantages of the NSM, flexibility remains perhaps its greatest strength. The model can be effectively utilized to plan nursing care for chronically ill clients in extended care facilities as well as for clients with a wide range of acuities in short-term care facilities. The model encourages incorporation of families and significant others into the planning process, which research has found to be highly significant in achieving optimal levels of wellness (Campbell, 1986).

The community-as-client approach (Lancaster and Whall, 1989) provides another avenue for application of the model. Effective utilization of the NSM in the systematic assessment and planning necessary for community-based nursing practice or in leadership/management positions, however, requires some manipulation of the concepts of basic structure, normal line of defense, flexible line of defense, and lines of resistance. Lack of definition by the theorist for these concepts in community or management situations requires determination of "goodness of fit" by the user. Each instructor must guide students in correct interpretation and analysis of their data.

Faculty Evaluation

Faculty support the value of the model as a teaching tool. Incorporation of the five dimensions of the client system (physiological, psychological, sociocultural, developmental, and spiritual) into the assessment phase of the nursing process upholds the philosophical view of the client as a wholistic being, encouraging the student to incorporate the family and significant others into the care planning process. Neuman strongly emphasizes that both the nurse's and the client's perceptions must be assessed in order to maintain a therapeutic level of care.

The level of abstraction of the NSM allows generalization to a wide variety of practice settings. The model's flexibility permits use of the same assessment and care planning tools for all clinical courses, thereby facilitating the transfer of knowledge and increasing the student's acceptance of theory-based nursing practice.

The model reinforces the student's commitment to health promotion and maintenance of wellness as appropriate goals for professional nursing practice. Faculty advisors refer to intra-, inter-, and extrasystem stressors when discussing with students the personal and school-related issues facing them on a daily basis. Such discussions allow faculty to role-model the reality of theory-based nursing practice in education as well as in clinical settings and provides a basis for future research.

Student Evaluation

Students find the abstractness of the model both a blessing because of its generalizability and a burden due to the nonspecificity of some concepts. Both MINE and generic students find the concepts of basic structure, lines of resistance, and normal line of defense easy to understand with faculty support and guidance. The fluid nature of the flexible line of defense is problematic initially, but students resolve the difficulty as they become more comfortable with the nursing knowledge base and their levels of clinical skills.

The process of incorporating and internalizing professional behaviors occurs subtly and often cannot be appreciated until some time after graduation. Students returning to the MSN program identify that the NSM provided a more sophisticated practice base than that of their peers from associate degree and diploma programs. RN and LVN students, initially reluctant to reframe their practice from a new perspective, acknowledged that the NSM gave them a framework for their own practice and enhanced interfacing with departments. This has been a consistent finding (Hinton Walker and Raborn, 1989). Many identified that the care they provided was far more comprehensive due to the wholistic and comprehensive approach of the model, which facilitated the establishment of a detailed data base. They also expressed awareness of the potential involvement of other health care providers to facilitate the client's movement toward the highest level of wellness. Students recognized that the terms basic structure, flexible line of defense, normal line of defense, and lines of resistance potentiated their understanding of the client–environment interaction; however, their inability to clearly explain the terms to clients or other health care providers sometimes prevented full utilization of the model's terms in their practice.

Both groups of students found the model to be compatible with the nursing process and applied it throughout their educational experiences in a variety of settings. They readily formulated nursing diagnoses based on synthesis on knowledge derived from the model and the client factor data base.

The NSM allows graduate students to conceptualize and utilize the nursing process for nursing practice within their own unique philosophies and styles of nursing. The impact of the model on continuing professional growth for students is somewhat difficult to define, as the students themselves are not always able to articulate clearly what motivated them to continue their formal and informal educational processes. Most faculty believe that theory-based learning in the undergraduate arena exposed the students to a large number of perspectives and convinced them of the value of the systems approach for a wide, varied, and continually updated knowledge base for providing quality nursing care. The increasing interest of both undergraduate and graduate students in qualitative research may be related, in part, to the model's emphasis on understanding the clients' experiences from their own perspectives. The NSM facilitates application of the philosophy of human caring through recognition of the fact that the nurse–client relationship demands high levels of trust and existential presence.

FUTURE IMPLICATIONS FOR USE OF THE NEUMAN SYSTEMS MODEL

Involvement in health care reform marks an exciting era for the nursing profession. As the health care system becomes even more complex and societal changes continue to influence nursing practice, the need for a theoretical base for organizing professional practice becomes increasingly evident. The strength of the NSM in curriculum planning and evolution has been proved over the years in numerous schools of nursing encompassing all levels of nursing education, as well as continuing education for practicing nurses. A systems approach to assessment is consistent with nursing's philosophical practice base and is also relevant to most practice settings. The systems approach has also facilitated the adoption of the model in other cultures.

In *Megatrends 2000,* Naisbitt (1990) identified one trend as the movement of consumers toward nontraditional approaches to health care and the movement of nursing practice away from the traditional formal acute-care institutions into the community. The political and economic pressure for collaboration to provide the highest quality of health care for the greatest number of people at the lowest cost mounts steadily. The flexibility and adaptability of the NSM provides health caregivers enormous strength and potential for use is a number of nursing and health care specialties and settings to meet the needs of the 21st century.

Scientific development and testing should, indeed, validate the model as efficacious and appropriate for multidisciplinary collaboration in international, community-based, and entrepreneurial practice applications. Further research and development of model concepts will find the model relevant to the future organizational structuring and delivery of health care reform mandates. Present health care complexity requires a broad and flexible organizing structure that the model well provides.

Congruence exists between consumer movement into the New Age and the NSM's addition of the spiritual dimension and the created environment. These concepts opened new vistas in mental health, counseling, and behavioral modification practice for nurses. Further definition and development of the new concepts will expand their use for group work in community and managerial settings.

Other trends identified by futurists include involvement of the consumer and expansion of nursing practice roles. Neuman clearly anticipated these trends in 1970 by structuring the client into the assessment and planning process, a recognition of the nursing profession's ethics and the rights of the consumer. Levels of prevention as intervention clearly guide movement of nursing professionals into expanded and nontraditional roles, increasing the relevancy of model usage in the 21st century.

In summary, the model proved very efficacious in education and clearly shows the potential to be equally effective in the guiding clinical practice with further development through nursing research. The NSM enhances the public call for more comprehensive approaches to health promotion and maintenance and allows for both diversity and specificity within nursing education in order to meet health care needs in the local and global arenas.

REFERENCES

Campbell, L. 1986. Hopelessness and uncertainty as predictors of psychosocial adjustment for newly-diagnosed cancer patients and their significant others. Unpublished dissertation, The University of Texas at Austin.

Hinton Walker, P., and Raborn, M. 1989. Application of the Neuman Model in nursing administration and practice. In *Dimensions of Nursing Administration,* edited by B. Henry, C. Arndt, M. DiVicenti, and A. Marriner-Tomey. Boston: Blackwell Scientific Publications.

Lancaster, D. R., and Whall, A. L. 1989. The Neuman Systems Model. In *Conceptual Models of Nursing: Analysis and Application,* edited by J. J. Fitzpatrick and A. L. Whall. Norwalk, Conn.: Appleton & Lange.

Naisbitt, J., and Aburdene, P. 1990. *Megatrends 2000.* New York: William Morrow and Company, Inc.

Neuman, B., and Young, R. 1972. A model for teaching the total person approach to patient problems. *Nursing Research* 21(3): 264–269.

Neuman, B. 1980. The Betty Neuman Health Care Systems Model: A total person approach to patient problems. In *Conceptual Models for Nursing practice,* 2d ed., edited by J. P. Riehl and C. Roy. New York: Appleton-Century-Crofts.

Neuman, B. 1982. *The Neuman Systems Model: Application to Nursing Education and Practice.* Norwalk, Conn.: Appleton & Lange.

Neuman, B. 1989. *The Neuman Systems Model,* 2d. ed. Norwalk, Conn.: Appleton & Lange.

APPENDIX A

Courses for the Neuman-Based Baccalaureate Program, University of Texas at Tyler, Division of Nursing

CURRICULUM SCHEMA (NURSING COURSES ONLY)—GENERIC

Semester I	Semester II
NURS 3205 (Concepts and Theories I)	NURS 3611 (Medical-Surgical)
NURS 3210 (Health Assessment)	NURS 3613 (Psychiatric)
NURS 3401 (Community Health)	CHEM 3108 (Pharmacology II)
NURS 3403 (Competencies)	
CHEM 3107 (Pharmacology I)	

Semester III	Semester IV
NURS 4621 (Obstetrical)	NURS 4333 (Concepts and Theories II/Research)
NURS 4623 (Pediatric)	NURS 4432 (Nursing Leadership)
	NURS 4134 (Advanced Nursing Process Seminar)
	NURS 4434 (Advanced Medical-Surgical)

CURRICULUM SCHEMA (NURSING COURSES ONLY)—MINE TRACK

Semester I	Semester II
NURS 3205 (Concepts and Theories I)	NURS 4625 (Clinical Applications II)
NURS 3210 (Health Assessment)	
NURS 3401 (Community Health)	
NURS 3415 (Clinical Applications I)	

Semester III
NURS 4333 (Concepts and Theories II/Research)
NURS 4432 (Nursing Leadership)
NURS 4134 (Advanced Nursing Process Seminar)
NURS 4434 (Advanced Medical-Surgical)[a]

[a]This is a required course for LVNs. RN students may take this course or an elective as preferred.

APPENDIX B
Case Study

Mr. R, a 55-year-old Caucasian, presents with a history of mild hypertension with progressive lung scarring and arthritis. He is married with a grown son and daughter no longer living at home and has recently been promoted to president of his company. Mr. R experienced a weight gain of 20 pounds over a six-month period with a resultant decrease in mobility and expresses greatest distress about his continuing physical and emotional fatigue. He uses logic and aggression strategies to cope with life problems and expects respect and support from family and other resources.

INTRAPERSONAL FACTORS

Physiological: Sharp stabbing headaches with bilateral eye pain at least once a month, related to eyestrain and fatigue; has had trouble sleeping for the past 12 years and "wake[s] up worrying about work and can't go back to sleep"; skips breakfast but eats two large meals a day including all food groups; has frequent indigestion after eating spicy foods; takes Maalox on a daily basis; has pain and swelling in both knees especially after exertion like climbing stairs for last five years.

Psychological: Pleasant, self-assured; projects positive self-image; rates ability to cope with stress on a scale of 1 to 10 as 10.

Sociocultural: French-American heritage, upper-middle-class background; values honesty, fairness, loyalty, hard work, and determination.

Developmental: Behavior appropriate to age; has experienced increased workload and stress before and is determined and confident that he will do his job well.

Spiritual: Methodist with strong belief system.

INTERPERSONAL FACTORS

Wide and supportive network of family and friends. Strong relationship with wife and best friend.

EXTRAPERSONAL FACTORS

Financially secure with health and life insurance. Operates investment business in addition to job. Enjoys job, fishing, mowing lawn.

SUMMARY OF ASSESSMENT FINDINGS[a]

SYSTEMS STRENGTHS (normal line of defense, flexible line of defense, lines of resistance)	STRESSORS (risk factors for potential nursing diagnoses or abnormal assessment data)	SYSTEM RESPONSES (abnormal assessment findings)
Values health and wellness in order to accomplish job.	"Sharp stabbing pain directly behind my eyes." Pain occurs at least once monthly. Has had this pain on and off for 10 years, mostly when glasses needed changing.	Recent increased workload due to death of company president and promotion to fill that role. Increased paperwork as a result of decreased staff. "I guess I really don't know how to take care of my eyes–not to strain them, you know." (intra)
Alert and well-oriented		
Tries to have regular eye examinations. Last eye exam two years ago.		
Two meals/day from all food groups. No food allergies or dislikes. Wife enjoys cooking and prepares his favorites as he likes them.	Increased weight gain of 20 pounds over last six months, with a 10-pound gain in last month.	Decreased exercise last six months. (intra)
		"I don't have time for breakfast; we're short-handed and I need to get into the office early. I usually have lunch sent in from a nearby fast food restaurant, and have a working lunch." (intra and extra)
General good health, with no family or financial worries. Children away from home and successful, stable home life with wife of 30 years. History of coping with work-related stress well in the past.	"I haven't slept well in months. I go to sleep quickly and easily, but then I wake up worrying about some problem at work and I can't go back to sleep."	Has gotten out of regular routines of exercise, etc. due to increased workload. Does not feel comfortable delegating work. "I want my employees to see me as a working hands-on kind of boss." (intra, inter, and extra)

[a]This is strictly a worksheet to be used by the student in identifying the client's responses and stressors. No grade will be assigned.

NURSING DIAGNOSES FOR Mr. R

Priority #	Diagnosis	Resolved
1	Pain: head and eye pain related to lack of knowledge about prevention of eyestrain	
2	Nutrition, altered: more than body requirements related to lack of knowledge about proper diet and exercise	
3	Sleep pattern disturbance related to ineffective coping with work-related psychological stress	
4	Mobility, impaired physical related to pain and swelling in knees	

12

NEUMAN-BASED ASSOCIATE DEGREE PROGRAMS
Past, Present, and Future

Lois W. Lowry
Grace G. Newsome

Neuman-based associate degree programs were unique entities to nursing one decade ago. Today 12 programs report using the model as a conceptual framework for curriculum development (personal communication, Betty Neuman, 1993). This chapter will present past and future relevance of the model as a guide for associate degree education and highlight findings from the first evaluation study of graduates of one of the programs.

Nursing education in the '90s is characterized by *accountability, changing paradigms, critical thinking,* and *evaluation* criteria. All levels of nurse educators are being challenged to reevaluate their teaching programs in relation to the above factors. Educators are asking questions such as:

1. What do nurse graduates need to know to best function within the health care system today and tomorrow?
2. As more nurses will be needed in home and community settings, how does this affect education of the associate degree nurse?
3. How must the associate degree curriculum be revised and enhanced to best prepare the student for practice in the 21st century?

These questions and more are being considered by associate degree educators across the country. Educators look to the National League for Nursing

(NLN) for guidance as they consider plans for curriculum revision. One future vision of the NLN (1993) is that graduates be competent to function within a health care system in which individuals and families are the primary decision makers in their own health care. This implies that graduates must be able to mutually plan with their clients to prepare them for management of health and illness at home. It further implies that graduates need an organizational structure to guide them as they provide optimal care and offer anticipatory guidance and discharge planning. Thus educators must revisit their curricula to determine if overall content, structures, and processes are appropriate to produce graduates who can function adequately in the future proposed health care system. Programs that had selected the Neuman's Systems Model were revisited to determine their perceptions of the efficacy of the model for the future of associate degree nursing.

The six programs contributing to this chapter are Athens Area Technical Institute, Athens, Georgia; Cecil Community College, North East, Maryland; Indiana University–Purdue University at Fort Wayne, Indiana; Los Angeles Valley College, Van Nuys, California; Santa Fe Community College, Gainesville, Florida; Yakima Valley Community College, Yakima, Washington. Three of the above adopted the model in the early '80s to guide curriculum development (Lowry and Green, 1989) and now report greater breadth, depth, and creativity in developing teaching/learning strategies, internalization by faculty, the development of articulation strategies, and a greater involvement in curriculum evaluation.

Each program stated that the Neuman Systems Model was selected because model constructs were congruent with their stated philosophy (Athens, Indiana–Purdue, Santa Fe, Yakima) and provided a nursing, as opposed to medical, focus. All programs value the concept of clients as wholistic beings. Further, the Neuman definitions of environment, health, and nursing are accepted and used to cluster curricular content. Faculty claim the model also affords flexibility in the arrangement of content and the conceptualization of program needs (Los Angeles Valley, Yakima Valley). Associate degree students, neophytes at the basic level of education, are open to new ideas and able to be socialized into a wholistic view of nursing. When neophytes are taught from a sound, logical, and flexible nursing framework, they are prepared with a strong foundation for practice and continuing education. Programs using the Neuman Model claim that the constructs are sufficiently comprehensive to accommodate all the approaches to care suggested by health care reform. In other words, the model was not only able to structure relevant educational programs in the past, but also has the breadth to accommodate the changes of care expected in the future. The NLN (1991) has characterized the practice of associate degree nurses as including skills in critical thinking, clinical competency, accountability, and commitment to the value of caring.

COMMONALITIES AMONG PROGRAMS

More similarities exist than differences among the six contributing associate degree programs. The concepts of wholism, persons as composites of the five Neuman Model interrelating variables, stressors and reactions to stress, wellness and illness on a continuum, and the three prevention as intervention modes become the vertical and horizontal threads of the curriculum content. Each program has developed course outlines and sequencing that they are willing to share with other schools upon request. All the programs focus primarily on the individual client and his or her reaction to stressors. The family is considered as the context within which the individual lives rather than the unit of care. Further, the client as community is not considered at the associate degree level. However, Cecil Community College reports that students conduct teaching projects for groups of individuals who receive care from community agencies based on the Neuman framework. Also, Athens Area Technical students have compiled a list of community resources for use by clients who attend clinics. The link between hospital and community is especially strong in the rural areas where these programs are located and where client knowledge about resources is scarce. The concept of hospital discharge planning, however, is strongly emphasized in all programs.

All programs have incorporated the spiritual variable into their assessment of clients. This is a unique characteristic of the Neuman Model compared to other nursing models, which subsume spirituality under sociocultural areas. The fact that spirituality is assessed as a distinct variable is appealing to the programs adopting the model. They state that considering spirituality as a specific entity provides a clearer focus for teaching the concepts of hope, grief, loss, death, and dying. Students are expected to assess the spiritual variable and to design interventions that buffer reactions to stressors.

The concept of created environment is introduced as one of the concepts of environment. The programs define the terminology, but none of the client assessment tools are designed to tease out the created environment of clients. This is a complex concept requiring greater sophistication and experience than demonstrated by basic students.

Differences among programs occur according to the emphasis placed on specific concepts. For example, most associate degree programs place emphasis on secondary and tertiary nursing interventions since students attain their clinical experience in acute and chronic care settings. Until recently, most graduates are initially employed in these settings as well. The Santa Fe Community College curriculum has given equal emphasis to primary prevention with the expectation that students will implement primary prevention strategies at all levels of caregiving. With the advent of shorter lengths of hospital stay and focus on discharge planning, there is a trend toward increased emphasis on primary prevention strategies. The Neuman Model provides a comprehensive approach to nursing care, applicable to all types of clients and all levels of wellness or illness. As associate degree programs now begin to increase emphasis on primary prevention, the model continues to remain relevant to changes occurring in the health care system.

CREATIVE MODEL APPLICATIONS

One of the advantages of the Neuman Systems Model is its flexibility in supporting the use of creative teaching strategies. In programs using the model the longest (7 to 14 years), faculty have become "professional" in understanding the model concepts, propositional statements, and guiding structure for the curriculum. To the degree faculty have internalized the model, experimentation with strategies that illustrate the dynamism of the model is forthcoming.

Indiana University–Purdue University Fort Wayne faculty share their orientation strategies for new faculty. They write that senior faculty are responsible for mentoring new faculty. This is accomplished by review of the literature, review of course materials that include the model, viewing the faculty-made video presentation about the model, and continuing discussions with senior faculty members. A more comprehensive internalization of the model increases over time through teaching students and receiving support from faculty peers. Responsibilities of new faculty in charge of courses include the orientation of part-time associate clinical faculty; thus the introduction and coverage of the model falls potentially to a new learner of the model (Beckman, Bruick-Sorge, and Boxley-Harges, 1993). What better way to truly learn than by becoming the teacher.

Yakima Community College has developed a gerontology course, one of the first of its kind in the United States, evolving from its use of the Neuman Systems Model. Evans (1993) writes,

> I believe I understand why the Model is particularly useful in the care of elders. Neuman's definition of developmental stage is left open to interpretation. This feature of openness that often occurs in the Neuman work permits evolution in thought and results in theory adaptability. Therefore, as gerontological nursing evolves from reliance on developmental stage theory toward the more fluid notion of person–environment dialectics, Neuman's work remains significant.

Common to both the Neuman Model and the dialectical study of change is the concept of reciprocal causality, that is, a nonlinear effect on each system variable by every other variable. Neuman concentrates on matching environmental stress and competence in order to achieve system stability. As we move beyond a basic understanding of a perfectly ordered, homeostatic world into a dialectical milieu in which change is the valued order of the day and asynchrony is a source of growth, we are able to accept contradiction and are better able to function more effectively by synthesizing a wealth of life experiences. Older persons, cognitively more mature and able to act upon and be acted upon by their environment, demonstrate this change and synthesis. The content of the gerontology course becomes more meaningful to students taught within the theoretically based Neuman Model conceptualization.

Beckman, Bruick-Sorge, and Boxley-Harges (1993) reports several creative teaching strategies using the model at the Indiana–Purdue Fort Wayne campus. The first selected example by Harges concerns the intraoperative component of the perioperative unit in a 100-level course. Focus for this classroom presentation is on use of client personal stressors to demonstrate application of the model with clients undergoing surgery (Figure 12–1). The method of teaching is interactive with student-directed participation. Students identify stressors and clarify whether or not each stressor is intra-, inter-, or extrapersonal in nature. As a stressor is identified, the lecturer defines how it impacts the client and which interventions may help to minimize the stressor. Surgical props are used to create the reality of the operating room. On the chalkboard, the client is represented as a stick figure with concentric circles. According to the potential degree of risk to the client's core structure, an arrow for each stressor is drawn penetrating the lines of defense and resistance. Through the use of stressors and pathology, preoperative measures and postoperative complications and potential risk factors can be effectively discussed and correlated. Students are challenged to identify appropriate nursing preventive interventions. The lecturer assists students in identifying both secondary and primary preventions. The lecturer also promotes active participation through positive and/or corrective feedback. By the end of this interactive session, students view all five variables and the wholism of the client during the intraoperative phase. Active discussion of both client and nurse perceptions is integrated throughout this activity.

The second selected example for these faculty concerns the student nurse case project presentation in the clinical component of a 200-level nursing course (Beckman and Bruick-Sorge, 1993). The project integrates model concepts and critical thinking skills with an actual case scenario of a client whom a student has cared for during the clinical experience. The student presents the case project in pre- or postconference. Specific criteria for assignment and evaluation are included in the course manual. Each student is required to submit a typed project content outline, nursing care plan, and bibliography. Students are encouraged to use multiple audiovisual aides to best make the project an effective teaching/learning experience for both the presenter and their peers in the clinical group. Self- and peer evaluations are an integral part of the assignment. The clinical faculty member role-models a previous student presentation utilizing the model as a framework to guide practice. Students are encouraged to be creative in their presentations; consequently, this activity has been successful in guiding students to view the model as having multiple possibilities for application of the nursing process.

Students from Athens Area Technical Institute develop family teaching plans

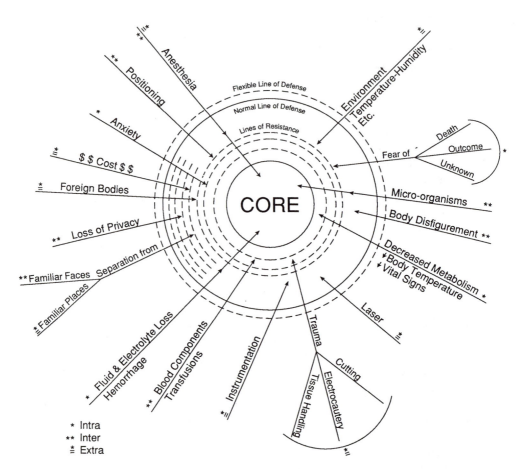

Figure 12–1 Intraoperative stressors based on Neuman as depicted by arrows impacting lines of defense and resistance of the client undergoing surgery. The arrows further indicate varying degrees of stressor penetration through lines of defense and resistance with the ultimate possibility of penetrating the core/basic structure energy resources. Potential or actual stressors are identified as intra-, inter-, or extrapersonal.

for various health promotion and care activities. This project was developed from student awareness of family needs when they were conducting pediatric assessments. The project was so successful that pediatric clinics have adopted the family teaching plan as part of their routine protocol.

Another unique aspect of the Athens program is an emphasis on student self-assessment during the first semester of the program. As each Neuman concept is introduced, students assess their own stressors and their physiological, psychological, sociocultural, developmental, and spiritual level of wellness. Various assessment inventories are used to elicit student data. Students reflect on how they have been cared for and how they care for others. They evaluate their support networks. By learning to assess themselves using the Neuman work, they become more sensitive to the needs of clients and the relevancy of using the Neuman Model. At graduation they measure their personal growth during the program by completing an instructor-developed instrument.

These unique examples are but a few successful learning strategies reported by programs for this chapter. As faculty increase their expertise in understanding and internalizing the model, to this degree students will be led to experience the "Aha" of new learning that fosters creativity and excitement to practice what they have learned within the classroom setting.

ARTICULATION TO HIGHER EDUCATION

Educational mobility between associate and baccalaureate degree nursing programs is imperative for advancement of the nursing profession and for individual nurses who strive to reach their highest potential. Several education articulation models have been developed within specific states that claim to maintain standards of excellence within each program, protect the integrity of each degree, and facilitate progression of students (Bowles, Lowry, and Turkletaub, 1987). The most successful articulation agreements occur between contiguous programs in which the upper division is able to build on knowledge gained in the lower division.

Two programs (Indiana–Purdue Fort Wayne and Cecil Community College) report that their successful articulation agreements between associate degree and baccalaureate programs stem from the foundation they provide in the concepts courses. Neuman Model concepts, supporting theories, and relational statements are the core of the concepts course. Baccalaureate programs tend to give more articulated credit to programs that demonstrate separate and distinct "concepts" courses. At Cecil Community College the philosophical conceptualization of client as a wholistic being, the understanding of stressors, reaction to stress, high-level or optimal wellness, and primary, secondary, and tertiary preventions as interventions provide the framework from which all curricular content flows throughout the curriculum. Not only is this educationally sound for the basic program but also for the baccalaureate program to which the student progresses. Further, when both associate and baccalaureate programs are based on the same nursing model, articulation is easier. For example, the Neuman-based baccalaureate program at Neuman College, Aston, Pennsylvania, articulates well with the associate program at Cecil Community College. Students can move from one program to the other knowing that the philosophy, model terminology, concepts, and definitions are the same. Students receive credit for former work and proceed to more in-depth study within the baccalaureate program. Graduates of the ADN program at Indiana–Purdue Fort Wayne enter the BS completion program with previous learning and practice of the model, which facilitates additional learning of this model as well as other selected nursing models presented in the first required nursing course, Concepts in Nursing, within the BS program.

ASSOCIATE DEGREE PROGRAM EVALUATION

Educators agree that evaluation is an important component of the educational process. Too often, however, it is given the least attention because of the difficulty in collecting and analyzing evaluative data. Programs based on nursing models could increase their credibility if they conducted studies to evaluate the efficacy of using models as conceptual frameworks.

A plethora of literature supports evaluation. Program evaluation is defined as a systematic collection of information in order to make decisions about the program (Bower, Line, and Denega, 1988). It encompasses all internal and external forces and constraints that impact a program and is a means for determining worth, effectiveness, and needed future direction. (Bevis and Watson, 1989).

The National League for Nursing through the accreditation process is the standard-setter for nursing education programs. Initial guidelines for their accreditation evaluation process compares program performance to predetermined standards to identify discrepancies. Originally, one standard explicitly stated that each program must be based on a philosophy or nursing model from which a conceptual framework could be developed for content organization. The latest criteria (1990) eliminated this standard.

The first associate degree Neuman-based program to develop an instrument to evaluate efficacy and use of the model in practice was Cecil Community College (Lowry and Jopp, 1989). Following validity and reliability testing, the Lowry-Jopp Neuman Model Evaluation Instrument (LJNMEI) was used to investigate perceptions of new graduates in relation to their internalization and use of the model in practice. A five-year longitudinal study of graduates of Cecil Community College was completed in 1990. The following questions were asked in the study:

1. Is there a significant difference within and between classes related to *internalization* of Neuman Model concepts at graduation and eight months after graduation?
2. Is there a significant difference within and between classes related to the *use* of the Neuman Model in practice at graduation and eight months after graduation?

It was hypothesized that there would be no difference either in graduates' internalization of Neuman Model concepts or in model usage within and between classes at graduation and over time. In other words, if graduates had internalized and used the model as students, they would continue to use it in practice.

The target population included all graduates from five classes (1985 through 1989), a total number of 128. The study sample numbered 104; 24 graduates who did not return the second questionnaire were dropped from the study. All but five subjects were female, ranging from ages 18 to 55. (Age did not significantly affect responses [Lowry, 1991].)

STUDY FINDINGS

All students (classes of 1985 to 1989) internalized well the major concepts of the Neuman Model as evidenced by mean scores ranging from 3 (most of the time) to 4 (always) both at graduation and eight months later. Students tended to be more consistent in their perceptions of client, nursing, and nursing process than in their perceptions of stressors and wellness. This could be due to their individual experiences with stress, health, and illness. T-tests of means within and between classes were not significant, indicating that there was no difference in perceptions over time. These findings lend support to the hypothesis that students internalize the model during the educational process and maintain their perceptions months after graduation.

More variation existed among classes in their use of the model through the four practice roles. For example, graduates from all classes used the model when providing client care sometimes or most of the time, both at graduation and eight months later. There was more variation among individual scores for the teacher and communicator roles, but no statistical difference before and after graduation.

Statistical differences did occur in responses to the last factor in section two, perceptions of how well colleagues in practice accepted and encouraged use of the model. At graduation three of the five classes responded that colleagues rarely encouraged model use. Two classes (1988 and 1989) indicated that sometimes colleagues encouraged its use. However, eight months after graduation, all classes claimed that colleagues rarely knew, accepted, or encouraged model use.

In summary, this study has demonstrated that associate degree graduates, educated within a Neuman-based curriculum, internalize the model concepts very well. Graduates use the model most of the time when fulfilling the roles of care provider and teacher. When students are socialized into a model, they tend to continue to practice from the model. Colleaguess in work settings tend to have a negative effect on the use of models.

Implications from this study are that nurses who are educated from a nursing model consciously assess and plan client care comprehensively. However, more communication and collaboration are needed between educators and agency nurse managers to enhance understanding of the value of nursing models and to encourage their use by nursing staff.

EVALUATION IN OTHER PROGRAMS

Santa Fe Community College and Athens Area Technical Institute have been developing evaluation instruments in relation to their own philosophies and program needs. Indiana–Purdue faculty made editorial revisions of the LJNM evaluation instrument and added six questions under a subheading entitled "Manager of Client Care." Alpha reliability and pilot tests were conducted with two classes of graduatess in 1993. Findings from the pilot study will enable the faculty to begin a longitudinal study with their graduates.

In addition to evaluating many aspects of their educational program, Athens Area Technical Institute also has developed for community agencies an evaluation of their program. They wish to know how well the nursing program has met community needs. This type of evaluation is innovative and will be critical in the future as the health care system changes and graduates from associate degree programs move into primary care areas.

FUTURE IMPLICATIONS FOR USE OF THE NEUMAN SYSTEMS MODEL AS AN ORGANIZING STRUCTURE FOR ADN PROGRAMS

We will now answer the rhetorical questions posed at the beginning of this chapter. First, associate degree graduates will need to know how to organize a large amount of assessment data and to critically analyze and synthesize the data into a meaningful whole. Second, the education of the associate degree nurse must expand its breadth. For example, primary prevention must be emphasized as much as secondary and tertiary prevention so that graduates will be better prepared to teach clients and families about health promotion and disease prevention. Neuman-based associate degree programs have demonstrated success in preparing graduates who practice in a wholistic and logically consistent manner. The model provides the structure wherein data can be organized and the preventions as interventions provide the processes for implementing care. The model's comprehensiveness includes all aspects of client care and permits educators to emphasize a selected nursing focus that is most needed by society at any given time.

Structured communication is imperative between education and service so that nurse managers can be made aware of the utility of nursing models and encourage staff to practice from a nursing model perspective. Graduates and faculty from Neuman-based programs are often invited to prepare in-service events that demonstrate use of the model for their colleagues in practice. Indiana—Purdue Fort Wayne faculty have very successfully set the standard for this type of involvement, collaborating with practice colleagues to demonstrate theory-based practice.

Articulation agreements with baccalaureate programs should emphasize the theoretical foundation provided by Neuman-based programs. Graduates report that having familiarity with one nursing model facilitates learning about other models in baccalaureate programs. Advancing from one Neuman-based program to another is the epitome of efficient and effective nursing education.

More research is needed from associate degree program faculty. Evaluation studies are critical to illustrate program and model strengths and weaknesses. The LJNM evaluation instrument (see Appendix A) provides a place to begin evaluation of the model as a framework for associate degree programs. The instrument can be revised and tested for continuing validity and reliability. Only through continuous evaluation will educators be able to keep programs dynamic and relevant to changing social needs. In its short history the Neuman Systems Model has proved to be very successfully used as a base for high-quality associate degree programming. The future is especially bright for continued Neuman Model usage in the 21st century within associate degree nursing education.

ACKNOWLEDGMENTS

The authors wish to thank the following faculty for sharing essential program information for the chapter.

Sarah J. Beckman, RN, MSN, Assistant Professor

Cheryl Bruick-Sorge, RN, MA, Assistant Professor

Sanna Boxley-Harges, RN, MA, Associate Professor
    Indiana University–Purdue University
    Fort Wayne, Indiana

Bronwynne Evans, RN, PhD, Assistant Professor and Clinical

Nurse Specialist
    Yakima Valley Community College, Yakima, Washington

Sue Johnson, RN, MSN, Professor and Director Cecil
    Community College
    North East, Maryland

Carole Rosales, RN, MS, Assistant Chairperson
    Health Sciences Department
    Los Angeles Valley College
    Van Nuys, California

Donna Forest, RN, MSN, Assistant Professor

Patricia Aylward, RN, MSN, Nursing Coordinator
    Santa Fe Community College
    Gainesville, Florida

Gloria Buck, MSN, Program Director

Grace Newsome, MSN, EdD, Educational Consultant
Athens Area Technical Institute
Athens, Georgia

REFERENCES

Beckman, S. T., Bruick-Sorge, C., and Harges, S. 1993. Summary of associate-degree program at Indiana University–Purdue University. Unpublished manuscript.

Bevis, E. M., and Watson, J. 1989. *Toward a Caring Curriculum: A New Pedagogy for Nursing.* (Pub #15–2278). New York: National League for Nursing.

Bower, D., Line, L., and Denega, D. 1988. *Evaluation Instruments in Nursing.* New York: National League for Nursing.

Bowles, J. G., Lowry, L. W., and Turkletaub, M. 1987. Background and trends related to nursing articulation in the United States. in *Collaboration for Articulation: RN to BSN,* edited by M. F. Rapson. New York: National League for Nursing.

Brady, L., and Netusil, A. 1988. A national study of nursing education's use of a model of program evaluation. *Journal of Nursing Education* 27:225–226.

Evans, B. 1993. Summary of associate degree program at Yakima Valley Community College. Unpublished manuscript.

Lowry, L. W. 1991. Perceptions of newly graduated RN's concerning internalization and application of the Neuman Systems Model. Unpublished raw data.

Lowry, L. W., and Green, G. H. 1989. Four Neuman-based associate degree nursing programs: Brief description and evaluation. In *The Neuman Systems Model,* 2d ed., edited by B. Neuman. Norwalk, Conn.: Appleton & Lange.

Lowry, L. W., and Jopp, M. C. 1989. An evaluation instrument for assessing an associate degree nursing curriculum based on the Neuman Systems Model. In *Conceptual Models for Nursing Practice,* 3d ed., edited by J. Riehl-Sisca. Norwalk, Conn.: Appleton & Lange.

National League for Nursing. 1990. *Educational Outcomes of Associate Degree Nursing Programs: Roles and Competencies.* (Pub #23–2348). New York: NLN.

National League for Nursing. 1991. *Criteria and Guidelines for the Evaluation of Associate Degree Programs in Nursing.* (Pub #23–2439). New York: NLN.

National League for Nursing. 1993. *A Vision for Nursing Education.* New York: NLN.

APPENDIX A ———————

Evaluation of the Neuman Systems Model

The following questionnaire was used by all graduates of the associate degree nursing program at Cecil Community College, North East, Maryland from 1985 through 1989. Graduates responded to the questionnaire three weeks before and eight months after graduation. Responses to the following statements assisted faculty in evaluating the Neuman Systems Model as a basis for their curriculum development.

The author invites readers to make further inquiry at the following address:

Lois W. Lowry, DNSc, RN
College of Nursing
University of South Florida
Tampa, FL 33612-4799

Instructions: Please circle the word that best describes your understanding of each numbered item.

	Section I:	Concepts of the Neuman Model			

A. Perception of Person

		0	1	2	3	4
		Never	*Rarely*	*Sometimes*	*Mostly*	*Always*
1.	I view persons as wholistic beings	*Never*	*Rarely*	*Sometimes*	*Mostly*	*Always*
2.	I assess persons as composites of the five variables (physiological, psychological, sociocultural, developmental, and spiritual)	*Never*	*Rarely*	*Sometimes*	*Mostly*	*Always*
3.	I relate to persons as open systems in dynamic interaction with the environment	*Never*	*Rarely*	*Sometimes*	*Mostly*	*Always*
4.	I consider persons as closed systems	*Never*	*Rarely*	*Sometimes*	*Mostly*	*Always*
5.	I consider persons as unique individuals, all of whom have a normal range of responses	*Never*	*Rarely*	*Sometimes*	*Mostly*	*Always*

		0 *Never*	1 *Rarely*	2 *Sometimes*	3 *Mostly*	4 *Always*
6.	I think of a person's normal range of responses as the normal line of defense	*Never*	*Rarely*	*Sometimes*	*Mostly*	*Always*
7.	I evaluate the client's potential for reconstitution	*Never*	*Rarely*	*Sometimes*	*Mostly*	*Always*
8.	I consider the interrelationships among the five variables when assessing the degree of an individual's reaction to stress	*Never*	*Rarely*	*Sometimes*	*Mostly*	*Always*

B. Perception of Stress/Stressors

1.	I assess stressors as internal and external stimuli that have the potential to cause disequilibrium or crises	*Never*	*Rarely*	*Somtimes*	*Mostly*	*Always*
2.	I categorize stressors as intrapersonal, extrapersonal, and interpersonal forces	*Never*	*Rarely*	*Somtimes*	*Mostly*	*Always*
3.	I evaluate the client's flexible line of defense, which acts as a protective buffer from stress	*Never*	*Rarely*	*Somtimes*	*Mostly*	*Always*
4.	I evaluate the stressors that affect a client's normal line of defense	*Never*	*Rarely*	*Somtimes*	*Mostly*	*Always*
5.	I identify the stressors that affect my client's condition	*Never*	*Rarely*	*Somtimes*	*Mostly*	*Always*
6.	I attempt to reduce the effect of stressors on the client	*Never*	*Rarely*	*Somtimes*	*Mostly*	*Always*
7.	I assess the processes of interaction and adjustment between the internal and external environments of persons	*Never*	*Rarely*	*Somtimes*	*Mostly*	*Always*

C. Perception of Wellness/Illness

1.	I assist individuals to become involved in planning their care to achieve the maximum state of wellness	*Never*	*Rarely*	*Sometimes*	*Mostly*	*Always*
2.	I view wellness/illness as a continuum between which individuals fluctuate	*Never*	*Rarely*	*Sometimes*	*Mostly*	*Always*
3.	I analyze illness in relation to the stressors that cause it	*Never*	*Rarely*	*Sometimes*	*Mostly*	*Always*
4.	I view clients as passive recipients of nursing care	*Never*	*Rarely*	*Sometimes*	*Mostly*	*Always*
5.	I assist clients to reconstitute from illness	*Never*	*Rarely*	*Sometimes*	*Mostly*	*Always*
6.	I view clients as active participants in their care	*Never*	*Rarely*	*Sometimes*	*Mostly*	*Always*
7.	I perceive illnesses as breakdowns of the lines of defense	*Never*	*Rarely*	*Sometimes*	*Mostly*	*Always*

D. Perception of Nursing

1.	I believe that the *primary* focus on nursing is to follow doctors' orders for treatments and medications	*Never*	*Rarely*	*Sometimes*	*Mostly*	*Always*

	0 Never	1 Rarely	2 Sometimes	3 Mostly	4 Always
2. As a nurse, I function to assist individuals, families, and groups to attain and maintain maximum wellness	Never	Rarely	Sometimes	Mostly	Always
3. When providing nursing care, I evaluate the relationships and reactions between clients and their environment	Never	Rarely	Sometimes	Mostly	Always
4. As a nurse, I prefer to provide care without assistance from the client	Never	Rarely	Sometimes	Mostly	Always
5. I function on the premise that the Neuman Model views persons as fragmented beings	Never	Rarely	Sometimes	Mostly	Always
6. As a nurse, I function to provide purposeful interventions aimed at reducing stress factors that interfere with optimal functioning	Never	Rarely	Sometimes	Mostly	Always
7. In my practice, I interpret the meaning of stress to clients so that appropriate interventions can be planned	Never	Rarely	Sometimes	Mostly	Always
8. I collaborate with clients to assess, plan, implement, and evaluate care	Never	Rarely	Sometimes	Mostly	Always
9. I attempt to involve my clients in planning of their care	Never	Rarely	Sometimes	Mostly	Always

In my experience to date, I have utilized:

10. Primary intervention	Never	Rarely	Sometimes	Mostly	Always
11. Secondary intervention	Never	Rarely	Sometimes	Mostly	Always
12. Tertiary intervention	Never	Rarely	Sometimes	Mostly	Always
13. I attempt to involve families/significant others in planning client care	Never	Rarely	Sometimes	Mostly	Always
14. I utilize the nursing process in my practice and/or further education	Never	Rarely	Sometimes	Mostly	Always

I utilize each step of the nursing process:

15. Assessment	Never	Rarely	Sometimes	Mostly	Always
16. Nursing diagnosis	Never	Rarely	Sometimes	Mostly	Always
17. Priority setting	Never	Rarely	Sometimes	Mostly	Always
18. Goal writing	Never	Rarely	Sometimes	Mostly	Always
19. Implementation	Never	Rarely	Sometimes	Mostly	Always
20. Evaluation	Never	Rarely	Sometimes	Mostly	Always
21. I encourage my clients to participate in goal setting	Never	Rarely	Sometimes	Mostly	Always
22. I function on the premise that nursing focuses on diagnosis and planned objectives for client care	Never	Rarely	Sometimes	Mostly	Always

Section II: Application of Model to Practice/Education

A. Provider of Care

1. Increases the probability that I will select care modalities from a wider range of relevant behaviors	Never	Rarely	Sometimes	Mostly	Always

		0	1	2	3	4
2.	Enables me to be more flexible when implementing care	Never	Rarely	Sometimes	Mostly	Always
3.	Enables me to develop new ideas/methods for application to clinical practice	Never	Rarely	Sometimes	Mostly	Always
4.	Increases my awareness for analysis and planning of nursing strategies when confronted with a new situation	Never	Rarely	Sometimes	Mostly	Always
5	Provides a consistent way of interpreting clinical situations	Never	Rarely	Sometimes	Mostly	Always

The Neuman Systems Model enables me to communicate effectively through:

6.	Nurses' notes	Never	Rarely	Sometimes	Mostly	Always
7.	Kardex	Never	Rarely	Sometimes	Mostly	Always
8.	Nursing care plan	Never	Rarely	Sometimes	Mostly	Always
9.	Nursing assessment/history	Never	Rarely	Sometimes	Mostly	Always

The Neuman Systems Model:

10.	Limits my creativity and flexibility	Never	Rarely	Sometimes	Mostly	Always
11.	Provides a basis for thinking ahead proactively rather than reactively	Never	Rarely	Sometimes	Mostly	Always
12.	Hinders my ability to function efficiently and effectively	Never	Rarely	Sometimes	Mostly	Always
13.	Serves as a checklist to encourage thoroughness in providing client care	Never	Rarely	Sometimes	Mostly	Always

The Neuman Systems Model enables me to improve my:

14.	Diagnostic skills	Never	Rarely	Sometimes	Mostly	Always
15	Observation skills	Never	Rarely	Sometimes	Mostly	Always
16.	Writing skills	Never	Rarely	Sometimes	Mostly	Always
17.	Performance skills	Never	Rarely	Sometimes	Mostly	Always
18.	The Neuman Systems Model makes no difference in my client care	Never	Rarely	Sometimes	Mostly	Always

I have utilized the following components of the Neuman Model:

19.	Person as a composite of five variables	Never	Rarely	Sometimes	Mostly	Always
20.	Subconcepts under the variables	Never	Rarely	Sometimes	Mostly	Always
21.	Stressors	Never	Rarely	Sometimes	Mostly	Always
22.	Degree of reaction	Never	Rarely	Sometimes	Mostly	Always
23.	Flexible lines of defense	Never	Rarely	Sometimes	Mostly	Always
24.	Normal line of defense	Never	Rarely	Sometimes	Mostly	Always
25.	Reconstitution	Never	Rarely	Sometimes	Mostly	Always

IIB1. Communicator/Teacher (Related to Client)

The Neuman Systems Model:

1.	Enables me to be consistent when mutually planning and implementing client care	Never	Rarely	Sometimes	Mostly	Always
2.	Hinders positive client responses	Never	Rarely	Sometimes	Mostly	Always
3.	Provides the structure for client teaching/learning activities	Never	Rarely	Sometimes	Mostly	Always

		0 *Never*	1 *Rarely*	2 *Sometimes*	3 *Mostly*	4 *Always*
4.	Makes my teaching plans more complex	*Never*	*Rarely*	*Sometimes*	*Mostly*	*Always*
5.	Promotes a positive client response to my nursing care	*Never*	*Rarely*	*Sometimes*	*Mostly*	*Always*

IIB2. Communicator/Teaching (Related to Self)

1.	The Neuman Systems Model provides structure for categorizing of new information	*Never*	*Rarely*	*Sometimes*	*Mostly*	*Always*

The Neuman Systems Model enables me in new learning environments to:

2.	Analyze	*Never*	*Rarely*	*Rarely*	*Mostly*	*Always*
3.	Synthesize	*Never*	*Rarely*	*Sometimes*	*Mostly*	*Always*

The Neuman Systems Model:

4.	Confuses my understanding of new information	*Never*	*Rarely*	*Sometimes*	*Mostly*	*Always*
5.	Makes no difference in my communication	*Never*	*Rarely*	*Sometimes*	*Mostly*	*Always*
6.	Increases my understanding of new information	*Never*	*Rarely*	*Sometimes*	*Mostly*	*Always*
7.	Makes a difference in my communication	*Never*	*Rarely*	*Sometimes*	*Mostly*	*Always*

IIC. Coordinator/Member of Discipline of Nursing

1.	I am able to articulate the Neuman concepts	*Never*	*Rarely*	*Sometimes*	*Mostly*	*Always*
2.	I feel comfortable sharing the Neuman Systems Model with my colleagues at work	*Never*	*Rarely*	*Sometimes*	*Mostly*	*Always*
3.	My colleagues encourage me to use the Neuman Model for planning and implementing client care	*Never*	*Rarely*	*Sometimes*	*Mostly*	*Always*
4.	My colleagues are using the Neuman Model in their clinical practice	*Never*	*Rarely*	*Sometimes*	*Mostly*	*Always*
5.	Nursing administration is aware that I am utilizing the Neuman Model	*Never*	*Rarely*	*Sometimes*	*Mostly*	*Always*
6.	Nursing administration encourages the use of the Neuman Model	*Never*	*Rarely*	*Sometimes*	*Mostly*	*Always*
7.	Utilization of the Neuman Model has enabled me to adapt to new responsibilities	*Never*	*Rarely*	*Sometimes*	*Mostly*	*Always*
8.	My colleagues discourage the use of the Neuman Model	*Never*	*Rarely*	*Sometimes*	*Mostly*	*Always*
9.	Is there anything else about the Neuman Model you would like to share? (Please describe any unique opportunities you have had to use the model.)					

10. What is your present position in the work setting?

Thank you very much for your contribution to this effort. If you would like a summary of the results, please print your name and address for future mailing.

Name: _____

Address: _____

_____

13

THE NEUMAN SYSTEMS MODEL IN CLINICAL EVALUATION OF STUDENTS

Victoria Strickland-Seng

In 1988 the Department of Nursing at The University of Tennessee initiated the process for change from an Associate of Arts (AA) program in nusring to a Bachelor of Science in Nursing (BSN) degree program in response to a regional need for baccalaureate education. In developing a framework for the program (see Appendix A), faculty decided to admit students to clinical nursing courses at the sophomore level and design a program with three levels (sophomore, junior, and senior). As faculty began working on the curriculum for the new program, they decided to select a single nursing model for the curriculum framework rather than continue with the eclectic approach used in the AA program. After careful study and discussion, the faculty determined that the Neuman Systems Model (NSM) corresponded best with the program's philosophy and began work on creating the new curriculum based on the NSM.

EVALUATION INSTRUMENTS

As a part of curriculum development the faculty determined the need to retain a nursing process-focused clinical evaluation package used in the AA program but to adapt it to include additional expectations for BSN graduates and the NSM. The instruments expanded from 20 to 24 items initially. One additional item was added following implementation of the evaluation package to bring the total number of items to 25.

The evaluation instruments used for evaluating student behavior in the clinical setting consist of a package including Clinical Evaluation, Summary of Clinical Evaluation, and Profile of Clinical Evaluation forms. All of the forms encompass 25 student behaviors and use a four-level rating scale consisting of Unsatisfactory (failing performance), Dependency (below expected performance), Satisfactory (expected performance), and Intradependency (optimal performance). Students receiving any Unsatisfactory ratings are not allowed to continue in the nursing program. Expectations for student performance increase as the student progresses through each of the three levels of the BSN program, so the number of Dependencies students can earn while receiving an overall Satisfactory rating in clinical lab decreases by one each semester from six in the first clinical nursing course to two for graduating seniors.

The first of the forms included in the evaluation instrument package, the Clinical Evaluation form, defines each of the four ratings for all 25 of the behaviors embodied by the instrument and grouped by a five-step nursing process. As students begin each level of the clinical program, they receive a copy of the Clinical Evaluation form for that level showing the progression of emphasis on the NSM concepts for that level. A sample of the ratings for one behavior at all three levels appears in Table 13–1.

At the end of each clinical nursing course for that level, faculty complete the Summary of Clinical Evaluation form indicating the rating for each of the 25 behaviors and providing anecdotal notes of observations influencing the selection of the ratings. The Summary form is reviewed by faculty and students and placed in the individual students' files as a part of their permanent records.

As faculty used the first two parts of the evaluation package, they recognized a need to communicate to other faculty documented areas of weaknesses to allow for follow-up during subsequent semesters. A Profile of Clinical Evaluation form was developed to provide an overall picture of each student's performance throughout the program. The Profile form is updated by faculty at the end of each semester and placed in the individual students' files.

Behavioral Definitions

The 25 specific behaviors evaluated are placed under the assessment, analysis, plan, intervention, and evaluation categories of the nursing process and defined in NSM terminology. Assessment includes three behaviors in the areas of therapeutic communication and knowledge of the client/client system. Analysis includes the two areas of problem identification and nursing diagnostic statement, each with one behavior defined. The plan section contains the areas of client/client system objectives with one behavior, nursing interventions with two behaviors, and scientific principles and rationale with one behavior. In the area of intervention, students are evaluated on individual/family/group care, individual/family/group education, therapeutic relationships, and personal responsibil-

TABLE 13–1. SAMPLE BEHAVIOR RATINGS BY LEVEL

Intradependency (Optimal)	Satisfactory (Expected)	Dependency (Below Expected)	Unsatisfactory (Failure)
Plan: Develops individualized plan of care with realistic objectives and goals.			
Level 1			
Develops individualized plan of care shared with the individual including specific information about the situation with realistic priorities, objectives, and optimal goals for physiological aspects.	Develops general plan of care shared with the individual including priorities, objectives, and optimal goals for the situation.	Develops plans of care using general standards for the given condition and/or diagnosis.	Identifies some measures of care needed by any individual without recognizing the priorities, objectives, and/or goals for the situation.
Level 2			
Develops individualized plan of care shared with the individual/family including specific information about the situation with realistic priorities, objectives, and optimal goals for physiological, psychological, sociocultural, and spiritual aspects.	Develops general plan of care shared with the individual/family including priorities, objectives, and optimal goals for the situation.	Develops plans of care using general standards for the given condition and/or diagnosis.	Identifies some measures of care needed by any individual/family without recognizing the priorities, objectives, and/or goals for the situation.
Level 3			
Develops individualized plan of care shared with the individual/family/group including specific information about the situation with realistic priorities, objectives, and optimal goals for physiological, psychological, sociocultural, developmental, and spiritual aspects.	Develops general plan of care shared with the individual/family/group including priorities, objectives, and optimal goals for the situation.	Develops plan of care using general standards for the given condition and/or diagnosis.	Identifies some measures of care needed by any individual/family/group without recognizing the priorities, objectives, and/or goals for the situation.

TABLE 13–2. COMPARISON OF AA BEHAVIORS WITH BSN BEHAVIORS USING NEUMAN TERMINOLOGY

AA Behaviors	BSN Behaviors Using Neuman Terminology
Assessment	**Assessment**
Interviewing Techniques	*Therapeutic Communication*
1. Communicates with patients using therapeutic technique and communicates pertinent information to health team.	1. Uses therapeutic communication to gather assessment data, reflecting knowledge of stressors and protecting confidentiality.
Knowledge of Patient	*Knowledge of Client/Client System*
1. Obtains comprehensive data base of patient's status.	1. Develops a comprehensive data base and organizes data reflecting synthesis of knowledge of interactions of variables and stressors.
2. Interprets patient's current status and significant changes.	2. Summarizes assessment information, identifying position on wellness–illness continuum and updating data as needed.
Analysis	**Analysis**
Problem Identification	*Problem Identification*
1. Based upon individual's norms and deviations, identifies existing and potential problems.	1. Clusters defining characteristics of variables, identifying actual or potential variances and resources.
2. Formulates nursing diagnoses, setting priorities.	*Nursing Diagnostic Statement*
	1. Formulates nursing diagnoses, setting priorities.
Plan	**Plan**
Patient Objectives	*Client/Client System Objectives*
1. Develops individualized plan of care with realistic patient objectives for nursing diagnoses.	1. Clusters defining characteristics of variables, identifying actual or potential variances and resources.
Nursing Activities	*Nursing Interventions*
1. Plans and identifies supplies for maintenance of functions to meet basic needs.	1. Plans care and identifies supplies needed for optimal health, incorporating the health care regime.
2. Organizes nursing and patient activities.	2. Organizes interventions, according to priorities, preferences, and health status to obtain objectives and goals.
Scientific Principles/Rationale	*Scientific Principles and Rationale*
1. Bases selection of nursing measures on scientific knowledge.	1. Uses scientific principles and rationales to select appropriate nursing measures for diagnoses and client/client system health status.

AA Behaviors	BSN Behaviors Using Neuman Terminology

Implementation

Patient Care

1. Performs comprehensive nursing care.

2. Safely performs therapeutic treatments for individual.

Intervention

Individual/Family/Group Care

1. Implements wholistic nursing actions as needed by client/client system.
[a]2. Implements nursing interventions according to expenditures and conservations of energy in reaction to stressors to promote optimal health.
3. Implements nursing interventions safely for client/client system's health status.

Patient Teaching

1. Provides therapeutic teaching/explanations.

Individual/Family/Group Education

1. Initiates education/reeducation using therapeutic teaching principles and knowledge of client/client system's health status.
[a]2. Selects mode of education based on client/client system's level of knowledge, variables, and energy expenditures to obtain optimal health.

Therapeutic Communication

1. Maintains therapeutic relationships.

Therapeutic Relationships

1. Uses therapeutic relationships, modifying interventions according to coping behaviors and interactions.

Personal Responsibilities

1. Demonstrates personal accountability and responsibility for quality patient care.
2. Follows appropriate policies for lab attendance and dress code.

Personal Responsibilities

1. Demonstrates accountability and responsibility for providing care.
2. Follows appropriate policies for lab attendance and dress code.
[a]3. Includes social, economic, ethical, and legal considerations in delivery of nursing interventions.

Evaluation

Health Team Communication

1. Documents use of nursing process.

2. Promptly documents significant data.

3. Reports significant data promptly and accurately to appropriate team members.

4. Interaction with peers and team members facilitates optimal patient care.

Evaluation

Health System Communications

1. Documents use of nursing process specific to client/client system.
2. Documents promptly and in sequence significant data and related interventions.
3. Reports significant data promptly and accurately to appropriate member of health care system.
4. Facilitates optimal care of client/client system(s) and cohesive work environment through interactions with peers and health care personnel.

TABLE 13-2. (continued)

AA Behaviors	BSN Behaviors Using Neuman Terminology
Patient Care Modifications	*Individual/Family/Group Modifications*
1. Modifies nursing care as indicated, based upon scientific principles/rationales.	a1. Elicits client/client system's perspectives on outcome of nursing interventions, validating feedback. a2. Identifies stability achieved, using scientific basis for interventions. 3. Modifies priorities and nursing interventions as needed to obtain optimal stability.

aIndicates behavior added to BSN evaluations.

ities. A total of nine behaviors are involved. The final area, evaluation, embodies health system communications and individual/family/group modifications with a total of seven behaviors. Table 13–2 provides samples that compare behaviors from the AA evaluations with behaviors in the BSN evaluations.

Relationship Between the Instruments and the NSM

In working with the NSM and placement of courses, the faculty decided that the entire model would be introduced in the first semester of the clinical nursing program, but that application of the model's concepts could be taught best in a progressive manner throughout the three levels of the program with different concepts receiving greater emphasis in certain courses of the program. For example, students in Level 1 of the program take foundations courses and focus on physiological aspects of nursing for individuals. In Level 2, the students continue to concentrate on physiological variables with clients experiencing acute and chronic illnesses but expand their learning to include emphasis on psychological, sociocultural, and spiritual variables in courses covering health assessment, pharmacology, and mental health nursing. They also enlarge the client concept to emphasize families. Senior students in Level 3 build on their earlier knowledge base as they incorporate developmental variables through family health and community health nursing courses and emphasize the client as individual, family, and/or group. The faculty acknowledged the importance of the Neuman wholistic view of the system; however, introduction of the NSM as a whole while practicing its application in a progressive manner has diminished anxiety and fostered confidence among the students. Table 13–3 shows the levels of emphasis used in the program to teach application of the NSM.

OUTCOMES OF IMPLEMENTATION OF THE INSTRUMENTS

Both students and faculty expressed positive viewpoints regarding utilization of the instruments and made suggestions for improvements.

TABLE 13–3. LEVELING OF CONCEPTS EMPHASIS

Concepts	Level 1	Level 2	Level 3
Person			
Basic Structures			
Individual	Individual	Individual	Individual
Family		Family	Family
Group			Group
Variables			
Physiological	Physiological	Psychological	Physiological
Psychological		Physiological	Psychological
Sociocultural		Sociocultural	Sociocultural
Developmental			Developmental
Spiritual			Spiritual
Environment			
Intrapersonal	Intrapersonal	Intrapersonal	Intrapersonal
Interpersonal	Interpersonal	Interpersonal	Interpersonal
Extrapersonal	Extrapersonal	Extrapersonal	Extrapersonal
Health			
Lines of Defense			
Normal	Normal	Normal	Normal
Flexible	Flexible	Flexible	Flexible
Lines of Resistance			
Nursing			
Modes of Prevention			
Primary	Primary	Primary	Primary
Secondary	Secondary	Secondary	Secondary
Tertiary		Tertiary	Tertiary

Student Responses

A review of the instrument is included at the beginning of clinical laboratory experiences for each level to highlight progression in application of the NSM. Sophomore students are particularly overwhelmed by the amount of detail when they first receive the 14-page instrument. As students become familiar with the instrument, they express a preference for the clear descriptions of acceptable and unacceptable behaviors included. The behavioral descriptions are also used as guides for clinical laboratory performance.

Use of NSM terminology in the instruments provides additional reinforcement of the model's application. By reviewing the behavioral descriptions, students are able to identify how the model can function in a clinical setting.

Utilization of the instruments for a variety of clinical experiences in hospitals, public health departments, home health agencies, and mental health centers further expands applications of the model.

The Profile of Clinical Evaluation form is popular with students. They enjoy watching their progress in clinical performance and take great pride in achieving higher ratings as they move through the program.

Faculty Responses

The evaluation instruments provide invaluable guidance to new faculty. The clear descriptions of student behaviors serve as guides for supervision and evaluation in the clinical laboratory setting. Faculty unfamiliar with the NSM are assisted in application of the model to clinical practice as they use the evaluation instruments.

Use of the instruments allows all faculty greater effectiveness in guiding the development of students as practitioners. The Profile of Clinical Evaluation ensures that students no longer reach the senior level with the same weaknesses identified in their early clinical laboratory experiences. Faculty can select clinical laboratory assignments that permit students to focus on behaviors that need improvement.

Revisions

Since implementation of the instruments in the BSN program, two revisions have occurred. The initial instrument package consisted only of the Clinical Evaluation and the Summary of Clinical Evaluation forms. As mentioned earlier, the need to follow the progress of students, particularly in areas where weaknesses were identified, prompted development of the Profile of Clinical Evaluation form.

The original BSN instruments contained 24 behaviors. A second revision resulted from a need to address student responsibilities related to social, economic, ethical, and legal considerations in the delivery of nursing interventions. A 25th behavior was added to the instrument. At that time faculty noted that with four ratings and 25 behaviors, numerical grades could be assigned easily if the need arose.

FUTURE IMPLICATIONS FOR USE OF THE NEUMAN SYSTEMS MODEL

The clinical evaluation instrument package incorporating the NSM holds a number of implications for the nursing profession now and in the future. The instruments currently foster application of the NSM to students' clinical practice by demonstrating specific situations and settings appropriate for use of the model. As students use the model in all of their clinical laboratory experiences, integration of the model into their knowledge base becomes enhanced.

Future implications and impacts encompass practice, research, and education. In the practice area, graduates of nursing programs using the evaluation instruments will naturally approach nursing practice with the NSM viewpoint. Adoption of the NSM by clinical agencies will be fostered by employment of an increased number of nurses familiar with the model as well as promotion of those nurses into management positions. Changes in nursing care incorporating the NSM should follow.

Research will benefit in a number of ways. Graduates from the BSN program focused on the NSM will use the model's perspective to guide practice. As employees the graduates will be involved in developing and conducting research within clinical agencies, thereby increasing the number of studies based on the model. The graduates who pursue master's and doctoral education may decide to usse the NSM in research because of their familiarity with the model.

Nursing education perhaps stands to gain the most from use of the instruments. Nursing curricula could be strengthened if clients, as students, are educated in programs that clearly define desired behaviors for students and provide a means for evaluating achievement of those behaviors. By demonstrating to students that the NSM can be applied to their clinical laboratory practice, students can learn to think critically with the NSM perspective.

SUMMARY

Clinical evaluation plays a major role in the education of students in nursing. Use of a clinical evaluation package that provides clear direction to students and faculty fosters effective development of the student as a practitioner. Relating the instruments to the NSM enhances application of the model to practice by students. The clinical evaluation instruments described in this chapter have critical implications to nursing practice, research, and education.

APPENDIX A ⎯⎯⎯⎯⎯⎯⎯⎯⎯

The University of Tennessee at Martin BSN Curriculum Plan

Freshman Year

Fall Semester

Biol 101 Principles of Biology (4)
Chem 121 General Chemistry (4)
Eng 111 English Composition (3)
Math 140 College Algebra & Elementary Functions (3)
Psych 210 General Psychology (3)

Spring Semester

Chem 122 General Chemistry (4)
Eng 112 English Composition (3)
Micro 251 General Bacteriology (4)
Nutr 100 Introduction to Nutrition (3)
Psych 220 Generall Psychology (3)

Sophomore Year

Fall Semester

Health 320 Advanced First Aid & CPR (3)
Nurs 211 Foundations in Nursing I (4)
Nurs 211 Concept & Theories in Nursing (3)
Zool 251 Human Physiology (4)
Elective[a] (3)

Spring Semester

CompSci 201 Intro to Computer Applications (3)
Nurs 231 Foundations in Nursing II (4)
Soc 202 Social Problems (3)
Zool 252 Human Physiology (4)
Elective[a] (3)

Junior Year

Fall Semester

Nurs 300 Pharmacology (3)
Nurs 311 Health Assessment (4)
Nurs 321 Acute Health Care Nursing (6)
Psych 313 Developmental Psychology (3)

Spring Semester

Nurs 331 Chronic Health Care Nursing (5)
Nurs 341 Mental Health Nursing (5)
Psych 315 Statistical Methods (3)
Elective[a] (3)

Senior Year

Fall Semester

Nurs 400 Family Health Nursing (7)
Nurs 421 Trends & Issues in Nursing (2)
Nurs 431 Community Health Nursing (5)
Elective[a] (3)

Spring Semester

Nurs 411 Advanced Health Care Nursing (4)
Nurs 441 Leadership & Management in
Nursing (5)
Nurs 451 Research in Nursing (3)
Elective[a] (3)

[a]Four of the electives must be selected from guidelines of specified courses and include 6 hours from humanities, 3 hours from multicultural, and 3 hours from communications courses.

14

THE NEUMAN SYSTEMS MODEL IN COOPERATIVE BACCALAUREATE NURSING EDUCATION
The Minnesota Intercollegiate Nursing Consortium Experience

Rita S. Glazebrook

In 1986 the College of St. Catherine, St. Paul; Gustavus Adolphus College, St. Peter; and St. Olaf College, Northfield, entered into a formal agreement to establish the Minnesota Intercollegiate Nursing Consortium. Over the next five years, the independent programs of three private, church-related, liberal arts, Phi Beta Kappa institutions in Minnesota developed and implemented a cooperative baccalaureate nursing program. These institutions, with a combined history of over 100 years in baccalaureate nursing education, used the Neuman Systems Model as the organizing framework for a new nursing curriculum (Mrkonich et al., 1989).

In 1991 the College of St. Catherine withdrew from this cooperative agreement in order to reestablish an independent nursing program. Gustavus Adolphus College and St. Olaf College reaffirmed their commitment to cooperative nursing education and continued as the Minnesota Intercollegiate Nursing Consortium (MINC). The change in consortium membership presented the continuing MINC faculty with the opportunity for reexamination of the philosophical foundations of the nursing program and evaluation of the utility of the Neuman Systems Model as the organizing framework for the curriculum.

After evaluation of the present curriculum, the faculty of the two ongoing MINC institutions made the decision to continue to utilize the Neuman Model. The development of a wholistic, systems-oriented, and futuristic educational program and practice model had been established, not only in the consortium, but elsewhere as reported in the literature. The model facilitated a client-oriented approach through emphasis on the continuous assessment of the client's perspective. The faculty believed the Neuman Model continued to demonstrate congruence with the program philosophy, applicability to all client systems, and opportunities for research in both educational and practice settings.

The Neuman view of the client was influential in the selection of courses that are prerequisite to the nursing major. These liberal arts courses were found to contribute positively to the student's understanding of client factors as described by Neuman. Since both colleges are coeducational liberal arts institutions of the church in the Lutheran tradition (ELCA), the spiritual dimension continued to be viewed as important and independent from, yet equivalent to, the physiological, psychological, developmental, and sociocultural dimensions (see Table 14–1).

Students were able to demonstrate the ability to use the nursing process effectively from a wholistic perspective. The identification of intra-, inter-, and extrapersonal stressors and the identification of the perceptions of both the client and the nurse facilitated the student's ability to view clients as dynamic and integral partners in the nurse–client relationship. The model facilitated the

TABLE 14–1. MINC PROGRAM REQUIREMENTS

Prerequisite College Course	Course Value
Biology: Anatomy & Physiology	2
Biology: Microbiology	1
Chemistry: Inorganic	1
Nutrition	1
Psychology: General	1
Psychology: Lifespan Development	1
Sociology: General or Marriage & Family	1
Total	8
Supporting Course	
Ethics	1
General College Requirement	
Religion	1–3[a]

[a] Varies by college

use of nursing interventions at all levels of prevention: primary, secondary, and tertiary.

The faculty of the continuing member colleges determined that only minor modifications of the existing MINC curriculum were desired. Course content was organized by the client systems of individual, family, and community and by client factors. This continued to give the curriculum a wholistic wellness orientation rather than a fragmented or illness focus. Additional considerations in course development included the availability of desired clinical learning opportunities and a progression of content from simple to complex, from general to specific, and from single to multiple stressors.

The nursing major continues to be comprised of a six-course sequence (10 course value) of upper division courses offered over four semesters. The first semester, or level one, consists of two courses with a three course value. Health Assessment and Nursing Concepts (two course value) introduces the student to the Neuman Model and to the concepts, processes, and skills basic to the curriculum and to nursing. The well person and the individual experiencing simple variances from wellness are introduced as the client system in Application of Nursing Concepts (one course value). Clinical experiences in long-term care and acute care facilities are provided. The nursing process is introduced with major emphasis placed on assessment skills.

In the second semester, or level two, one course with a two course value is offered that incorporates both theory and clinical experiences. In Alterations in Adult and Child Health, a wholistic perspective is maintained with the individual client across the life span as increasingly complex variances from wellness are explored. Major emphasis is placed on physiological and developmental factors, and clinical experiences are provided with adults and children. The process focus of the course encourages students to expand upon the knowledge and skill acquired in the previous courses. The major emphasis in the use of nursing process is data analysis and identification of a variety of appropriate nursing interventions.

Level three consists of one course with a two course value offered in the third semester of the major. In Family Health, the focus shifts to the family and community as client systems. The major emphasis is on family and community assessment, the childbearing family, and families experiencing variances in wellness. Clinical experiences are provided in both acute care facilities and the community. Major emphasis is placed on sociocultural factors. The application of the nursing process emphasizes use of nursing interventions at all levels of prevention.

The final semester of the major, level four, consists of two courses with a three course value. In Alterations in Mental Health (one course value), students focus on psychological variances, multiple stressors, and the concept of chronicity. The nursing profession as part of the health care system and the nursing profession studied from the perspective of intra-, inter-, and extrapersonal stressors are explored in Nursing in Complex Systems (two course value). The role of the

TABLE 14–2. MINC CURRICULUM

Junior Year—Fall Semester	Junior Year—Spring Semester
Nu 41/310—2 course value Health Assessment and Nursing Concepts Nu 42/320—1 course value Application of Nursing Concepts	Nu 45/330—2 course value Alterations in Adult and Child Health
Senior Year—Fall Semester	Senior Year—Spring Semester
Nu 93/350—2 course value Family Health	Nur 95/360—1 course value Alterations in Mental Health Nu 99/384—2 course value Nursing in Complex Systems

nurse as leader and manager is explored as students direct the care of a group of clients with multiple stressors and complex variances. The use of the nursing process emphasizes evaluation and replanning. Table 14–2 summarizes the MINC nursing curriculum.

Over time, MINC faculty have continued to engage in discourse regarding varying interpretations of the use of systems theory. Ongoing curriculum development has clarified the meaning and use of the Neuman Model, and faculty have continued to affirm their belief in the value of the model as a framework for the MINC curriculum.

With society's demand for health care reform and the increased attention placed on prevention activities to reduce health care costs, the nursing profession is faced with more opportunities than ever before in history. The Neuman Model has provided the consortium with a useful framework for organizing nursing content within courses and preparing professionals to deliver wholistic, client-centered nursing care. The model has assisted the MINC program to build a nursing curriculum that is logical, consistent with the program philosophy, and influenced by beliefs about learning and learners, and that prepares graduates for a future-oriented practice in a variety of settings.

REFERENCE

Mrkonich, D., Miller, M., and Hessian, M. 1989. Cooperative baccalaureate education: The Minnesota Intercollegiate Nursing Consortium. In *The Neuman Systems Model,* 2d. ed., by B. Neuman, 175–182. East Norwalk, Conn.: Appleton & Lange.

15

THE NEUMAN SYSTEMS MODEL AND PHYSICAL THERAPY EDUCATIONAL CURRICULA

Jane L. Toot
Beverly J. Schmoll

Physical therapy has become an increasingly complex health profession over the past 70 years.

> Physical therapists are key members of the health care team, whose education and clinical experience uniquely prepare them to manage care related to functional improvement to relieve pain and to prevent the onset of disease and functional disability. Through evaluation, diagnosis and individualized treatment programs, physical therapists both treat existing problems and provide preventive health care for people with a variety of needs.
>
> Physical therapist care, provided at the acute, rehabilitative, or preventive stages strives to achieve increased functional independence and decreased functional impairment. Through timely and appropriate intervention, the physical therapist frequently reduces the need for costlier forms of care such as surgery, as well as shortens the length of institutional stays. Physical therapists preventive care forestalls or prevents the development of functional deterioration and the need for more intense care through hospitalization or extended care facilities. (APTA, 1993)

Involvement of the physical therapist may occur in the acute care setting, rehabilitation center, extended care facility, sports medicine or private clinic, public health department, patient's home, hospice, industry, or school setting.

As the demands on the profession have become more extensive and the standards for practice have been elevated, educational programs have been subject to considerable revision. While physical therapy programs exhibit a variety of organizational designs, they generally choose to seek accreditation by the Commission on Accreditation in Physical Therapy Education (CAPTE). Physical therapists must graduate from an approved program and pass a state licensing examination in order to practice. At present, an approved program is defined as one accredited by CAPTE in all 50 states.

To bring the academic programs in line with the standards of practice, curricula have added courses in the areas of neurology, orthopedics, cardiac rehabilitation, administration, and geriatrics to name a few. The result has been an increasingly unwieldly content course curriculum model that presents students and faculty with an overwhelming amount of information. Although physical therapy educators have been careful to build curricula from the basic sciences to the clinical and from the simple disabling conditions to the more complex disease ramifications, a coherent wholism has been lacking.

Since the current approach to health care in general is to compartmentalize diagnosis and patient needs, it is not surprising to find a lack of evidence of wholism in physical therapy curricula. Indeed allied health professionals are described as (1) reactive to changes in medicine, (2) problem solvers for short-term problems, (3) learners after graduation to external certification, (4) communicators primarily within disciplines, and (5) owners of a hospital perspective of health care narrowly defined within one's own discipline (Bruhn, 1992). While this list is not typical of every health care professional, it does represent current practice for many. Indeed, Bruhn in the same article indicates what will characterize the future allied health professional. He describes allied health professionals as (1) critical, proactive thinkers who can choose appropriate solutions from a number of options, (2) managers who not only can foresee and avoid long-term problems but also have the skills to manage those that do arise, (3) lifelong learners who are internally motivated rather than externally driven, (4) communicators who can demonstrate an ability to work through discipline parameters, and finally, (5) leaders who understand the broad perspective of health. Of course, today it is possible to identify clinicians who demonstrate some or all of these qualities. There are too few clinicians, however, to assure consistent optimal and integrated health care. Bruhn (1992) contended that to bring about necessary change, educators of allied health care professionals should consider revision of curricula to focus on problem-based learning. He believes that this would force faculty and students to utilize systematic approaches toward patients and their needs.

The call for education to develop a clinician fitting Bruhn's description is reflected in recent publications. In 1991 and 1992 two extensive reports were developed to consider future trends, possibilities, and potential problems faced by health care. The contributors for these reports came from the health care professions; educational institutions, such as medical schools and colleges of allied health; and health administrators. The two reports—the Belmont Vision (1992) developed by the Institute for Alternative Futures and the PEW Report (1991) from the Pew Health Profession Commission—are thought-provoking, challenging, and to some audiences, controversial. Both reports, however, make it clear that wholistic approaches to health care education and practice will demand new alliances, increased accountability, cost-effectiveness, and increased awareness of the Gestalt of all involved entities. These documents reportedly allude to the need for the use of systems thinking when discussing education practice and administration relating to health care. The Pew Report (1991) emphasizes that the teaching/learning process should promote inquiry skills and the ability to handle large volumes of information. The need for developing skills to make informed decisions is overwhelming for traditional strategies based on content course models focusing on memorization.

Although these two reports are intriguing, they are not the first to advocate systems science when looking at health care practice and education. In 1973 Brody wrote an article based on the work of Lazlo (1972) in which he explored the complexities of studying man, health, and disease and urged the use of systems science. Brody drove his point further when he wrote of medical curricula that, while being redesigned to be better integrated, are still not understood within any coherent philosophical overview. The systems approach helps to provide that overview. It can complement current curricular design by examining in a wholistic manner the multilevel problems presented by patients.

The concepts of wholism, inquiry, and scientific approach are familiar to physical therapy. Many in this profession have written of these concepts in regard to physical therapy education and practice.

From a practitioner came a proposal to apply a wholistic health model to physical therapy (Gee, 1984). This model followed a definition of wholistic health as defined in Dorland's Medical Dictionary.

> A system of preventive medicine that takes into account the whole individual, his own responsibility for well-being and the total influences—social, psychological, environmental—that affect health.

The five principles included in the model were:

1. Self-responsibility for health
2. Prevention
3. Wellness
4. Looking at a whole person
5. Looking at illness as a learning experience

Several educators in physical therapy have presented problem-solving approaches utilizing disciplined inquiry to integrate information and to design treatment interventions. McKeough and Perry (1990), and Rothstein and Echternach (1986) recognized the need for the use of an organized methodology that relies not on rote memory but rather on a thoughtful analysis of presenting problems when dealing with complex patient needs. Jensen and Denton (1992) wrote on reflective thinking and included Davey's belief that the use of reflection in time of doubt leads to purposeful inquiry and problem solving.

Beissner (1992) described the use of concept mapping as a spatial learning strategy to aid in dealing with clinical problems. She depicted relationships between concepts with dotted lines. Maps are developed that help learners to mentally construct bridges between new information and prior knowledge by including concepts from prior knowledge on the map. Such a strategy does contribute to continuity in a curriculum.

Hislop (1978) presented physical therapy with a model using a structure ranging from cell to family in a hierarchical plot to analyze human structure and function in relation to physical therapy.

The scientific methods briefly noted indicate the direction in which physical therapy has been moving. Many in education and practice recognize the need for practitioners to consistently and thoughtfully address care interventions as complex issues. However, while Hislop's model could be identified as having the capability of isomorphism, there have been no efforts to incorporate general systems theory to physical therapy education, practice, and administration. Physical therapy educators need to heed the words of Marilyn Ferguson (1980):

> General Systems theory, a related modern concept (to wholism), says that each variable in any system interacts with the other variables so thoroughly that cause and effect cannot be separated. A single variable can be both cause and effect. Reality will not be still and it cannot be taken apart. You cannot understand a cell, a rat, a brain structure, a family, or a culture if you isolate it from its context. *Relationship is everything.*

This is true for physical therapy curricula. The profession of physical therapy, as any other health provider, cannot function in isolation. No profession can be effective unless it works in collaborative arrangement with clients and a multitude of colleagues. The complexities of health care delivery today demand interdisciplinary wholistic interventions. Accordingly, models must be provided for students through curricular designs: classroom, laboratory, and clinical instruction that demonstrate the role of physical therapy within health care and within society.

There are several directions one can take to apply a systems perspective to a professional curriculum/program. One can consider the structural resource aspect and analyze its position, organizational support system, and financial and human resources. Another aspect is to study the elements of the curriculum such as basic preparation, physical therapy theory and practice, and the role and contributions of physical therapy in the greater context of health care delivery.

Ideally, a curriculum is a dynamic entity that meets current and future needs of learners within a program of study. The concept of curriculum development is greater than the initial development of a curriculum. It encompasses the development, review, and revision of a curriculum. This multifaceted view of curriculum development is comprehensive and facilitates the dynamic nature of a curriculum. Physical therapy educators hold the challenge of designing a curriculum that is conceptually sound and capable of being responsive to changes within the profession, health care, and society while being solidly grounded in clinical practice. This challenge can best be met by assuming a "systems" perspective. An adaptation of the Neuman Systems Model (1989) can be used to ensure a dynamic physical therapy curriculum subject to a comprehensive review and revision process that leads to graduates of the curriculum being prepared for current and future physical therapy practice.

A SYSTEMS REVIEW OF A PHYSICAL THERAPY PROGRAM

Physical therapy curricula are reviewed as part of the accreditation process by evaluative criteria established by the Commission on Accreditation in Physical Therapy Education (CAPTE, 1990), which became effective in January 1992. Table 15–1 provides an overview of the components of evaluative criteria used for accreditation of physical therapy education. The Evaluative Criteria are organized into four sections in the accreditation documents. Section 1 focuses on the organization in which a physical therapy program of study resides. Section 2 focuses on resources—human and nonhuman—available to support a physical therapy program. Section 3 focuses on the curriculum. The curriculum evaluative criteria address liberal arts, basic and clinical sciences, clinical experiences, and research experiences. Section 4 addresses the performance of program graduates. The performance of graduates is assessed from the perspectives of patient care, delivery of physical therapy, and physical therapy in the context of health care and society. The Evaluative Criteria encompass a systems view of physical therapy education by virtue of the criteria and by identifying the intrasystems, intersystems, and extrasystems that have an impact on physical therapy education.

The Neuman Systems Model has been adapted in Figure 15–1 to depict Sections 1 and 2 of the CAPTE Evaluative Criteria, which address the organization and resources associated with a physical therapy program. The mission and philosophy of the curriculum are the core of the system. The lines of resistance include the curriculum, faculty, staff, and the students. The department represents the normal line of defense. The flexible lines of defense include the school or college within which the department resides, the institution, and the state higher education system within which the institution resides. This adaptation of the Neuman Systems Model highlights the subsystems that have impact on the department. The intrasystems reflect the relationships among the department,

TABLE 15–1. EVALUATIVE CRITERIA FOR ACCREDITATION OF EDUCATION PROGRAMS FOR THE PREPARATION OF PHYSICAL THERAPISTS (CAPTE, 1990)

Inputs	Section 1:	External environment—institute of higher education
	Section 2:	Internal environment—PT department resources
	Section 3:	Curriculum design
		• Mission/philosophy
		• Content
		• Liberal arts
		• Didactic PT (basic and clinical sciences, clinical experiences, research experiences)
		—Patient care
		—Delivery of PT
		—PT in context of health care and society
Process	{	Teaching/learning strategies
Outcomes & Evaluation	{Section 4:	Performance of program graduates

school or college, other schools or colleges, and the institution. The extrasystems include the system within which the institution exists and the broad scope of influences on physical therapy education.

Similarly, Figure 15–2 depicts Sections 3 and 4 of the Evaluative Criteria using an adaptation of the Neuman Model. The mission and philosophy of the curriculum are the core of this system. The lines of defense represent the components of the curriculum addressed in the evaluative criteria. The normal line of defense represents the curriculum in its totality and the performance of the graduates expected as an outcome of the curriculum. The flexible lines of defense are the institution and clinical facilities, both of which are essential for the implementation of the curriculum. The intrasystems are comprised of the normal line of defense, curriculum, and the lines of resistance. The intersystems are represented by the curriculum, institution, and clinical facilities. The extrasystems are comprised of a wide array of influences having impact on the implementation of a physical therapy curriculum.

The adaptation of the Neuman Model for the Evaluative Criteria used by CAPTE for accreditation of physical therapy education programs provides a graphic representation of the criteria from a systems perspective. This is extraordinarily useful for a program undergoing a self-study for either curriculum development or accreditation. Such a review done in the context of the subsystems—intra-, inter-, and extrasystems—provides insights into the strengths or weaknesses of a program. The model also helps in identifying strategies that are responsive to multiple layers of influence on the program and for targeting where in the system it is best to introduce strategies for change. Importantly, the systems view of the evaluative criteria we present emphasizes the role of a program's mission and philosophy. All aspects of curriculum development, review, and revision must center around the mission and philosophy of a curriculum.

A SYSTEMS REVIEW AND REVISION OF A CURRICULUM

The Neuman Model is also useful for designing and assessing curricular goals and sequencing of learning in a curriculum. Physical therapy curricula generally are constructed as a course of study with predetermined sequencing of learning activities. Curriculum designs vary widely with some focusing on subject

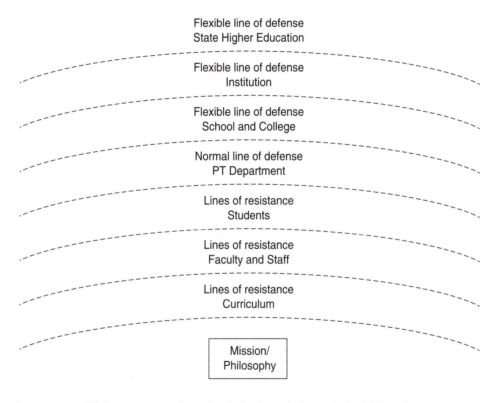

Intrasystems: PT department, students, faculty/staff, curriculum, mission/philosophy

Intersystems: PT department, school or college, other schools, colleges, institutions

Extrasystems: state higher education system, legislature, profession, health care, federal funding for research

Figure 15–1. Systems View of Organization and Resources: Evaluative Criteria for PT Education. *(Adapted from Neuman, 1989; Schmoll and Toot, 1993.)*

matter, while others focus on courses, problem solving, or experiential experiences. Regardless of a particular curriculum design, typically physical therapy
curricula are comprised of strands or threads of content that represent vertical
bands within a curriculum. For physical therapy the vertical bands commonly
are represented by major categories such as orthopedics or neurological aspects

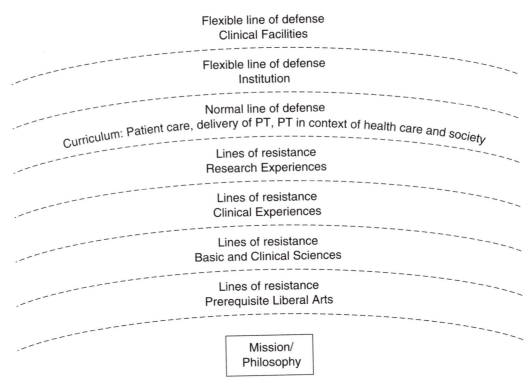

Intrasystems: curriculum, research experiences, clinical experiences, basic and clinical sciences,
prerequisite liberal arts

Intersystems: curriculum, institution, clinical facilities

Extrasystems: health care reimbursement, POPTS, utilization of students, profession, legislative
actions, federal funding for research

Figure 15–2. Systems View of Curriculum and Performance of
Program Graduates: Evaluative Criteria for PT Education. *(Adapted
from Neuman, 1989; Schmoll and Toot, 1993.)*

of physical therapy practice. Table 15–2 lists several vertical bands or major categories of content common in physical therapy curricula. The fabric of a curriculum is made whole by the horizontal threads or sequencing of learning activities across the curriculum that address the major bands or categories of content across time.

A useful concept for tracking the vertical and horizontal strands within a curriculum is that of an instructional unit (Schmoll, 1990). An instructional unit represents repeated inclusion of an instructional focus within a course or multiple courses within a given term or semester as well as within several courses or organized learning activities across a curriculum. The concept of the instructional unit enables faculty and students to track the introduction and sequencing of key concepts or instructional focus in a curriculum. Instructional units represent incremental demands for learner performance and can be expressed in terms of taxonomies for levels of cognitive, affective, and psychomotor behavior.

TRACKING CURRICULAR INSTRUCTIONAL UNITS

Although faculties devise numerous mechanisms for depicting their curricula and tracking the instructional units or vertical and horizontal threads within the curriculum, they are challenged when they must review their curricula in the context of evaluative criteria used for the purpose of accreditation. The tracking of key concepts or major categories within a curriculum does not necessarily ensure that the curriculum is sound from a systems perspective. That is, the curriculum may address several major categories of instructional focus, but they may not be addressed from a wholistic perspective.

An adaptation of the Neuman Systems Model has been devised for use by physical therapy faculty to aid in tracking instructional units and to determine if the units are addressed in the curriculum from a wholistic perspective while also being consistent with the CAPTE Evaluative Criteria. The matrix depicted in Table 15–3 can be used to review instructional units within a curriculum. The

TABLE 15–2. CATEGORIES OF CURRICULAR BANDS OF INSTRUCTIONAL UNITS

Orthopedics
Neurology
Pediatrics
Geriatrics
Cardiopulmonary
Wellness and health promotion
Motor learning
Research
Growth and development

TABLE 15–3. MATRIX FOR REVIEW OF CURRICULUM INSTRUCTIONAL UNITS

	Physiological	Psychological	Sociocultural	Spiritual	Developmental
Primary Level Research					
Clinical Education					
Basic/clinical science					
Pre-PT					
Secondary Level Research					
Clinical education					
Basic/clinical science					
Pre-PT					
Tertiary Level Research					
Clinical education					
Basic/clinical science					
Pre-PT					

vertical columns are adapted from the Neuman Model. The horizontal rows represent the CAPTE Evaluative Criteria. The major horizontal categories are the three categories of graduate performance addressed in the criteria. The categories represent three levels of intervention by a graduate. These are present levels of preparation that are akin to the levels of prevention in the Neuman Systems Model. The primary level is in the context of the health care system and society. The secondary level is in the context of the physical therapy delivery system. The tertiary level is patient care.

Each category of graduate performance has been uniformly subdivided into pre-PT, basic and clinical services, clinical education, and research. These represent four aspects of curricular instructional focus that are expected to be present in all physical therapy curricula.

Application of this systems model for curriculum development, review, or revision must begin with the mission of a program of study. Let us assume a mission statement for a physical therapy program of study includes the following key concepts:

- Graduates are prepared to assume roles within various practice patterns.
- Graduates are prepared to promote optimal health and function.
- Graduates are prepared to exercise professional judgement and clinical decision making.
- Graduates are prepared to serve as the entry point into the health care system.
- Graduates are prepared to serve in the roles of practitioner, teacher, and clinical researcher.
- The curriculum embraces a humanistic and wholistic philosophy and value system.
- The program of study strives to meet the needs of the community in which it serves.

The mission statement should provide the philosophical framework for a curriculum. The goals and design of a curriculum should emanate from the mission of the program.

Next, assume the faculty choose to review the instructional unit related to health promotion. The inclusion of an instructional unit on health promotion within the curriculum is both within the scope of physical therapy practice and consistent with the mission statement of this program of study. In addition, there are evaluative criteria for the accreditation of physical therapy education programs that relate to curricular attention to health promotion and wellness.

Evaluative criteria exist for all three levels of graduate performance: patient care, physical therapy delivery system, and the health care system and society. The specific evaluative criteria related to wellness and health promotion appear in Table 15–4.

Tracking the instructional unit for wellness and health promotion is depicted in Figure 15–3 in terms of its being the core of a basic structure and in relation to lines of defense, lines of resistance, a normal line of defense, and a flexible line of defense. This figure clearly shows the complexity of the curriculum and the significance of the subsystems for being able to effectively provide an instructional unit on wellness and health promotion within this curriculum. Such a system review can be useful when a faculty assesses the strengths and weaknesses of curriculum. In this case illustrated in Table 15–5, it becomes apparent through review of the instructional unit matrix that the efficacy of the instructional unit of wellness and health promotion within the curriculum is dependent on courses offered by other departments, schools, or colleges and thus will be influenced by the curricula of other departments, schools, or colleges.

TABLE 15-4. ACCREDITATION EVALUATIVE CRITERIA RELATED TO WELLNESS AND HEALTH PROMOTION

Patient Care

4.1.2. The program graduates are able to screen individuals to determine the need for physical therapy examination for referral to other health professionals by:
    4.1.2.1. Identifying potential health problems
    4.1.2.2. Recognizing patient problems that may require other professional attention in addition to that from a physical therapist
4.1.4. The program graduates design a comprehensive physical therapy plan of care that includes:
    4.1.4.4. Concepts of health maintenance and promotion and prevention of disease and disability

Physical Therapy Delivery System

4.2.5. The program graduates are able to plan and implement programs designed to promote and maintain health and wellness

The Health Care System and Society

4.3.2. The program graduates are able to participate in developing methods to meet the physical therapy needs of society

---

An application of the matrix to review the instructional unit of wellness and health promotion has been noted with each level of graduate performance.

Courses in the curriculum are plotted for each aspect of the curriculum appearing in the evaluative criteria in relation to five dimensions of curricular focus. The arrows indicate that a course addresses more than one dimension represented in the vertical columns. This provides a view of the instructional unit in relation to its fulfillment of the evaluative criteria and in relation to the scope of attention given to wellness and health promotion in this curriculum. It becomes readily apparent if an instructional unit receives attention at one or more subsystem levels and if this occurs from one or more instructional dimensions.

The matrix could also be built with course objectives, module titles, or other designations of instructional focus rather than course titles, depending on the design of a curriculum. Such a matrix can be readily adapted for use by any physical therapy curriculum. This is an important feature since there is considerable variation in the design of physical therapy curricula. The matrix is also useful for developing curricula or for review of curricula. Programs in a state of initial development can use this method or an appropriate variation to build a curriculum, or the method can be used with existing curricula whether or not they were designed using a systems perspective. With the matrix a faculty determines if various instructional units are addressed from a systems perspective that is comprehensive both in terms of evaluative criteria and in terms of dimensions the faculty has identified to be important.

PROJECTED USE OF THE NEUMAN SYSTEMS MODEL FOR CURRICULUM DEVELOPMENT

The present application of the Neuman Systems Model has been limited to physical therapy education in the context of accreditation evaluative criteria and the tracking of instructional units within a curriculum. Future adaptations of the

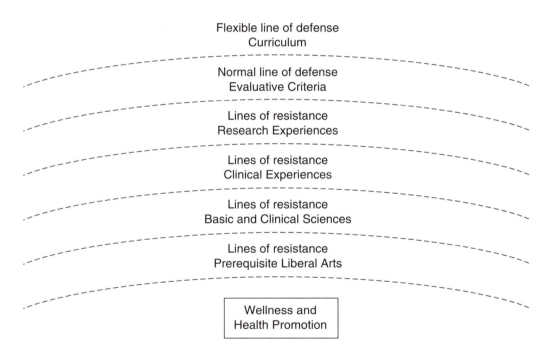

Intrasystems: instructional unit, prerequisite liberal arts, basic and clinical sciences, clinical experiences, research experiences, and specific evaluative criteria

Intersystems: achievement of evaluative criteria in context of entire curriculum

Extrasystems: PT department, school or college, other schools, colleges, institutions

Figure 15–3. Systems View of Tracking an Instructional Unit. *(Adapted from Neuman, 1989; Schmoll and Toot, 1993.)*

TABLE 15–5. MATRIX FOR REVIEW OF THE INSTRUCTIONAL UNIT ON WELLNESS AND HEALTH PROMOTION

Health Care System & Society Primary Level 4.3.2					
Research	Research Practicum→ → → → → → → → → → →				
Clinical education	Clinical Education II → → → → → → → → → → → →				
Basic/clinical science	Health Promotion & Wellness	→ → → →	Health Ed & Comm Resource → → →	Prof Orientation → → →	→ → →
Pre-PT				Ethics of Health Care	

PT Delivery System Secondary Level 4.2.5					
Research	Current Research in PT → → → → → → → → → → → →				
Clinical education	Clinical Correlations → → → → → → → → → → → → →				
Basic/clinical science	PT Mgmt Cplx Clin Problems	Found Teaching/Learning → → → → → → → →		→ → →	→ → → →
Pre-PT					

Patient Care Tertiary Level 4.1.2 & 4.1.4.4					
Research	Intro to Res				
Clinical education	Clinical Education I → → → → → → → → → → → → → → →				
Basic/clinical science	Anatomy Kinesiology Ther Ex III Eval Proc I Neuroanatomy Clin PT Exer Physio Dev & Mat T/O Life Stages →	→ → → →	Impact Phy Dis on Psych-Soc Dynamics I → → → →	Found of Teaching/ Learning → → →	→ → →	Clin Embryo → → → →
Pre-PT	4 Biology Courses	PSY 100 Social Sciences	SOC 100	Humanities	

Wellness and Health Promotion					
	Physiological	Psychological	Sociocultural	Spiritual	Developmental

model could span total curriculum review to more finite investigation of learner performance levels in relation to Bloom's Taxonomy.

It is intended to extend this effort to relate the curriculum development, review, and revision to total quality management. At a time when there is an emphasis on outcome performance and demonstrations of accountability, it will be highly useful to regard curricular activities in a context of internal and external influences. The relationship of faculty endeavors and the efficacy of a curriculum will be better identified.

Presenting Neuman's conceptual framework to students in their final year of the professional curriculum will initiate them to a systems approach that they can apply to clinical problems in each content area. Before this can be successful, extensive faculty education will be necessary. Bringing Neuman to the faculty through curricular review would provide the necessary foundations.

Students, faculty, and practitioners will benefit in the utilization of an isomorphic systems model not only to master content unique to physical therapy but also to understand the Gestalt of the provision of health care. Such knowledge is crucial as we come upon the crossroads of health care reform.

REFERENCES

American Physical Therapy Association. Recommendations for health care reforms. Position paper, January 1993.

Beissner, K. 1992. Use of concept mapping to improve problem solving. *Journal of Physical Therapy Education* 6(1):22–27.

Brody, H. 1973. The system view of man: Implications for medicine, science, and ethics. *Perspectives in Biology and Medicine* Autumn:71–92.

Bruhn, J. G. 1992. Problem-based learning: An approach toward reforming allied health education. *Journal of Allied Health* 21(3):161–174.

Commission on Accreditation of Physical Therapists. April 1990. Evaluative Criteria for Accreditation of Education Programs for Preparation of Physical Therapists.

Ferguson, M. 1980. *The Aquarian Conspiracy, Personal and Social Transformation in the 1980's*. Boston: Houghton Mifflin Co.

Gee, R. 1984. The physical therapist as a holistic health practitioner. *Clinical Management* 4(1):18–21.

Hislop, H. 1975. The not-so-impossible dream. *Physical Therapy* 55(10):1069–1080.

Institute for Alternative Futures. August 1992. *Healthy People in a Healthy World: The Belmont Vision for Health Care in America*. Alexandria, Virgo. The Institute for Alternative Futures.

Jensen, G., and Denton, B. 1992. Teaching physical therapy students to reflect: A suggestion for clinical education. *Journal of Physical Therapy Education* 6(1):22–27.

Lazlo, E. 1972. *The Systems View of the World: The Natural Philosophy of the New Development in the Sciences*. New York: Braziller.

McKeough, D. M., and Perry, J. 1990. A model for integrating patient-care positions of the curriculum. *Journal of Physical Therapy Education* Spring:41–44.

Neuman, B. 1989. *The Neuman Systems Model*. Norwalk, Conn.: Appleton & Lange.

Pew Health Profession Commission. October 1991. PEW Report.

Rothstein, J., and Echternach, J. 1986. Hypothesis-oriented algorithm for clinicians. *Physical Therapy* 66(9):1388–1394.

Schmoll, B., and Darnell, R. 1990. Incorporating clinical practice into education. *Physio Therapy Theory and Practice* 6(4):193–201.

Section III

Application of the Neuman Systems Model to Nursing Practice

16

COGNITIVE IMPAIRMENT
Use of the Neuman Systems Model

Patricia Chiverton
Jeanne C. Flannery

Our society is highly mechanized, stressful, fast-paced, and complex. Clients who are cognitively impaired are greatly limited in their ability to function in this type of society. Cognitive impairment affects both the young and old. It is estimated that there are more than 8.1 million head injuries in the United States every year, with more than one-fourth resulting in brain damage (Harmon, 1985). The number of elderly cognitively impaired clients is steadily growing. An estimated 1.5 million Americans suffer from severe dementia, and this number is expected to increase 60 percent by the year 2000 (Light and Lebowitz, 1989).

Nurses in all settings need to be better prepared to assess cognitive impairment and to develop interventions that assist clients to function at the highest possible level of independence. The Neuman Systems Model provides a framework to guide the assessment of cognitively impaired clients and to plan appropriate interventions to achieve optimal functioning.

RELATIONSHIP OF COGNITION TO THE NEUMAN MODEL

The Neuman Systems Model is a comprehensive, wholistic, and systemic approach to the client/client system. The importance of cognition is a component that has not previously been discussed in relation to the Neuman Model, yet it is crucial to the functioning of the client system. Cognition is defined as the organism's awareness of self and environment with a readiness to react and

Reviewed by Patricia Hinton Walker.

interact appropriately, through analysis of sensation and perception of the internal and external stimuli. Cognitive responses are wholistic and utilize judgment, learning, motor ability, and language skills, all of which depend upon interaction with memory (Brooks, 1984; Brown, 1977; Eliot, 1971; Goldstein and Ruthven, 1983).

The Client/Client System

In the Neuman Model, the client system is comprised of the basic structure, lines of resistance, normal line of defense, and flexible line of defense. In a cognitively impaired client all areas are affected.

Basic Structure. The basic structure is composed of factors common to all organisms. The client's cognitive function fits this description. Damage to the basic structure, such as a traumatic brain injury, may disrupt an individual's cognitive function for a period of time. Repeated assessments by the nurse provide data on which improvement can be evaluated. The importance of a baseline cognitive assessment is evident. In the case of gradually progressive or irreversible cognitive impairment, the assessment process becomes crucial to the development of nursing interventions.

Flexible Line of Defense. The flexible line of defense cannot function optimally in an individual who is cognitively impaired. As shown in Figure 16–1, this line acts as a buffer system for the client's stable state. The dynamism of the flexible line of defense is best illustrated in the following examples. A delirious client often experiences periods of lucidity alternating with periods of confusion (Lishman, 1978). During the lucid periods the line of defense expands away from the normal defense line, providing greater protection. Increased confusion causes the flexible line of defense to draw closer to the normal line of defense. In a client with a progressive dementia the flexible line of defense gradually draws closer to the normal line of defense. When the normal line of defense is penetrated, the client's symptoms increase.

Nursing interventions must be developed to strengthen the flexible line of defense and prevent or slow penetration of the normal line of defense. For example, the development of memory aids strengthens the client's ability to function in day-to-day activities and prevents penetration of the defense lines. The effectiveness of interventions must be continually assessed, and interventions must be revised based on the assessment.

Client Variables. Not only can cognitive impairment result in damage to the basic structure, but it may occur as a result of changes to client variables. Stress reduces cognitive ability (Fry, 1986). Psychological stress may disrupt a client's ego structure and result in changes in cognition. For example, the cognitive ability of a client experiencing a severe depression is often slowed, and thus the

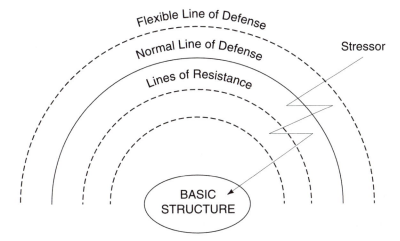

Figure 16–1. Cognitively impaired client system.

lines of defense may be weakened or ineffective. Physiological causes, such as metabolic imbalance or toxicity, can result in a delirium and affect cognitive function.

While spiritual belief and sociocultural variables do not directly impact on cognitive ability, there is an indirect relationship. A client's spiritual belief may provide the calming influence that enables him or her to function at a higher level. A client who is unable to draw from spiritual strength may not deal as effectively with the impairments. The sociocultural variable includes psychosocial resources, such as family support, that may strengthen the lines of defense and enhance functional ability. Cognitive changes related to the client variables cross all concentric circles shown in Figure 16–1.

Normal Line of Defense. The normal line of defense is weakened in clients with a cognitive impairment. This may be a gradual weakening over time, as in a client with a progressive dementia, or a sudden shift, such as following a traumatic brain injury. The extent of the change to the normal line of defense is influenced by other factors, such as coping patterns and support systems. The normal line of defense is dynamic over time; it varies with age and development.

Internal Lines of Resistance. The internal lines of resistance surround the basic structure and are activated following invasion of the normal line of defense by stressors. They protect the basic structure by controlling the degree of reaction. Cognitively impaired clients faced with stressors may have a greater initial reaction and may not rebound as quickly as cognitively intact individuals. This reaction is often seen when a patient with a dementing illness is hospitalized with an acute illness or injury. Additional stressors further deplete the internal lines of resistance and worsen the client's cognitive impairment.

The system's ability to reconstitute depends on the effectiveness of the lines of resistance in reversing the reaction to stressors. Ineffectiveness leads to energy depletion and death.

Environment

The environment of the client system refers to all internal or external factors, that is, all influences surrounding the client. In cognitively impaired individuals the environment plays a major role in the ability of the client system to function adequately to relearn information.

Internal Environment. The internal environment consists of forces contained within the boundaries of the client system. Intrapersonal factors are part of the internal environment. Clients who are cognitively impaired may or may not realize they are impaired. Severely impaired brain-injured clients are at first unresponsive to any stimuli, then later are responsive only to their own inner confusion. It may be months postinjury before they realize their loss. Early stage dementia clients may be aware of cognitive loss and become depressed, increasing the intrapersonal stress. As the cognitive impairment increases, the demented client becomes less interactive and more a closed system.

External Environment. The external environment plays a major role in the rehabilitation and functioning of cognitively impaired individuals. External exchanges are diminished in a client who is cognitively impaired. Stressors add to the impairment and increase isolation. This is often seen with demented clients who become isolated and withdrawn, fearful of participating due to increased memory loss. Another example is the brain-damaged individual who may become disinhibited and demonstrate hypersexual behavior. In this instance the client has no awareness of his or her behavior and must rely on the external environment to improve or correct the behavior. Environmental exchanges become crucial to the improvement of outcomes for the client or the client system.

Created Environment. According to Neuman (1989), the created environment is dynamic and represents the client's unconscious mobilization of all system variables, including the basic structure energy factors, toward system integration, stability, and integrity. It is inherently purposeful, though unconsciously developed, since its function is to offer a protective shield for system function. It encompasses both the internal and external environment.

However, cognitively impaired clients may not be able to develop unconsciously a created environment or an open system exchanging energy with both the internal and external environment. For example, the brain-injured client who has lost short-term memory function cannot process anything other than immediate stimuli and therefore cannot synthesize information. In this instance it is up to the care provider to assist the patient to maintain system integrity. Environmental factors can be used to assist the cognitively impaired client to function at the highest optimum level.

Cognitively impaired clients may not be able to adjust to reach a wellness state. The caregiver's role is to assist the client to conserve and use energy to preserve and enhance the client's functional level. The cognitively impaired client may be unaware of the created environment and its relation to health. Another missing component in the care of cognitively impaired individuals may be the interpersonal relationship that develops between client and care provider. Cognitively impaired clients may no longer recognize those individuals who provide for their well-being. Nurses must be aware of the stress this imparts to the family and/or care provider. They must also work with care providers to educate them and develop individualized plans of care based on cognitive assessment. The interpersonal factors may take such a toll on the client system, and caregivers may become so exhausted, that extrapersonal factors are not given adequate attention. Often family members become so absorbed with the client's problems that their jobs, health, and spirituality may suffer.

Health

Health is viewed as being on a continuum and dichotomous with illness. A client's health changes throughout the life span because of basic structural changes and adjustment to environmental stressors. In order to maintain a cognitively impaired client's "optimum system stability," other existing stressors must be reduced. Often additional stressors may result from unrealistic expectations from nurses and/or care providers. The client with a cognitive impairment may look physically healthy, and thus expectations may be too high. This results in additional energy use by the client with a resulting increase in impairment, as well as increased frustration and disappointment among caregivers.

Nursing

The focus of nursing is to maintain client system stability through accurate cognitive assessments and interventions. However, if this is to be accomplished, nurses must be able to accurately assess cognitive function. Although nurses routinely collect data, most nurses do not know how to interpret the data to make a cognitive level diagnosis. Without this formulation, the cognitively impaired client is unlikely to have prescribed a nursing care plan that promotes function at the highest level possible. The following example demonstrates the importance of a cognitive assessment.

> Barry S., age 19, who was attending a well-known university on a prized football scholarship obtained for his place-kicking ability, was doing well in his sophomore year. He had helped the team win the Conference, had maintained

a 3.5 GPA, and had been selected for the baseball team. His parents were very proud of their son's success. The family history went back to the pioneer days as farmers; they had always struggled to survive. Barry was the first of their family to attend college. Without the scholarship it would have been impossible. His parents were eager to sacrifice the help Barry would have been on the farm and even to accept not seeing him throughout the year, for he could not afford to fly home often.

Thus it was a tragedy on multiple levels when his parents were notified by the university hospital that Barry had been seriously injured. The family, including Barry's sister, drove to the university as soon as they were able to make arrangements. Their church helped raise money, and friends assisted with running the farm while they were gone.

Upon arrival, they found Barry barely responsive to intense stimuli but stable physiologically. When they inquired what had happened, the physician explained that Barry had been in the back of a truck with his teammates, going home from a party, when the truck veered to miss a dog, causing Barry to tumble out, striking his head on the concrete. He had received a diffuse brain injury that had left him comatose for 36 hours. He was now beginning to respond and was to be moved out of ICU to a regular room. The parents inquired when Barry would be well enough to return to school, and the physician informed them that he didn't know.

As the days passed and Barry seemed to improve little by little, it was easy for his parents to expect him to recover completely. When Barry deliberately struck his father with his foot, which had a heavy splint to prevent contractures and spasticity, Mr. S. was shocked. Mrs. S. attempted to reason with Barry, and her efforts only intensified Barry's agitation. He cursed, threw his food, ripped the sheet, and spoke as if he were hallucinating. He refused to obey requests to remain in bed and fell each time he got up because of his splint. He was placed in leather restraints and a posey vest and was sedated with intravenous medication around the clock.

Mrs. S. had to leave, since she could not bear to see her son treated like this. Mr. S. verbally attacked the physician and staff for allowing his son to get worse and threatened to remove Barry from their care. Barry's sister, Alice, who was 17, remained with Barry but could only cry hopelessly as she watched Barry tear at his restraints and act "like a crazy person." Secretly she assumed Barry must have been on drugs and was in withdrawal.

It was at this point that Laura, a nurse who was used to assessing clients who had alterations in cognitive functioning, was assigned as Barry's nurse. In Laura's initial assessment she discounted the Glasgow Coma Scale, for Barry had already reached the ceiling for that instrument. She then applied the Levels of Cognitive Functioning Assessment Scale (LOCFAS).

Laura, in her assessment of Barry, utilized the LOCFAS tool. This assessment tool is discussed in *Appendix A*. In order to help Barry, Laura needed to know to what extent the stressor had penetrated the basic structure to measure the degree of reaction. Secondary intervention with Barry was the first priority.

Relationship to Interventions

Primary Prevention. In the case of Barry's family, primary prevention did not occur. Primary prevention would have strengthened each family member's normal line of defense. Ideally, Barry's family should have received education and support from the nurse prior to their interactions with Barry. Since this did not occur, each family member experienced a weakening of their internal lines of resistance. When Laura began to work with Barry, she also instituted a secondary intervention with family members.

Secondary Prevention for the Client. Secondary prevention protects the basic structure by strengthening the internal lines of resistance. In the cognitively impaired client the goal is to treat the symptoms to achieve the highest level of function possible. Table 16–1 illustrates the progression of the nursing assessment process and the development of interventions for a cognitively impaired client utilizing the LOCFAS tool.

The continuation of the case example demonstrates the use of this assessment process to develop a nursing care plan for the client.

So it was that Laura, having observed Barry during her visits to his room, had checked the behaviors present on the LOCFAS, which showed the majority of his behaviors falling in Level IV.

With an understanding of where Barry was on the continuum of brain injury manifestations from injury to recovery, Laura began to coordinate a different plan of care with Barry's neurosurgeon and the treatment team, including Barry's parents and sister. First Laura explained, particularly to Barry's family, that the change from the quiet, frequently sleeping compliant state that Barry had been in just the day before to this violent, uncontrolled behavior, so foreign to Barry's behavior prior to the injury, was progress. He had progressed in his level of consciousness from occasional wakefulness in Level III to constant awareness in Level IV, even though he was not alert and oriented to his external environment. Laura described this stage as expected and self-limiting, to ease the fright of Barry's family and help them appreciate their responsibility at this time.

Laura then explained that with his severe short-term memory impairment Barry could not remember long enough even to get to the end of a sentence, let alone remember a command and explanation such as, "Don't pull on your catheter. That's to empty your bladder so that you won't get the bed wet."

Further, the agitation Barry was demonstrating, she explained, was resulting from his internal confusion, which he could not explain. Barry was not able to reason; therefore, when those around him provided him with elaborate rationales as to why he should or should not do something, his agitation only increased.

Since Barry was not oriented to place or time, he blended all memories of distant past, recent past, and present and could not be expected to be a reliable historian. In fact, if his conversation were intelligible, it would most cer-

TABLE 16–1. COGNITIVE ASSESSMENT AND INTERVENTIONS BASED ON LOCFAS LEVELS

LOCFAS Levels	Assessment	Interventions
Level I: Limited response to stimuli	• Elicit and document response to stimuli	• Prevent physiological complications • Prevent sensory deprivation • Stimulate to move to next level of recovery
Level II: Generalized response	• Assess for response to all sensory stimuli • Monitor pupil and eye movements in response to light • Orientation	• Reduce environmental distractions • Stand directly in front of client and remain calm and soothing in all interactions • Always explain actions
Level III: Localized responses	• Orientation • Memory deficits • Language ability	• Provide consistent reorientation • Explain purpose of any intervention • Allow extra response time because processing skills are slow
Level IV: Confused— agitated	• Behavioral status • Sleep/wake cycle • Orientation • Gross motor tasks (ability to perform self-care) • Language ability (ability to process information)	• Use safety precautions • Continue reorientation • Explain all actions • Decrease stimulation • Increase attention to external environment
Level V: Confused— inappropriate, nonagitated	• Orientation • Language ability—verbal, written • Memory deficits (ability to learn new information)	• Maintain constancy in environment • Provide memory aids (clock, calendar) • Reorient to condition (e.g., "You have a head injury") • Instruct with short, simple sentences

tainly be inappropriate. From his own created environment he would be likely to confabulate—create explanations—when he could not find the real answers.

Laura felt that a very important behavior to explain was Barry's aggression, which could cause harm to those who tried to control his activity, and his abusive language. Caretakers could easily be driven to anger when he refused to participate in self-care, even though physically he was capable. Barry was functioning on drives from basic needs and was without normal inhibitions. If his bladder is full, he will walk to the bathroom, but not to take a shower. If he is hungry he will eat, but will toss the tray if he wants sleep at that moment. No one should take personally any of Barry's behavior.

Since the restraints caused discomfort, particularly if Barry wished to turn over, get up, get a drink, or scratch his leg, he fought without rest to escape until he was exhausted. Not only did this inhibit his recovery through expenditure of excessive energy, but it added to his confusion, heightened his agitation, and could cause physical injury. Without the ability to attend to environmental stimuli as normal brain function directs, Barry used all of his momentary thought and will in such intensity that the probability of getting loose was high. Generally, because of such a danger, particularly on the night shift when staffing is less, Barry was likely to be prescribed a sedative. Of course, such medication reduces cognitive function, prolongs confusion, and delays recovery.

Secondary Interventions for the Family. The interventions that are required for families of cognitively impaired clients is shown in Figure 16–2.

When Laura explained the intrapersonal factors generating Barry's reaction to stressors, it automatically changed the effects of intrapersonal factors among his family and the caregivers on the unit. When the family's fear, anger, revulsion, confusion, suspicion, and inability to accept what they needed to deal with were alleviated, tension was reduced. The father no longer believed that the hospital personnel caused his son to get worse. Mrs. S. saw how important her role was in Barry's recovery and no longer found it difficult to be around him. Once the assessment was explained to all the staff, a plan was developed that, through collaboration, softened the effects of extrapersonal factors on Barry, such as confusing medications, restraints, unrealistic explanations, and sensory overload.

The plan that Laura, the team, and Barry's family created focused on what Barry could do, not what he could not do, thereby enhancing his strengths. Once the family was educated, they were able to be realistic in their expectations and reduce the stress on Barry. Tertiary prevention was also used to maintain the wellness of each family member. As a result of these interventions Barry's improvement occurred in a more timely and effective manner with a partnership between the family and health care providers.

FUTURE IMPLICATIONS FOR THE USE OF THE NEUMAN SYSTEMS MODEL

With the growing number of cognitively impaired individuals in our society, nurses must be taught the skills necessary to perform a cognitive assessment and

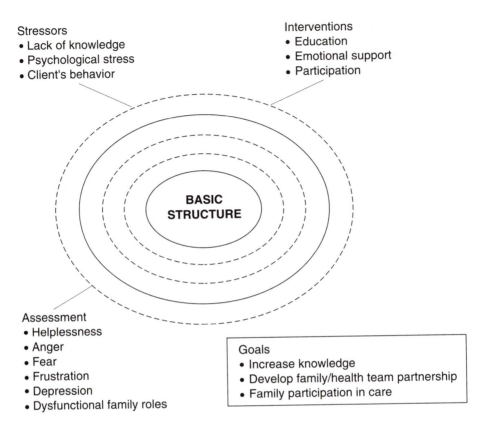

Figure 16–2. Client's family.

arrive at a nursing diagnosis. Curricular content in all nursing education programs must be examined and students prepared to complete cognitive evaluations in the practice setting.

Nursing must assume responsibility for providing theory-based rationale for interventions. The use of the Neuman Systems Model as the framework for studies will enhance the quality of care and provide for consumer satisfaction. In order to ensure that appropriate interventions are provided, tools such as the LOCFAS must be tested, and specific tools may need to be developed for specialty populations.

Nurses in all settings who are well trained in cognitive assessment and familiar with the Neuman Systems Model will be able to maximize the functional ability of their clients.

REFERENCES

Brooks, N. 1984. Cognitive deficits after head injury. In *Closed Head Injury: Psychological, Social and Family Consequences,* edited by N. Brooks, 43–73. New York: Oxford University Press.

Brown, J. 1977. *Mind, Brain, and Unconsciousness.* New York: Academic Press.

Eliot, J. ed. 1971. *Human Development and Cognitive Processes.* New York: Holt, Rinehart & Winston.

Fry, P. S. 1986. *Depression, Stress and Adaptations in the Elderly: Psychological Assessment and Intervention.* Rockville, Md.: Aspen Publications.

Goldstein, C., and Ruthven, L. 1983. *Rehabilitation of the Brain Damaged Adult.* New York: Plenum Press.

Hagan, C. 1982. Language-cognitive disorganization following a closed head injury: A conceptualization. In *Cognitive Rehabilitation: Conceptualization and Intervention,* edited by L. Drexler, 131–151. New York: Plenum Press.

Harmon, A. R., ed. 1985. *Critical Care Nursing Series: Nursing Care of the Adult Trauma Patient.* New York: John Wiley & Sons.

Light, E., and Lebowitz, B. 1989. *Alzheimer's Disease Treatment and Family Stress: Directions for Research.* DHHS Publication No. (ADM) 89–1569.

Lishman, W. A. 1980. *Organic Psychiatry: The Psychological Consequences of Cerebral Disorder.* Boston: Blackwell Scientific Publications.

Malkmus, D., Booth, J., and Kodimer, C. 1980. *Rehabilitation of the Head-Injured Adult: Comprehensive Cognitive Management.* Downey, Calif.: Professional Staff Association of Rancho Los Amigos Hospital, Inc.

Neuman, B., ed. 1980. *The Neuman Systems Model.* Norwalk, Conn.: Appleton & Lange, 10–40.

APPENDIX A

Levels of Cognitive Functioning Assessment Scale

The Levels of Cognitive Functioning Assessment Scale (LOCFAS) was developed by Jeanne Flannery, DNS, from the Rancho Los Amigos Levels of Cognitive Functioning (Malkmus, Booth, and Kodimer, 1980), using only Levels I through V of the eight original levels. The client at these lower levels of the scale cannot or will not participate in specific neuropsychological assessments or is an unpredictable or inefficient participant. When a client is functioning at Level V or higher, more sophisticated diagnostic batteries are appropriate for planning the details of the rehabilitation program (Hagen, 1982). However, knowledge of the client's cognitive functioning at or below Level V is critical for the development of appropriate care plans for ensuring optimal functioning.

DESCRIPTION OF THE INSTRUMENT

The Rancho Los Amigos Levels of Cognitive Functioning is a behavioral rating scale for assessment of cognitive functioning in adults with traumatic brain injury (TBI). It was developed by an interdisciplinary team based on their observations of 1,000 patients during recovery following TBI (Malkmus, Booth, and Kodimer, 1980). The tool provides a way of systematically describing and categorizing the patient's present level of cognitive functioning into one of eight levels. Malkmus et al. (1980) adopted Luria's model (1973), which postulates that changes in the patient's behavior will provide indices of changes in cognitive recovery. Subsequent studies have provided empirical support for these assumptions (Brooks, 1984; Craine, 1982; Eames and Wood, 1985; Lewin, Banton, and Grossman, 1982; Warren and Peck, 1984).

The Levels of Cognitive Functioning Assessment Scale (LOCFAS) was adapted and extended by this investigator from the Rancho Los Amigos Levels, using only Levels I through V of the eight original levels. These selected levels include behaviors more commonly seen in the earliest stages of recovery, when the TBI patient is more likely to be in an inpatient acute care setting.

On the LOCFAS a grid beside each behavior allows the nurse simply to make a check to indicate the presence of that behavior. Once completed, a summary grid allows the nurse to designate the cognitive level in which most behaviors were observed. This outcome reveals the patient's maximum capacity at the time of each observation. Repeated use of the instrument also provides a common interdisciplinary language to describe a patient's progress in recovery. More importantly, by identifying the patient's current level of cognitive functioning, the tool can serve as a basis for the development of an appropriate plan of care to facilitate cognitive recovery.

Initial psychometric data with the LOCFAS were reported by Flannery (in press). Construct and content validity were established by expert opinion. Three reliability studies were conducted using five written vignettes developed to request each of the five LOCFAS levels. Interrater reliability, with raters experienced in assessing cognitive functioning for care-planning purposes, was supported with high agreement among cognitive levels (coefficient Kappa = 1.00) and individual items (mean coefficient Kappa = .871). A second interrater reliability study with nurses who varied in educational preparation and neuroscience exposure yielded a mean coefficient Kappa of .98 among cognitive levels and .925 for individual items. Test–retest reliability yielded a mean coefficient Kappa of .991 for all levels.

The LOCFAS tool continues to be revised based on ongoing research. Further information about the instrument can be obtained from the investigator, Jeanne Flannery, RN, DNS, CNRN.

17

APPLYING THE NEUMAN SYSTEMS MODEL TO PSYCHIATRIC NURSING PRACTICE

Gail W. Stuart
Lore K. Wright

PARAMETERS OF PSYCHIATRIC NURSING PRACTICE

The nature of psychiatric nursing practice has changed greatly in the past decade in response to three recent trends in the mental health field. The first is the increasing number of individuals in this country who are experiencing mental illness, particularly severe mental illness. Other vulnerable groups also have pressing mental health needs, such as substance-exposed infants; children and adolescents with behavioral, developmental, and learning disabilities; women with depressive and anxiety disorders; individuals with substance-abuse problems; and elderly patients with psychiatric disorders. These and other population groups have increasing and often unmet needs for mental health promotion and psychiatric intervention. The second major trend is the shift in the mental health field to a more biological and neurochemical model of understanding and treating mental illness. For psychiatric nurses this requires a sophisticated understanding of biological and neurochemical processes and greater proficiency in rapidly emerging technology, while continuing to emphasize wholistic, biopsy-

Reviewed by Barbara Stambaugh, Jan Russell.

chosocial psychiatric nursing care. The third trend is the change in the organization and delivery of mental health services. Patients who are hospitalized for psychiatric treatment are more acutely ill and present the nursing staff with complex behavioral management problems. In addition, patients are often treated more aggressively due to a limited length of stay. At the same time, early discharge, changing reimbursement structures, and public sector initiatives are moving less acute mental health care into the community at a rapid pace, with increased emphasis being placed on the continuum and continuity of psychiatric care. Thus there are new demands and roles for psychiatric nurses in community health centers and home health agencies, and in clinical case management initiatives.

These trends present exciting opportunities for psychiatric nursing practice. They also suggest the need for psychiatric nurses to have an organizing conceptual framework that reflects current knowledge about the etiology, nature, and course of psychiatric illness, as well as the types of nursing interventions that will be associated with positive outcomes for individuals and their families. The Neuman Systems Model (1989) presents a nursing process format that can be used by psychiatric nurses as a conceptual map to describe, guide, and study the components of contemporary psychiatric nursing practice.

A foundational concept of the Neuman Model is the understanding that health and illness occur on a continuum. This is an essential concept since psychiatric nurses also view behavior on a continuum from healthy, adaptive responses to unhealthy, maladaptive responses. Psychiatric illness is seen as multicausal and contributed to by genetic vulnerability, physiological stressors, developmental events, and psychosocial stressors (Stuart and Sundeen, 1991). Thus all persons are vulnerable to mental illness and may react to stress with maladaptive behaviors.

Psychiatric nurses also recognize that one's highest level of wellness is rarely reached, and plateaus occur as individuals aspire to reach their optimal level of wellness. Neuman defines optimal wellness as a state when system needs are met. While this concept of homeostasis is highly relevant at the cellular level, a more dynamic view is required when talking about mental well-being. For example, a prolonged state where all of a person's needs are met may lead to inertia and apathy. Individuals may express this as boredom, and health professionals may label it as "lack of motivation" to change. But motivation arises from recognizing unmet needs, specifying desired outcomes, and setting realistic goals. Thus it is important to recognize that unmet needs provide the energy for an individual to strive toward a goal or an ideal, and it is this striving, with incremental experiences of success, that creates a sense of mental well-being (Wright, 1993). In contrast, repeated and multiple experiences of failure and self-defeating and unrealistic thinking deplete energy and propel individuals towards the illness end of the continuum (Ellis, 1987).

Also inherent in this conceptualization is the notion that mental health and illness are subjectively experienced and always in flux. This dynamic view of mental health and illness addresses Fawcett's (1989) recommendation that health and illness in the Neuman Model be viewed as polar ends of the continuum and not as dichotomous conditions. Death, or entropy in the Neuman Model, has to be acknowledged, but as long as a person is alive, neither health nor illness ever reach the polar end points.

Finally, all of the components of the nursing process—assessment, diagnosis, planning, implementation, and evaluation—are represented in the Neuman Model, and thus it presents an integrated and wholistic framework for guiding psychiatric nursing practice, regardless of setting (Herrick and Goodykoontz, 1989; Herrick et al., 1992; Moore and Munro, 1990; Mynatt and O'Brien, 1993).

PSYCHIATRIC NURSING ASSESSMENT

When a psychiatric nurse meets an individual, the initial assessment focuses on two critical concepts identified in the Neuman Model: the person's basic structure, and known, unknown, and universal stressors. While each person is unique, the nurse needs to assess the various predisposing factors contained within the individual's basic or core structure. These predisposing elements are conditioning factors that influence both the type and amount of resources the person can elicit to handle stress (Stuart and Sundeen, 1991). From the perspective of psychiatric care, biological predispositions include genetic background and family history of physical and psychiatric illness, nutritional status, biological sensitivities, general health status, exposure to toxins, and comorbid medical conditions. Psychological factors include intelligence, verbal skills, morale, personality, past experiences, self-concept, motivation, and sense of mastery over one's own fate. Sociocultural characteristics include age, education, income, occupation, cultural background, religious beliefs, and level of social integration or relatedness. Together these factors provide the psychiatric nurse with important information about vulnerabilities and risk factors and have implications for deciding among various treatment modalities.

Neuman classifies stressors as known or possibilities. Known precipitating stressors can be directly linked to presenting problems, which require excess energy and produce a state of tension within the individual (Stuart and Sundeen, 1991). Neuman suggests that it is useful to think about stressors as occurring at three levels: the intrapersonal, interpersonal, and extrapersonal. For example, an individual's chronic back pain can be a biological, intrapersonal stressor located in the client's endowed structure. If the pain leads to loss of self-esteem, it then becomes a psychological and interpersonal stressor. If the pain leads to loss of a significant relationship or a job, it may then represent a sociocultural or extrapersonal stressor. In addition to assessing the nature and origin of the stressor, psychiatric nurses should also assess the timing and the number of the stressors, because vulnerability to psychiatric illness increases when stressors are more frequent, enduring, and intense.

A critical question for the psychiatric nurse's assessment of an individual is: How do these known or potential stressors affect the client? In the Neuman Model this is assessed by noting the client's "reaction to stressors." Several protective systems surround the basic structure. These are the flexible line of defense, a normal line of defense, and lines of resistance. All lines of defense have within them five key variables related to the client's functioning: physiological, psychological, sociocultural, developmental, and spiritual. These variables are consistent with the multicausal nature of psychiatric illness and are useful constructs for the psychiatric nurse.

In the Neuman Model the "flexible line of defense" acts as a buffer system. It is accordion-like in function and can expand away from the "normal line of defense," thus providing more protection, or it can draw closer and provide less protection. For psychiatric nurses the flexible line of defense can be thought of in two ways—as the client's appraisal of the stressor and as the range of available coping resources (Stuart and Sundeen, 1991).

An individual's appraisal of a stressor refers to the processing and comprehension of the stressful situation that takes place on the cognitive, affective, physiological, behavioral, and social levels. It is an evaluation of the significance of the event for one's well-being. The stressor assumes its meaning, intensity, and importance by the unique interpretation and affective significance assigned to it by the person at risk (Lazarus and Folkman, 1984). It is important, therefore, for the psychiatric nurse to assess an individual's perception of the stressor or event because it is the psychological key to understanding a person's coping efforts and the nature and intensity of the stress response. Too often nurses and other health care providers assume they know the meaning of an event or stressor for an individual and fail to ascertain the client's perception of the situation. These unvalidated assumptions jeopardize subsequent mutual treatment planning and future goal attainment.

Assessing coping resources, options, or strategies is also important, since the more resources a client has, the more protection there will be against stress. Examples of coping resources include social support, material resources, strong ego identity, cultural stability, constitutional strengths, positive beliefs, and problem-solving and social skills (Antonovsky, 1979; Kadner, 1989; Mechanic, 1977; Lazarus and Folkman, 1984). Coping resources are a critical concept in psychiatric nursing practice, since nurses are the only mental health professionals who routinely assess individuals' and families' strengths, in addition to the presenting problems. For example, the nurse assessing a client whose stressor was the loss of a significant relationship would ask: "What makes it better for you?" "What other people can support you at this time?" "What else have you tried?" "What has worked for you in similar situations in the past?" If the client answers "working longer hours, tackling projects around the house, and doing more volunteer work so that I don't have to think about it," the nurse would interpret these behaviors as the client's effort to expand the flexible line of defense. The nurse would then assess whether the flexible line of defense is effective or if it needs strengthening.

The "normal line of defense" in the Neuman Model represents the usual wellness or the state to which the client has evolved over time. The normal line of defense protects the innermost "lines of resistance." The normal line of defense is invaded when the flexible line of defense is unable to buffer stressors. In the example cited above, the client may continue to be involved in volunteer activities claiming "they need me," but if these behavioral responses have not been effective in dealing with the loss, the client may report crying spells, feelings of worthlessness, sleeplessness, loss of appetite, and inability to concentrate at work (behaviors associated with depression). Such changes in one's normal level of wellness activate the "lines of resistance," which in turn protect system integrity by supporting the client's basic structure as well as the normal line of defense. Neuman cites the activation of the body's immune system in response to insult as an example of this idea.

Environment is the final key concept in the nurse's assessment, and it is important to the formulation of nursing diagnoses. Neuman broadly defines environment as including all internal and external factors surrounding the client system, and she proposes that the client and environment are in reciprocal relationship. More recently, Neuman (1990) has coined the term "created environment," a concept that represents the client's unconscious mobilization of all system variables. It encompasses both external and internal environments but may not necessarily represent the actual environment or "reality" as perceived by others. The created environment's function is to offer a protective shield for system function. Neuman further proposes that it is spontaneously created and that it increases or decreases as warranted by the client's needs. Importantly, however, this protection binds and uses energy, thus making less energy available for other system needs.

From a slightly different perspective, psychiatric nurses can view the created environment more wholistically as the psychological and sociocultural components of an individual's "lines of resistance." Specifically, this component of Neuman's Model is assessed in the three main types of coping mechanisms used by individuals experiencing stress (Stuart and Sundeen, 1991). The first type, problem-focused coping mechanisms, involves tasks and direct efforts to cope with the threat itself, such as through negotiating, confrontation, and seeking advice. Cognitively focused coping mechanisms are attempts to control the meaning of the problem and thus neutralize it. Examples include positive comparisons, selective ignorance, substitution of rewards, and the devaluation of desired objects. The third type of coping mechanisms are intrapsychic and emotion-focused. They are also referred to as ego defense mechanisms. For example, a client's denial or "blocking" of hurtful events can be interpreted as activating emotion-focused lines of resistance to block further trauma. Thus Neuman's examples of a client's created environment (the use of denial, rigidity, continuation of earlier developmental patterns, requiring a certain amount of social space, and sustaining hope) can more precisely be conceptualized as the psychological and sociocultural variables considered by the psychiatric nurse when assessing the degree to which lines of resistance have been activated and their capacity for protecting system homeostasis.

Finally, lines of resistance and associated coping mechanisms may be constructive (moving the system toward evolution) or destructive (moving the system to entropy). They can be considered constructive when the individual accepts the challenge to resolve the problem and acquires control over the stressor. Destructive coping mechanisms use evasion instead of resolution and impede the individual's progress toward restoring equilibrium and regaining health. The psychiatric nurse should thus assess five specific areas related to a client's normal lines of defense and lines of resistance, or coping mechanisms:

1. The types of mechanism and behavior exhibited
2. The frequency with which they are used
3. The degree to which they promote health
4. How much more (or less) is needed for protection
5. The reason the individual is using them

This will require that the psychiatric nurse observe clusters of response patterns, use intuition, display empathy, and validate all inferences. In the example previously cited involving the client's loss of a significant relationship, the nurse might infer that the client is coping with the intense emotional pain that would be felt when thinking about the loss by functioning as an "indispensable volunteer." This client may not yet be ready to deal with the pain and may require additional protection and new experiences to feel safe.

In summary, the application of the Neuman Systems Model to psychiatric nursing practice suggests a number of areas that should be included in a psychiatric nursing assessment. These include the individual's basic structure or predisposing factors; precipitating and possible stressors; the flexible line of defense, characterized by the client's appraisal of the stressor and coping resources; and the individual's lines of resistance, or coping mechanisms, which ideally maintain the normal line of defense and preserve system integrity.

PSYCHIATRIC NURSING DIAGNOSIS

A client's basic or core structure, the duration or time of encounter with the stressor, and one's resistance to it all influence the degree of reaction to the stressor. Thus the conceptual flow of Neuman's Model from assessment to psychiatric nursing diagnoses becomes apparent. Reactions in the Neuman Model are congruent with the definition of nursing diagnoses—responses to actual or potential stress. Psychiatric nursing diagnoses identify problems that may be overt, covert, existing, or potential, and the psychiatric nurse assumes responsibility for therapeutic decisions regarding the client's health responses. The diagnosis of these reactions or responses is always specific to the individual, and NANDA nursing diagnoses should be used to complement DSM-III-R (American Psychiatric Association, 1987) diagnoses in a psychiatric setting. The important point here is that nursing diagnoses complement DSM-III-R diagnoses; they are not contingent upon them. Neither should DSM-III-R diagnoses or medical models be substituted for nursing models of care. It is particularly important for psychiatric nurses to practice from a nursing conceptual framework and utilize nursing diagnoses, rather than to base their practice solely on a medical model of psychiatric care and its diagnostic classification system. It is only by identifying the phenomena of concern to nursing that psychiatric nurses will be able to articulate their role, prescribe nursing orders, and implement nursing care in true collaboration with other mental health professionals.

PLANNING AND IMPLEMENTING PSYCHIATRIC NURSING INTERVENTIONS

Accurate and in-depth assessments form the basis for planning and implementing psychiatric nursing care. In acute care situations, with individuals exhibiting severely maladaptive responses, management of life-threatening behavior is the immediate priority. For example, a client with self-inflicted burns and slashed wrists alerts the nurse that lines of resistance have been penetrated and that immediate intervention is necessary to restore system integrity. Initial assessment data will thus be focused on safety issues, with other information being obtained once the individual is safe from immediate harm. In nonacute situations, psychiatric nurses can complete assessments of their clients' stressors and level of response. Planning and implementation activities flow naturally from this knowledge. Contemporary psychiatric nursing practice also requires that the nurse consider the integration of biological, psychological, and sociocultural interventions in designing a wholistic plan of care. Nursing intervention can then be aimed at counteracting entropy and restoring and maintaining homeostasis.

Conceptually, it is helpful to separate assessment from planning and implementation; however, in reality, interactions between the psychiatric nurse and the client during the assessment mark the beginning of negotiation for mutual goal setting and interventions. When the psychiatric nurse asks a client, "What have you done to make it better?" and "Has it helped?", the client is becoming engaged in a therapeutic alliance with the nurse. The nurse's nonthreatening questions not only provide critical assessment data, but they also set the stage for helping clients evaluate their own coping mechanisms. This may lead to clients' willingness to modify thinking and behavior in the pursuit of more adaptive and satisfying outcomes.

One of the psychiatric nurse's goals is to provide new experiences for the client's external and internal environments. In the example of the client experiencing the loss of a relationship, the nurse might initially provide an environment for the client that assures safety and the provision of basic needs. Understanding the biological components of the client's basic structure (such as a family history of major depressive illness) might also suggest the need for specific somatic treatments (such as an antidepressant medication). The next activity would be to engage the client in a one-to-one relationship that can provide the client with an opportunity to explore fears, feelings, and hopes. Slowly, the underlying question of "What am I without the person whom I have lost?" will emerge. The psychiatric nurse can then mobilize the synergy and encourage the client to continue to explore options and to view this life event as a challenge instead of a threat. As the client begins to express grief openly, there will be a release of bound energy, and the psychiatric nurse can now mobilize this energy to help the client set new life goals.

In planning nursing care, the psychiatric nurse can also find the Neuman Model useful in its focus on primary, secondary, and tertiary preventions that are congruent with Caplan's (1964) classic work, *Principles of Preventive Psychiatry*. At the primary level there is total resistance to the penetration of the client's normal line of defense, and no symptoms are evident. Nursing activities can be directed, however, to identifying individuals and populations who may be at risk for stress. At this level the focus of care is on helping clients retain their level of functioning, avoid stressors, strengthen their resistance factors, and promote their mental health. Community-based activities that focus on strengthening the flexible and normal lines of defense can be directed toward such groups as single mothers, adolescents, crime victims, or children of the mentally ill, with the psychiatric nurse's goal being to prevent mental illness and promote mental health.

Secondary level responses occur when the line of defense has been penetrated and symptoms are evident. Nursing interventions are required to strengthen the defenses, intervene in maladaptive processes, and assist the client to use resources to attain optimal wellness. Nursing care at this level may require more intensive interventions as symptoms can be severe. Often a protected inpatient environment is indicated, but psychiatric nursing care can also be delivered in a variety of community settings with an emphasis on the "least restrictive" environment, such as outpatient centers, day treatment, home care, or intensive day treatment.

Tertiary level responses rehabilitate the individual experiencing stress. Psychiatric nurses assist clients to readapt, maintain an optimal level of functioning, and become educated to prevent future recurrences. The goal here is recovery, and psychiatric nursing interventions may include social skills training, reality orientation, behavior modification, progressive goal setting, and psychoeducation programs. In the Neuman Model, client system stability is facilitated through all three modes of intervention.

EVALUATING PSYCHIATRIC NURSING OUTCOMES

The Neuman Model identifies the goal of "reconstruction" and notes that the range of outcome possibilities may extend beyond the client's normal line of defense. Outcomes, therefore, are evaluated at the intrapersonal, interpersonal, and extrapersonal levels. Goals that have been mutually formulated between the nurse and client are also mutually evaluated. For the client to realize "how far he or she has come" provides positive feedback and the possibility of integrating the experience into his or her developing repertoire of coping mechanisms.

Too often, however, mental health services focus exclusively on symptom remission in the measurement of psychiatric outcomes. This is a limited and restricted evaluation of the client's total life experience. Rather, in addition to symptom remission, psychiatric nurses also need to evaluate the client's functional status, quality of life, and satisfaction with care received. Wholistic psychiatric nursing care must focus on the integrated experience of individuals in their internal and external environment and not merely target symptomatic relief.

Thus an evaluation of outcomes involves consideration of continuity of care issues as well. At discharge, scheduling a follow-up appointment is no longer sufficient. Support from family members may need to be elicited, help from community agencies may need to be arranged, and for the psychiatric nurse case manager, home visits may be planned to support the family and further stabilize the client in his or her home environment.

IMPLICATIONS FOR PSYCHIATRIC NURSING PRACTICE AND RESEARCH

The current health care environment characterized by managed competition, prescriptive authority for psychiatric clinical nurse specialists, and capitated funding for individuals with psychiatric illness suggests new settings and new roles for conceptually based psychiatric nurse clinicians (Scheter, 1993). The renewed interest in preventive care is an opportunity for psychiatric nurses to use their knowledge of mental health, understanding of the biological and neurochemical components of mental illness, and therapeutic and teaching skills in caring for individuals at all points of the health—illness continuum.

An important development for community-based psychiatric nursing is that a single role often spans responsibilities for all three levels of intervention. Psychiatric nurses currently employed in secondary and tertiary prevention settings increasingly practice as clinical case managers. Because of their wholistic perspective of the person, health, and environment, psychiatric nurses are critical to multidisciplinary treatment planning. For example, a psychiatric nurse may work with an individual with schizophrenia during an acute episode in an inpatient setting, facilitate subsequent rehabilitative care in a partial hospitalization or supervised living program, and then facilitate the person's return back to family and the community. At the same time the nurse may work with the family members in primary prevention interventions that will help them deal with the problems of stigma, altered family relationships, or fears about the individual's relapse. Such situations provide tremendous opportunity for primary prevention, and psychiatric nurses in the future must be prepared to work in fluid boundaries and across treatment settings to provide the highest quality psychiatric nursing care.

The application of the Neuman Systems Model to psychiatric nursing practice also suggests some areas for future nursing research. Clearly, the greatest need is for research documenting the outcomes of psychiatric nursing care. Nurses must be able to demonstrate the effectiveness and efficiency of the services they provide. This is a priority for all nursing research in the next decade. There are also numerous clinical questions that can be studied based on the Neuman Model. Some of these include:

- What is the relationship between coping resources and ego strength?
- What role does a basic structure of hardiness and resilience play in protecting one from illness?
- What risk factors from one's basic structure place a person at higher risk for the development of specific psychiatric illnesses?
- What early psychiatric nursing interventions can delay or impede the development of psychiatric illnesses?
- What role does the assessment of an individual's coping resources play in mutual goal setting?
- How does functional status relate to psychiatric nursing diagnosis and intervention?
- Is an individual's quality of life significantly improved by psychiatric case management services?
- Do nurses make effective case managers for selected psychiatric populations, such as those with high recidivism or medical comorbidity?
- What impact does the nurse–patient therapeutic alliance have on patient satisfaction and self-efficacy?

These and other questions will elucidate the present parameters of psychiatric nursing practice and create windows of opportunity for psychiatric nursing practice in the year 2000 and beyond.

REFERENCES

American Psychiatric Association. 1987. *Diagnostic and Statistical Manual of Mental Disorders,* 3d ed., revised. Washington D.C.: The Association.
Antonovsky, A. 1979. *Health, Stress and Coping.* San Francisco: Jossey-Bass.
Caplan, G. 1964. *Principles of Preventive Psychiatry.* New York: Basic Books.

Ellis, A. 1987. The impossibility of achieving consistently good mental health. *American Psychologist* 42:364–375.

Fawcett, J. 1989. Hallmarks of success in nursing practice. *Advances in Nursing Science* 11:1–8.

Herrick, C., and Goodykoontz, L. 1989. Neuman's system model for nursing practice as a conceptual framework for a family assessment. *Journal of Child and Adolescent Psychiatric and Mental Health Nursing* 2:61–67.

Herrick, C., Goodykoontz, L., and Herrick, R. 1992. Selection of treatment modalities. In *Psychiatric and Mental Health Nursing with Children and Adolescents,* edited by P. West and C. Evans. Gaithersburg, Md.: Aspen Publications.

Kadner, K. 1989. Resilience: responding to adversity. *Journal of Psychosocial Nursing* 27:20–24.

Lazarus, R., and Folkman, S. (1984). *Stress, Appraisal and Coping.* New York: Springer Publishing Co.

Mechanic, D. 1977. Illness behavior, social adaptation, and the management of illness. *Journal of Nervous and Mental Diseases* 165:79–82.

Moore, S., and Munro, M. 1990. The Neuman Systems Model applied to mental health nursing of older adults. *Journal of Advanced Nursing* 15:293–299.

Mynatt, S. L., and O'Brien, J. 1993. Partnership to prevent chemical dependency in nursing: Using Neuman's Systems Model. *Journal of Psychosocial Nursing* 31:27–32.

Neuman, B. 1989. *The Neuman Systems Model,* 2d ed. East Norwalk, Conn.: Appleton & Lange.

Neuman, B. 1990. Health as a continuum based on the Neuman Systems Model. *Nursing Science Quarterly* 3:129–135.

Scheter, R. 1993. Ten trends in managed care and their impact on the biopsychosocial model. *Hospital and Community Psychiatry* 44:325–327.

Stuart, G., and Sundeen, S. 1991. *Principles and Practice of Psychiatric Nursing.* St. Louis, Mo.: Mosby Yearbook.

Wright, L. 1993. *Alzheimer's Disease and Marriage: An Intimate Account.* Newbury, Calif.: Sage Publications.

18

THE NEUMAN SYSTEMS MODEL FOR CRITICAL CARE NURSING
A Framework for Practice

Maureen McCormac Bueno
Kathi Kendall Sengin

This chapter describes how the Neuman Systems Model can be applied to a highly complex and rapidly changing critical care environment. Since critical care nurses manage, coordinate, and deliver care to clients and client systems in highly specialized and technological environments, the systems approach of the Neuman Model is a good approach for nursing practice. This model provides a comprehensive and flexible guide for nurses to assist clients and their families in attaining an optimal level of wellness from physiological, psychological, sociocultural, developmental, and spiritual systemic perspectives.

The nursing requirements of the critically ill client have become dramatically more complex, interdisciplinary, and technologically sophisticated over the last several decades. Within this context, it is important to provide a conceptual framework in which intensive care nursing is practiced as both an art and a science. In respect to the art aspect, Thoreau wrote, "It is something to be able to paint a picture or to carve a statue, and so to make a few objects beautiful. But it is far more glorious to carve and paint the atmosphere in which we work, to affect the quality of the day—this is the highest of the arts" (Donohue, 1985, ix). Nightingale described nursing as "the finest of the arts"

Reviewed by Barbara Shambaugh.

(Donohue, 1985, ix), whereas Nutting described it as "one of the most difficult" (Kinney, Packa, and Dunbar, 1988, 4). More often, nursing has been identified as both an art and a science. "The science of nursing is the knowledge base for what is done and the art of nursing is the skilled application of that knowledge" (Taylor, Lillis, and Lemone, 1993, 5). Conceptual nursing models provide the framework for the application (i.e., art) of nursing's knowledge base (i.e., science).

In recent years the focus has often been placed on the science aspect. The American Nurses Association (1980) defined nursing as "the diagnosis and treatment of human responses to actual or potential health problems" (p. 9). This definition fostered the development of the science side of nursing knowledge, often in the context of the nursing process to meet the actual or potential health needs of clients.

CONCEPTUAL MODELS IN CRITICAL CARE

In order for a conceptual model to be useful, it must be relevant to clinical practice (Stevens, 1984). An ideal conceptual model within the critical care environment provides a focus on physiological needs while also providing a framework for addressing psychological, sociocultural, developmental, and spiritual needs. It is essential that this model be reasonably easy to understand in terms of concepts, contain a manageable language, and provide a structure for application of the nursing process (Fulbrook, 1991). Kinney (1988) suggests that critical care nursing may be the most complex of all nursing specialties, identifying the scope of critical care nursing as being the "dynamic interaction of the critically ill patient, the critical care nurse and the critical care environment" (p. 4). The integration of these elements requires an organized, systematic view of the client/client system. Neuman's systemic views offer nursing and the health care system what von Bertalanffy's (1968) systems theory provided as a structural framework in systems applications for other scientific disciplines. Hazard (1971) suggests that the systems approach provides a necessary context for nursing practice as it embraces the theory of organized complexity, wherein all components interact. "Systems science has demonstrated its capacity of effectively attacking highly complex and large-scale problems. . . . To adapt systems thinking to nursing demands a high degree of flexibility that allows for much creativity" (Neuman, 1989, 5–6).

THE NEUMAN SYSTEMS MODEL IN CRITICAL CARE

The Neuman Model, as related to von Bertalanffy's work, is a systems model based on open systems thinking. The model provides a systemic approach to the care of critically ill clients as they interact with the critical care environment (Taylor, 1993). The purpose of the Neuman Systems Model "is to help nurses organize the nursing field within a broad systems perspective as a logical way of dealing with its growing complexity" (Neuman, 1989, 23). Nowhere is that complexity more evident than in the critical care environment. In addition to physiological variables, the Neuman Model provides structure for critical care nurses as they manage psychological, sociocultural, developmental, and spiritual issues of the client and client system.

The model supports a wholistic concept of person, is easily understood, and has manageable terms. It utilizes the nursing process and a systems approach to health care management. A wholistic concept of man involves viewing clients within the context of this environment, within which there is constant interaction and, ideally, dynamic equilibrium. The environment can be defined as both internal (intrapersonal) and external (interpersonal and extrapersonal). Stressors arise from the environment and interact with the system. Neuman (1989) considers stressors to be neutral. The response of a system to these stressors is individualized and largely dependent upon their type, number, magnitude, and the condition of the system with outcome determined by whether the stressors are positive or noxious for the client.

"Critical care units are characterized by a multiplicity of stressors affecting patients, nurses and patients' families, and the ability of the patients to attain wellness is greatly influenced by their ability to counteract both internal and external stressors. With its emphasis on stressors, the Neuman's System Model seems especially suited to the critical care setting" (Fawcett, Cariello, Davis, Farley, Zimmaco, and Watts, 1987, 206–207).

In the Neuman Model, the client is believed to exist along a wellness continuum. The goal of the critical care stay is to advance clients along this continuum, ultimately returning them to their maximum state of wellness or achievable functioning. The American Hospital Association (1980) described wellness not merely as illness avoidance but life enhancement through the improvement of physical, mental, emotional, and spiritual dimensions of the client's life. Taylor (1993) identified two additional dimensions that compose the whole person: the sociocultural and the environmental. Neuman (1989) defines the client/client system as composed of five interactive variables: physiological, psychological, sociocultural, developmental, and spiritual. A significant feature of the Neuman Systems Model is that it uniquely provides a framework in which these variables are applied. The utility of the framework relates to its ability to guide and direct the caregiver in the application of the nursing process.

Critical care nursing is the specialty within nursing that deals with life-threatening problems and subsequent responses (AACN, 1984). In the critical care environment, progress toward wellness is dependent upon a complex, interrelated network of systems that are both internal and external to the client/client system. Viewing the critically ill client within a systems context allows the caregiver to examine the part while managing the whole. In the

Neuman Systems Model "nursing is viewed as a unique profession concerned with all variables affecting the client system's response to stressors" (Fawcett, Cariello, Davis, Farley, Zimmaco, and Watts, 1987, 205).

The physiological needs of the client in critical care settings cannot be overstated. Examples include breathing and gas exchange, the exchange of food and nutrients, fluid and electrolyte balance, thermal regulation, cardiac function, and movement. These needs are often the most significant reason for admission to critical care units. What must not be lost in the midst of a technologically advanced environment are the remaining variables, which require careful assessment and intervention for their impact on the client/client system. These Neuman-defined client system variables (psychological, sociocultural, developmental, and spiritual) are inseparable from the physical component.

The psychological variable refers to the client's mental and emotional process, interrupted and potentially altered by critical illness or injury. Nurses in high-intensity environments frequently manage clients with a variety of stress manifestations: fear, sadness, psychosis, anxiety, grief, problems with self-concept, loss of control, and loneliness.

Sociocultural variables involve the relationships the client has with family, friends, significant others, and community members. "Health practices and beliefs are strongly influenced by a person's economic level, lifestyle, family and culture" (Taylor, 1993, 25). In the critical care environment, the relationships, role enactment, personal patterns of care, and life-styles are often altered. Each caregiver assessment and plan of treatment needs to be congruent with these client variables. Teaching plans, for example, must be designed according to the language, culture, and method of learning that is appropriately identified by the client, significant others, and nurse.

The ability to conceptualize and to respond to changes in health status on the part of the client is related to developmental age (Kozier, 1989). The developmental variable encompasses cognitive abilities, educational achievements, and life experiences. All of these components play an important role in the critically ill client's ability to interpret and cope with the current crisis and plan for recovery. The explanations chosen by the caregiver for client education need to be consistent with current developmental stage and cognitive ability.

The spiritual dimension is related to religious beliefs and human values, which may be heightened, diminished, or unchanged as a result of critical illness or injury. Critical care nurses assess this dimension for each of their clients and subsequently develop plans of care to address their needs. For instance, they consult pastoral care representatives in the hospital and religious representatives in the community according to the needs of the client/client system.

An assessment of the five variables provides the foundation for nursing diagnosis, goal setting, interventions, outcome management, and evaluative processes. Neuman (1989) uses the nursing process to provide an organized, systematic, and deliberate framework for nursing actions within the model.

THE NEUMAN NURSING PROCESS

Critical care nurses use all phases of the nursing process in their daily management of cardiac, pulmonary, renal, surgical, trauma, and other critically ill clients to develop:

- Nursing assessment and diagnosis
- Nursing goals
- Nursing intervention
- Nursing outcomes and evaluation

Nursing Assessment and Diagnosis

Critical care nurses collect tremendous amounts of data from a variety of clients and include family environmental sources through physical assessment, chart review, verbal and nonverbal communication, and many more methods. Table 18–1 lists a sample of data elements identified by critical care nurses as well as a sample of the numerous data sources they use. The experienced and proficient nurse rapidly synthesizes, analyzes, and evaluates these data for variances from the expected norms. Within the Neuman nursing process format, nurses indentify and evaluate potential or actual stressors that pose a threat to the stability of the client/client systems (Neuman, 1982, 1989). That is, they develop nursing diagnoses through the identification of health variances from normal that may threaten the client's basic structure.

The following case study demonstrates the application of the first phase of the Neuman nursing process format: nursing diagnosis.

Mr. C., a 30-year-old Hispanic male, presented to the emergency department following a high-speed motorcycle crash in which he lost control of his vehicle. In the resuscitation and in surgery, he was diagnosed and treated for bilateral femur fractures, pelvic fractures, 30 percent pneumothorax, and concussion.

The primary nurse received the client directly from the operating suite into the surgical intensive care unit and immediately began her assessment. While the assessment incorporates all five variables (i.e., physiological, psychological, sociocultural, developmental, and spiritual), the physiological assessment takes precedence on admission to the unit. The nurse works collaboratively with physicians and other members of the trauma team to provide systematic, high-quality care in an efficient and effective manner. While the goal is to prevent complications, this is not always possible in the immobile client with multiple trauma.

Approximately 30 hours after injury, the primary nurse identified several new manifestations:

TABLE 18–1. SAMPLE DATA COLLECTION SOURCES AND ELEMENTS IN CRITICAL CARE

- Cardiac monitors:
Heart rate
Cardiac rhythm
Diagnosis of dysrhythmias
- Hemodynamic monitors:
Pulmonary artery catheters:
—Pulmonary artery pressures (systolic, diastolic, mean)
—Pulmonary capillary wedge pressures (PCWP)
—Systemic vascular resistance (SVR)
—Continuous mixed venous oxygen saturation (SVO_2)
Central venous lines:
—Central venous pressure (CVP)
Arterial lines:
—Arterial pressures (systolic, diastolic, mean)
- Pulse oximeters:
Oxygen saturation
End tidal carbon dioxide ($ETCO_2$)
- Mechanical ventilators:
Tidal volume (TV)
Peak end expiratory pressure (PEEP)
Respiratory rate
- Intracranial pressure monitors:
Intracranial pressures
- Chest tubes:
Amount and color of drainage
- Foley catheters:
Amount and color of urine
Temperature if catheter senses temperature
- Nasogastric and rectal tubes:
Amount and color of drainage
- Intravenous infusions:
Colloids
Crystalloids
- Patient's chart:
History and physical
Laboratory data
Radiology reports
Multidisciplinary progress notes
- Patient and/or family/friends:
Previous illness or injury
General health status
Past health practices
Values
Beliefs
Education
Mental capacity
- Members of the team:
Nurses (e.g., trauma nurse coordinator)
Physicians
Social Workers
Clergy
Dieticians

Manifestations	Data Collection Source
Tachypnea	Physical assessment
Hypoxemia	Blood gas analysis
Respiratory alkalosis	Blood gas analysis
Lethargy, slight confusion	Assessment, patient and family interview
Increased temperature	Thermometer

The nurse used assistance from the family to evaluate mental status since the client spoke primarily Spanish. Since this client sustained chest, extremity, and head trauma, these signs and symptoms are not necessarily specific to any one particular condition. The experienced critical care nurse, however, suspected the presence of fat embolism and looked for additional signs of this syndrome. On further assessment she noted petechiae developing across the chest and axillae.

The manifestations of fat embolism syndrome and subsequent nursing diagnoses (Figure 18–1) posed a serious threat to the client's basic structure factors and energy resources. This client's flexible lines of defense were unable to protect the client/client system, and the stressor invaded the normal line of defense or normal range of response to the environment (neuman, 1982, 1989). The lines of resistance surrounding the inner core then functioned to stabilize and return the client to the optimal state of wellness following the stressor reaction.

Although the physiological variable has been highlighted thus far, the critical care client/client system is a composite of all five interacting variables: physiological, psychological, sociocultural, developmental, and spiritual. The interaction of these variables in the internal (i.e., intrapersonal) and external environment (i.e., interpersonal and extrapersonal) is simultaneous and complex in nature. Sample stressors and their interactions in a trauma client/client system are summarized in Table 18–2. The scientific nursing literature has documented common stressors for clients in critical care environments through the use of research strategies. Wilson (1987), for example, ranked 22 stressors in a surgical intensive care unit, including having pain, not being able to move freely, frequent interruptions of sleep, being thirsty, and having too many tubes. Client/client system stressors in critical care are numerous and complex and require the mobilization of internal and external resources for management.

The critical care nurse identifies the actual and potential internal and external resources necessary to attain an optimal state of wellness. Table 18–3 provides common internal and external resources that would be mobilized in Mr. C.'s case. As in many critical situations, the number of external resources mobilized exceeds internal resources since the client is in a compromised and potentially life-threatening situation.

Nursing Goals

The critical care nurse systematically integrates symptom manifestations, variance from normal data, nursing diagnoses, stability needs, and available re-

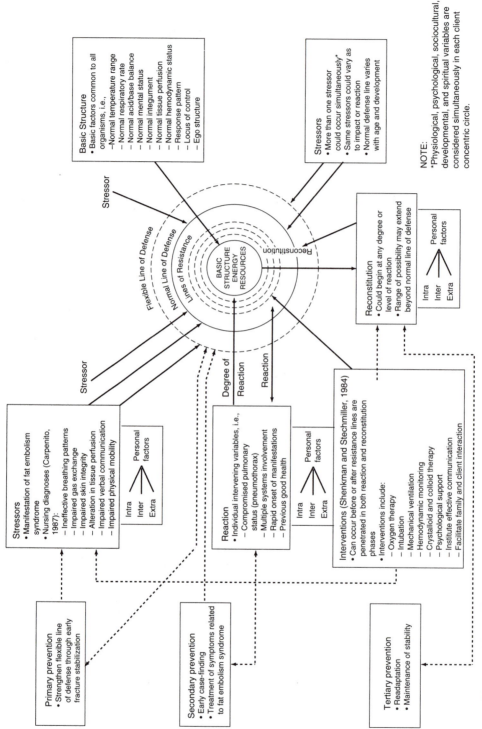

Figure 18–1. The Neuman Systems Model applied to a critically ill trauma client with fat embolism syndrome. *(Adapted with permission from B. Neuman, PhD, FAAN.)*

sources to determine goals for the client/client system. Common goals in critical care include the following:

- The client will demonstrate absence of physiological complications from immobilization: atelectasis, pneumonia, pressure sores, contractures, etc.
- The client will demonstrate a return to baseline hemodynamic function by day three of the intensive care unit stay.
- The client will maintain a regular pattern of interaction with the family.
- The client will acquire information regarding risk behaviors and prevention strategies.

Nursing Interventions

Critical care interventions are derived from nursing diagnoses and goal statements. Nursing interventions in critical care are numerous, including medication administration, blood transfusion, hemodynamic monitoring, enteral feeding, titration of medicated drips, suctioning, education, cardiopulmonary resuscitation, intraaortic balloon pump timing and augmentation, emotional support, family support, and airway management. Figure 18–1 illustrates specific interventions required following the diagnosis of fat embolism syndrome. Consistency exists between assessment data, stressors, variance data, nursing diagnoses, nursing goals, and interventions.

Nursing Outcomes and Evaluation

In the Neuman Model, nursing interventions are accomplished through the use of one or more of three prevention modes:

1. Primary prevention (action to retain system stability)
2. Secondary prevention (action to attain system stability)
3. Tertiary prevention (action to maintain system stability), following secondary prevention as intervention (Neuman, 1989, 20)

Interventions in the critical care environment for Mr. C. will focus on secondary and tertiary prevention since the basic structure has already been comprised. Although these two forms of prevention are common in intensive care environments, critical care nurses also use primary prevention. The prevention of pressure sores and other complications of immobility, for example, represents primary prevention. Other types of primary prevention include the prevention of pneumonia, respiratory distress syndrome, pulmonary embolism, deep venous thrombosis, sensory overload, and intensive care psychosis.

Nursing outcomes are evaluated continuously to determine if the plan of care needs to be changed. For instance, a client who develops sacral redness despite meticulous skin care and repositioning may need a different kind of mattress and other physiological assessments such as nutritional status to prevent skin breakdown. Systematic evaluations are more likely to result in positive and expected outcomes.

TABLE 18-2. SOURCES OF STRESSORS FOR CRITICALLY ILL TRAUMA CLIENT

VARIABLES	Intrapersonal	Interpersonal	Extrapersonal
Physiological	• Type and severity of traumatic injury: —Bilateral femur fractures —Pelvic fracture —30% pneumothorax —Concussion • Effects of trauma: —Acidosis —Hypoxemia —Electrolyte disturbance —Hypovolemia • Complications: —Fat embolism —Pneumonia —Acute renal failure —Multiple system organ failure • Risk factors: —Alcohol ingestion —Illegal drug ingestion	• Nosocomial infections • Hypothermia induced through interventions (fluid resuscitation, body surface exposure)	• Effects of sleep disturbance • Safety/environmental risk factors: —Mechanical —Electrical —Thermal —Chemical —Adjunctive restrictive equipment
Psychological	• Past psychiatric illness • Self-blame • Denial • Anxiety • Depression • Intrusion • Fear • Powerlessness	• Support systems: —Family members —Friends —Trauma coordinator —Bereavement specialists —Trauma team members • Dependency on caregivers • Nurse/patient interactions	• Intensive care psychosis • Environmental overload: —Noise —Lights —Temperature —Odors —Colors

Sociocultural		

• Values
• Cultural impact:
  —Pain management
• Risk behaviors:
  —Seat belt use
  —Helmet use
  —Speeding
• Insurance coverage
	• Language barriers
	• Financial issues
	• Locus of control
	• Interruption in plans
	• Restrictive visitation
	• Separation of significant other
	• Life-style changes
	• Role alterations (temporary or permanent):
	  —Familial
	  —Occupational
	  —Sexual
		• Lack of education related to trauma prevention
		• Lack of ability to pay for hospitalization
		• Guardianship determination through judicial system

Developmental		

• Age of the trauma patient:
  —Children
  —Elderly
• Education
• Gender differences
• Cognitive abilities
	• Initiation and maintenance of relationships according to expected developmental stage	• Disability affecting development

Spiritual		

• Spiritual beliefs affecting trauma management:
  —Altered worship practices
  —Heightened awareness of life/death
  —Jehovah's Witnesses refusing blood transfusions
  —Advanced directives
  —Resuscitation
  —Organ donation
  —Hope/hopelessness
	• Family differences in spiritual decisions	• Lack of support from clergy or other spiritual representatives

TABLE 18–3. SAMPLE INTERNAL AND EXTERNAL RESOURCES FOR A CRITICALLY ILL TRAUMA CLIENT

Resources	
Internal	*External*
Previous good health	**Activation of personnel:**
No previous hospitalization or major illness	
Young age	Trauma physician
Mental health	Pulmonologist
Good coping skills	Anesthesiologist
Works well with hospital personnel	Trauma nurse coordinator
Spiritual beliefs	Respiratory therapist
Value system	Social worker
Education	Nursing personnel
Risk behaviors	Family members/friends
Health practices	Clergy
	Utilization equipment/supplies:
	Oxygen and intubation equipment
	Mechanical ventilator
	Intravenous fluids
	Blood products
	Medications
	X-ray machine
	Blood sampling tubes, syringes, etc.

Family Needs

Admission to a critical care environment is considered more threatening than a routine, noncritical care admission and creates a potential for significant disruption of family structures (Lewandowski, 1992). Leske (1992) suggests that families of the critically ill client are affected by three major stressors: "realization the family member is extremely ill, the critical care environment and the disruption in family roles, routines and future plans" (p. 590). As a result, critical care nurses integrate family and/or significant others in the care of clients.

Scientific research and investigation provides the basis for understanding and classifying family needs. Several authors have clustered needs into categories for application to practice settings (see Table 18–4). Hickey (1990) conducted an extensive literature search and found two family needs were consistently identified: "to have questions answered honestly" and "to know specific facts regarding what is wrong with the patient and the patient's progress" (p. 406).

Literature on family needs provides the basis for planning family-centered intervention strategies (Caine, 1989; Cray, 1989; Halm, 1992; Leske, 1992; McClowry, 1992; Norris and Grove, 1986). "To offer complete care to clients, it is vital for healthcare providers, including critical care nurses, to be aware of the diversity of families as they exist today and to assess the nature and well being of the family of which each client is uniquely a part" (McCool, Tuttle, and Crowley, 1992, 549). Family members experience many of the same feelings as clients, including threat, fear, hopelessness, powerlessness, anxiety, and loss of control (Titler and Walsh, 1992). These responses are worsened by limited contact with the client and caregivers. The need for regular and frequent updates from a consistent caregiver is extremely important. Family members will benefit from liberal visiting practices that are guided, but not restricted, by the caregiver (Titler and Walsh, 1992). Often staff are concerned that liberal visiting practices may interfere with the delivery of care and adversely affect the client. However, Titler and Walsh (1992) assert that more liberal visitation has resulted in positive client outcomes (e.g., increased orientation, improved sleep, decreased anxiety), positive family outcomes (e.g., decreased anxiety), and enhanced job satisfaction for caregivers. This illustration depicts the interrelatedness of the client, caregiver, and family in the critical care environment.

Critical care nurses are involved in the implementation of many creative strategies to address family needs. For instance, families in some critical care units rent portable radio pagers to maintain communication with caregivers (Titler and Walsh, 1992). This allows family members to leave the institution for rest, nourishment, and other activities of daily living. These needs are often neglected when family members remain in the hospital setting for long periods of time. Pager systems reduce family stress and prevent illness in family members as a result of being in the hospital for prolonged periods of time.

The Neuman Systems Model provides a framework for identifying and addressing family needs of the critically ill client. The critical care provider can adapt the prevention as intervention strategies (primary, secondary, and tertiary) to the family (Table 18–5). Many primary intervention strategies are aimed at retaining family system integrity and reducing stressor encounters. Secondary intervention focuses on both utilizing and strengthening the existing family structure. Reconstitution of the client/client system is the principal aim of tertiary prevention.

Family-focused care is the trend for future health care. Families will demand

TABLE 18–4. FAMILY NEEDS OF CRITICALLY ILL CLIENTS

Simpson (1989)	Hickey (1990)	Henneman & Cardin (1992)	Leske (1992)
Information	Information	Information	Information
Visitation	Visitation	Visitation and	Proximity
Reassurance interventions	Emotional support	convenience	Assurance
Supportive interventions	Supportive interventions	Reassurance	Support and comfort
Environmental comforts	Empathy		

TABLE 18–5. PREVENTION AS INTERVENTION FOR THE FAMILIES OF CRITICALLY ILL CLIENTS

Interventional Category	Goal of Intervention	Intervention Strategy
Primary		
Intervention as prevention	• Retain family stability • Reduce stressor encounter • Desensitize family to stressors	• Develop family-focused critical care environment —Support team planning —Communication system —Convenient waiting/phone —Liberal visitation • Anticipate/plan family needs —Client data supplement —Illness/support response • Family and staff education
Secondary		
Intervention as treatment	• Attain family system stability • Utilize family's resources	• Utilize support teams to assist family (psychosocial/spiritual) • Establish family communication with consistent personnel —Answer questions honestly —Update family regularly • Support client/family interaction (liberal visitation) • Establish family involvement in care planning • Provide assurance regarding treatments/prognosis
Tertiary		
Intervention as reconstitution	• Maintain the family system • Avoid additional reactions to stressors	• Involve family in ongoing care • Maintain family contact with support teams • Maintain effective communication • Provide education for planned transfer/discharge

greater involvement in decisions about treatment modalities and options for care. Critical care nurses are uniquely positioned to represent and address family needs.

Management Patterns Under the Neuman Systems Model

The Neuman Model suggests many managerial directions in critical care. The model can be adapted to professional practice and alternate care delivery models that exist in many critical care settings. Case management, a major component of these care delivery models, focuses on the achievement of optimal care outcomes within efficient time frames and with appropriate use of resources.

Case managers, critical care technicians, and support personnel work with the primary nurse and other team members to meet quality and cost targets. The case manager in critical care often coordinates and integrates quality and cost for successful outcome by:

- Promoting collaborative team effort among multidisciplinary team members
- Encouraging autonomy and accountability of professional practice by ensuring that information is shared by all disciplines
- Identifying variances from the standard protocols and working with team members to resolve variances
- Promoting coordinated care through the hospital system
- Promoting client and caregiver satisfaction
- Ensuring that all client/client system needs are met (Brett and Tonges, 1990; Cohen and Cesta, 1993; Conti, 1989; Olivas, Del Togno-Armanasco, Erickson, and Harter, 1989; Tonges, 1989; Zander, 1988)

Nurse case managers can well utilize the systems approach to organize and deliver health care as it supports wholism through a logical organization of the client, client system, and care providers. This is extremely important in critical care settings where practitioners have a tendency to focus on parts or subparts of the client/client system. For example, the orthopedic surgeon focuses on stabilization of fractures, while cardiologists focus on management of heart conditions. Nurses have traditionally focused primarily on physiological variables when clients are in unstable condition, leading to the possibility of fragmentation in intense care environments. Flexible scheduling patterns, such as 12-hour shifts and per diem programs in critical care, have made the continuous flow of client/client system information and the coordination of care more difficult to accomplish (Ritter, Fralic, Tonges, and McCormac, 1992).

The nurse case managers ensure that all parts of the system are comprehensively integrated and managed. They provide structure, organization, and direction for nursing action in intense environments. The role of nurse case manager is consistent with the Neuman Systems Model, which promotes a comprehensive approach to client care.

THE FUTURE OF CRITICAL CARE

The clear challenge for the future in health care will be to do more with less. The health care industry is experiencing financial constraints, competition for resources, an emphasis on outpatient services, sophisticated technology, and increased consumer involvement in care. In the hospital of the future there will be a shift from routine care to more critical or monitored care. As hospitals have shorter lengths of stay, patients will be discharged to family members with significant requirements for further care (Leske, 1992). The client/client system will demand and will be entitled (i.e., self-determination act) to greater involvement in decision making and outcome determinations.

The dramatically increased use of inpatient technology, compressed length of stay, and increasing demand for family-centered services will influence the delivery of nursing care. To facilitate this evolutionary health care system, a paradigm shift will be necessary to provide a comprehensive structure that guides and directs critical care nursing practice. The Neuman Systems Model provides a framework that will work extremely well.

REFERENCES

American Association of Critical Care Nurses. 1984. *Definition of Critical Care Nursing.* Calif.: American Association of Critical Care Nurses.

American Hospital Association. 1980. Wellness: What is it? *Promoting Health* 1(1):1–5.

American Nurses Association. 1980. *Nursing: A Social Policy Statement.* Kansas City, Mo.: American Nurses Association.

Anderson, K. H., and Tomlinson, P. S. 1992. The family health system as an emerging paradigmatic view for nursing. *Image: Journal of Nursing Scholarship* 24:57–63.

Brett, J. L., and Tonges, M. C. 1990. Restructured patient care delivery: Evaluation of the ProACT™ model. *Nursing Economics* 8(1):36–44.

Caine, R. M. 1989. Families in crisis: Making the critical difference. *Focus on Critical Care* 16(3):184–189.

Carpenito, L. J. 1987. *Nursing Diagnosis: Application to Clinical Practice,* 2d ed. Philadelphia: J. B. Lippincott.

Cohen, E. L., and Cesta, T. G. 1993. *Nursing Case Management: From Concept to Evaluation.* St. Louis: C. V. Mosby.

Conti, R. 1989. The nurse as case manager. *Nursing Connections* 2(1):55–58.

Cray, L. 1989. A collaborative project: Initiating a family intervention program in a medical intensive care unit. *Focus on Critical Care* 16(3):212–218.

Donohue, M. P. 1985. *Nursing: The Finest Art.* St. Louis: C. V. Mosby.

Fawcett, J. 1989. *Neuman's Systems Model. Analysis and Evaluation of Conceptual Models of Nursing,* 2d ed. Philadelphia: F. A. Davis.

Fawcett, J., Cariello, F. P., Davis, D. A., Farley, J., Zimmaco, D. M., and Watts, R. J. 1987. Conceptual models of nursing: Application to critical care nursing practice. *Dimensions of Critical Care Nursing* 6(4):202–213.

Fulbrook, P. R. 1991. The application of the Neuman Systems Model to intensive care. *Intensive Care Nursing* 7(1):28–39.

Halm, M. A. 1992. Support and reassurance needs: Strategies for practice. *Critical Care Nursing Clinics of North America* 4(4):633–643.

Hazard, M. E. 1971. An overview of systems theory. *Nursing Clinics of North America* 6(3):385–393.

Henneman, E. A., and Cardin, S. 1992. Need for information. *Critical Care Nursing Clinics of North America* 4(4):615–621.

Hickey, M. 1990. What are the needs of families of critically ill patients? A review of the literature since 1976. *Heart & Lung* 19(4):401–415.

Hickey, M. L., and Leske, J. S. 1992. Needs of families of critically ill patients. *Critical Care Nursing Clinics of North America* 4(4):645–649.

Kinney, M. R., Packa, D. R., and Dunbar, S. B. 1988. *AACN's Clinical Reference for Critical Care Nursing.* New York: McGraw-Hill.

Kozier, B., Erb, G., and Bufalino, P. M. 1989. *Introduction to Nursing.* Men Lo Park, Calif.: Addison-Wesley.

Leske, J. S. 1992. Needs of adult family members after critical illness. *Critical Care Nursing Clinics of North America* 4(4):587–596.

Lewandowski, L. A. 1992. Needs of children during the critical illness of a parent or sibling. *Critical Care Nursing Clinics of North America* 4(4):573–585.

McClowry, S. G. 1992. Family functioning during a critical illness. *Critical Care Nursing Clinics of North America* 4(4):559–564.

McCool, W. F., Tuttle, J., and Crowley, A. 1992. Overview of contemporary families. *Critical Care Nursing Clinics of North America* 4(4):549–558.

Neuman, B. 1982. *The Neuman Systems Model.* East Norwalk, Conn.: Appleton-Century-Crofts.

Neuman, B. 1989. *The Neuman Systems Model,* 2d ed. East Norwalk, Conn.: Appleton & Lange.

Norris, L. O., and Grove, S. K. 1986. Investigation of selected psychosocial needs of family members of critically ill adult patients. *Heart & Lung,* 15(2):194–199.

Olivas, G. S., Del Togno-Armanasco, V., Erickson, J. R., and Harter, S. 1989. Case management: A bottom line care delivery model. Part 1: The concept. *Journal of Nursing Administration* 19(11):16–20.

Ritter, J., Fralic, M. F., Tonges, M. C., and McCormac, M. 1992. Redesigned nursing practice: A case management model for critical care. *Nursing Clinics of North America* 27(1): 119–128.

Rowe, M. A., and Weinert, C. 1987. The CCU experience: Stressful or reassuring? *Dimensions of Critical Care* 6(6):341–348.

Shenkman, B., and Stechmiller, J. 1984. Fat embolism syndrome: Pathophysiology and current treatment. *Focus on Critical Care* 11(6):26–35.

Simpson, T. 1989. Needs and concerns of families of critically ill adults. *Focus on Critical Care* 16(5):388–397.

Stevens, B. 1984. *Nursing Theory: Analysis, Application, and Evaluation.* Boston: Little, Brown.

Taylor, C., Lillis, C., and Lemone, P. 1993. *Fundamentals of Nursing.* Philadelphia: J. B. Lippincott.

Titler, M. G., and Walsh, S. M. 1992. Visiting critically ill adults. *Critical Care Nursing Clinics of North America* 4(4):623–632.

Tonges, M. C. 1989. Redesigning hospital nursing practice: The Professionally Advanced Care Team (ProACT™) model, Part 1. *Journal of Nursing Administration* 19(7): 31–38.

Von Bertalanffy, L. 1968. *General Systems Theory: Foundations, Developments, Applications.* New York: George Braziller.

Wilson, V. S. 1987. Identification of stressors related to patients' psychologic responses to the surgical intensive care unit. *Heart & Lung* 16(3):267–273.

Zander, K. 1988. Nursing case management: Strategic management of cost and quality outcomes. *Journal of Nursing Administration* 18(5):23–30.

19

APPLICATION OF THE NEUMAN SYSTEMS MODEL TO GERONTOLOGICAL NURSING

Anne Griswold Peirce
Terry T. Fulmer

Gerontological nursing involves the study of the process and problems of aging and care of the elder person. As a group the elderly are diverse, so frameworks used in gerontological nursing must be flexible and adaptable to a wide range of groups and situations. The Neuman Systems Model provides the needed flexibility, allowing the nurse to conceptualize elders within an organizational framework without negating important differences found within each age cohort. This chapter will illustrate how the Neuman Model can be used by gerontological nurses to improve elder care.

DEMOGRAPHICS OF AGING

The American population is aging. At the turn of the century the average life expectancy was 40 years, with less than 5 percent of the population reaching the age of 65 (US Senate, 1988). As the century nears its end, the average life expectancy is 79 years, and over half of the population will live to age 65 or beyond (Healthy People 2000, 1992).

The size of the elderly population is also growing relative to other age groups. In the 1980s about 12 percent of the population was over 65. This percentage is rising, and by 2030, when today's "baby boomers" are elderly, they will account for approximately 18 percent of the population. Even more important is the fact that the oldest old are also increasing in numbers, with those over 85 years showing the most growth. It is estimated that people aged 75 and older will see a 70 percent increase by the year 2000 (US Senate Special Committee on Aging, 1988).

GERIATRIC IMPERATIVE

There are many reasons for the increasing longevity, including better standards of living, nutrition, control of infectious diseases, and the progress in health care (Alford and Futrell, 1992). Yet normal aging involves inevitable and irreversible changes, such as diminution in muscle tone, bone density, endurance, and so forth. The increasing numbers of elderly have had a profound influence on the health care system, with 40 percent of all hospital beds and 46 percent of intensive care beds occupied by the elderly (Campion et al., 1981).

However, not all the changes attributed to aging are in fact age related. For example, many elders and their caregivers attribute incontinence to the inevitable changes of aging and consequently don't seek help from health care providers. Yet the majority of incontinence problems are reversible with treatment. The task of gerontologic nursing is to discern which changes are intrinsic and which are extrinsic and what nursing actions can be brought to bear on both. This chapter will concentrate on the physiological variables as exemplars of the theory's relationship to the nursing care of the elderly.

THE NEUMAN SYSTEMS MODEL AS AN APPROACH TO GERONTOLOGICAL NURSING CARE ACROSS THE CONTINUUM

The Neuman Systems Model provides a logical, systematic way of looking at the total client. Especially important to the gerontological nurse is that the client can be conceptualized as an individual, family, or community. Many elder problems may in fact be problems of the family constellation or of the community. It is also important that the Neuman Model be considered a wellness model, and as such, aging will be seen as a normal process, rather than an abnormal disease state.

The Neuman Model illustrates how system stability is maintained when encroached upon by stressors. Neuman depicts the client system as a set of interrelated subsystems with a unique central core called the *basic structure*. The core includes factors common to all life, such as genetic structure, organ strengths and weaknesses, ego structure, and response patterns. Surrounding the core are lines of defense. The outer boundary is a flexible line of defense that protects the normal level of wellness by providing a buffer zone. For example, an individual elder may sleep from five to eight hours per night without compromise because the sleep line of defense is flexible. The normal line of defense represents the client's usual level of wellness. Wellness is conceptualized as stability within the client system's physiological, psychological, sociocultural, developmental, and spiritual variables. The inner boundaries, or lines of resistance, protect the core when the normal line of defense is broken by stressors, such as in infection when white blood cell counts rise.

Aging, as noted above, brings with it inevitable, irreversible change. These changes vary from individual to individual but almost always represent loss of function in the Neuman physiological wellness variable. Conceptualized as a loss of flexibility and buffering ability in the lines of defense, these losses represent a change in the ability to fend off the effects of stressors (see Table 19–1). The other variables—psychological, sociocultural, developmental, and spiritual—may or may not vary in the elderly. For example, self-concept may continue to develop, but self-esteem may decline, reflecting a loss of function and diminished social status seen in many elders (Atchley, 1984). As Markides (1983) notes, spirituality is important to many elders and has been associated with a sense of well-being. Using a framework such as Erikson's, developmental growth (see Table 19–2) as well as decline can be seen until death (Erikson, Erikson, and Kivnik, 1986). Thus the changes of aging can be seen as both pos-

TABLE 19–1. SOURCES OF STRESSORS IN THE ELDERLY

	Intrapersonal	Interpersonal	Extrapersonal
Physiological	Aging organ systems Chronic disease	Transmission of infection	Lack of easily accessed health care
Psychological	Anxiety Loss of self-esteem	Problematic or ineffective support systems	Lack of support from community organizations
Sociocultural	Loss of role Cultural beliefs about aging	Differences in beliefs about aging Role expectations	Lack of financial security Lack of support from cultural group
Developmental	Developmental tasks of aging	Developmental differences between significant others	Environmental factors that decrease needed stimuli
Spiritual	Spiritual beliefs	Disagreements with family about matters of spirituality	Lack of spiritual support Access difficulties

TABLE 19-2. DEVELOPMENTAL TASKS OF ERIKSON'S PSYCHOSOCIAL STAGES

Stage	Developmental Task
Infant	Basic trust versus basic mistrust
Toddler	Autonomy versus shame and doubt
Preschooler	Initiative versus guilt
School-ager	Industry versus inferiority
Adolescent	Identity versus role confusion
Young adult	Intimacy versus isolation
Middlescent	Generativity versus stagnation
Older adult	Ego integrity versus despair

itive and negative. The nurse who uses the Neuman Model can maintain the positive wellness variables and reduce the effects of the negative, thus stabilizing the client system toward optimal wellness.

Acute Care

Within the acute care setting, the nurse may use the Neuman Systems Model to conceptualize the care needed for the individual elder client. According to the model, the elderly client is hospitalized because the usual lines of defense and resistance have failed to protect the normal lines of defense and core structure. For example, the elder client may be hospitalized with pneumonia, a common problem in this age group (Kane, Ouslander, and Abrass, 1989). In fact, pneumonia and influenza are the fourth leading cause of death in the elderly (National Center for Health Statistics, 1990). The normal line of defense may reveal an elder person who lives at home and until this point was in his or her usual state of wellness (see Figure 19–1). The physiological wellness variable includes hypertension controlled by medication but no other known health problems. The stressor is the bacterial or viral organism that broke the normal line of defense. The lines of resistance include white cell mobilization to fight infection, cough to remove secretions, increased body temperature to weaken infective agents' cellular walls, and quick diagnosis. In the elderly the lines of defense and resistance may be weakened because there is a loss of immune defense, weakened ability to cough, and a tendency to late diagnosis (Matteson and McConnell, 1988). The elder may not present with "typical" symptoms of fever, productive cough, and elevated white blood cell counts. Instead the elder may exhibit changes in consciousness, increased respiratory rate, chest pain, and dehydration (Rowe and Besdine, 1987). When the flexible line of defense, the normal line of defense, and the lines of resistance fail to protect the basic structure, then hospitalization for pneumonia may result.

Neuman emphasizes prevention as intervention at three levels: primary, secondary, and tertiary. When a client is hospitalized for pneumonia, the nursing actions for that problem are directed toward strengthening the lines of resistance in order to promote secondary prevention and achieving system stability. The nurse utilizes the external resources available, such as antibiotics, nutritional

Core
• All physiological functions
• Genetic endowment

Threatened core
• Pneumonia
  (secondary prevention necessary)

Normal line of defense (NLD)
• Usual coping response to
  environment developed over time
• Normal respiratory function

Invaded NLD
• Compromised respiratory status
  (secondary prevention necessary)

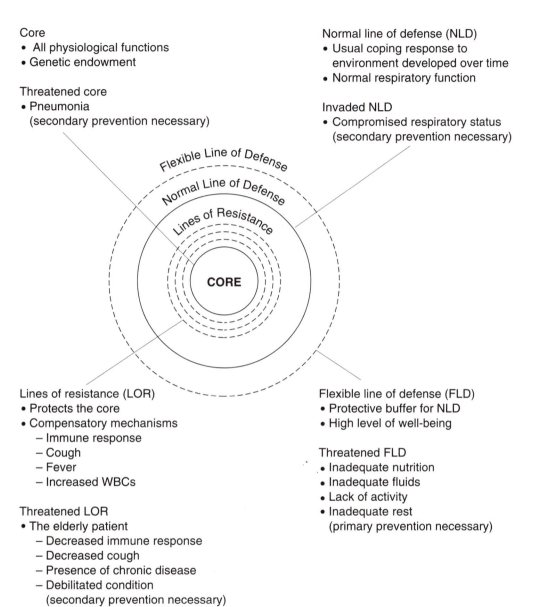

Lines of resistance (LOR)
• Protects the core
• Compensatory mechanisms
  – Immune response
  – Cough
  – Fever
  – Increased WBCs

Threatened LOR
• The elderly patient
  – Decreased immune response
  – Decreased cough
  – Presence of chronic disease
  – Debilitated condition
    (secondary prevention necessary)

Flexible line of defense (FLD)
• Protective buffer for NLD
• High level of well-being

Threatened FLD
• Inadequate nutrition
• Inadequate fluids
• Lack of activity
• Inadequate rest
  (primary prevention necessary)

Figure 19–1. Pneumonia.

supplements, fluids, oxygen, chest physiotherapy, and adequate rest and sleep. The nursing assessment is important because it enables the nurse to support activities that the client deems important in systems restoration. For example, the assessment may reveal that the client believes that lung congestion is aided by drinking citrus juice and avoiding milk-based drinks. Other cultural beliefs may also be important to the elder client. Elderly Filipino Americans may believe that certain spices will aid their healing (DiMatteo and DiNicola, 1982). The nurse can incorporate this information into the plan of care.

Tertiary prevention as intervention is directed toward reeducation and maintenance of gains made. For an elderly client with pneumonia the nurse may want to encourage the client to receive the pneumococcal vaccine as a preventive measure. The client will also need education about getting adequate rest, activity, nutrition, and follow-up care after hospitalization.

Within the hospital primary prevention as intervention can be directed toward preventing iatrogenic problems. For example, the nurse realizes that elderly clients are at risk for problems such as pressure ulcer formation, sleep problems, and incontinence. The care plan will identify the clients' usual state of resistance, coping strategies, and potential areas of instability in the lines of resistance. For examples, see the following sections on pressure ulcers, incontinence, and elder mistreatment.

Home Care

Individual as Client. Within the home the influences of the community are more apparent. For example, the elder whose normal line of defense in maintaining nutrition is altered from such things as loss of physical strength, mobility, or sensory changes may rely on community resources such as congregate meal programs and home-delivered meals (see Table 19–3). In this case the boundaries of the lines of resistance are expanded to include community resources.

Family as Client. The family is also important to the elder client. Many families supply care to elders when they cannot do so themselves. According to Brody (1978), responsible caregiving includes physical, emotional, social, and economic support corresponding to the wellness variables of the Neuman Systems Model. All of the caregiving variables have stressors inherent within them. For example, the social needs of the family may be subsumed by the time spent with the elder. Thus the family as client can also be addressed within the Neuman Model. When there is care dependency, the nurse must care for the wellness of the family in order to maintain its structural integrity (Peirce, Wright, and Fulmer, 1992).

Community as Client. In considering the community as the client in terms of the geriatric population, the nurse must be familiar with the many subsystems that provide services and how they relate to one another. For example, the fiscal health of the community may relate to the crime rate, transportation services, recreational offerings, health services offered, and availability of educational programs. An assessment of the community system using the Neuman Systems Model can be used to identify elder needs, services available, and services needed to maintain structural integrity.

TABLE 19–3. CONTINUUM OF COMMUNITY SERVICES FOR ELDERLY

Short to Mid-Range Housing	State mental hospital
	Acute care general hospital
	Chronic care hospital
	Rehabilitation
	Skilled nursing facility
	Intermediate care facility
Long-Range Housing	Hospice
	Group home
	Personal care home
	Foster home
	Domiciliary care home
	Boarding home
	Congregate care home
	With meals
	With social services
	With medical services
	With housekeeping
	Retirement villages
Community-based and In-Home Geriatric Services	Hospice in home
	Respite care
	Geriatric day rehabilitation hospital
	Adult day care
	Sheltered workshop
	Congregate meals
	Community mental health
	Senior citizen center
	Geriatric medical services
	Dental services
	Podiatry services
	Home health
	Legal services
	Protective services
	Visiting nurse
	Homemaker
	Home health aide
	Chore services
	Meals on Wheels

From S. J. Brody and C. Masciocchi (1980). Data for long-term care planning by health systems agencies. *American Journal of Public Health* 10:11.

THE APPLICATION OF THE NEUMAN SYSTEMS MODEL TO COMMON PHYSIOLOGICAL GERIATRIC SITUATIONS

Pressure Ulcers

Pressure ulcers are a common problem in hospitalization and bedridden elders. The estimates of incidence vary, but one large study of acute care facilities gave a prevalence rate of 9.2 percent (Meehan, 1990). The rate may be even higher for elderly patients hospitalized with hip fractures; one study found an incidence of 66 percent in this group (Versluysen, 1986). The basic structure in this case is normal intact skin, a factor common to all organisms. The common stressors known to be risk factors are increased pressure on the skin, shear forces, friction, poor nutrition, immobility, moisture, incontinence, and altered consciousness (AHCPR, 1992). The skin is normally protected by its flexible line of defense. Aging brings about skin changes that increase the propensity for breakdown and reduced ability to heal. These changes include thinning of the dermis, thickening of the epidermis, decreased collagen, reduced elasticity, and vascularity (McConnell, 1988). The normal line of defense includes the structures of the skin and ability to move, stay dry, and eat sufficient calories, vitamin C, zinc, and protein. When serious illness or movement deficits occur, the flexible and normal lines of defense are no longer able to protect the structural integrity of the aging skin. After identifying at-risk clients who are either nutritionally compromised or have impaired mobility, the nurse may institute a plan of care aimed at primary prevention to avoid a reaction to the identified stressors and resultant breakdown. The primary measures, designed to support the lines of defense and resistance, are shown in Table 19–4. Secondary prevention is directed toward the treatment of ulcers that have developed (see Table 19–5). Finally, for those clients who have recovered from a pressure ulcer, nursing activity is directed toward avoiding further breakdown using the preventive measures outlined in Table 19–4.

TABLE 19–4. PRIMARY PREVENTION: SKIN CARE OF THE ELDERLY

Assess skin daily
Keep the skin clean and dry
Maintain adequate ambient humidity
Keep the client hydrated
Maintain activity and movement or ensure the client is moved
    at least every two hours
Ensure adequate nutrition
Keep bony surfaces from contact with each other
Keep the heels elevated off the bed
Don't massage bony prominences
Use pressure-reducing mattresses and chair cushions

Adapted from: Pressure Ulcers in Adults: Prediction and Prevention. Clinical Practice Guideline, Number 3. US Department of Health and Human Services, Agency for Health Care Policy and Research, No. 92–0047.

TABLE 19–5. SECONDARY PREVENTION: CARE OF PRESSURE ULCERS

Stage 1

- Remove causative stressor
- Institute primary prevention measures

Stage 2

- Keep wound clean with normal saline
- Cover wounds with nonstick dressing or use hydrocolloid dressing

Stage 3

- Keep wound clean with normal saline
- Cover shallow wounds with a hydrocolloid dressing
- For deeper wounds, use wet saline dressings. Keep moist if wound is pink and clean. For wounds with eschar, allow to dry between changes.
- For very moist wounds, use chemical absorber

Stage 4

- Clean and irrigate wound with normal saline
- Pack wound with wet dressing, allow to dry
- Evaluate for other aides such as special mattresses, nutritional supplements, chemical debridement agents

Adapted from: Pressure Ulcers in Adults: Prediction and Prevention. Clinical Practice Guideline, Number 3. US Department of Health and Human Services, Agency for Health Care Policy and Research, No. 92–0047.

Urinary Incontinence

Urinary incontinence is the problematic, involuntary loss of urine, affecting up to 30 percent of noninstitutionalized elderly (AHCPR, 1992). There are multiple causes, including environmental problems from inaccessible toilets to internal causes such as medications and structural damage of the genito-urinary system. In the elderly, bladder capacity diminishes and there is an increase in involuntary bladder contractions. In elderly women there are the added problems of loss of bladder outlet and urethral resistance as a result of decreased estrogen and muscle tone loss from childbirth (Kane, Ouslander, and Abrass, 1989). While common, incontinence is not a normal part of aging. The basic structure is a urinary system that is emptied on a voluntary basis and where urination does not interfere with normal activities (see Figure 19–2). The client's flexible lines of defense may include frequent toileting, fluid restriction, and avoiding stimulants such as caffeine and alcohol. These activities may reduce incontinence in the client, but a stressor such as hospitalization breaks through the line and results in incontinence. Primary prevention techniques may include a regular and usual toileting regime, providing easy access to toilets, adequate lighting, keeping fluid consumption at a normal level (eight 8-ounce glasses), and avoiding tea, coffee, caffeine drinks, and alcohol. Secondary prevention may include treatment for

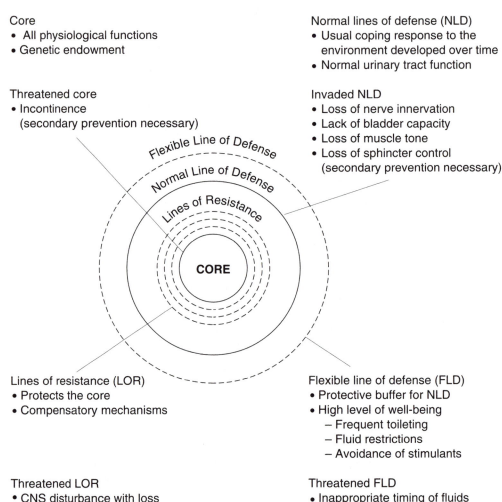

Core
- All physiological functions
- Genetic endowment

Threatened core
- Incontinence
  (secondary prevention necessary)

Normal lines of defense (NLD)
- Usual coping response to the environment developed over time
- Normal urinary tract function

Invaded NLD
- Loss of nerve innervation
- Lack of bladder capacity
- Loss of muscle tone
- Loss of sphincter control
  (secondary prevention necessary)

Lines of resistance (LOR)
- Protects the core
- Compensatory mechanisms

Threatened LOR
- CNS disturbance with loss of normal stimuli
- Use of diuretics with increased urine production
  (secondary prevention necessary)

Flexible line of defense (FLD)
- Protective buffer for NLD
- High level of well-being
  - Frequent toileting
  - Fluid restrictions
  - Avoidance of stimulants

Threatened FLD
- Inappropriate timing of fluids
- Difficulty in locating or getting to toilet
- Loss of self-esteem about loss of urine
  (primary prevention necessary)

Figure 19–2. Urinary Incontinence.

urinary tract infections, reduction of hypervolemic states, surgical removal of obstructions such as enlarged prostrate glands, bladder suspension operations for stress incontinence, and use of certain medications such as estrogen and bladder relaxants. For some clients the secondary interventions may include incontinence undergarments, external collection devices, and intermittent catheterization. Tertiary prevention may include teaching pelvic floor (Kegel) exercises, biofeedback, and bladder training.

Sleep Disturbances

Sleep disturbances are a common problem of aging and may affect over half of all elderly persons (National Commission on Sleep Disorders Research, 1992). While sleep problems are common, they are not a normal part of aging, and most will respond to treatment.

The key basic structure factor to be considered is that all humans require sleep (see Figure 19–3). The flexible lines of defense may include nighttime rituals, daily activity, comfortable bed, quiet surroundings, and avoidance of stimulating fluids and alcohol (Matteson and McConnell, 1988). The normal line of defense is the quantity and quality of sleep required by that client. The internal lines of resistance include the compensation factors of daytime sleepiness and naps. Internal stressors that may break the line of defense include the physical aging process of the central nervous system (causing circadian rhythm disturbance), illness, anxiety, nocturia, and depression. External stressors might include changes in sleep environment and noise levels. Primary prevention of sleep disturbances includes maintaining nighttime rituals and assuring adequate, normal daytime activity. Besides rectifying external causes of sleep disturbances, secondary prevention may include the treatment of sleep-disturbing disease symptoms such as orthopnea, sleep apnea, nocturia, and angina. Psychological disturbances such as grief, anxiety, and depression must also be treated. Tertiary prevention includes teaching so the individual can avoid future problems and for certain individuals may include sleep-time behavior modification (National Commission on Sleep Disorders Research, 1992). Behavior modification techniques include such strategies as getting out of bed if sleep does not come in a specified period of time, using the bedroom only for sleep and sex, and setting and adhering to set bedtime and rising schedules.

Elder Mistreatment

Elder mistreatment, which includes abuse and neglect, is a serious and common problem in this country, with up to 10 percent of all elders being affected (JAMA, 1987). Fulmer and O'Malley (1987) define abuse as the actions of a caregiver that create unmet needs for the elder and neglect as the failure of the caregiver to respond to established needs for care. Whatever its definition, it affects both sexes and cuts across all socioeconomic, ethnic, and religious groups. The same is true of those who abuse the elderly. There are many theories to explain mistreatment, but none have proved fully explanatory.

Elder mistreatment affects the basic structure (psychological) that addresses affiliation. A core assumption of humans is that those who care for others will not harm them. When the caregiver becomes an abuser, there is a basic loss of trust, which is even more traumatic when the abuser is a family member.

The flexible line of defense against abuse or neglect is the ability of the elder to avoid the abuser or the abuser's actions or to seek support in removing

Core
- All physiological functions
- Genetic endowment

Normal line of defense (NLD)
- Usual coping response to environment developed over time
- Normal sleep pattern

Threatened core
- Sleep disturbance (secondary prevention necessary)

Invaded NLD
- Altered sleep pattern (secondary prevention necessary)

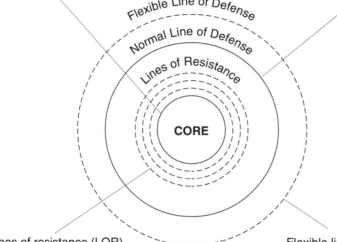

Lines of resistance (LOR)
- Protects the core
- Compensatory mechanisms
  - Fatigue
  - Naps

Flexible line of defense (FLD)
- Protective buffer for NLD
- High level of well-being

Threatened LOR
- The elderly patient
  - Changes in circadian rhythms
  - Depression/grief
  - Presence of chronic disease
  - Debilitated condition (secondary prevention necessary)

Threatened FLD
- Loss of comfortable bed
- Inability to perform sleep-time rituals
- Lack of activity
- Stimulating fluids and alcohol (primary prevention necessary)

Figure 19–3. Sleep Disturbance.

the abuser (see Table 19–6). The normal line of defense can be conceptualized as the actions taken to ward off harm, such as striking back. The internal lines of resistance may include denial on the elder's part, withdrawal, and going along with the abuse to avoid further trouble.

The primary prevention of abuse may include awareness of escalating stress

TABLE 19–6. FACTORS CONTRIBUTING TO MISTREATMENT

Interpersonal

Elderly person is:
  Vulnerable target
  Scapegoat
  Isolated
  Powerless
  Not able to fight back
  In poor health
  In poor physical condition
  Increasingly dependent
Lack of social and emotional support systems
Poverty/financial stress
Poor housing
Lack of options for help

Intrapersonal

Family stress or crisis, including economic, housing, marital
Family member's unemployment
Substance abuse in family
Longstanding problems between family members and elder
Pathology of family/breakdown of family pattern
Changing roles/role reversals
Unrealistic role expectations
Issues of power
Financial control

Extrapersonal

Inadequate community resources, social services, and planning
Lack of skilled practitioners to provide help
Lack of commitment and concern for elderly
Negative attitudes of the public, including stereotypes
Insufficient follow-up by practitioners or others

Adapted from P. N. Chen, S. L. Bell, D. L. Dolinsky, et al. (1981). Elderly abuse in domestic settings: A pilot study. *Journal of Gerontologic Social Work* 4(1):3–17.

in a caregiver. The stressed caregiver theory of abuse says that as stress levels in the caregivers rise so does abuse (O'Malley, Everett, O'Malley, and Campion, 1983). Another preventive measure is to identify, if possible, caregivers who themselves have been abused, have psychopathology, or will gain from the abusive situation. These preventive measures are based on other explanatory theories of mistreatment including transgenerational violence, which posits that those who have been abused will themselves abuse. The exchange theory explains abusers who gain from the abuse (e.g., psychologically or financially) and so will continue to abuse (Pillemer, 1986). Abusers have also been identified as dependent (dependency theory) upon those they abuse for housing, repairs, finances, and transportation (Pillemer and Wolfe, 1986). And caregivers who exhibit signs of psychiatric illness, substance abuse, or mental retardation (psychopathology theory) may be more prone to mistreat than others (Pillemer and Finkelhor, 1989).

Secondary prevention must include the identification of abuse. It is often the case that the signs of abuse are subtle, confused with normal conditions of aging or accidents and unreported by the elder. Detection is often very difficult (Peirce, Ryan, and Fulmer, in press). Once assessed, the abused elder should be referred to an appropriate service, such as police, adult protective services, lawyers, clergy, and abuse programs (Pratt, Koval, and Lloyd, 1983).

Tertiary prevention is then aimed at restoring the elder to a state of wellness. Tertiary care may involve individual and family counseling, finding new housing for the elder, and ensuring that any protective services put in place are maintained (see Table 19–6).

Elder mistreatment was considered from the level of the individual, but this problem could also be effectively analyzed in the systems model at the family or community level.

RESEARCH, GERIATRICS, AND THE NEUMAN SYSTEMS MODEL

The Neuman Systems Model can provide the conceptual framework needed to support a wide range of research studies on the nursing care, and other needs, of the elderly. The following examples illustrate the many possibilities for future studies:

1. What nutritional factors best protect the flexible and normal lines of defense of the elderly's skin?
2. What hospital-induced stressors can be modified to reduce the invasion of elders' sleep lines of defense?
3. What client variables of the five identified by Neuman are most influenced when elders are mistreated?

FUTURE IMPLICATIONS FOR GERIATRIC USE OF THE NEUMAN SYSTEMS MODEL

Escalating changes in the health care system are mandating nursing structures and activities that are comprehensive, effective, and adaptable. The features of the Neuman Systems Model make it reasonable to assume that it will play an increasing role in the future of nursing, especially in the care of the elderly. The Neuman Model allows the nurse to conceptualize the elderly client as an individual as well as part of a family and community.

REFERENCES

Alford, D. M., and Futrell, M. 1992. AAN working paper: Wellness and health promotion of the elderly. *Nursing Outlook* 40(5):221–226.

Atchley, R. C. 1984. *The Social Forces in Later Life*. Belmont, Calif.: Wadsworth Publishing Company.

Beljan, J., Bertozzi, G., Estes, S., et al. 1987. Council of Scientific Affairs: Elder abuse and neglect. *JAMA* 257:966–971.

Brody, S. 1978. The family unit: A major consideration in the long term care support system. *Gerontologist* 25(1):556–560.

Campion, E. W., Mulley, A. G., Folstein, R. L., et al. 1981. Medical intensive care for the elderly: A study of current use, costs and outcomes. *JAMA* 246:2052–2056.

DiMateo, M. R., and DiNicola, D. D. 1982. *Achieving Patient Compliance: The Psychology of the Medical Practitioner's Role*. New York: Pergamon Press.

Erikson, E. H., Erikson, J. M., and Kivnik, H. Q. 1986. *Vital Involvement in Old Age*. New York: W. W. Norton.

Fulmer, T. T., and O'Malley, T. A. 1987. *Inadequate Care of the Elderly*. New York: Springer Publishing Company.

Kane, R. L., Ouslander, J. G., and Abrass, I. B. 1989. *Essentials of Clinical Geriatrics,* 2d ed. New York: McGraw-Hill.

Markides, K. S. 1983. Aging, religiosity and adjustment. *Journal of Gerontology* 38(5): 621–625.

McConnell, E. S. 1988. Nursing diagnoses related to physiological alterations. In *Gerontological Nursing: Concepts and Practice,* by M. A. Matteson and E. S. McConnell, 331–428. Thorofare, N.J.: W. B. Saunders.

Meehan, M. 1990. Multisite pressure ulcer prevalence survey. *Decubitus* 3(4):14–17.

National Center for Health Statistics: Health United States. 1990. DHHS Pub. No. 90–1232, Public Health Service. Washington, D.C.: US Government Printing Office.

National Commission on Sleep Disorders Research. 1992. Wake up America: A National Sleep Alert. Washington, D.C.: US Printing Office.

O'Malley, T. A., Everett, D. C., O'Malley, H. C., and Campion, E. W. 1983. Identifying and preventing family-mediated abuse and neglect of elderly persons. *Annals of Internal Medicine*. 98(6):998–1005.

Peirce, A. G., Ryan, M., and Fulmer, T. T. In press. Elder mistreatment. In *Nursing Issues in the 90's,* edited by D. Fishman and O. Strickland. Albany, N.Y.: Delmar.

Peirce, A. G., Wright, F., and Fulmer, T. T. 1992. Needs of the family during critical illness of elderly patients. *Critical Care Nursing Clinics of North America* 4(4):597–606.

Pillemer, K. A. 1986. Risk factors in elder abuse: Results from a case-control study. In *Elder Abuse: Conflict in the Family,* edited by K. A. Pillemer and R. S. Wolfe. Dover: Auburn House.

Pillemer, K. A., and Finkelhor, D. 1988. The prevalence of elder abuse: A random sample survey. *The Gerontologist* 28:51–57.

Pillemer, K. A., and Wolfe, R. S., eds. *Elder Abuse: Conflict in the Family*. Dover: Auburn House.

Pratt, C., Koval, J., and Lloyd, S. 1983. Service workers responses to abuse in the elderly. *Social Casework* 64(3):147–153.

Rowe, J. W., and Besdine, R. W. 1987. *Geriatric Medicine*. Boston: Little, Brown, & Co.

US Department of Health and Human Services; Agency for Health Care Policy and

Research. 1992. Pressure Ulcers in Adults: Prediction and Prevention. Clinical Practice Guideline: Number 3. Washington, D.C.: US Printing Office.

US Department of Health and Human Services; Agency for Health Care Policy and Research. 1992. Urinary Incontinence in Adults. Clinical Practice Guideline. Washington, D.C.: US Printing Office.

US Department of Health and Human Services Staff. 1992. *Healthy People 2000: National Health Promotion and Disease Prevention Objectives.* Boston: Jones and Bartlett Pub.

US Senate Special Committee on Aging in Conjunction with the AARP, FCOA, and the USAA. 1988. Aging America: Trends and Projections. Washington, D.C.: US Printing Office.

Versluysen, M. 1986. How elderly patients with femoral fracture develop pressure sores in hospital. *British Journal of Medicine* 292:1311–1313.

20

APPLICATION OF THE NEUMAN SYSTEMS MODEL TO PERINATAL NURSING

Marie-Josée Trépanier
Sandra I. Dunn
Ann E. Sprague

Perinatal nursing is one of a growing number of specialized areas of practice. Because of the complexity of perinatal care, nurses who work in this area require education beyond the basic level. In this chapter we will stress how the Neuman Systems Model can guide perinatal nursing education and practice. To demonstrate the utility of the model, we will draw on the example of low birthweight, one of the most pressing problems in perinatal care today.

USE OF THE NEUMAN SYSTEMS MODEL IN PERINATAL NURSING EDUCATION

The University of Ottawa School of Nursing, in collaboration with the Perinatal Education Program of Eastern Ontario, offers three courses in its post-RN baccalaureate program's perinatal concentration. Using the Neuman Systems Model as their theoretical framework, these courses focus on the identification and management of the mother, fetus, neonate, and family at risk during the antepartum, intrapartum, and neonatal periods. The courses emphasize not only the wholistic assessment of strengths and stressors that influence clients' well-being but also the primary, secondary, and tertiary intervention strategies that help attain and maintain wellness. The clinical component of the courses allows the students to enhance their knowledge and to use the model while caring for perinatal clients in a variety of settings. In the remainder of the chapter, we will summarize how we adapted the Neuman Model in these courses to help the students learn its value in perinatal care.

VIEW OF THE PERINATAL CLIENT

The perinatal client, by definition, is the pregnant woman and fetus, or the neonate. In Neuman's terms they each consist of five variables (physiological, psychological, sociocultural, developmental, and spiritual), and they are constantly exposed to stressors from within (intrapersonal), from others (interpersonal), and from their environment (extrapersonal). The mother, fetus, or newborn can be viewed separately, but they are also considered interdependent units influencing each other. In addition, the role of the family in contributing to the client's well-being can never be overlooked.

Figure 20–1 illustrates fetal growth and development through the use of the model's concentric circles. At this point, a brief review of these circles will help interpret the diagrams. The flexible line of defense (FLD), comprised of the client's strengths, reflects the degree of protection for the normal line of defense (NLD). Lack or absence of strengths exposes the NLD to stressor penetration. The NLD represents the normal state of client functioning that has developed over time. The lines of resistance (LOR) refer to the resources that the client mobilizes to fight the stressors that have penetrated the NLD and threaten the core.

Following conception, the fetal core (made up of the organ systems) develops within the maternal core. At this point, the fetal lines of resistance and defense are virtually nonexistent. The fetus totally depends on the mother for survival and for protection from stressors (Figure 20-1A). As much as the mother protects the fetus, she can also be a stressor. Conversely, the fetus can become one of the various stressors that the mother adapts to during pregnancy.

As gestation advances and fetal and maternal cores gradually separate, the fetus develops its own lines of resistance, which continue to strengthen throughout gestation. The LORs provide the growing fetus with compensatory mechanisms to combat stressors. However, before the 24th week of gestation, the fetus remains totally dependent on the mother and is greatly affected by stressors that they both may encounter. Survival is unlikely if birth occurs before this point (CPS and SOGC, 1993) (Figure 20–1B).

If the fetus is born prematurely, its lines of defense and resistance are weak. Survival is possible, but varying degrees of support are required, depending on the extent of prematurity. Moreover, the mother is still completing the develop-

THE MATERNAL-FETAL UNIT

About 8 – 12 Weeks Gestation

A

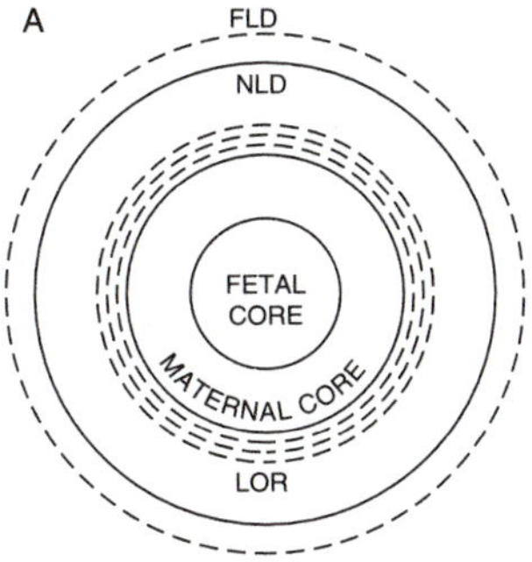

FLD
NLD
FETAL CORE
MATERNAL CORE
LOR

- Physiological function of all organ systems develop
- Fetus totally dependent on mother for protection from stressors
- Fetus can be a stressor to mother (i.e., hyperemesis)
- Mother can be a stressor to fetus (i.e., infection)

About 12 – 24 Weeks Gestation

B

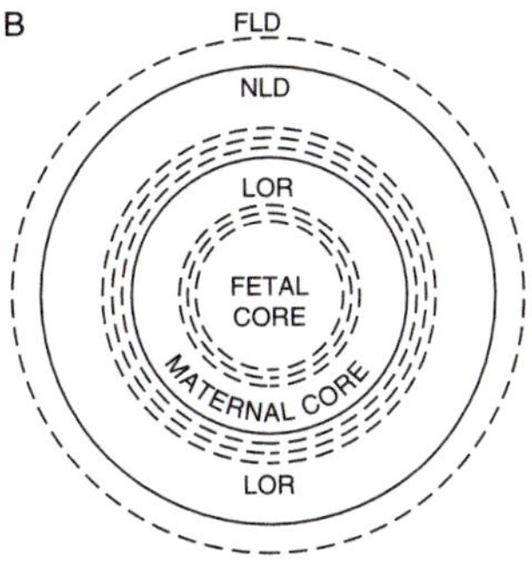

FLD
NLD
LOR
FETAL CORE
MATERNAL CORE
LOR

- Fetal LOR developing
- Some compensatory mechanisms established (i.e., fetal tachycardia with hypoxia)
- Stressors affecting mother affect the fetus
- Fetus totally dependent on mother
- Survival unlikely if born at this point

About 24 – 37 Weeks Gestation

C

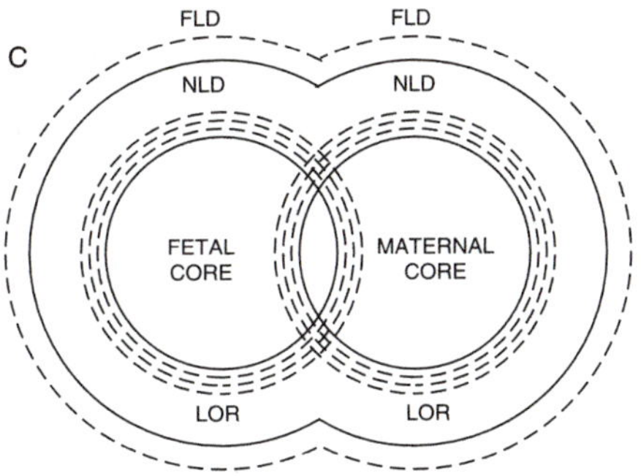

FLD   FLD
NLD   NLD
FETAL CORE   MATERNAL CORE
LOR   LOR

- The maternal unit provides NLD and FLD:
  - Protection from infection
  - Oxygenation
  - Nutrition
- Maternal developmental tasks not achieved
- Survival may be possible if born now
- Varying degrees of support will be required dependent on level of prematurity

D

FLD
NLD
LOR
INFANT CORE

THE FULL-TERM NEONATE AND MOTHER

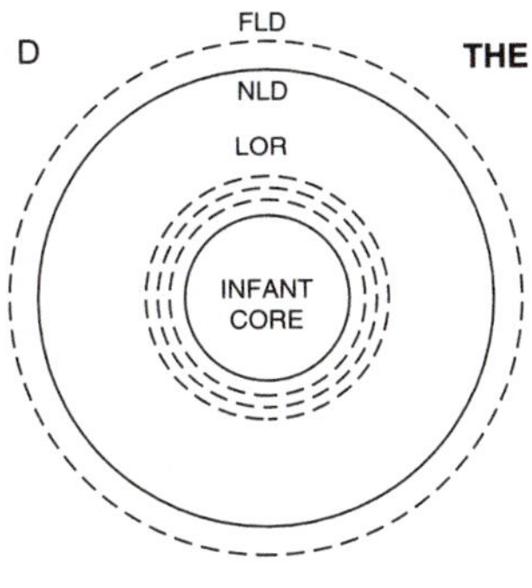

- Following birth, the neonate is a separate individual
- Still dependent on family and caregivers

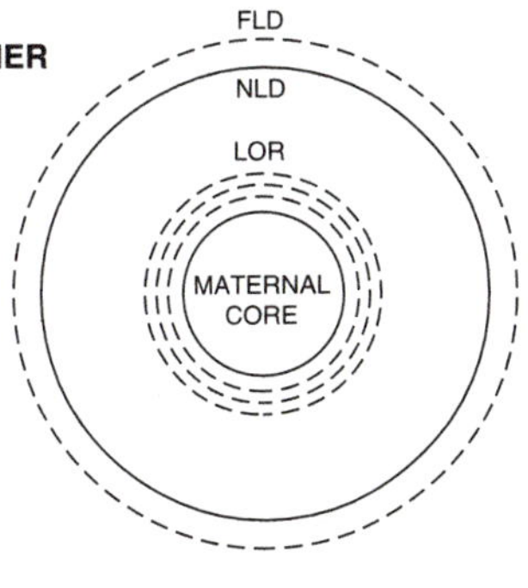

FLD
NLD
LOR
MATERNAL CORE

Figure 20–1. Growth and Development of the Fetus.

mental tasks of pregnancy. Nurses must therefore carefully consider gestation and stage of development when planning care (Figure 20–1C).

At birth the infant and the mother become separate individuals (Figure 20–1D). The full-term neonate is born with its own resistance and defense mechanisms. However, the flexible line of defense is weak, and the baby's well-being depends on support from others (mother, family, caregivers). To survive, the neonate needs a sturdy normal life of defense (e.g., strong and stable respiratory and cardiovascular functions).

ASSESSMENT OF PERINATAL CLIENTS

Nurses working in perinatal settings have early and frequent contact with pregnant women, neonates, and their families. This places them in an ideal position to thoroughly assess the clients' strengths and stressors, a crucial component of comprehensive perinatal care. The Neuman Systems Model provides a foundation for this thorough assessment.

We have designed maternal/fetal and neonatal/family assessment tools to help the nurse collect and concisely organize client data. Table 20–1 shows the abbreviated version of the Maternal/Fetal Assessment Tool, and Table 20–2 shows the Neonatal/Family Assessment Tool. Nurses can integrate information from the three sources of strengths/stressors (intra-, inter-, and extrapersonal) with each of the five variables (physiological, psychological, sociocultural, developmental, and spiritual) in a grid format. Each tool therefore comprises 15 sections, and the items outlined in each section list key factors to explore with the client. The examples offered are suggestions only. We recognize that overlapping can occur in the categorization of findings, and this is acceptable as long as the nurse assesses all facets and explores those requiring further investigation. On request the authors will provide a detailed version of both tools.

RISK GRADING

After completing the initial client assessment, the nurse must determine priorities for care. This involves grading the risk or the degree of stressor penetration, in other words, the extent of client stability or instability. The Perinatal Risk-Grading Tool (Figure 20–2) was designed for just this purpose. Relevant data from the assessment tool goes onto a one-page form that highlights strengths and stressors from all five variables. This distinguishes it from risk-grading tools in the medical model, which focus mainly on detecting physiological stressors. It uses four risk categories (AA, A, B, C) to determine the extent of protection from stressors and/or the degree to which the normal line of defense has been penetrated (Figure 20–3).

A strong FLD is reflected by an AA rating in the Perinatal Risk-Grading Tool.

TABLE 20–1. NEUMAN SYSTEMS MODEL ASSESSMENT OF THE MATERNAL/ FETAL UNIT

Sources of Stressors		
Intrapersonal	*Interpersonal*	*Extrapersonal*
Physiological Variables		

Maternal
Weight and weight gain
Nutritional status
Pregnancy-related
  complications
Labor progress/complications
Systems assessment
Lab results
	Maternal
	Family health history
	Relationships that influence
	  maternal physiological
	  status
		Maternal
		Environmental hazards
		Invasive tests/procedures

Fetal Estimated weight FHR characteristics Fetal blood sampling Fetal assessment results	*Fetal* Maternal life-style factors Maternal conditions affecting fetal status	*Fetal* Environmental hazards Invasive tests/procedures
Psychological Variables		
Maternal Developmental tasks of pregnancy Self-concept Stress Normal coping mechanisms Major stressors	*Maternal* Support Significant relationships Communication patterns Bereavement Family violence Responses to crisis	*Maternal* Transfer/separation Hospitalization Tests, procedures, situations
Sociocultural Variables		

Maternal
Marital status
Occupation
Cultural/ethnic background
Language(s)
Cultural beliefs/values
  regarding:
• Health practices
• Pregnancy
• Birth
• Infant nutrition
• Postpartum period
• Child care
• Father's role
	Maternal
	Father's/partner's
	• Occupation
	• Cultural background
	• Language
	Other children
	Roles/tasks within the family
	Social support
		Maternal
		Socioeconomic status
		Financial problems
		Social service involvement
		Effect of pregnancy on pat-
		  terns of living

Developmental Variables		

Maternal
Age
Developmental tasks
Education level
Knowledge deficits
Previous experience
	Maternal
	Prenatal classes
	Planned feeding method
		Maternal
		Environmental factors
		  influencing growth and
		  development

Fetal
Gestational age
Genetic/congenial anomalies
	Fetal
	Maternal factors affecting
	  growth and development
		Fetal
		Environmental factors
		  influencing growth and
		  development

Spiritual Variables		

Maternal
Religion or religious beliefs
	Maternal
	Parental or partner spiritual
	  belief that may influence
	  maternal/fetal health
		Maternal
		Spiritual support

TABLE 20–2. NEUMAN SYSTEMS MODEL ASSESSMENT OF THE INFANT AND FAMILY

Sources of Stressors		
Intrapersonal	*Interpersonal*	*Extrapersonal*
Physiological Variables		

Infant
Physical assessment
Organ system weakness/
  disease
Lab x-ray findings
Diagnostic tests
Nutritional status
	Maternal Conditions Affecting
	  Fetal Development and
	  Status at Birth
	Health:
	• Past OB history
	• Pregnancy (present)
	• Labor and delivery
	Lifestyle habits:
	• Smoking/alcohol/drugs
	• Family violence
		Environmental Hazards to
		  Infant
		Transport
		Cold stress
		Invasive tests/procedures

Psychological Variables		

Infant
Behavioral assessment
Signs of stress/coping
	Parental Interactions and
	  Coping
	Self-concept
	Bonding and attachment
	Bereavement
	Family violence
	Responses to crisis:
	• Communication patterns
	• Anxiety/stress
	• Interpersonal relationships
	• Problem solving/decision
	  making
	• Role conflict
	• Support systems
		Environmental Stressors to
		  Infant and Family
		ICU environment
		Hospitalization
		Transfer/separation
		Tests/procedures

Sociocultural Variables		

Infant's Family Composition
Marital status
Siblings
Cultural/ethnic background
Language(s)
	Family Functioning that May
	  Influence Acceptance/
	  Coping
	Cultural beliefs/values
	  regarding:
	• Health practices
	• Pregnancy/birth/postpartum
	• Infant nutrition
	• Critical care
	Decision-making mechanisms
	Patterns of daily living
	Conflict resolution ability
	Task allocation/role conflict
		Environmental Factors That
		  May Influence Family
		  Functioning
		Occupation
		Socioeconomic status
		Financial problems
		Social service involvement
		Community resources

Developmental Variables		

Infant Development
Gestational age
Birthweight
Genetic/congenital anomalies
Developmental status
	Family Development and
	  Parenting Ability
	Parental age
	Developmental tasks of
	  parenting
	Education level
	Knowledge deficits
	Previous experience
		Environmental Factors That
		  May Influence Infant's
		  Development
		Excessive/inadequate stimuli
		Educational programs for
		  parents
		Community resources

Spiritual Variables		
Family Religion or religious beliefs	*Religious Beliefs That May* *Influence Infant Care* Circumcision Blood transfusion Conflicts with religious beliefs	*Spiritual Support*

Following completion of the assessment tool, transfer the identified strengths/stressors within the five variables, according to the following grading system.

Client has a high functional level that provides extra buffer against stressors. (Normal perinatal care required.)
List *strengths* here:

FLD   Physical   _____

       Psychological   _____

AA   Sociological   _____

       Developmental   _____

       Spiritual   _____

Client is in usual steady state of wellness and is at no predictable risk. (Normal perinatal care required.)
List *normal findings* here:

NLD   Physical   _____

       Psychological   _____

A   Sociological   _____

       Developmental   _____

       Spiritual   _____

Client is experiencing stressors that put the mother/fetus/neonate at risk. (Basic or advanced perinatal care required.)
List *mild to moderate stressors* here:

       Physical   _____

B   Psychological   _____

       Sociological   _____

       Developmental   _____

       Spiritual   _____

LOR   Client is experiencing stressors that are so overwhelming that the mother/fetus/neonate are obviously in danger. (Critical perinatal care required.)
List *severe stressors* here:

       Physical   _____

       Psychological   _____

       Sociological   _____

C   Developmental   _____

       Spiritual   _____

Figure 20–2. A Guide to Perinatal Risk Grading.

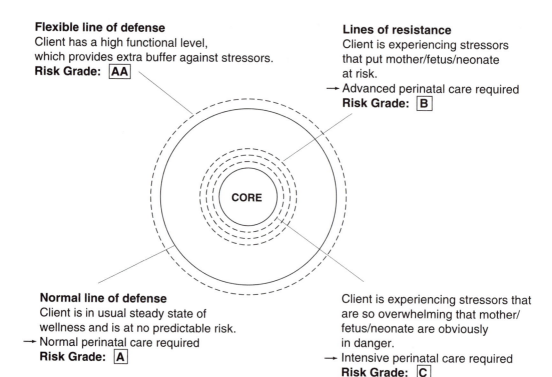

Flexible line of defense
Client has a high functional level,
which provides extra buffer against stressors.
Risk Grade: AA

Lines of resistance
Client is experiencing stressors
that put mother/fetus/neonate
at risk.
→ Advanced perinatal care required
Risk Grade: B

Normal line of defense
Client is in usual steady state of
wellness and is at no predictable risk.
→ Normal perinatal care required
Risk Grade: A

Client is experiencing stressors that
are so overwhelming that mother/
fetus/neonate are obviously
in danger.
→ Intensive perinatal care required
Risk Grade: C

CORE

Figure 20–3. Neuman Systems Model—Degree of Stressor Penetration:
A Guide to Perinatal Risk Grading.

The client's *strengths,* identified in any of the five variables, are recorded here
(e.g., supportive family and community environment, excellent nutrition, previous experience). This tells the nurse that the client has resources to prevent or
minimize the effects of stressors. Supportive primary interventions can then help
the client maintain a high level of wellness.

An A rating applies to a client who is in a steady, usual state of wellness,
indicating an intact NLD. *Normal findings* (e.g., normal weight gain, lab values,
and vital signs; absence of signs and symptoms) in the five variables are noted
here. Nurses should provide both primary interventions and secondary interventions for early stressor identification.

When a client's NLD has been penetrated and LORs are mobilized (indicating a client's response to stressors), a risk grade of B or C is assigned. If
moderate stressors appear in any of the variables, but the client's life is not immediately threatened (e.g., controlled insulin-dependent diabetes, hyperbiliru-
binemia), a B risk is given. However, when *stressors are so overwhelming*
that life is endangered (e.g., severe hemorrhage, extreme prematurity, refusal

of treatment due to spiritual or cultural beliefs), a C risk is assigned. Differentiating between a B and C risk involves judging how stressors affect the client (based on either the number or severity of stressors, or the client's perception of the stressors). Secondary interventions are required in various degrees, depending on whether the client needs basic or advanced care (B risk), or critical care (C risk).

Once the nurse has identified the stressors and assigned a risk grade, he or she can develop an individualized plan of care. The first step involves formulating and ranking nursing diagnoses in order of priority. In the second step, the client and the nurse work together to determine the client goals, or desired level of wellness, for each problem identified. In the third step, the nurse plans the appropriate levels of intervention (primary, secondary, or tertiary). Finally, to determine whether the plan of care was effective, the nurse must evaluate goal attainment. This completed process represents a comprehensive approach to nursing care.

FUTURE IMPLICATIONS: USING THE NEUMAN MODEL TO ADDRESS THE PROBLEM OF LOW BIRTHWEIGHT

Because the Neuman Systems Model provides a truly comprehensive approach to health promotion and maintenance, it is the perfect tool with which to address the most pressing problem in perinatal care today: low birthweight (LBW). In fact, approximately 16 percent of all infants worldwide have LBW (Kramer, 1987), a problem that accounts for about 75 percent of early neonatal mortality in both Canada (Silins et al., 1985) and the United States (McCormick, 1984, 1985). LBW also contributes significantly to both infant and childhood morbidity (Aylward, Pfeiffer, Wright, and Verhulst, 1989; Dunn, 1981; Hack and Fanaroff, 1984, 1989; Kramer, 1987; Millar, Strachan, and Wadhera, 1992; Mitchell and Najak, 1989; Paton and Yacoub, 1987; Teberg, Walther, and Pena, 1988).

Over the years, advances in perinatal medical technology have led to a dramatic decrease in the rate of infant mortality; however, the rate of LBW has decreased only slightly (Watters and Avard, 1992). The two major contributors of LBW are preterm birth and intrauterine growth restriction. Therefore, as we move toward the 21st century, we must concentrate on decreasing the modifiable risk factors for these problems: poverty, smoking, alcohol and drug use, young maternal age, prepregnancy and prenatal nutrition, low education level, stress, working conditions, violence, environmental toxins, and lack of prenatal care (Kramer, 1987; Watters and Avard, 1992).

Currently, LBW prevention focuses on identifying and treating medical risk factors. Women found to be at risk are followed more closely and may, in fact, be referred to a high-risk-prevention program. However, this approach has limited impact on LBW because it does not always address the many social and environmental factors mentioned above, nor does it consider the impact of the family and the community on pregnancy and birth (Stewart and Nimrod, 1993). On the other hand, by using the Neuman Model to conduct a client assessment, the nurse can easily identify many of the modifiable risk factors for LBW (see examples in Table 20–3).

The risk-grading tool, which lists client stressors and strengths, helps to determine the degree of instability (threat to the core) and the type of care required. Let us use as an example a woman carrying twins: she is at higher risk of LBW. If this woman is threatened by other stressors such as smoking, family violence, and poverty, the risk of LBW would increase even more; as a result, she would be considered more unstable and in need of many more secondary interventions. Conversely, if she has none of these stressors, benefits from ample social support, and truly perceives these as strengths, she now has resources that increase her ability to cope with the risk of LBW infants; this means that primary interventions may suffice in maintaining her stability and preventing stressor invasion. Therefore, nurses must consider the strengths, as well as the stressors, to individualize care and plan the appropriate primary, secondary, and/or tertiary interventions.

A supportive family and community, along with the individual's willingness to change behavior and participate in care, play a vital role in decreasing the effects of the modifiable risk factors for low birthweight. When developing LBW prevention strategies, nurses can rely on the Neuman Model to help them view the client as an entire family or community, a broader perspective that increases the diversity of prevention approaches. Furthermore, because the health care dollar is increasingly limited, health promotion and illness prevention are becoming the most logical approaches to care. So, not only does the Neuman Model provide a framework for wholistic assessment, it also helps nurses focus on prevention and health promotion—the very tenets of optimal perinatal care.

TABLE 20–3. MATERNAL/FETAL STRESSORS ASSOCIATED WITH LBW

	Intrapersonal	Interpersonal	Extrapersonal
Physiological	Malnutrition, smoking, drug and alcohol use	Battering	Environmental toxins
Psychological	Stress	Family violence	Work environment
Sociocultural	Poverty	Lack of social support	Isolated cultural group
Developmental	Young maternal age	Lack of antenatal care	Low education level
Spiritual		Religious conflict	

These are provided only as examples and are not all-inclusive.

SUMMARY

This chapter demonstrates how the Neuman Systems Model can be adapted for use in perinatal care settings. Because nursing the perinatal client requires highly specialized skills, nurses can only benefit from a structured framework that guides their care. The Neuman Systems Model provides such a framework, allowing nurses to:

- Develop more effective and thorough assessment skills, leading to a wholistic view of the client
- Gain expertise in identifying risk factors (potential and actual)
- Improve their skills in gathering and organizing data on client strengths and stressors
- Improve the planning of interventions and identify the proper level of prevention
- Increase their awareness of discrepancies that exist between the client's perception of the situation and their own

Improved assessment tools and a risk-grading tool, presented here for the first time, provide a means of determining priorities of care based on an assessment of strengths and stressors. We have shown that the Neuman Model is flexible enough to cover the entire spectrum of perinatal nursing, from health promotion to critical care. To demonstrate the utility of the model, we have examined the issue of low birthweight. This structured framework should not only help nurses provide the best possible perinatal care but also improve their professional satisfaction and accountability.

REFERENCES

Aylward, G., Pfeiffer, S., Wright, A., and Verhulst, S. 1989. Outcome studies of low birthweight infants published in the last decade: A meta-analysis. *Journal of Pediatrics* 115(4):515–520.

Canadian Pediatric Society (CPS) and Society of Obstetricians and Gynecologists of Canada (SOGC). 1993. *Approach to the Woman with Threatened Birth of an Extremely Low Gestational Age Infant (22–26 Completed Weeks)*. Publication pending.

Dunn, H. 1981. *Residual Handicaps in Children of Low Birth Weight*. Ottawa: Author.

Hack, M., and Faranoff, A. 1984. The outcome of growth failure associated with preterm birth. *Clinical Obstetrics and Gynecology* 27(3):647–661.

Hack, M., and Faranoff, A 1989. Outcome of extremely low birthweight infants between 1982 and 1988. *The New England Journal of Medicine* 321(24):1642–1647.

Kramer, M. S. 1987. Determinants of low birth weight: Methodological assessment and meta-analysis. *Bulletin of the World Health Organization* 65 (5):663–737.

McCormick, M. 1985. The contribution of low birth weight to infant mortality and childhood morbidity. *The New England Journal of Medicine* 312:82–90.

McCormick, M., Shapiro, S., and Starfield, B. 1984. High-risk young mothers: Infant mortality and morbidity in four areas in the United States. *American Journal of Public Health* 74(1):8–23.

Millar, W., Strachan, J., and Wadhera, S. 1991. Trends in low birthweight Canada, 1977–1989. *Health Reports 1991* 3(4):311–325.

Mitchell, S., and Najak, Z. 1989. Low birthweight infants and rehospitalization: What's the incidence? *Neonatal Network* 8(3):27–36.

Paton, T., and Yacoub, W. 1987. *The Risk Register Approach to Observation of Children's Development: A Review of the Literature from 1980–1986.* Edmonton: Board of Health.

Silins, J., Semenciw, R., Morrison, H., Lindsay, J., Sherman, G., Mao, Y., and Wigle, D. 1985. Risk factors for perinatal mortality in Canada. *Canadian Medical Association Journal* 133:1214–1219.

Stewart, P., and Nimrod, C. 1993. The need to use a community-wide approach to promote healthy babies and prevent low birthweight. *Canadian Medical Association Journal* in press.

Teberg, A., Walther, F., and Pena, I. 1988. Outcomes of SGA infants. *Seminars in Perinatology* 12(1):84–87.

Watters, N., and Avard, D. 1992. *Prevention of Low Birthweight in Canada: Literature Review and Strategies.* Ottawa: Canadian Institute of Child Health.

21

USING NEUMAN FOR A STABLE PARENT SUPPORT GROUP IN NEONATAL INTENSIVE CARE

Leigh Ann Ware
Mary K. Shannahan

In the past, critically ill and premature infants died, usually within the first 24 to 48 hours of life. By the early 1980s the death rate was 13 to 14 for every 1,000 of these infants (Harrison and Kositsky, 1983). The increased survival rate of these infants is the result of the biomedical and technological advances in neonatology, including the establishment of neonatal intensive care units (NICUs). Survival does not guarantee health or a problem-free status, however. Due to long-term sequelae of being critically ill or premature at birth, a child may have disabilities requiring long-term parental and professional care. Generally, parents have neither anticipated the challenges to be faced nor planned how to meet these challenges. Therefore, they experience significant psychological stress. Without adequate support during and after an infant's discharge from the NICU, parents may face "burn-out" due to parenting a less mature and/or less responsive infant. This can result in an abusive or neglectful situation for the child (Yoos, 1989). Parent support groups (PSGs) can be effective in assisting with

The authors thank R. Shawn Coughlin for assistance with graphics.

the resolution of these issues by providing parent-to-parent support services (Steele, 1987).

PSGs fill a real need, but not all groups become stable. Group stability can be conceived of as involving three dimensions: (1) length of time in existence; (2) provision of basic services such as regular meetings, newsletter/printed materials, and postdischarge follow-up care; and (3) provision of innovative activities such as lobbying for supportive legislation and satellite services in outlying communities (Ware, 1992a, 1992b). Nurses are in a unique position to enhance group stability through use of the Neuman Systems Model and conceptualization of the PSG as client system.

APPLICATION OF THE NEUMAN SYSTEMS MODEL

An adaptation of the Neuman Systems Model (NSM) was used in developing the Parent Support Group as Client (PSGC) Model. The NSM includes the individual, families, groups, and/or the community as a client system (Neuman, 1989). Within this model the PSG is the client system having the following interrelated subsystems: parent-to-parent support, group parent support, parent education and information sharing, financial ability to support group functioning, and advocacy for PSG services.

According to Fawcett (1983), any conceptual model of nursing must address four central concepts: person, health, environment, and nursing. Each is defined below to provide the foundation for the PSGC Model. *Person* is the parent support group, which includes all family members who have preterm or critically ill NICU infants and who participate in a parent support group. The *environment* is all intra-, inter-, and extrasystem forces affecting and affected by the PSG, which is itself part of each family's environment. Unique to the Neuman Model is the created environment, which is protective and unconsciously derived. It acts as a "shield or 'safety net' against the reality of the environment" (Neuman, 1990, 130). Table 21–1 identifies the internal, external, and created environments for the PSGC Model. *Health* is the ability of the PSG to function effectively. It is a state of equilibrium in which the subsystems are in harmony so that the whole can perform at its maximum potential and sustain itself over time. A healthy PSG is stable. *Nursing* is a profession that contributes to the health of the PSG by providing professional assistance.

The NSM identifies five variables common to all client systems: *physiological, psychological, sociocultural, developmental,* and *spiritual* (Neuman, 1989). These variables, as identified in the PSGC Model, are found in Figure 21–1.

Within the NSM, the client system is conceptualized as a *basic structure (core)* surrounded by a series of broken and solid concentric circles, which are the lines of resistance and defense. The *flexible line of defense* is the PSG's first line of defense, or buffer zone, against stressors. A temporary response, it prevents stressors from invading the system and causing instability (Neuman, 1989).

TABLE 21–1. IDENTIFICATION OF INTERNAL, EXTERNAL, AND CREATED ENVIRONMENTS OF THE PARENT SUPPORT GROUP BASED ON THE NEUMAN SYSTEMS MODEL

Internal	External		Created
Intrasystem	*Intersystem*	*Extrasystem*	
1. Composition of the PSG (new parents, veteran parents, professionals)	1. Relationship with nursing, medical, and social work professionals	1. Relationship of PSG with non-NICU hospital departments and hospital administration	1. Motivation of the PSG
2. Processes of the PSG in relation to how it functions	2. Communication patterns with nursing, medical, and social work professionals	2. Established standards for PSGs (e.g., Parent Care, Inc.)	2. Normalization of the NICU experience
3. Communication patterns among members	3. Structure of the NICU	3. Requirements or training needed to gain approval to function from hospital or Parent Care, Inc.	3. Positive affect
4. Resources available to achieve goals	4. Professionals' time and resources		
5. Group values and norms	5. Hospital facilities for group		
6. Perception of the PSG as to its position in the health care facility and community	6. Hospital funds and resources		
7. Change over time			
8. History and experience of group members			

The next protective barrier is the *normal line of defense,* which is the level of health the PSG has reached over time. The final buffer surrounding the PSG is composed of the *lines of resistance,* which support the PSG's basic structure and normal line of defense, stabilizing the PSG and allowing reconstitution when stressors break through the normal line of defense (Neuman, 1989). Figure 21–2 shows the basic structure and lines of resistance and defense for the PSGC Model.

Stressors are "tension-producing stimuli or forces occurring within both the internal and external environmental boundaries of the client/client system" (Neuman, 1989, 70) that have the potential for causing disequilibrium in the system. In the PSGC Model, stressors are classified as intraorganizational, interorganizational, and extraorganizational. *Intraorganizational stressors* are internal environmental forces, *interorganizational stressors* are external environmental forces that interact outside the boundary of the client at proximal range, and *extraorganizational stressors* are external environmental forces that interact outside the boundaries of the client at distal range (Neuman, 1989). These stressors are identified in Table 21–2.

When the flexible and normal lines of defense are penetrated by stressors,

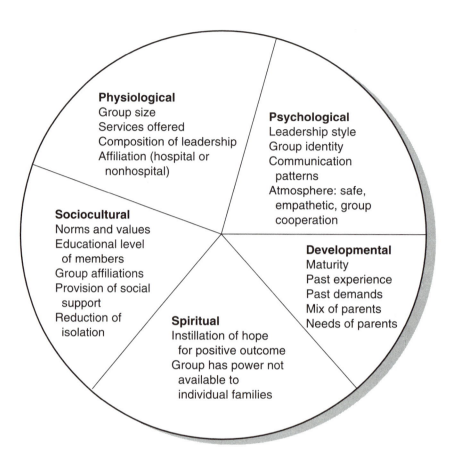

Figure 21–1. The five client variables for the Parent Support Group based on the Neuman Systems Model.

the result is disruption of the PSG system. The amount of disequilibrium or disruption that results is the *degree of reaction*. The degree of reaction is reflected in decreased effectiveness and disorganization (entropy), or even the disbanding, of the PSG. There may be a failure to (1) maintain or increase membership, (2) retain active member participation, (3) maintain or increase level of services, (4) maintain current funding or attract new funding sources, and/or (5) maintain or increase community/legislative support.

Reconstitution is the "return and maintenance of system stability following treatment of stressor reaction" (Neuman, 1989, 71). Reconstitution can lead to a level of stability that is the same as, greater than, or less than it was prior to the stressor reaction (negentropy).

Nursing interventions are activities that strengthen flexible lines of defense, strengthen resistance to stressors, and maintain system adaptation. Interventions, described in terms of primary, secondary, and tertiary levels of prevention, are

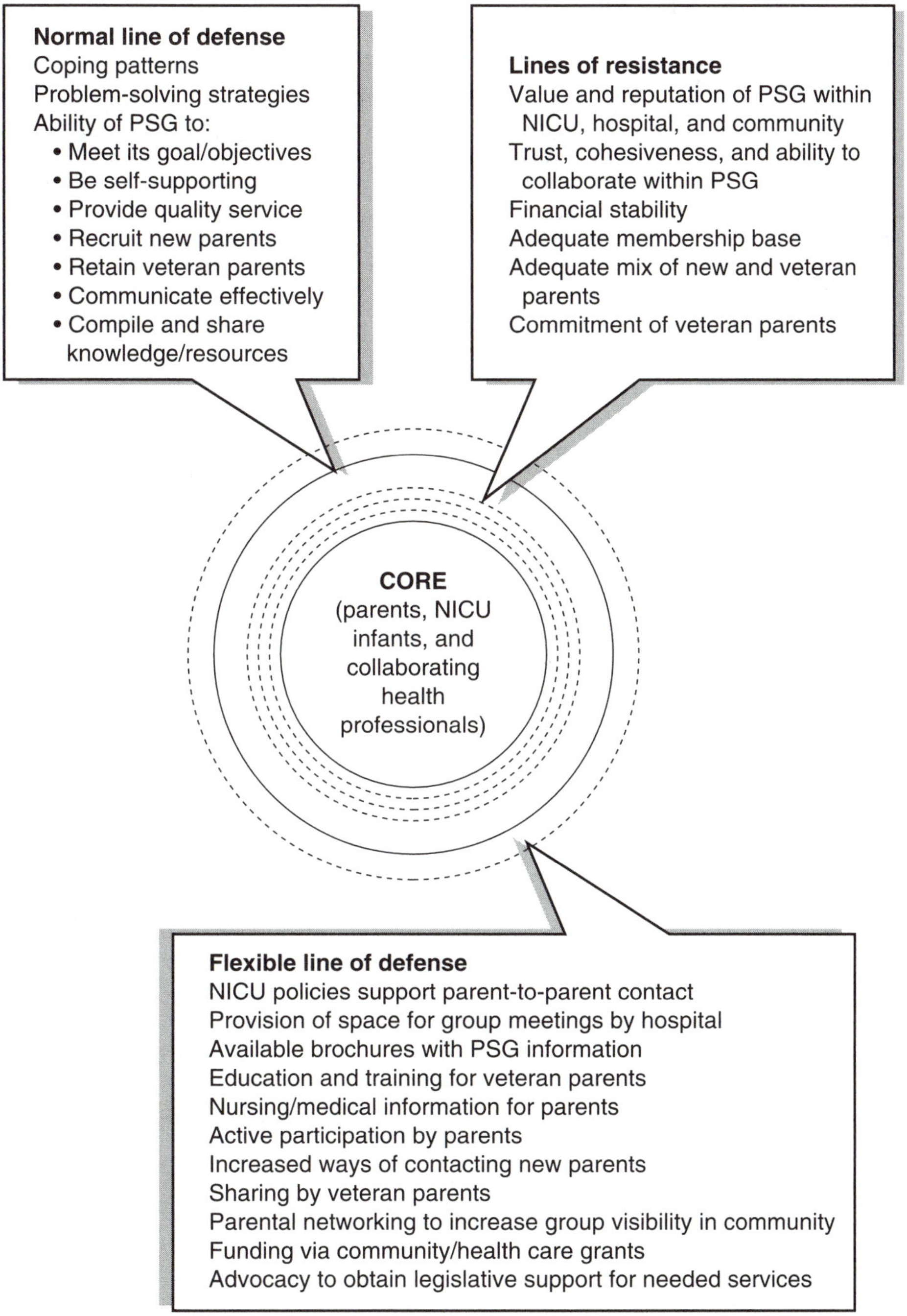

Normal line of defense
Coping patterns
Problem-solving strategies
Ability of PSG to:
• Meet its goal/objectives
• Be self-supporting
• Provide quality service
• Recruit new parents
• Retain veteran parents
• Communicate effectively
• Compile and share
  knowledge/resources

Lines of resistance
Value and reputation of PSG within
  NICU, hospital, and community
Trust, cohesiveness, and ability to
  collaborate within PSG
Financial stability
Adequate membership base
Adequate mix of new and veteran
  parents
Commitment of veteran parents

CORE
(parents, NICU
infants, and
collaborating
health
professionals)

Flexible line of defense
NICU policies support parent-to-parent contact
Provision of space for group meetings by hospital
Available brochures with PSG information
Education and training for veteran parents
Nursing/medical information for parents
Active participation by parents
Increased ways of contacting new parents
Sharing by veteran parents
Parental networking to increase group visibility in community
Funding via community/health care grants
Advocacy to obtain legislative support for needed services

Figure 21–2. The Parent Support Group as Client, adapted from the Neuman Systems Model.

TABLE 21–2. CLASSIFICATION OF PARENT SUPPORT GROUP STRESSORS USING THE NEUMAN SYSTEMS MODEL

Intraorganizational	Interorganizational	Extraorganizational
1. Not enough people planning and carrying out activities	1. Collaboration and professional support not available/present	1. Insufficient funds to support PSG activities
2. Autocratic leadership style	2. Refusal of PSG access to NICU	2. Hospital policies that are not supportive of PSG or PSG goals
3. Inability or failure of parents and professionals to collaborate	3. Refusal of PSG access to parents with infants currently in NICU	3. Legislation indifferent or antithetical to PSG goals
3. Group focus changing because balance between new and veteran parents not maintained	4. Inadequate support or involvement of families (siblings, grandparents, significant others)	4. Geographical distances served by PSG
5. Not enough veteran parents to provide parent-to-parent support	5. Lack of professional assistance to train veteran parents	5. Number of hospitals served by PSG
6. Format of meetings or selected topics not helpful to parents	6. Poor communication between PSG and staff	6. Meeting space difficult to find, unavailable, or is lost
7. Imbalance in informational, educational, and emotional support services	7. Inadequate methods of contacting new parents	7. Public awareness of NICU infant and parent needs is low
8. Leader burn-out	8. Fluctuation of patient population	

intended to reduce the possibility of a client reaction or to reduce the severity of a reaction following its occurrence and can begin at any point at which a stressor is either suspected or identified.

Nursing diagnoses for the PSGC Model derive from assessment of the PSG's basic structure (core), normal and flexible lines of defense, and lines of resistance, and identification of stressors, along with any degree of reaction. Some examples of nursing diagnoses that may be appropriate for the PSGC Model are (1) alteration in PSG function related to lack of collaboration with health care professionals; (2) alteration in PSG function related to decreased or inactive membership; (3) knowledge deficit of members about development, maintenance, and growth of PSGs related to inadequate educational offerings; and (4) ineffective individual coping of PSG members related to inadequate PSG parent-to-parent or group parent support services.

The goal of nursing is to help the PSG to attain, maintain, or restore system stability, thereby achieving optimal effectiveness and health. Specific *nursing goals* are derived from the nursing diagnoses. Using the nursing diagnosis of alteration in PSG function related to lack of collaboration with health professionals, a nursing goal might be to promote professional awareness of the value of PSG services. An intervention for this goal would be to coordinate a seminar for professionals to educate them on the need for, and benefits of, PSGs.

Primary prevention identifies potential stressors before they occur and strengthens the lines of defense. Assisting a PSG in becoming well organized, with the establishment of goals; making hospital contacts; and helping the group find meeting facilities are examples of primary prevention.

Secondary prevention, applied after a stressor has penetrated, supports the lines of defense and resistance to minimize the degree of reaction. Assisting the PSG with communication skills training and problem-solving techniques after group problems arise are examples of secondary prevention.

Tertiary prevention is used after stressor penetration has caused a degree of reaction, and is aimed at preventing further disequilibrium and supporting reconstitution. For example, when a leader faces "burn-out," tertiary prevention may involve assisting with group maintenance until a new leader is found or the previous leader is re-energized. Assisting the leadership with dispersement of the work load might also be included.

Using the Neuman Systems Model with the PSGC Model, nursing interventions might include (1) describing the availability and benefits of PSGs to new parents, (2) assisting the group to develop a variety of methods for informing parents about PSG services, (3) assisting in recruitment of veteran parents, (4) encouraging member participation, (5) serving as a resource for PSG members, and (6) allowing veteran parents access to the NICU and new parents.

CASE STUDY

A hospital-affiliated Parent Support Group (PSG) was initiated by a nurse, herself a former NICU parent. The hospital appointed her as Parent Support Coordinator (PSCo), and over three years her role expanded from three to 32 hours per week. PSG officers were elected who worked closely with the PSCo. Basic services provided through collaboration were parent-to-parent support, weekly group support for current NICU parents, a monthly group for veteran parents, and a monthly newsletter. Additionally, a Parent Lending Library and a decorated parent lounge were provided by the hospital. The PSCo-provided services included (1) providing premature baby clothes, burial gowns, and memory bags for all infants who died; (2) providing holiday gifts and pictures; and (3) maintaining the "NICU Gallery," beautiful photographs in the hallway to "gently introduce parents to the world of the NICU."

Several changes took place over the next five years. The parent lounge was converted to a "Step Down Unit," leaving parents no place to wait or to talk to health care providers privately. The PSCo's time was gradually decreased to eight hours per week because of budgetary constraints and beliefs that the group was well established.

The PSG struggled to maintain system stability for a few years. A positive affect and parent–professional social activities were maintained, but with the decreased collaboration of the PSCo, the PSG ceased feeling safe and supported. PSG energy became increasingly bound up in supporting the illusion of stability. As energy was depleted, members responded with negative, angry interactions. After three years of struggling to maintain services, PSG attendance declined and recruitment of veteran parents decreased, as did referrals for parent-to-parent support.

Finally, the PSG decided not to meet over the summer. In the fall the PSCo took a three-month leave of absence, and the PSG subsequently held no meetings. Upon return the PSCo found that the library had few books in it, slide and video presentations on NICU issues had not been shown to parents for months, veteran parents were not meeting or visiting the NICU, no newsletter had gone out for six months, and no parent-to-parent referrals had been made in three months. Based on PSG system assessment, the PSCo convinced the hospital to again expand her time allotment to 20 hours per week to re-establish the group and its services. Reorganization began with an emphasis on recruitment of both current and veteran NICU parents and manageable dispersement of responsibilities among members.

ANALYSIS

The stressors of reduced and inconsistent amount of professional collaboration resulted in inadequate training of veteran parents, ineffective communication between the PSG and NICU staff, reduced means for the PSG to contact current NICU parents, veteran parent leader burn-out, and reduced services. Other concurrent stressors included decreased funding for group activities and fluctuations in NICU patient population. Increasingly, PSG energy had become bound in maintaining the illusion of stability in order to avoid the reality of the environment.

With increased and consistent professional collaboration, total parent responsibilities for group maintenance was eliminated, and bound energy necessary for maintaining the created environment (Neuman, 1989, 33) was released for supporting needed positive changes. To support the PSG's existing strengths, the PSCo assumed responsibility for (1) describing availability and benefits of the PSG to new parents, (2) collaborating with parent leaders in provision of PSG services, (3) assisting with recruitment and training of veteran parents, (4) encouraging member participation, (5) serving as a resource person, and (6) being an advocate for the PSG with the hospital and community. Thus both the wellness level and quality of PSG services were re-established (reconstitution).

Research by Cherniss (1987) and Ware (1992a, 1992b) suggests that PSG survival and growth is enhanced by a working relationship between parents and professionals. Additionally, Ware found that PSG stability was related to having (1) two or more methods of informing parents about the availability of a PSG and (2) 10 or more members active in planning and carrying out PSG activities.

FUTURE IMPLICATIONS FOR USE OF THE NEUMAN SYSTEMS MODEL

The implications for nursing are that the total environment must provide adequate support before, during, and after the establishment of a PSG. The group is unlikely to function without the collaboration of health care professionals. The NSM—with its broad systems concepts and physiological, psychological, sociocultural, developmental, and spiritual variables—provides nurses with a unique framework for working wholistically with clients as they interact with their environment.

The NSM also provides nurses with an effective framework for an expanded, advanced practice role with the group as a client system. Using the NSM with the PSG as client, primary prevention nursing interventions might include enhancement of group skills to (1) work collaboratively with the interdisciplinary health team, (2) initiate successful parent-to-parent support, and (3) develop and maintain an effective PSG.

Also within the context of primary prevention, nurses might work with parents and local, state, and/or national policy makers to implement health care policies that help prevent neonatal problems and that provide comprehensive interdisciplinary health care services (e.g., medical, nursing, social work, and rehabilitation) for premature/critically ill infants and their families. Furthermore, wholistic assessment of the intra-, inter-, and extraorganizational environments would help nurses identify and advocate for families who traditionally have not been well served by the health care system because of race, culture, ethnicity, socioeconomic status, or the nature of their child's illness.

The concepts of the Neuman Model, with its systems perspective, provide an excellent basis for structuring appropriate nursing intervention strategies for parent support groups as client systems. Furthermore, while working within the NSM framework to enhance PSG stability, nurses have the very real potential to strengthen the individual family systems that make up the PSG.

REFERENCES

Cherniss, D. S. 1987. Stability and growth in parent support services: A national survey of peer support for parents of premature and high risk infants. In *Research on Support for Parents and Infants in the Postnatal Period* edited by C. F. Z. Boukydis, 161–196. Norwood, N.J.: Ablex.

Fawcett, J. 1983. *Analysis and Evaluation of Conceptual Models of Nursing.* Philadelphia: F. A. Davis.

Harrison, H., and Kositsky, A. 1983. *The Premature Baby Book.* New York: St. Martin's Press.

Neuman, B. 1989. *The Neuman Systems Model,* 2d ed. Norwalk, Conn.: Appleton & Lange.

Neuman, B. 1990. Health as a continuum based on the Neuman Systems Model. *Nursing Science Quarterly* 3:129–135.

Steele, K. H. 1987. Caring for parents of critically ill neonates during hospitalization: Strategies for health care professionals. *Maternal Child Nursing Journal* 16(1):13–27.

Ware, L. A. 1992a. Results of research on the stability of parent support groups in neonatal intensive care units—Part 1. *Neonatal Intensive Care,* 5(2):28–32.

Ware, L. A. 1992b. Results of research on the stability of parent support groups in neonatal intensive care units—Part 2. *Neonatal Intensive Care* 5(3):52–56.

Yoos, L. 1989. Applying research in practice: Parenting the premature infant. *Applied Nursing Research* 2(1):30–34.

22

ASSESSING AND MEETING THE NEEDS OF HOME CAREGIVERS USING THE NEUMAN SYSTEMS MODEL

Jan Russell
Judy Willis Hileman
Joan S. Grant

Although the Neuman Systems Model was first developed in 1970 for the purpose of teaching analysis of client care, it has been used in a variety of ways for a variety of reasons (Neuman, 1982, 1989). For instance, application of the Neuman Model has been effective and efficient with the care of the community as client (Beddome, 1989); to organize the curriculum within a school of nursing (Conners, 1989); and to organize nursing practice in a hospital setting (Burke, Capers, O'Connell, Quinn, and Sinnott, 1989). Therefore it seems logical to use the model to assess and meet the needs of the caregivers of homebound clients.

TRANSITION TO HOME CARE

The precarious state of the American economy and mounting health care costs have compelled health care agencies to provide home-based care to more clients

Reviewed by Gail Stuart.

who have higher acuity levels than ever before (Katoff, 1992; Miller, 1985; Morris, 1984). This national trend has been identified by the United States General Accounting Office (1981), which projected an increase in the demand for home health care throughout the 1990s.

The types of clients needing care at home are expanding (Bader, 1985). For example, along with the homebound acutely ill client is a rapidly increasing number of older Americans with chronic diseases such as Alzheimer's disease, dementias, cancer, cardiovascular disease, and multiple injuries needing home care (Rabins, Fitting, Eastham, and Fetting, 1990). In addition, younger Americans are homebound with HIV/AIDS (Katoff, 1992), and Americans of all ages are homebound with head traumas (Brooks, Campsie, Symington, Beattie, and McKinlay, 1986). The homebound clients discussed in this chapter are those with cancer, HIV/AIDS, and head traumas.

The primary caregiver for a homebound client is most often a lay home caregiver who is a family member or a close friend (Morris, 1984; Rabins, Fitting, Eastham, and Fetting, 1990). Therefore, not only are the numbers of homebound clients rising, but the numbers of lay home caregivers are rising and are expected to continue to rise for the next 50 years (Bader, 1985).

The caregivers discussed in this chapter are lay individuals who care for clients with cancer, HIV/AIDS, or head traumas. Cancer has become a manageable chronic disease in the home as diagnoses and treatments have improved (Frank-Stromborg and Wright, 1984). The lay caregivers for this group of clients are predominantly female family members (Hileman and Lackey, 1990; Hileman, Lackey, and Hassanein, 1992). Like those with cancer, an increasing number of clients with HIV/AIDS are being cared for at home by lay caregivers (Katoff, 1992). However, in these cases, a role reversal phenomenon has evolved in relation to the AIDS epidemic, as many older parents have become caregivers of their young adult children (O'Donnell and Bernier, 1990).

Head injury is the "silent epidemic" of our time, resulting from fast-paced life-styles and advanced technology that increases survival rates. Adults with head injuries tend to be individuals less than 35 years of age, which is similar to the age group infected with HIV/AIDS (Adamovich, Henderson, and Averbach, 1984). Caregivers tend to be family members, usually female, as they are with cancer patients; but given the ages of clients with head traumas, many caregivers are the same age or older than the homebound clients, which is similar to the case of caregivers of homebound clients with HIV/AIDS (Grant and Bean, 1992).

NEUMAN AND THE NURSING PROCESS

More and more, nurses are providing direction, support, and education for lay caregivers (Brackley and Meadows, 1989; Hoke, 1985). To provide wholistic structure to meet caregivers needs, the nursing process as developed by Neuman (1989) can be used. Step 1, nursing diagnosis, includes assessment of the client, acquisition of a data base, evaluation of the dynamic interaction among the variables within the client, and the formulation of one or more nursing diagnoses. Step 2, nursing goals, incorporates negotiated client perception of goals between the health care professional and the client. Primary, secondary, and/or tertiary interventions are formulated during this stage as well. Step 3, nursing outcomes, involves the implementation and evaluation of the proposed plan in Step 2.

USING THE NEUMAN MODEL TO MEET LAY CAREGIVER NEEDS

Step 1: Nursing Diagnosis

The caregiver needs to be assessed within the context of the home environment and in relation to the homebound client. Therefore, the environment in relation to the client system or the caregiver becomes the focus for the nurse. "The *environment* is broadly defined as all internal and external factors or influences surrounding the identified client . . . system" (Neuman, 1974, 103). The client system in this context is considered the lay caregiver and the homebound client. The client system and the environment have a reciprocal relationship whereby the feedback input from the environment produces an adjustment by the system. The focus of the system's adjustment is to retain or maintain a balance that is perceived by the system as acceptable.

Assessing Caregivers of Clients with Cancer. Family structure is vitally important for protection and strength in the face of a serious illness such as cancer (Nordlicht, 1982). Each family member relationship affects the stability of the entire family unit (Googe and Varricchio, 1981). Thus families should be included in the treatment plans (McCorkle and Germino, 1984). This is critical in cancer patients' care as this diagnosis disrupts family functioning and the emotional well-being of family members (Freidenbergs, Gordon, Ruckdeschel, and Diller 1980; Lovell, 1984; Nathanson and Monaco, 1984). Most family members are ill prepared for the extra duties, stresses, and frustrations of the caregiving role (Brandt, 1984). Eventually, almost all families with a homebound client with cancer seek outside help to supplement their efforts in order to function (Oberst, Thomas, Gass, and Ward, 1985).

Assessing Caregivers of Clients with HIV/AIDS. Ben Thomas (1989) described the difficulty for significant others (e.g., parents, partners) in caring for a family member with a life-threatening illness. "Caring for a partner who has AIDS is not met with such respect or sympathy" as most other caregiving situations (Thomas, 1989, 33). Therefore these home caregivers may need even more help from professionals. Affirming the worth of clients with AIDS and their home caregivers is a critical role for nurses dealing with this population. Supporting home care and home caregivers is critical to maintaining the quality of life for clients with AIDS (Rose and Catanzaro, 1989). The caregivers of these patients, who usually lose jobs, income, health insurance, and support systems, desperately need the supportive resources of nursing professionals.

Assessing Caregivers of Clients with Head Traumas. Head-injured adults (HIAs) who return home commonly have both physical and psychological sequelae. While physical sensorimotor and gait disturbances are well documented, literature also indicates that long-term morbidity is associated with cognitive, behavioral, and social and family problems (Brooks, Campsie, Symington, Beattie, and McKinley, 1986). In addition, traumatic head injury often occurs in young adults. Therefore this can affect the family's primary source of income (DeFazio, Kelly, and Flynn, 1989).

Postinjury, HIAs may become self-centered, rigid, impulsive, emotionally labile, and depressed (DeFazio, Kelly, and Flynn, 1989). In a five-year follow-up of 42 adults with severe blunt head injury, Brooks et al. (1986) found personality change, slowness, poor memory, irritability, bad temper, tiredness, depression, rapid mood change, tension and anxiety, and threats of violence to be the 10 problems reported most frequently by relatives. Although self-care deficits were not reported frequently (14 percent), 21 percent of the adults needed supervision, while nearly 50 percent could not be left in charge of the household. In a larger study, Jacobs (1988) reported even more traumatic results. Only 20 percent of 142 HIAs were able to return to their former jobs one to six years after the injury; 66 percent had difficulty with higher order skills such as housework, managing money, and child care. In addition, approximately 25 percent reported severe behavioral and emotional problems.

The caregiver typically assumes major responsibility for managing these deficits. Family members play a significant role in the survival of the head-injured adult, and the demands of caregiving often result in complex, long-standing needs (Grant and Bean, 1992). The needs are multidimensional, and the ability or inability to address these needs may influence family stress and burden (McClellan, 1988). Brooks et al. (1986) found that the level of subjective burden experienced by the caregiver is significantly higher at five years postinjury than at one year postinjury.

Stressors and the Internal Environment. The internal environment is minimally composed of a caregiver and an individual needing care. Stressors or tension-producing stimuli found in this environment are considered intrapersonal for the client as a system. Many examples of all three targeted groups can be gleaned from the information given earlier. For instance, intrapersonal stressors common for caregivers of all the targeted homebound patients is the diagnosis itself, which can cause family disequilibrium.

Stressors and the External Environment. The external environment exists outside of this system. Stressors found here are interpersonal and extrapersonal in nature. For instance, for all caregivers and their homebound clients a lack of adequate health insurance would be an extrapersonal stressor, whereas an interpersonal stressor might be the social isolation each has to endure because of the chronic illness of the homebound client.

Stressors and the Created Environment. The created environment is seen as dynamic by Neuman (1989). It encompasses both the other environments and provides insulation through which client system responses must travel. It serves to protect the system as a whole. For example, if the caregiver is told that the client is terminal, then, through the mechanism of the created environment, the caregiver maintains hope that there will be a cure. The extrapersonal stressor of the negative prognosis for the client has been interpreted through the protective insulation of the created environment. The client system response is based on the reality of that knowledge mixed with an exaggerated hope.

Assessment of Caregiver Needs. Prior to 1989 there were no instruments to assess the needs of lay caregivers of homebound clients. Therefore the Home Caregiver Need Survey (HCNS) was developed by Hileman and used in a study that identified, categorized, and assessed the importance of needs expressed by 492 home caregivers in a statewide study conducted in Kansas (Hileman, Lackey, and Hassanein, 1992). The investigators identified six categories of caregiver needs: information, household, patient care, personal, spiritual, and psychological. Moreover, in general, findings suggest that most clients, caregivers, and nurses identify the greatest needs of caregivers as psychological, informational, and physical. The outcome in this study was supported by previous studies that focused on caregiver needs (Hileman and Lackey, 1990; Wingate and Lackey, 1989). The Home Caregiver Need Survey was then modified to be used with lay caregivers of *any* client population at home and is now being used to collect data from lay caregivers of HIV/AIDS homebound clients.

The needs of lay caregivers for homebound HIAs has been of concern too. In an attempt to address this concern, Oddy, Humphrey, and Uttley (1978) asked family members to identify areas not addressed adequately by health professionals since the injury. Relatives expressed a need for more information on head injury and services available to HIAs. In a subsequent study, Campbell (1988) identified the perceived needs of 14 relatives of HIAs. Family members specified educational, emotional, and social support needs. Honest answers to questions and information on the effects of head injury, community resources, financial aid, physical care, methods for addressing psychological sequelae, and respite care were educational needs identified by family members. Psychological needs involved the need to know what the future held for their relatives, to have emotional support, to be able to communicate feelings, to have assistance with marital adjustments, and to feel hope. Social needs were those involving personal time for self and activities outside the home, assistance in reorganizing family responsibilities and communicating with family members, and support from religious institutions. Caregivers were concerned over what would happen to the HIA if something happened to them.

The most recent study in this area was conducted in 1992 by Grant and Bean, who used Neuman as the theoretical framework for the study. Lay caregivers identified 110 different needs, with an average of 4.6 needs per individual caregiver. Of the 110 needs, 37 were intrapersonal, 24 were interpersonal, and 49 were extrapersonal. Intrapersonal stressors identified were needing time for self and social activities, assurance of care of the HIA if the lay caregiver was unable to provide care, physical and emotional rest, and meeting the needs of the HIA. Intrapersonal stressors spanned both physiological and psychosociocultural variables (e.g., physical and emotional rest). Interpersonal stressors most commonly reported were the lack of support groups, friends to assist with housekeeping chores, supportive family/friends, and health professionals. Again, these stressors spanned physiological and psychosociocultural variables. Extrapersonal stressors identified most frequently were the lack of respite care, financial support for physical and psychosocial care of the HIA, day care programs addressing both physical and psychosocial needs, alternative living arrangements, transportation, information on head injury, psychosocial care of the HIA, resources for psychosocial care of the HIA, and individuals to care for the HIA.

In conclusion, the stressors (needs) of the caregivers are intrapersonal, interpersonal, and extrapersonal. Moreover, the stressors should be readily categorized into the variables as described by Neuman (1982, 1989): physiological, psychological, sociocultural, developmental, and spiritual.

Assessment Process. The created environment of the caregiver needs to be assessed first by the nurse. the following information needs to be gathered: What is the nature of the perceived created environment for the system; what is the value placed on that perception; what is the ideal outcome for the system or any of its members; how are the unmet needs prioritized; and what is the effect of the bound energy on the system.

The internal and external environments can then be evaluated in terms of stressor potential and effects. However, the examination of both of these environments must be within the context of the created environment. The caregiver's needs can be used to clarify and validate any system instability identified when the examination of the created environment was conducted.

Diagnostic Conclusions. Based on the data gathered for these caregivers, several diagnoses can be identified to guide nursing practice (see Tables 22–1, 22–2, and 22–3). These diagnoses must be developed with the lay caregiver.

Step 2: Nursing Goals

Since the target group is individuals who are essentially well themselves but who are caring for individuals who are not well, the emphasis for the group is to

TABLE 22–1. DIAGNOSTIC STATEMENT AND RELATED PRIMARY PREVENTION STRATEGY

Anxiety related to knowledge deficit about progression of the disease for the homebound client, about the current condition of the client, about meeting the needs of the client, about being the only one who can meet those needs "properly."

Primary Strategy:

Reduce stressors—discuss information about all of the above, give informational pamphlets, discuss perception of "Proper Care." Strengthen FLD—provide resources that would give "proper care."

retain system stability. Therefore nursing actions should be focused in the primary prevention mode for the caregiver. In this mode the nursing goal is to reduce possible stressor encounters or to strengthen the caregiver's flexible lines of defense (see Tables 22–1, 22–2, and 22–3). When developing interventions, health care professionals must remember the fears, stigmas, varying life-styles, and complexity of the needs of caregivers (Gwyther and Allers, 1990).

Step 3: Nursing Outcomes

The interventions within the plan of care should be evaluated as to effectiveness and efficiency. Then the plan is modified based on the evaluation.

Case Example

A case example might be that although continuous care is needed for the client, the caregiver may feel that only he or she can give "proper care" to the client. Data collection would include the definition of "proper care" as defined by the caregiver (the perceived created environment). The nurse would seek supportive services that correspond with this perception. Together, the nurse and the caregiver would develop a schedule to provide an opportunity for the caregiver to be relieved from direct care, thus conserving the caregiver's energy. With this intervention plan the created environment has been preserved, and the level of wellness for the system has been enhanced.

TABLE 22–2. DIAGNOSTIC STATEMENT AND RELATED PRIMARY PREVENTION STRATEGY

Physical and emotional exhaustion related to constant care for homebound client.

Primary Strategy:

Reduce stressors—discuss nurse's perception of exhaustion with caregiver to validate; have caregiver discuss exhaustion and possible solutions. Strengthen FLD—schedule resources that would give care for client and refer caregiver to counselor for emotional support.

TABLE 22–3. DIAGNOSTIC STATEMENT AND RELATED PRIMARY PREVENTION STRATEGY

Social isolation related to lack of personal time, lack of activities outside of the home, lack of contact with other people.

Primary Strategy:

Reduce stressors—discuss the isolation with caregiver to validate, have caregiver discuss possible solutions. Strengthen FLD—schedule resources that would allow personal time for the caregiver, and provide possible support groups, which could be attended by the caregiver.

FUTURE RESEARCH

Even though there is literature on the needs of lay caregivers during the acute care experience, there is minimal research related to the needs of caregivers in the home setting (Grant and Bean, 1992). Nolan and Grant (1989) aptly state that addressing the needs of informal caregivers is a neglected area of nursing practice. Continued research is greatly needed in this area of caregiving, to determine not only needs but also effective strategies for problem resolution.

FUTURE CARE FOR LAY CAREGIVERS

A major problem confronting the health care system today is the effects of long-term illness on the family. One must try to balance the needs of both the client and the family simultaneously. As more families become involved in the health care of ill members, nurses must move to a family-centered nursing role (Wright and Dyck, 1985). Families able to identify their needs are more likely to use health services (Romsass and Juliani, 1983). Illness, adjustment, and acceptance become easier when the family learns how to properly give home care and cope with situations that arise (Lovell, 1984).

FUTURE ROLE OF THE NEUMAN SYSTEMS MODEL WITH LAY CAREGIVERS

The Neuman Systems Model can and should be used to organize a specific assessment instrument that guides nursing care for clients at home and their lay caregivers. In this way a systematic method would be developed for examining the many complex stressors facing these homebound clients and their caregivers. Effective and efficient interventions can then be developed that are grounded in accurate client system data for implementation using the Neuman three preventive intervention modalities.

CONCLUSION

Preliminary studies indicate that lay caregivers have many unmet needs; however, common needs must be identified prior to developing useful interventions. The Nueman Systems Model (1989) provides a comprehensive structure for gathering critical data and developing valid plans of client care.

REFERENCES

Adamovich, B., Henderson, J. A., and Averbach, S. 1984. *Cognitive Rehabilitation of Closed Head Injury.* San Diego: College Hill Press.

Bader, J. E. 1985. Respite care: Temporary relief for caregivers. *Women's Health* 10(2–3): 39–52.

Beddome, G. 1989. Application of the Neuman Systems Model to the assessment of community-as-client. In *The Neuman Systems Model,* edited by B. Neuman. Norwalk, Conn.: Appleton & Lange.

Brackley, M. H., and Meadows, R. F. 1989. Nursing support of family caregivers. *Dimensions in Oncology Nursing* 3(1):14–20.

Brandt, M. A. 1984. Consider the patient part of a family. *Nursing Forum* 21(1):19–31.

Brooks, N., Campsie, L., Symington, C., Beattie, A., and McKinley, W. 1986. The five year outcome of severe blunt head injury: A relative's view. *J Neuro Neurosurg Psychiatry* 49:764–770.

Burke, S. M. E., Capers, C. F., O'Connell, R. K., Quinn, R. M., and Sinnott, M. 1989. Neuman-based nursing practice in hospital setting. In *The Neuman Systems Model,* edited by B. Neuman. Norwalk, Conn.: Appleton & Lange.

Campbell, C. (1988). Needs of relatives and helpfulness of support groups in severe head injury. *Rehab Nurs* 13:320–325.

Conners, V. 1989. An empirical evaluation of the Neuman Systems Model: The University of Missouri–Kansas City. In *The Neuman Systems Model,* edited by B. Neuman. Norwalk, Conn.: Appleton & Lange.

DeFazio, A., Kelly, M., and Flynn, J. 1989. The head injured outpatient: Presentations and rehabilitation. *MMJ* 38:1035–1041.

Frank-Stromborg, M., and Wright, P. 1984. Ambulatory cancer patients' perception of the physical and psychosocial changes in their lives since diagnosis of cancer. *Cancer Nursing* 7(2):117–130.

Freidenbergs, I., Gordon, W., Ruckdeschel, A. H., and Diller, L. 1980. Assessment and treatment of psychosocial problems of the cancer patient: A case study. *Cancer Nursing* 3(4):111–119.

Googe, M., and Varricchio, C. G. 1981. A pilot investigation of home health care needs of cancer patients and their families. *Oncology Nursing Forum* 8(4):24–28.

Grant, J., and Bean, C. 1992. Self-identified needs of informal caregivers of head-injured adults. *Fam Community Health* 15(2):49–58.

Gwyther, L. P., and Allers, C. T. 1990. AIDS and the older adult. *The Gerontologist* 30(3):405–407.

Hoke, J. 1985. Charting for dollars. *American Journal of Nursing* 85(6):658–660.

Hileman, J., and Lackey, N. 1990. Self-identified needs of patients with cancer at home and their home caregivers: A descriptive study. *Oncology Nursing Forum* 17(6): 907–912.

Hileman, J., Lackey, N., and Hassanein, R. 1992. Identifying the needs of home caregivers of patients with cancer. *Oncology Nursing Forum* 19(5):771–777.

Jacobs, H. 1988. The Los Angeles head injury survey: Procedures and initial findings. *Arch Phys Med Rehab* 69:425–431.

Katoff, L. 1992. Community-based services for people with AIDS. *Primary Care* 19(1):231–243.

Lovell, B. 1984. A family affair. *Nursing Mirror* 158(2):19–21.

McClellan, R. 1988. Psychosocial sequelae of head injury—anatomy of a relationship. *Brit J Psychiatry* 153:141–146.

McCorkle, R., and Germino, B. 1984. What nurses need to know about home care. *Oncology Nursing Forum* 11(6):63–69.

Miller, A. 1985. When is the time ripe for teaching? *American Journal of Nursing* 85(7): 801–804.

Miller, W. G. 1986. The neuropsychology of head injuries. In *The Neuropsychology Handbook,* edited by D. Wedding, A. Horton, and J. Webster, 347–375. New York: Springer Publishing.

Morris, E. 1984. Home care today. *American Journal of Nursing* 84(3):341–345.

Nathanson, B. A., and Monaco, P. G. 1984. Meeting the educational and psychosocial needs produced by a diagnosis of pediatric/adolescent cancer. *Health Education Quarterly* 10(1):67–75.

Neuman, B. 1974. The Betty Neuman health-care systems model: A total person approach to patient problems. In *Conceptual Models for Nursing Practice,* edited by J. P. Riehl and C. Roy, 103. New York: Appleton-Century-Crofts.

Neuman, B. 1982, 1989. *The Neuman Systems Model.* Norwalk, Conn.: Appleton-Century-Crofts.

Nolan, M. R., and Grant, G. 1989. Addressing the needs of informal careers: A neglected area of nursing practice. *J Adv Nurs* 14:950–961.

Nordlicht, S. 1982. The family of the cancer patient. *New York State Journal of Medicine* 82(13):1845–1846.

Oberst, M. T., Thomas, S. E., Gass, K. A., and Ward, S. E. 1985. Caregiving demands and appraisal of stress among family caregivers. *Cancer Nursing* 12(4):209–215.

Oddy, M., Humphrey, M., and Uttley, O. 1978. Stresses upon the relatives of head-injured patients. *Brit J Psychiatry* 133:507–513.

O'Donnell, T. G., and Bernier, S. L. 1990. Parents as caregivers: When a son has AIDS. *Journal of Psychosocial Nursing* 28(6):14–17.

Rabins, P., Fitting, M., Eastham, J., and Fetting, J. 1990. The emotional impact of caring for the chronically ill. *Psychosomatics* 31(3):331–336.

Romsass, E. P., and Juliani, L. M. 1983. Resource utilization in an outpatient setting. *Oncology Nursing Forum* 11(3):45–48.

Rose, M. A., and Catanzaro, A. M. 1989. AIDS caregiving crisis: A proactive approach. *Holistic Nursing Practice* 3(2):39–45.

Thomas, B. 1989. Supporting the carers of people with AIDS. *Nursing Times* 85(16):33–35.

United States General Accounting Office. 1981, Dec. 7. The elderly should benefit from expanded home health care, but increasing these services will not ensure cost reduction. *Report to the Chairman of the Committee on Labor and Human Resources.* United States Senate, GAO/IPE-83-1; 1–61.

Wingate, A., and Lackey, N. 1989. A description of the needs of noninstitutionalized cancer patients and their primary caregivers. *Cancer Nursing* 12(4):216–225.

Wright, K., and Dyck, S. 1985. Expressed concerns of adult cancer patients' family members. *Cancer Nursing* 7(5):371–374.

Section IV

Nursing Administration and the Neuman Systems Model

Introduction

This section of the third edition of the Neuman Systems Model provides an excellent variety of applications of the model in administration. The use and value of nursing models in nursing administration is emphasized in a number of chapters in *Dimensions of Nursing Administration* by Henry et al. (1988). While other nursing models are frequently thought of primarily for direct care roles, the Neuman Systems Model has grown significantly beyond applications in practice to administration. Many administrators have recognized that in order to facilitate the use of conceptual models in direct care, a framework at the organizational level is necessary. Also, as more health care agencies work toward common language and develop plans for information systems, it will become more critical for organizations to find a common conceptual framework for administration of care within the agency or institution. As health care reform unfolds, integrated systems are being promoted that will facilitate care across settings, serving a variety of populations. This will stimulate the nursing progression to look at ways to define and approach care in similar ways, and use of nursing models is one way to find common ground between and among nurses in a variety of settings.

The wealth and variety of settings using the Neuman Systems Model at the organizational level confirms the positioning of the model for the 21st century and for global reforms in the health care systems. Wisely selected chapters for this section provide future-oriented administrators with rich examples of how a nursing model can be adapted organizationally. Additionally, this section is enhanced by inclusion of international applications from Canada and the United Kingdom, as well as from the United States.

A detailed conceptualization of the use of the Neuman Systems Model and the management process (Kelly and Sanders) provides a basic framework for the use of the model by any administrator in any setting. Next, Hinton Walker's chapter using the model in the context of TQM brings the model into focus with the latest emphasis in health care management. The TQM chapter reinforces the use of the theoretical material covered by Kelly et al. (Neuman, 1989) and describes how this approach was used to teach administration to nurses and other disciplines. For practical application, use of the model in a variety of practice settings with a wide variety of populations is also included in this section. Two chapters describe the use of the model in Canada. Felix, Hinds, and Martin present use of the model in a chronic care facility; and a chapter written by Coulter and Craig describes an application of the model in psychiatric hospitals in Canada. Another chapter by Scicchitani et al. highlights application of the model in a psychiatric hospital (Friends Hospital) in the United States.

As our nation and other countries try to care for the increasing needs of the mentally and chronically ill across the age span, new applications of the Neuman Systems Model discussed here provide global perspectives beyond use in one agency. In a community and public health use of the model is growing. The model is integrated into a statewide public health department in Oklahoma (Frioux, Butler, and Roberts) and in the United Kingdom by Damant. These chapters clearly build on the chapter in the previous edition by Drew, Craig, and Beynon (Neuman, 1989), who introduced application of the model in community health administration. Future directions in community-based care across the wellness–illness continuum are topics addressed by Rodriguez's chapter on care of elderly residents in a retirement community and in Hinton Walker's chapter on community nursing centers. The chapter on nursing centers explores emerging trends for the future with descriptions of nurse-managed primary care in urban and rural settings across populations and settings by nurse practitioners. Clearly, this section demonstrates the breadth and scope of the use of the Neuman Systems Model organizationally and internationally.

Patricia Hinton Walker

23

A SYSTEMS APPROACH TO THE HEALTH OF NURSING AND HEALTH CARE ORGANIZATIONS

Jean A. Kelley
Nena F. Sanders

In the previous edition (Neuman, 1989), our chapter was entitled, "A Systems Approach to the Role of the Nurse Administrator in Education and Practice." In that chapter the Neuman Systems Model was integrated with the management process (planning, organizing, directing, and controlling). This integrated model offered an assessment tool for the nurse administrator to assess, analyze, and evaluate stressors in the environment and the three client systems (personal, nursing, and organizational), with the intended outcome being the maintenance or re-establishment of health for the client systems.

The integrated systems-management model provides the nurse administrator with a multidimensional framework for assessing, identifying, and directing needed and quality management practices; the environmental factors impacting on nursing practice, education, research, and the delivery of health care; and the reaction–response of the nurse administrator, the nursing system, and the organization to environmental factors that are reshaping the delivery of nursing practice, education, research, and health care. The framework furnishes the nurse administrator with a systematic strategy for further improving the quality of nursing education, practice, and research.

While the chapter in the previous edition focused on the personal client system, the current chapter focuses on the nursing and organizational client systems. Although numerous applications of the Neuman Systems Model have been made to the personal client system, only limited application and testing have been made to the nursing and organizational client systems. A notable limitation of much organizational analysis is the lack of interest that has been shown, despite a commitment to an open system in much of the work concerned, in the impingement of role expectations arising in extraorganizational statuses upon the definition and performance of organizational roles (Silverman, 1971).

OPERATIONALIZATION OF THE NEUMAN SYSTEMS MODEL FOR THE NURSE ADMINISTRATOR

Based on a systems approach to understanding complex phenomena, the Neuman Model provides an organizing framework for guiding the practice of a nurse in an administrative role. The four core concepts from the Neuman Model have been operationalized for the nurse administrator role and are illustrated in Table 23–1. The table provides a concise summary of how each concept in the Neuman Systems Model can be utilized by nurse administrators to guide their practice explicitly and effectively.

Person or Client

According to the Neuman Model, the concept of "person" can be operationalized as a *personal system,* such as a nurse administrator at any level of manage-

TABLE 23–1. CORE CONCEPTS FOR THE ROLE OF THE NURSE ADMINISTRATOR IN EDUCATION AND PRACTICE

Concepts	Level of System		
	Personal system	Nursing system	Organizational system
Person Environment			
	Intrapersonal	Intranursing	Intraorganizational
	Interpersonal	Internursing	Interorganizational
	Extrapersonal	Extranursing	Extraorganizational
Health	Stability of normal line of defense	Stability of normal line of defense	Stability of normal line of defense
Nursing	Three levels of prevention	Three levels of prevention	Three levels of prevention
	Three levels of administrative practice	Three levels of administrative practice	Three levels of administrative practice
	Integration of management process with the Neuman Systems Model	Integration of management process with the Neuman Systems Model	Integration of management process with the Neuman Systems Model

ment: first-line, mid-level, or top-level manager (Figure 23–1). Each nurse administrator viewed as a system possesses a basic core of characteristics based on physiological, psychological, sociocultural, developmental, and spiritual variables. A nurse administrator's core characteristics are the result of his or her experiences, educational opportunities, values, and beliefs.

- *Physiological variables:* the personal or individual system core characteristics of a nurse administrator, including physical stamina, physical handicaps, level of health
- *Sociocultural variables:* family patterns, ethnicity, cultural background, work ethic, social and work status, age, sex, religion, role behaviors
- *Psychological variables:* level of emotional maturity, cognitive potential, conception of self, ego, satisfaction of role
- *Developmental variables:* stage of development as an individual, as a nurse, and as a nurse administrator; formal and informal educational

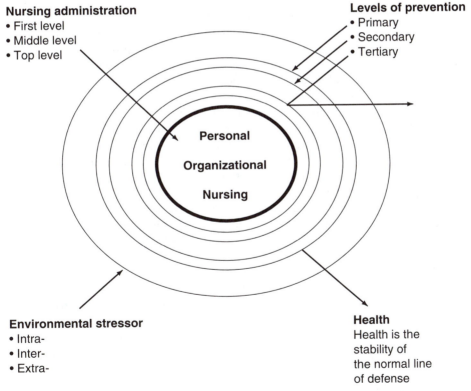

Nursing administration
- First level
- Middle level
- Top level

Levels of prevention
- Primary
- Secondary
- Tertiary

Personal

Organizational

Nursing

Environmental stressor
- Intra-
- Inter-
- Extra-

Health
Health is the
stability of
the normal line
of defense

Figure 23–1. The Neuman Systems Model: A framework for nurse administrators.

preparation as an administrator; past administrative and nursing experiences (Neuman, 1982)
- *Spiritual variables:* morals, beliefs, values, standards, decision making, and religious affiliations

According to Neuman, the stability of the core structure of a nurse administrator is protected from instability or disequilibrium by three lines of defense. The flexible line of defense for a nurse administrator includes those basic physiological, psychological, sociocultural, developmental, and spiritual variables that comprise his or her core structure. The flexible line of defense is particularly sensitive to situational conditions and serves to protect or prevent the nurse administrator from reaching a state of instability. The flexible line of defense is a nurse administrator's protective response to situations that have caused stress within and among the core variables.

The normal line of defense is the administrator's normal state of system stability or wellness and the administrator's potential to adapt to situations based on his or her ability to cope or solve problems. The strength of the administrator's normal line of defense is determined by his or her ability to assess a situation and restore the system to a state of balance or harmony. The nurse administrator depends on the management process to adapt and restore the situation to a desired stability state or functional condition.

While the line of defense mitigates stressors and retains the stable or system wellness condition, lines of resistance are a nurse administrator's resource or ultimate defense in returning the system to a stability state following a reaction to stressors. Both these lines resist attempts from stressors to cause system instability or unmanageable stress within the administrator. The interrelationship and interaction occurring among the five core variables—physiological, psychological, developmental, sociocultural, and spiritual—determine the general ability to resist stressors that cause system instability and help return it to a normal, adaptive steady state.

A major strength of the Neuman Model as a framework for the nurse administrator is that the focus of the concept of "person" can be viewed as a personal system, a nursing system, or an organizational system (Table 23–1). The systems perspective of the model allows the nurse administrator considerable flexibility in utilizing the framework as a guide to comprehensive practice. Instead of the nurse administrator serving as the core structure, the administrator can identify the core as the nursing system or the organizational system. The major focus of the nurse administrator can thus be on self; on a department, division, or unit within the nursing delivery system; or on the total health care organization. By operationalizing the system core in terms broader than the individual, a nurse administrator at the various levels of management—first, middle, and top—may use the Neuman Model as a framework to improve managerial practices.

In terms of the *nursing system,* the core structure can be interpreted as a nursing department, division, or unit within a health care organization. Based on their management level within the organization, nurse administrators may focus either on their personal system or on the nursing system for which they are responsible (see Table 23–1). This flexibility in operationalizing the model allows the nurse administrator various options or a wide range of options for assessing and managing stressors that could result or have resulted in instability or an unhealthy condition of stress reaction within the system.

The model allows for a third level of application to be made by administrators: the *organizational level.* As top-level nurse administrators become involved in and impacted by the total organization, they need an organizing framework to assess, evaluate, and adapt the activities of an organization to best influence its overall state of health.

Like the personal system, the nursing and organizational systems also have a set of core structure characteristics that determine the overall level of health or stability of the nursing system or total organization. Just as with the personal system, the nursing system and the organizational system depend on a set of core characteristics to maintain a steady state or to resist environmental stressors that could cause an unsteady, unhealthy system condition. These characteristics can be described using the Neuman Model's five client system variables—physiological, psychological, sociocultural, developmental, and spiritual. Examples of these variables for a nursing or organizational system follow:

- *Physiological variables* are variables that imply or indicate the overall health of the nursing system or organization. The structures and processes that enable a nursing system or organization to accomplish (or inhibit it from accomplishing) its mission or goals are considered physiological characteristics of a system or organization. These elements include the size of the organization or nursing system, number of employees and beds, types of services offered, urban or rural location, and composition of the leadership team.
- *Psychological variables* are characteristics of a nursing or organizational system that reveal the personality of the system or organization. Such variables include the nursing system's identity within the organization or the organization's identity within the community; channels and processes available for communicating within the nursing system or organization; the leadership style of the administrators involved in the nursing system or organization; and the general attitudes, cooperation, or atmosphere of the nursing system or organization.
- *Sociocultural variables* are viewed as the components that reflect social, cultural, economic, political, and technological viability of the nursing system or organization. These variables are the norms and values of the nursing system or organization, for example, loyalty, group affiliations, networks, economic and human resources, system or organization affiliations, and values.
- *Developmental variables* indicate the maturity level or degree to which the nursing system or organization has evolved, developed, or declined over

time and as a result improved its ability to accomplish its mission and goals. Such variables include life patterns of the nursing system or organization, past experiences and history, and previous demands placed on the nursing system or organization (Kelly, 1985).

- *Spiritual variables* are the purpose, mission, and philosophy of a nursing or organizational system. These variables reflect the standard and values that guide professional behavior within. They encompass the seven values endorsed by the nursing profession (AACN, 1986; ANA, 1976): (1) altruism, or the caring for the health care and welfare of people; (2) equality, or a commitment to improving access to nursing and health care; (3) esthetics, or the creation of a quality work environment; (4) freedom, or fostering a work environment that encourages open discussion on professional issues; (5) human dignity, or a respect for the worth and uniqueness of human beings; (6) justice, or professional practices that reflect moral and legal standards and beliefs; and (7) truth, or accountability for clinical judgment and professional activities related to the quality of nursing and health care.

In order to maintain the basic core structure of the nursing or organizational system, three levels of protection exist: lines of resistance, normal line of defense, and flexible line of defense. Each level provides mechanisms or responses that maintain or restore the system or prevent maladaptation or instability of the system. The lines of resistance are resources comprised of characteristics that protect an organization or nursing system by increasing its ability to prevent stressors from threatening the viability of the system or return it to a healthy state once an unsteady or unstable state exists. The strength or effectiveness of the lines of resistance is determined by the interactions occurring and interrelationships among the five core variables (Figure 23–2) and the environment. Examples of lines of resistance for an organizational or nursing system include the organization's position in the community; the nursing system's position in the organization; the amount, or lack, of trust, loyalty, cohesiveness, collaboration, and interaction among the group members; the economic position or financial viability of the organization or nursing system; how well the organization is positioned in the competitive marketplace; the number, type, and mix of clients available to use it; and the reputation of the organization in the community or the nursing system within the organization.

The normal line of defense is a state of wellness that is considered "normal" for the organizational or nursing system. It represents the organization's or the nursing system's level of health. Features of the normal lines of defense are developed over time and are refined with experience and knowledge. Therefore an organization or a nursing system's health is a composite of how well goals and objectives are attained, financial outcomes are achieved, an acceptable level of quality service is provided, and appropriate productivity levels are maintained. The decision-making process is critical to achieving organizational health. "The nature of the decision making process is directly related to the stability and growth of organizations" (Silverman, 1971). In addition, the health of an organization or nursing system is influenced by the staff's morale, motivation levels, interactive processes, ethnicity, life-style, and quality of work life, all of which affect the work groups' ability to accomplish the goals of the organization or nursing system.

The flexible line of defense reflects the dynamic state of health that exists or results from the introduction of a stressor into the organization or nursing system. The strength of the flexible line of defense is contingent upon the nature of the current situation and events occurring at that particular point in time. It is how a nursing system or organization responds to a stressor (i.e., problem) or issue having the potential to cause system instability that determines whether or not health or stability is retained.

Thus the concept of "client" or person in the Neuman Systems Model is operationalized as the personal system, nursing system, or organizational system (Table 23–1). The model provides an analytic framework for nurse administrators in education and practice and other nonnurse health care administrators to organize data for use in improving their management practices.

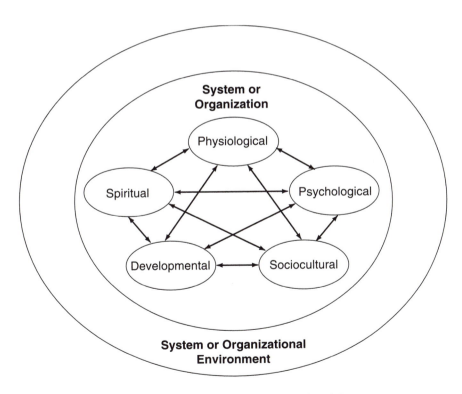

Figure 23–2. Organizational health.

Environment

Currently, the health care environment plays a vital role in an organization's ability and effectiveness as a health care provider. Because educational and health care environments are complex, in a state of constant change, and the source of most stressors affecting the nursing and organizational systems, major priority should be placed on assessing and understanding the environment of the nursing and organizational systems. The environment is viewed as being either internal or external to the core structure of the nursing system or organizational system. The internal environment refers to forces and stressors related to the intrapersonal system, intranursing system, or intraorganizational system. Intrasystem stressors occur within the person, nursing system, or organizational system. Intrapersonal stressors can be viewed as perceptions of one's role, length of time in that role, acceptability of that role by others, and the physical stamina to carry out the role. Intranursing system or intraorganizational system stressors include the perception the nursing system or organization has regarding its position in the marketplace; the amount of change that has or has not occurred in the nursing and organizational systems over time; the social, cultural, and spiritual norms and values of the nursing and organizational systems; the structures and processes that exist within the systems; and the amount and type of resources available for accomplishing the goals of the systems.

The external environment consists of two components: the intersystem and the extrasystem factors. The intersystem factor focuses on stressors among other influencing systems at close proximity. Interpersonal system stressors can occur as a result of conflict or forces exerted on the nurse administrator by other individuals, such as health care administrators, nurses, physicians, clients, and families. Internursing system stressors can be experienced as a result of forces or conflicts occurring among nursing units or nursing departments within an organization. Interorganizational stressors exist among entities that share like markets comprised of clients, physicians, and third-party payers. Interorganizational stressors are most commonly viewed as a result of competition for resources or markets.

Extrapersonal factors that introduce stress into the system are policies and procedures, job designs, standards, accreditation requirements, system design, social equity, and other forces outside the personal system that influence one's ability to implement the administrative role. Extranursing system factors that create stress for the nursing unit or department are conflicts that occur between the nursing department and another department. For example, pharmacy could be considered an extranursing system force or stressors. Numerous extraorganizational system forces that usually exist simultaneously can introduce stress into the organizational system; these need identification. Some examples are competition for market share and resources, reimbursement sources, methods of health care delivery, accreditation, and regulation requirement.

Five interrelated environmental dimensions (Silverman, 1971) that effect a nursing or health care organization are (1) *human relations,* or a person's commitment to the mission and goals of the organization and to his or her work group; (2) *culture,* or the structure, values, or beliefs of an organization that influence human relations; (3) *socio/technical,* or the impact of societal, techno-logical, and economic trends on organizational form and performance; (4) *struc-ture* and functions, or the dynamic stability of systems in adapting to their environment; and (5) *decision making,* or the rationality or irrationality of making choice related to the growth and development of the organization. Figure 23–3 illustrates the interrelatedness between and among the Neuman Model five core variables and the five environmental dimensions impacting orga-nizational health.

Health

The concept of organizational health presented in the Neuman Model is viewed as the adaptation, stability, or alignment between the nursing system or organi-

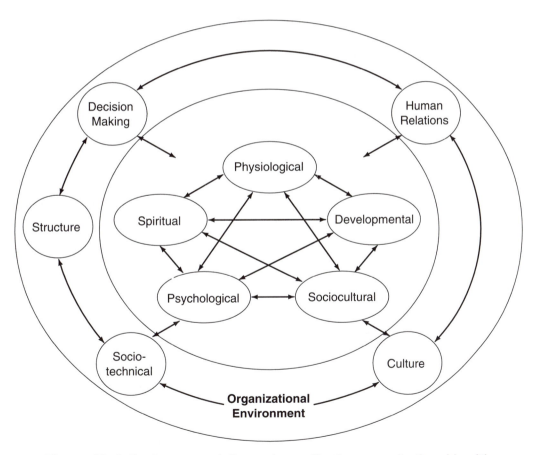

Figure 23–3. Environmental dimensions effecting organizational health.

zational system and the environment. Health of the system is relative and contingent upon the interrelationship of the physiological, psychological, sociocultural, developmental, and spiritual variables and the ability of the system to adapt to environmental stressors. Organizational illness or instability can occur when stressor events or forces cause such severe disruption within the system that the internal lines of resistance against stress are permeated, resulting in reduced effectiveness in mediating the reaction to stressors. Health of a nursing or organizational system is very dynamic, complex, and sensitive to all circumstances surrounding a particular stress situation. The ability to accurately survey and assess the environmental dimensions as stressors cited earlier and to select appropriate prevention as intervention strategies to maintain or reconstitute the system directly impacts the health of the organization. Where an unsteady state or instability exists between the system and the environment, reconstitution or restorative secondary prevention activities must be quickly instituted. Otherwise the health of the system will continue to deteriorate, culminating in the death of the system.

Nursing

Using the Neuman Model, nursing has been operationalized for a nurse administrator at any level of administration: first line, mid-level, or top level. The major responsibility of a nurse administrator is to create, maintain, and monitor relationships between oneself, the nursing system, or the organization and the environment. Traditionally, administrators have used the management process to adapt and properly realign themselves, or a system, with the environment. The management process allows the nurse administrator to plan, organize, direct, and control activities necessary to retain or reconstitute harmony between a system and its environment.

This multidimensional use of the model helps the administrator identify and implement preventive interventions that can increase any system resistance to stressors and lessen the possible or actual reaction of the system to a stressor. The level of prevention introduced can be primary, secondary, and/or teritary, depending upon the response of the nursing or organizational system. Primary prevention decreases the possibility of an encounter with stressors or strengthens the system flexible line of defense in the presence of stressors. When a system's normal line of defense has been penetrated by a stressor causing a reaction to occur, secondary prevention is required to treat symptoms. Tertiary prevention is reconstitution efforts to assist in restoring and maintaining optimal function of the system that has been altered or made maladaptive as a result of stressors penetrating the normal line of defense.

In summary, the basic structure of the administrative framework based on the Neuman Systems Model places the nurse administrator at the first, middle, or top level of management (Figure 23–1). The system core is viewed either as the person, the nursing system, or the organizational system at one of the three management levels. Whatever the nature of the environment, intra-, inter-, or extrapersonal stressors are always present. For example, as defense mechanisms, the nurse administrator might perform preventive interventions. The level of the prevention depends on the response of the nurse administrator to the environmental stressor; that is, if the stressor has not penetrated the normal line of defense, primary prevention would be appropriate. Where the stressor has penetrated the normal line of defense, secondary and tertiary preventive interventions must occur. By integrating an assessment of the environment with the Neuman Systems Model (Figure 23–3), nurse administrators have a framework to assess, plan, implement, direct, and evaluate their efforts to strengthen, reconstitute, or adapt a system to the environment once stressors have been anticipated, identified, or introduced.

Health of the personal, nursing, or organizational system depends on the stability of the normal line of defense. If the stressor penetrates the system core, the basic structure dies. Preventive interventions are thus needed to promote, treat, or maintain the client system. The purpose of the Neuman-based multidimensional framework (Figure 23–3) is to provide a more comprehensive approach to assessing and resolving problems in nursing and health care systems and to evaluate the total system outcome response to environmental stressors.

ROLE AND BEHAVIORS OF THE NURSE ADMINISTRATOR

Although this chapter primarily focuses on nursing and organizational systems, it is the role of the nurse administrator to maintain system integrity by realigning the nursing or organizational system to its environment. The role of the nurse administrator in education and practice settings is rapidly changing and subject to considerable stress, strain, conflict, and confusion. Role itself is a complex concept having many different connotations. Generally, it is equated with behavior or viewed as a behavioral pattern whose norms are established by society. A role is difficult to enact to everyone's satisfaction. Superiors, peers, subordinates, and self may have different perceptions and expectations of behavior for a given role. Neuman's interrelated concepts, however, provide a systematic framework for viewing the role and behavioral expectations of the nurse administrator. The concepts are independent classes of phenomena that interact to influence behavioral patterns for the nurse administrator.

The first of these concepts (client or person) may be translated into the *personal role*. A competent nurse administrator should be committed to and be held accountable for creating and maintaining a healthy environment within one's self, within the nursing education or practice system, and within the larger organizational system, such as a university or health care system. A healthy work environment ideally facilitates the delivery of quality nursing education and/or health care. In addition, a positive functional role carries with it the expectation that the nurse administrator will act to further the professional growth and development of a nursing faculty or staff. This requires the nurse administrator to be a human relations expert, sensitive to creating a challenging, nurturing climate and facilitating resource availability for nurse productivity and goal attainment. A competent nurse administrator must function in concert with the top management team of an educational or health care organization, and this requires cooperative and interdependent behaviors, understanding of and respect for the role and expertise of other team members, and skill in acquiring essential knowledge concerning the institution, its commitment to society, and how the goals of nursing interrelate and can be achieved. This aspect of the personal role requires the nurse administrator to be an expert in interdisciplinary relations (Kelley, 1977).

The second of Neuman's concepts may be converted into the interrelated role of an *environmentalist.* A competent nurse administrator must be cognizant of three different types of environments: internal, external, and lateral. The nurse administrator is expected to create an *internal climate* that establishes the standard that nurse faculty and/or staff will perform their functions using a research-based knowledge approach to educational and clinical practice. Arranging for support services, allocating sufficient resources, and providing opportunities for staff nurses to be relieved from everyday routines are essential to building a healthy internal environment. The *external environment,* on the other hand, may include the community, the region, the state, the federal government, and professional nursing and health-related organizations. The nurse administrator will be challenged to balance the mission and goals of the external environment with those of the internal environment. Often overlooked is the *lateral environment.* This is considered the peer climate. It involves the attitude of the president of a university or chief executive officer of a hospital toward nursing and the attitudes of other college administrators or department heads. The nurse administrator is expected to provide leadership in moving the nursing organization in the direction of collaborative, rather than competitive or suppressive, interorganizational relationships.

Based on Neuman Model concepts, the third critical role relates to the health system in education or practice. When the nurse administrator selects a model to guide in organizing a school of nursing or nursing practice department, the structure chosen may be impacted by multiple factors: (1) the mission and goals of the organization, (2) the type and kind of workers, (3) the nature of the work to be done, (4) the learning or health care needs of consumers, and (5) the resources available. A nurse administrator who is aware of structural enablers and who has the ability to neutralize or stabilize barriers to organizational health is more likely to foster quality output from nurse faculty and/or staff.

Based on Neuman concepts, the fourth crucial role is that of *nursing.* A competent nurse administrator facilitates and coordinates highly diverse work groups with a wide range of qualifications and work experiences. Today nurse administrators must be highly skilled and fully knowledgeable about the discipline of nursing in order to develop, deliver, and determine effective nursing practice. Additionally, the nurse administrator needs to integrate a broad view of management into collaborative interactions with the administrative team at the first, mid-, and top levels of management within an organization. A commitment to assessing, planning, organizing, leading, and controlling the quality of nursing education or practice within an institution rests with the nurse administrator. Active participation in program planning, policy development, and organizational restructuring that affect nursing education and health care delivery should be the real role, not just an ideal role, of the nurse administrator. In the final analysis, the work of a nursing organization in an educational or practice setting is measured in terms of its output: the observable results of its efforts and the extent to which it contributes to organizational effectiveness and efficiency.

The nurse administrator in nursing education and practice plays a major role in integrating nursing and managing processes with other units of an institution and for making quality decisions that affect the nursing education or practice system. As a knowledgeable worker (Drucker, 1976), the nurse administrator is an idea generator and information processor who uses a conceptual, analytic, and risk-taking approach to getting the goals accomplished and producing quality results.

APPLICATION OF THE NEUMAN SYSTEMS MODEL TO NURSING AND ORGANIZATIONAL SYSTEMS

A Synthesized Assessment Tool

The management process, the Neuman Systems Model, and the environmental dimensions can be intertwined to form a synthesized assessment tool. Through the use of such a tool, a nurse administrator can assess, resolve, prevent, and evaluate stressors. The usefulness of the Neuman Model becomes evident when the tool is used to assist in analyzing the reaction to stressors in any type of administrative setting. Based on the Neuman Systems Model, a modified assessment tool has been developed for nurse administrators, called the Neuman Systems-Management Tool for Nursing and Organizational Systems (Figure 23–4). Whether the nurse administrator is at the first, middle, or top management level, the tool may be readily used to assess and evaluate the total system response to a given environmental stressor.

As a nurse administrator uses the tool to analyze a management situation, a check mark or circle is placed at each relevant descriptor in categories A through D. Category B addresses stressors in the internal or external environment, or , both and the type of client system involvement. Category C focuses on the intra-, inter-, or extrapersonal factors and five classical variables. Category D directs formulation of the problem in relation to the five dimensions of the environment and the three levels of prevention. By checking or circling each appropriate descriptor in categories A through D, the nurse administrator achieves a

A. Intake Summary

Who?	What?	Where?	When?	Why?
Personal system	Structure dx	Education	Timing	Goals
Nursing system	Management dx	setting	Timeframe	Short-term
Organizational	Planning	Practice		Long-term
system	Organizing	Setting		
	Directing			
	Controlling			
	Outcome dx			

B. Stressors: _____

	Client System		
Environment	Personal	Nursing	Organizational
Internal	_____	_____	_____
External	_____	_____	_____

C. Factors

	Developmental	Psychological	PhysiologicaL	Spiritual	Sociocultural
Intrapersonal	_____	_____	_____	_____	_____
Interpersonal	_____	_____	_____	_____	_____
Extrapersonal	_____	_____	_____	_____	_____

D. Organizational Orientation to the Environment

	Environmental Dimensions				
Intervention	Human Resources	Culture	Socio/ Technical	Structure/ Function	Decision Making
Primary	_____	_____	_____	_____	_____
Secondary	_____	_____	_____	_____	_____
Tertiary	_____	_____	_____	_____	_____

E. Problem(s) Defined _____

_____

_____

_____

F. Problem Resolution (Goal) with Rationale

_____

_____

_____

G. Prevention (Action Plan)

_____

_____

_____

H. Outcomes (Evaluation)
    Predicted: _____
    Actual: _____

Figure 23–4. Neuman Systems Management Tool for Nursing and Organizational Systems.

quick, easy, and accurate assessment. Categories E through H require a short written statement about the goal to be achieved, the prevention needed, and the outcome desired.

The first category (intake summary) includes the biographical data of the administrative organization. The five W's are assessed in this category: who, what, where, when, and why. In the "who" subcategory, assessment of the core is performed to determine the boundary of the client system. The system may be personal, nursing, or organizational. Included in the category called "what" are the structure diagnosis, management diagnosis, and outcome diagnosis. The nursing management process is subdivided into four functions: planning, organizing, directing, and controlling. The nurse administrator decides what diagnosis or step of the process would indicate the stressor effect. Education and practice are the two labels in the "where" category. If the nurse administrator is a dean in the school of nursing but the decision affects the clinical rotations in a hospital, both labels would be checked. The "when" section is the timing element and time frame of the reaction to the stressor, and the "why" section is related to the goal of the nurse administrator regarding the stressor. Both the "when" and "why" sections require short behavioral statements.

In category B the stressors perceived by the nurse administrator are identified. The administrator specifies the stressor and classifies it according to the client system (personal, nursing, or organizational) and type of environment (internal or external). Only the major or most pressing stressor is assessed. If additional stressors need to be identified, the nurse administrator completes additional tools.

Category C allows the nurse administrator to classify the stressor into one of three environmental factors—intrapersonal, interpersonal, or extrapersonal—in relation to the five variables—developmental, psychological, sociocultural, physiological, and spiritual—of the client system. The nurse administrator chooses the variable that would be most affected by the stressor.

Under category D the nurse administrator assesses the organizational orientation in terms of five environmental dimensions—human resources, culture, socio/technical, structure/function, and decision making. The nurse administrator checks or writes in the dominant environmental dimension requiring primary, secondary, or tertiary prevention as intervention.

Under category E the nurse administrator formulates the specific organizational or nursing system problem to be resolved. A single concise phrase is written to clarify the problem based on findings from A, B, C, and D. The problem can be primary, secondary, or tertiary in nature and is classified by the client system, the core client system variables, and the environmental dimensions.

In category F the nurse administrator develops a behavioral goal for problem resolution. The goal should be stated with a rationale. Other goals may be listed but should be prioritized. Category G is the prevention or action plan proposed by the administrator. The prevention modality chosen should correlate with the type of problem formulated so that the primary, secondary, and tertiary categories are consistent. Category H is the outcome or evaluation stage. The predicted outcome is always written during the assessment; the actual outcome is written once the plan has been implemented. Once the predicted and actual evaluation is complete, the nurse administrator begins another tool based on the findings of the previously completed assessments.

SUMMARY

Conceptual models have been used for a number of years to guide the construction, implementation, and evaluation of nursing education programs (Fawcett, 1984). The use of models to guide planning and evaluation of nursing and health care organizations has been less evident. Conceptual models and related theories provide structure for the mission, goal, and objectives of nursing and organizational systems, and for the direction of administrative decisions. The use of a model as here proposed would contribute greatly to improvements for quality nursing practice, client care outcomes, and organizational effectiveness. In essence, conceptual–theoretical models provide criteria for standards of nursing practice and patient care, quality improvement initiatives, staffing, and resource allocation and utilization. The Neuman Systems Model framework for nursing and organizational systems discussed in this chapter has major future implications for nursing practice, education, and research as we move into the 21st century and health care reform.

Practice

The nurse administrator at each of three different levels of management is in a key position to assess work situations in educational and practice settings and to initiate interventions designed to maintain quality, influence change, and enhance performance of nurse faculty or staff. Through use of a conceptually based, analytic approach that combines a nursing model with environmental dimensions, the nurse administrator can consistently be an efficient and effective leadership risk taker in the face of anticipated rapid social change. The Neuman-based management tool for nursing systems and organizations provides the nurse administrator with a synthesized and systematic mechanism for shaping, managing, and positively changing the performance of an individual system, the productivity of a nursing system, and the outcomes of an organizational system (Deal, Kennedy, and Spiegel, 1983).

The more comprehensive use of nursing models, as here proposed, will be needed to respond to the health care reform movement. In particular, with the focus on quality care cost containment and anticipated expansion of health care delivery systems into the community, the Neuman management tool for nursing systems and organizations will prove most valuable for assessing, diagnosing, implementing, and evaluating the success of alternative health care delivery systems and in particular nursing services and community-based centers. Also, the tool provides nurse consultants with a comprehensive assessment instrument valuable for assessing the health of organizations and proposing strategies for reconstitution.

Education

The Neuman Systems Model combined with the environmental dimensions can be used for both formal and informal educational development of nurse administrators. Formally, the model can provide an organizing framework for developing and implementing a curriculum designed to prepare analytic nurse administrators. It serves as a guide to the identification and organization of essential content needed by the graduate student majoring in nursing service administration. Additionally, the model provides an efficient and practical framework for student use in acquiring the expected role behaviors of a nurse administrator.

Informally, the Neuman Systems Model can be used by a nurse administrator to identify personal learning needs related to the current nursing education system and/or health care delivery system and to assess self-performance in implementing the role of nurse administrator. As nurse administrators experience stressors and the inability to align or maintain stability among themselves, the nursing system, the organization, and the environment, continuing education programs may need to be developed and offered for nurse administrators to expand, update, and improve intervention skills (for example, to facilitate nurse administrators' intervention to prevent instability in their personal normal and flexible lines of defense as a result of impinging stressors).

Research

Use of a specific conceptual frame of reference helps a nurse administrator categorize information and identify themes or patterns in need of further study. As nurse administrators attempt to align themselves with the evolving nursing system, health care organization, and environment, research will become increasingly important in identifying and documenting the need for innovative, effective, and efficient approaches to providing nursing education and client care services. A number of doctoral dissertations focusing on the personal client system have been conducted (Flannery, 1987; Pierce, 1987; Thornhill, 1985; Williamson, 1989). Research using the Neuman Systems Model related to nursing and organizational systems is less developed. However, studies are being conducted in home health care and long-term care settings (Peoples, 1990; Rowles, 1992).

The integrated conceptual model presented in this chapter is important for future use by nurse administrators in education, practice, and research as it provides a systematic framework for assessing, planning, organizing, directing, and controlling work activities. Through use of an integrated systems model, work goals and prevention strategies can be more effectively formulated by a nurse administrator in response to faculty or staff reactions to major stressors. Such a reevaluation plan of goals and intervention outcomes allows a nurse administrator to continue to assess and improve the work environment and quality of health care provided.

REFERENCES

AACN. 1986. *Essentials of College and University Education for Professional Nursing*. Washington, D.C.

American Nurses' Association. 1976. *Code for Nurses*. Kansas City, Mo.: ANA.

Deal, T. E., Kennedy, A. K., and Spiegel, A. H. 1983. How to create an outstanding hospital culture. *Hospital Forum* 26(1):21–43.

Drucker, P. 1976. *The Effective Executive*. New York: Harper & Row.

Fawcett, J. 1984. *Analysis and Evaluation of Conceptual Models of Nursing*. Philadelphia: Davis.

Flannery, J. 1987. Validity and reliability of levels of cognitive function assessment scale for adults with closed head injuries. Doctoral dissertation, University of Alabama at Birmingham, School of Nursing.

Kelley, J. 1977. The role of the top level administrator. In *Nursing Administrator: Issues for the 80's—Solutions for the 70's*. Minneapolis: University of Minnesota.

Peoples, L. 1990. The relationship between selected client, provider, and agency variables and the utilization of health care services. Doctoral dissertation, University of Alabama at Birmingham, School of Nursing.

Pierce, J. 1987. Effects of two chest tube clearance protocols on chest tube drainage in myocardial revascularization surgical patients. Doctoral dissertation, University of Alabama at Birmingham, School of Nursing.

Rowles, C. 1992. Relationship of selected personal and organizational variables and the tenure of directors of nursing in nursing homes. Doctoral dissertation, University of Alabama at Birmingham, School of Nursing.

Silverman, D. 1971. *The Theory of Organizations*. New York: Basic Books, Inc.

Thornhill, B. 1985. A Q analysis of stressors in the primipara during the immediate postpartal period. Doctoral dissertation, University of Alabama at Birmingham, School of Nursing.

Williamson, J. 1989. The influence of self-selected monotonous sounds of the night sleep patterns of postoperative open heart surgical patients. Doctoral dissertation, University of Alabama at Birmingham, School of Nursing.

24

TQM AND THE NEUMAN SYSTEMS MODEL
Education for Health Care Administration

Patricia Hinton Walker

Total quality management (TQM) has taken the business and health care management world by storm. TQM and/or CQI (continuous quality improvement) training and processes are changing the paradigm of management and administration in the literature, in the organizational workplace, and in managers' actions and roles. At the same time, health care reform promises a significant shift from medical intervention to true health care, which involves primary care and prevention.

"Quality management is both a philosophy and a set of guiding principles that represent a foundation of a continuously improving organization, all the processes within the organization, and the degree to which present and future needs of the customers are met" (Brocka and Brocka, 1992). The Neuman Systems Model (NSM) is also seen as both a philosophy and a set of wholistic concepts to guide practice, education, research, and/or administration for those who use the model for these purposes. Betty Neuman's concepts—such as open systems, a wholistic view of the client system, and an emphasis on client involvement in the process of decision making toward health—are consistent with today's directions for health care reform. In addition, although Neuman's emphasis on prevention as intervention is not new, this perspective is developing as a major focus of health care reform and of new management approaches and roles in TQM.

The purpose of this chapter is to demonstrate how the Neuman Systems Model and TQM are used to prepare health care administrators for the future.

Reviewed by Pat Aylward.

This author blends the new TQM philosophy/approach and the Neuman Systems Model as a framework for teaching health care managers in the nursing administration master's program at the University of Rochester School of Nursing and in an administrative skills course to medical fellows program connected to the school of medicine in Rochester, New York. The term "health care administrator" is used instead of nurse administrator because this author views the Neuman Systems Model as an interdisciplinary model and because it is used to teach nurses and other health care providers in an administrative skills course for physicians and junior faculty in the school of medicine.

BACKGROUND, RATIONALE, AND CONCEPTUAL LINKAGES

The 1993 National League for Nursing's vision for nursing education, published as a guide for the future of education, practice, and research, emphasizes that nurses should be prepared as care managers. Central to "care management" of the client system for health and to the process of managing "healthy" organizations for delivery of care are Deming's 14 points, which are frequently cited as the backbone of TQM. Key administrative actions adapted from Deming's work include: creating constancy of purpose for improving the quality of the product or service; adopting the new philosophy; ending the practice of awarding business on price alone; eliminating fear; breaking down barriers; eliminating numerical quotas and doing it right the first time; increasing the focus of reeducation and training; and involving the customer (Walton, 1986). Another TQM advocate, Crosby (1979), emphasizes leadership, trust, cooperation, and creativity in management.

The parallel focus in the business world on the "customer as king" and in the new health care agenda on the "patient or client as an active participant" clearly creates new challenges for health care managers and impacts nursing administration education programs. When health care administration is taught, it is important to blend these new paradigm shifts with sound theoretical teaching in meaningful ways for future leaders and managers of health care delivery organizations.

Faculty (collectively speaking) in the University of Rochester School of Nursing administration program are interested in preparing students for health care management roles across settings, with knowledge, skills, and philosophies consistent with patient/client care and managerial approaches for the 21st century. Although the philosophy of the school of nursing and the curriculum as a whole is eclectic in nature, individual faculty provide guidance and education from a variety of theoretical perspectives. The nursing program at the University of Rochester School of Nursing includes course content in organizational development and role development for administration, consistent with other nursing administration master's programs. This content is considered the foundation of nursing administration practice and is taught in the first course. This author, as an advocate for the use of nursing theoretical models as frameworks for nursing administration, encourages students to integrate the Neuman Systems Model and TQM into an organizing framework for the study of organizations and the role of health care administrator.

This author's approach is consistent with the perspective that Carroll brings to the development of nursing administration education programs. She states that "the nature of administration and organization content . . . is dependent upon: (1) the faculty's philosophy regarding the importance and appropriateness of nursing adminstration as a valid field of study for nursing; (2) the faculty's view of nursing administration practice; and (3) the resources available in the educational institution" (Henry, 1988). As mentioned previously, this author's philosophy and views of nursing, using the Neuman Systems Model and the richness of expertise and resources at the University of Rochester, influence the program.

Because two of the three nursing administration courses are coordinated by two associate deans for practice, students experience firsthand a broad perspective of applied theory in nursing administration, based in the reality of practice. One associate dean is the director of nursing at Strong Memorial Hospital and the other (this author) is CEO of a community nursing center where the Neuman Systems Model is used as a conceptual base for care. Consequently, students are encouraged to view the organization as a client system with outcomes of sound health care administration resulting in quality patient/client care using a nursing model as a guide.

The use of nursing models as theoretical frameworks for nursing administration are explored in depth in *Dimensions of Nursing Administration* by Henry (1988). This very important contribution to the use of theory in nursing administration is used as one of the textbooks for the first nursing administration course. Three important chapters (the first by Meleis and Jennings, the second by Ference, and the third by Fawcett) provide the basis and rationale for blending nursing science and management science (Henry, 1988). Dienneman discusses five metaphors as analogies to theories for the study of organizations. These are: the organization as a machine, as a biological organism, as an information-processing unit, as a culture, and as a political system. She further writes that "each metaphor or image provides a partial, limited subjective view of objective reality" (Henry, 1988). In a subsequent discussion of epistemological approaches to interdisciplinary inquiry, Henry identifies the basic concepts in these metaphors and identifies the Neuman Systems Model in the view of the organization as a living organism. New management science perspectives are also using the living organism metaphor, with books on "healthy organizations" and "dysfunctional organizations," some of which even present the idea of managers as healers.

Viewing the organization as a living organism or system is a metaphor that assists health care providers in studying health care management. Because the expected outcome of "good organizational management" is quality, cost-effective care to clients/patients, using the same organizing framework makes good sense. Giovinco (Henry, 1988) reinforced this idea when discussing the relationship of philosophy to common sense. She stated that "common sense can be the beginning of philosophical inquiry . . . an ideal springboard for an epistemological journey." This author believes that the metaphor of organizations as living systems enhances learning by appealing to common sense and by building on the knowledge of the human system. This approach assists interdisciplinary health care-oriented students to blend theoretical concepts and content from management science with health care and nursing sciences in the study of health care administration.

Rationale and operational definitions for the use of the Neuman Systems Model in nursing administration have been articulated by Kelley, Sanders, and Pierce in the 1989 second edition of *The Neuman Systems Model*. Building on this important contribution to the use of the NSM in nursing administration, teaching strategies and assignments in the course reflect the explanations of major concepts of the NSM (client system, health, environment, and nurse). Content from the chapter on nursing administration from the second edition will be summarized here for clarification. Kelley, Sanders, and Pierce (1989) identified core concepts related to "person" as the personal system, nursing system, and the organizational system. Environment (internal and external) is subsequently described as intra-, inter-, and extrapersonal, intra-, inter-, and extranursing, and intra-, inter-, and extraorganizational.

Kelley, Sanders, and Pierce (1989) explained that "like the personal system, the nursing system and organizational systems also have a set of core characteristics that determine the overall level of health or stability of the nursing systems or total organization." Very briefly described, the following operational definitions of the five variables provided by Kelley et al. include:

- *physiological:* structures and processes such as size, number of employees, types of services offered, and composition of leadership team
- *psychological:* system's identity within organization and community, leadership style, general attitudes, and atmosphere
- *sociocultural:* norms, values, networks, and economic and political status
- *developmental:* maturity level, life and past experiences, and history

An operational definition of the spiritual variable was not clarified for nursing administration in the previous edition of *The Neuman Systems Model*. This author, using Hawley's (1993) book *Reawakening the Spirit in Work*, proposes the exploration of spiritual qualities at work in the organization as an operational definition for nursing administration. As a guide for students conducting a health systems organizational assessment, the *spiritual* variable includes, but is not limited to, sense of power, creative energy, hope and hopelessness or despair, love, and caring.

NEUMAN SYSTEMS MODEL IN A TQM ORGANIZATION

The use of the Neuman Systems Model as a conceptual approach to the study of organizations as "client systems" has been previously discussed as a logical shift for students (nurses, physicians, and other health care providers) who already understand assessment of a human client for care. Scalzi and Anderson have developed a systems view conceptual model for theory development in nursing administration. This dual-domain model facilitates the integration of nursing theory for patient care with nursing theory for organizational science in *Dimensions of Nursing Administration* (Henry, 1988). Uniting the approach to organizational effectiveness and quality care as an outcome brings the Neuman Systems Model and TQM together as a sound approach for addressing the increasing criticisms and pressures on the health care delivery system.

The national focus on quality health care for Americans will be a significant driving force for the need for total quality management in health care organizations for many years to come. Zeigenfuss (1993) describes nine pressures from the external environment that are impacting the organization as a system and the health care manager of today. These pressures are: sociological changes, technology, economics, politics, laws and regulations, educational demands, resources, cultural changes, and demographics.

Using the Neuman Systems Model and quality management approaches to deal with external environmental stressors, this author designed Figure 24–1 as an overriding framework for teaching the first nursing administration course. The core or structure of the organization and the external pressures or stressors, using total quality management and leadership principles, are represented.

The Neuman Systems Model is used in major course assignments, including a health systems organizational assessment and a personal managerial philosophy, which involves a self-assessment for the future role of the health care administrator. Students are assigned to a health care organization, with a nursing administrator as a mentor, for the health care systems assessment. Figure 24–2 provides a condensed version of the assignments for the organizational assessment and the personal managerial philosophy using the Neuman Systems Model. Generally, students have little difficulty assessing organizational characteristics in the physiological, psychological, and sociocultural variables. However, for the spiritual and developmental variables, additional references and guidance are needed. Hawley's book (1993) is recommended as a reference for spiritual aspects of leaders and organizations.

Students are able to assess the developmental variable and its relationship to organizational functioning after discussing Cribbin's explanation of the life cycle of an organization. In his book, *Leadership—Your Competitive Edge,* Cribbin (1991) provides a chart that describes the life cycle of an organization with a discussion of important factors related to developmental stages from birth through senescence and renewal. Factors influenced by developmental variables

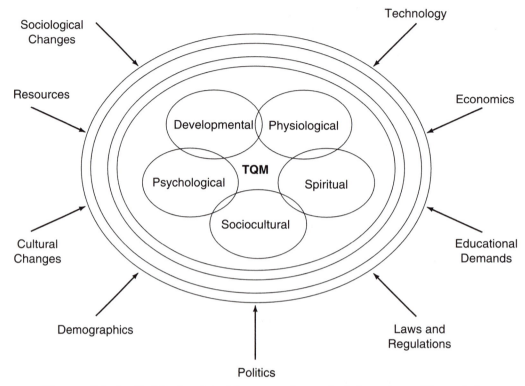

Figure 24–1. Guide for teaching nursing administration. *(Copyright 1993. All rights reserved, Patricia Hinton Walker.)*

include: primary objectives, organizational character, energy focus, central problem, type of planning, and leader/manager type. He also suggests some new types of leadership/management roles needed for different life stages of organizations. These leader/manager roles are: innovator, opportunist, consultant, participant, corporateur, statesman, and mover-shaker. As students learn about the role of the health care administrator and look for future employment, understanding what is needed in the life cycle of the organization is critical for a good fit in a new job.

NEUMAN SYSTEMS MODEL AND TQM ROLE SHIFTS FOR THE HEALTH CARE MANAGER

The role of the nursing or health care administrator is also taught in this first course from the TQM perspective. It is easy to relate TQM to the Neuman Systems Model, particularly with the focus on primary prevention. Crosby

University of Rochester
School of Nursing

NUR 481
Nursing Administration I

HEALTH CARE SYSTEM ANALYSIS—PART I

Part I: Assessment using Neuman Systems Model as an overall framework for a (Macro) Health Care Systems Analysis. This project is to be a typewritten project, integrating ideas from class discussions, textbook content, and other outside readings as appropriate to support your analysis of the health care system.

Introduction   [5 points]

VARIABLES

I.   Assessment of Client (Health Care System) Variables: [25 points]

    A. Physical: This variable includes the size of the organization or system, number of employees, number of beds, types of services offered, urban or rural location, and composition of the leadership team. This also includes assessment related to physical plant, working environment, and technology.

    B. Psychological: Such variables include system's identity within the organization or the organization's identity within the community; channels and processes for communicating; the leadership style of the administrators; and general attitudes, cooperation, or atmosphere of the system or organization. Additional assessment related to competencies, self-esteem, well-being, and satisfaction of managers and employees.

    C. Developmental: Review the life cycle of an organization and relate this to longevity of employees, whether the institution is new or old, and traditions. Also, assess the maturity of the organization according to Cribbin.

    D. Sociocultural: These variables reflect the overall social, economic, or political viability. These variables include norms, values, loyalty, group affiliations, religious affiliations, organizational culture, etc. Also included here is the sociocultural mix of staff and clients/patients, and relationship to the community.

    E. Spiritual: Hope vs. despair, spirit of the organization and/or the leadership. Positive energy or apathy? Impact of the leader on the "spirit" of the organization. Truth, belief, character, integrity, peace, love, and caring.

Figure 24–2. Sample course assignments for organizational assessment and personal managerial philosophy.

(1979), in his early writings on TQM, reinforces this when he states, "the entire world, it seemed, was convinced that prevention—at least on a grand scale—was highly desirable but completely unattainable and impractical." Although this statement was written in reference to business settings, it sounds as if health care discussions that call for a change, with emphasis on prevention instead of treatment, are coming in line with a basic premise of the Neuman Systems Model since its inception.

The focus of the nursing role in the NSM and of the leader/manager role in TQM is to maintain stability of the client system or organization. For the Neuman Systems Model this is realized by supporting and maintaining the normal line of defense; for TQM this is realized by maintaining stability and quality within the organization. Leebov and Scott (1990) propose 10 shifts in role for health care managers. These shifts are: "from provider to customer orientation; from getting by to raising standards; from directing to empowering staff; from employee as expendable resource to employee as customer; from reactive to proactive behavior; from busyness to results; from tradition and safety to experimentation and risk; from turf protection to teamwork across lines; from we-they thinking to organizational perspective; and from cynicism to new optimism."

In the context of the NSM, TQM shifts in role described by Leebov and Scott (1990) clearly support the lines of defense in the Neuman Systems Model and/or serve as primary prevention as intervention strategies in the face of pressures and stressors in the health care environment (see Figure 24–3). For teaching pur-

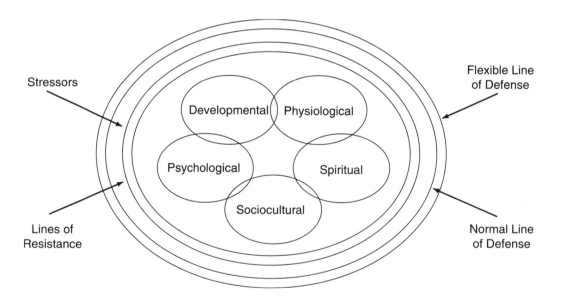

Figure 24–3. Client, nurse, nursing, and the organizational system. *(Copyright 1993. All rights reserved, Patricia Hinton Walker.)*

poses, these roles were placed into three categories, as interventions for the client/patient as customer, the employee/staff as customer, and the organization as a whole. Figure 24–4 depicts this blending of the Neuman Systems Model view of the client system and TQM management role shifts needed for effective administration.

The first category includes those role shifts that are directed to maintaining the stability and strengthening the normal line of defense of the client system (individual, family, or group) who is receiving care or services from the health care organization. Within this category are role shifts toward customer (client) orientation and satisfaction. This includes a "customer is first" orientation, with emphasis on providing quality, excellence, and high standards instead of "just getting by" and improving quality in response to customer complaints.

The second category includes those role shifts that are directed toward employees medical staff, and other staff as the client system. Use of management strategies in this category not only strengthens the normal line of defense against organizational system breakdown because of employee issues, problems, and/or stress, but also serves as a flexible line of defense to prevent stressor invasions of the employee as client system. Empowering employees and other staff, valu-

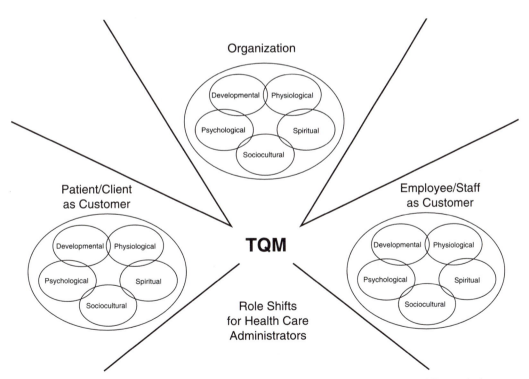

Figure 24–4. Role shifts for health care administrators. *(Copyright 1993. All rights reserved, Patricia Hinton Walker.)*

ing them as integral parts of the organization, and using a team approach allow them to address and solve their own problems. In addition, this encourages employees and staff to develop their own lines of defense against work stress, poor quality products, and customer complaints.

The third category includes role shifts directed toward maintaining stability in the organization as a whole and emphasizes the relationship of the health care administrator as a living organism to the organization as a living client system. Numerous management books and articles have been written about the new leadership and management approaches that bring life into organizations. Stephen Covey (1990) supports these critical shifts toward relationships and optimism, as does Burt Nanus (1992) in his book, *Visionary Leadership*. Both authors write about proactive versus reactive approaches, optimism communicated down through the organization, a philosophy of organizational caring, and willingness to experiment and take the risk of sharing responsibility, values, and leadership with organizational members. Table 24–1 summarizes the 10 role shifts according to the three categories presented here.

All the TQM role shifts discussed also become prevention as intervention strategies for addressing problems with patients as customers, employees and other staff as customers, and the organization as a client system. The focus of TQM is to establish an organizational culture and climate that foster strong relationships between and among all players in the organization, including the patient. By implementing TQM principles, the health care administrator has implemented primary prevention interventions to maintain the stability of the organization and its services. If the system breaks down and the patient as customer or employee as customer is dissatisfied, the same strategies become secondary prevention interventions. TQM advocates emphasize the critical nature of continued education, training, and retraining in order to prevent a return to former ways of dealing with management problems. Ongoing education of the patient and the employees as clients to healthy processes for problem solving and conflict resolution could be considered tertiary prevention strategies for the organization, according to Neuman. Philosophically, it seems that the Neuman Systems Model was ahead of its time, with its focus on the mutual determination of goals and prevention. The strengths of the model make it effective in

TABLE 24–1. TQM CHANGING MANAGEMENT ROLES FOR CLIENT SYSTEM(S) AS CUSTOMERS

Client/Patient as Customer	Employee/Staff as Customer	Organization as Customer
1. Customer orientation	3. Empower employees	6. Proactive behavior
2. Raising standards	4. Employee as customer	7. Experiment and take risks
	5. Teamwork across lines	8. Results oriented
		9. Organizational perspective
		10. New optimism

teaching students sound theoretical ways of viewing the patient, the employee, and the organization in order to apply current total quality management principles.

SUMMARY AND FUTURE IMPLICATIONS

The Neuman Systems Model's flexibility related to the targeted client system makes it a model of choice for nursing administration. The relationship of nursing systems and management systems is an easy relationship to build on for classroom teaching, because both are systems models. Viewing the client system as "patient customer," the employee or staff as "customer," and the total organization within a framework based on the Neuman Systems Model translates to continuity of care and effective administration. The total quality management movement in American business and health care calls for significant change in past management practices.

Although customer involvement and attention to the perceptions and goals of the customer (client system) are relatively new perspectives emphasized by TQM, these ideas are not foreign to users of the Neuman Systems Model. Neuman has historically advocated that the health care provider, through the assessment process, determine mutual goals and directions for care with the client or patient. This basic premise brings TQM and NSM together as the critical beginning point for the nursing and management process. For future health care administrators interested in a wholistic yet realistic path toward total quality management, this chapter offers the Neuman Systems Model as a sound, conceptual approach that is philosophically consistent with TQM principles.

REFERENCES

Brocka, B., and Brocka, M. S. 1992. *Quality Management.* Homewood, Ill.: Business One Irwin, 3.

Covey, S. 1990. *Principle-Centered Leadership.* London: Summit Books.

Cribbin, J. J. 1981. *Leadership—Your Competitive Edge.* New York: American Management Association Publishing Group, 48–49.

Crosby, P. B. 1979. *Quality Is Free.* New York: New American Library, 120–135, 4.

Hawley, J. 1993. *Reawakening the Spirit in Work.* San Francisco: Berrett-Koehler Publishers.

Henry, B., Arndt, C., Di Vincenti, M., and Marriner-Tomey, A, eds. 1988. *Dimensions of Nursing Administration.* Boston: Blackwell Scientific Publications, 497, 7–19, 121–133, 143–155, 161, 242, 247.

Leebov, W., and Scott, G. 1990. *Health Care Managers in Transition.* San Francisco: Jossey-Bass Publishers, 11.

Nanus, B. 1992. *Visionary Leadership.* San Francisco: Jossey-Bass Publishers.

National League for Nursing. 1993. *A Vision for Nursing Education,* 12–13. New York: National League for Nursing.

Neuman, B., ed. 1989. *The Neuman Systems Model,* 2d ed. Norwalk: Appleton & Lange, 115–126, 199, 121–122.

Walton, M. 1986. *The Deming Management Method.* New York: Putnam Publishing Group, 34–36.

Ziegenfuss, J. T. 1993. *The Organizational Path to Health Care Quality.* Ann Arbor: Health Administration Press.

25

CARE MANAGEMENT OF PREGNANT SUBSTANCE ABUSERS USING THE NEUMAN SYSTEMS MODEL

Victoria L. Poole

Juanzetta S. Flowers

This chapter provides a demonstration of how the Neuman Systems Model can be utilized to effectively guide nurse-managed care of the substance-abusing pregnant client. A case demonstration illustrates the nurse-managed care collaborative opportunities with the client, health care providers, and community agencies for the drug-abusing client during the prenatal, intrapartal, and post-partal periods.

Drug use during pregnancy is a social, economic, and health concern of national import. It has been shown to have adverse effects on the mother, fetus, newborn, and the child in later years. The possible effects differ depending on the drug used (such as marijuana, heroin, cocaine, or alcohol) and the frequency and intensity of use (Klerman, Brown, and Poole, 1993). The life-style behaviors of pregnant women using drugs are such that they receive little or no prenatal health care, are malnourished, often resort to prostitution, and abuse

Reviewed by Jean Kelley.

other substances such as tobacco and alcohol (Flandermeyer, 1987). Often born prematurely or suffering withdrawal symptoms, drug-exposed infants require extended hospital stays and expensive treatments in newborn nurseries and neonatal intensive care units (Phibbs et al., 1991). In addition, the life-style of a mother who continues to use drugs after delivery often results in inadequate parenting, abuse, and neglect for the child (Zuckerman and Frank, 1992; Mays et al., 1992).

THE NEUMAN SYSTEMS MODEL AND THE PREGNANT SUBSTANCE ABUSER

The interaction of psychological, physiological, sociocultural, and spiritual needs of the drug-using pregnant woman places increased demands on the perinatal nurse. The Neuman Systems Model as depicted in Figure 25–1 provides direction for determining appropriate primary, secondary, and tertiary nursing prevention as intervention strategies to reduce perinatal drug use. Primary intervention strategies include early identification of high-risk clients and implementation of teaching formats to improve life-style and dietary habits. Secondary interventions include strategies to assist the drug-using mother to stop the abuse as early as possible in the pregnancy. Tertiary interventions include intensified health education and behavior modifications prior to another conception as well as pregnancy planning.

THE NEUMAN SYSTEMS MODEL AND MANAGED CÁRE OF THE PREGNANT SUBSTANCE ABUSER

Wholistic perinatal nursing care of the drug-abusing pregnant client can be managed more effectively by the perinatal nurse through utilizing the client, nursing, and health care system as target subsystems of the Neuman Systems Model. Nurse-managed care fosters collaborative opportunities with the client, health care providers, and community agencies for the drug-abusing pregnant woman during the prenatal, intrapartal, and postpartal periods. Such nurse-managed care focuses on the tools and systems that support cost-effective, quality-oriented health care for pregnant substance abusers (see Table 25–1).

The Drug-Abusing Perinatal Client

The pregnant woman using cocaine, for example, is at risk for hypertension, stroke, and obstetric hemmorhage from placental abruption. Cocaine is a short-acting drug that is inhaled or injected. Because of its capacity to cause constriction of blood vessels, frequent inhalation can cause destruction of the nares or nasal septum. Concurrent problems are associated with use of dirty needles and anaerobic infection from local ischemia. Poor nutrition is a major concern due

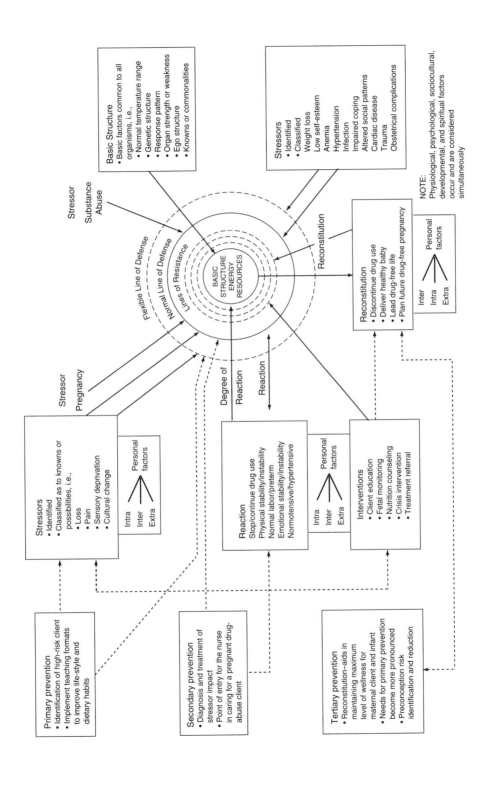

Figure 25–1. The Neuman Systems Model and Managed Client Care for Aggregate Pregnant Substance Abusers.

TABLE 25–1. NURSE-MANAGED PERINATAL CARE BASED ON THE NEUMAN SYSTEMS MODEL

Client System	Nursing System	Health Care and Other Community Agency System
Substance-abusing pregnant woman (utilize primary, secondary, and tertiary preventions as interventions)	(utilize primary, secondary, and tertiary preventions as interventions)	(utilize primary, secondary, and tertiary preventions as interventions)

I. Person
  Physical variables
  Psychological variables
  Spiritual variables
  Sociocultural variables
  Developmental variables
  Basic survival mechanism
	I. Prenatal period
	  A. Nursing assessment
	    1. Data gathering
	    2. Stressors identified
	      a. Intrapersonal
	      b. Interpersonal
	      c. Extrapersonal
	  B. Nursing diagnoses
	  C. Nursing goals
	  D. Nursing outcomes
		Obstetrical health care providers
		
		Neonatal/pediatric health care providers
		
		General medical care providers
		
		Psychiatric/psychological mental health care providers

II. Environment
  Intrapersonal factors
    Physiological
    Psychological
    Developmental
    Sociocultural
    Spiritual
 	
  Interpersonal factors
    Family
    Spouse/significant other
    Friends
    Caregivers
	II. Intrapartal period
	  A. Nursing assessment
	    1. Data gathering
	    2. Stressors identified
	      a. Intrapersonal
	      b. Interpersonal
	      c. Extrapersonal
	  B. Nursing diagnoses
	  C. Nursing goals
	  D. Nursing outcomes
		Social services
		
		Substance abuse counselors
		
		Nutritionist—WIC programs
		
		Group support systems (Narcotics Anonymous, Alcoholics Anonymous)

Extrapersonal factors
    Community resources
    Employment opportunities
    Health care agencies
    Society
 	
Stressors
  Physiological
  Psychological
  Sociocultural
  Developmental
  Spiritual
	III. Postpartal period
	  A. Nursing assessment
	    1. Data gathering
	    2. Stressors identified
	      a. Intrapersonal
	      b. Interpersonal
	      c. Extrapersonal
	  B. Nursing diagnoses
	  C. Nursing goals
	  D. Nursing outcomes
		Medicaid
		
		Vocational training
		
		Day care
		
		Job placement
		
		Housing
		
		Parenting support groups
		
		Family planning

to the starvation ketosis and dehydration associated with drug abuse. The neonate is at risk for intrauterine growth retardation, malformations of the genitourinary tract, altered neonatal behavior patterns, and small head circumference. There is also the risk for cerebral hemorrhage in utero, preterm delivery, an increased incidence of SIDS, and perhaps neural tube defects (Chasnoff, 1991; Hadeed and Siegel, 1989; Janke, 1990; Jones, 1991).

Furthermore, common complications of heroin or methodone use during pregnancy include first trimester spontaneous abortions, premature delivery, and maternal and fetal infections. Narcotic-exposed infants are at an increased risk for neonatal withdrawl syndrome characterized by irritability, poor sucking and swallowing, respiratory distress, tremors, and excoriation of the extremities (Torrence and Horns, 1989).

Alcohol consumption by the maternal client often results in poor nutritional intake of proteins, vitamins, and essential fats, exposing the infant to intrauterine growth reatrdation. The deleterious effects of alcohol on the developing fetus range from death to a variety of malformations related to dose, timing, and frequency of exposure (National Institute on Alcohol Abuse and Alcoholism [NIAAA], 1990). Fetal alcohol syndrome (FAS) is characterized by microcephaly, mild to moderate retardation, irritability, poor coordination, and physical anomalies (Abel and Sokol, 1991).

Because mothers who are involved with drugs are mentally and physically consumed by the need for them, they may not be able to care for a child adequately, particularly one that may be jittery or unable to respond to maternal cues. Such infants have been abandoned at the hospital, or abused or neglected if they are taken home.

Managing the care for the drug-abusing pregnant client includes attention to nutrition for prevention of iron and protein deficits and maternal ketosis; prevention and treatment of infection; psychological support to prevent or ameliorate depression or low self-esteem; and management of the substance abuse to promote withdrawal and to discover polydrug use.

A CASE ILLUSTRATION

The following case illustration is an example of how the Neuman Systems Model can guide the perinatal nurse in managing the care of a pregnant substance abuser during the prenatal, intrapartal, and postpartal periods.

Prenatal Period

Mary is a 22-year-old white female who presents at the health department for birth control. At this time she learns that she is already pregnant. Mary receives initial counseling from the family planning nurse regarding nutrition and how to set up appointments in the prenatal clinic. During the discussion the nurse learns that Mary is presently living in a small apartment with several friends, dropped out of college several months earlier, and is working during the day as a waitress. Mary is extremely upset over the positive pregnancy test and states it is against her religion to have an abortion, but she is too embarrassed to tell her parents about the baby. Mary is concerned about her frequent use of cocaine, marijuana, and alcohol but decides not to share this information with the nurse.

Although Mary wanted to go to a private physician, her problems with finances and transportation were such that the health department prenatal clinic was her only health care option. Leaving the clinic that day, she overheard several conversations where the women were complaining of long waiting times, no continuity in health care providers, difficulty finding transportation, and no one to help with the children when they were being seen by the doctor.

When Mary tells her friends the news of the pregnancy, she is told as soon as the baby is born she will have to move out of the apartment. Mary delays going for prenatal care and tries to block out her fears with alcohol and marijuana. She uses cocaine one day before going to work. At work she faints, and the other waitresses, who have agreed to keep her pregnancy a secret, are concerned and finally take Mary to the prenatal clinic. At this time her drug use is discovered. She has lost weight and is anemic. Although the nurse arranges for a social worker and makes an appointment with an agency to care for women who are drug abusers and pregnant, Mary continues to dismiss the counseling and frequently fails to keep her prenatal appointments.

Using the Neuman Systems Model, the nurse's initial prenatal assessment of Mary's health status was as follows:

Client System

Pregnancy unplanned
Fear of parental discovery
Concealment
Financial affairs in disarray
Altered social patterns
Lack of acceptance that drug use is a problem
Decreased ability to handle stress
Employment difficulties
Impaired problem solving
Alteration in personal, occupational, and social life
Ineffective coping
Weight loss
Megablastic anemia as a result of folic acid deficiency
Alcohol ketoacidosis as a result of heightened sensitivity to fasting hypoglycemia in
    pregnancy
Poly drug abuse—alcohol, marijuana, and cocaine
Knowledge deficit of pregnancy

Nursing System

Identify women at risk for drug abuse (e.g., family history of drug use, loss of child or spouse,
    absence of support system, history of depression, suicide attempt, high stress levels)
Maintain nonjudgmental attitude when interviewing the client
Obtain a complete data base about drug use, quality of life, and psychosocial history
Obtain a complete data base concerning type and route of drug use (e.g., illicit drugs, pre-
    scriptions, vitamins, over-the-counter drugs, caffeine, alcohol, and cigarettes)
Schedule prenatal appointments at least biweekly but make appointments available when-
    ever the patient comes to clinic even if she is late or comes on wrong day
Encourage client to come in whenever she feels the need

Praise any effort the client makes to comply with treatment regimen
Plan for client to see as few different providers as possible in the course of the pregnancy
Assist client to spend minimal time in a waiting room
Allow adequate time for client to talk about unfamiliar procedures and treatments
Coordinate hours and paperwork of prenatal services with other services needed by the
    client
Identify any social support system or personal resources

Health Care and Other Community Agency System

Prenatal care
WIC
Medicaid
Genetic counseling
Welfare and unemployment agencies
Churches and community service groups
Shelters for homeless
Substance abuse counselors

Intrapartal Period

Following a later episode of using cocaine and alcohol, Mary goes into labor at
34 weeks. She has attended no prenatal classes and presents at the emergency
room of a local hospital with no support system. Over the course of her pregnancy, Mary has only kept three of her clinic appointments for prenatal care.
The nurse's assessment of Mary revealed:

Client System

Behavior is dependent, needing constant gratification and lacking in a sense of responsibility
Very low level of self-care associated with low self-esteem
Poor nutritional state
Knowledge deficit of labor and delivery process
Poor tolerance for pain
Lack of family or others for social support
Fluid volume deficit
Anxiety/fear
Ineffective individual coping

Nursing System

Explain procedures
Encourage client to verbalize fears and concerns
Determine maternal drug intoxication at delivery and have drug antagonist available
If mother is positive, deal with reporting if state requires it
Monitor fetal status closely for deceleration of FHT and observe for meconium staining
Support the substance abuser's need for dependency and instant gratification
Provide for continuity of care and organize the efforts of the whole team—obstetrician,
    psychiatrist, social worker
Provide caring labor support by a trusted supportive person and lay the psychological
    groundwork for sound bonding and family integration
Provide communication with the mother about her progress in labor and about the baby
    during labor, at delivery, and following birth

Health Care and Other Community Agency System

Hospital or birthing center
Obstetrical caregiver
Substance abuse counselor
Social services
Medicaid

Postpartal Period

Mary delivers a low birthweight male infant with Apgar scores of 4 and 7. The baby is sent to the neonatal intensive care unit. The nursing assessment of Mary and her infant indicated:

Client System

Lack of knowledge of parenting skills
Lack of knowledge of self-care skills
Potential for child neglect/abuse
Lack of social support
Disturbance in body image
Ineffective individual coping
Grieving related to potential loss of infant or birth of an imperfect child
Potential for altered parenting

Nursing System

Monitor neonatal respiratory and neurologic status closely after birth
Make a special effort to relive the labor/delivery with the mother, praising her for any attempt to assist with the birthing process
Encourage the mother to hold baby and visit the intensive care nursery
Continue communication with all health team members to provide continuity of care during and after the hospitalization
Encourage all drug-abusing women to leave the hospital with a method of birth control and knowledge of how to use it
Encourage frequent and early newborn and postpartum check-up appointment, if at all possible on same day and at same facility
Give mother number of drug and parenting hotline and number of nursing staff

Health Care and Other Community Agency System

Family planning services, private and public
Parenting support groups
Substance abuse treatment programs, inpatient and outpatient
WIC
Social service
Health department
Unemployment/job services
Family court

SUMMARY AND FUTURE IMPLICATIONS

The purpose of this chapter is to provide a demonstration of how the Neuman Systems Model can be used to more effectively guide nurse-managed care of the substance-abusing pregnant client. The ideal situation is to have one nurse manage the care during the prenatal, intrapartal, and postpartal periods. However, in situations where that is not possible, the model can also be used by the various nurses involved in each phase to provide better continuity of care. The prenatal nurse would manage care utilizing the prenatal period plan, the intrapartal nurse would continue the care using that portion of the plan, and the postpartum nurse manager would provide in-hospital care using that portion of the plan. Ideally, the in-hospital postpartum nurse would refer the client to a community-based nurse who would manage the care of the client through reconstitution.

However it is utilized, by one nurse manager or by multiple nurse managers, the Neuman Systems Model provides an ideal guide for care of all types of clients. While this chapter focuses on the pregnant substance abuser, the model can be modified to provide a guide for care for any client with specialized needs, such as those with AIDS or the homeless client. The important thing to remember is that all three subsystems (client, nursing, health care system) in the model work as a whole. No one aspect could or should stand alone for a wholistic perspective. By using the model as a guide, client care will become less fragmented and more consistent in approach. More importantly, there is less chance of omitting vital therapeutic concerns, thus allowing for care continuity.

The current health care system reform movement is focused on three essential elements: quality, access, and cost. Nurse-managed care using the Neuman Systems Model as illustrated in this chapter is an ideal way to improve upon all three elements. Not only can the Neuman Systems Model assure that the quality of care is delivered, it can also help contain costs. With a prenatal client, for instance, care is under the guidance of a nurse who is responsible for making certain that clients have access to cost-effective quality health care without vital aspects of health care services getting overlooked.

As the health care reform movement is being formulated at present, future access to care will be provided through basic health insurance, which is supposed to provide the previously uninsured with choices for care (Webb, 1992; Gaffney and Mikulencak, 1993). Nurse-managed care under the guidance of the Neuman Systems Model can be an ideal choice for many of these clients.

It will also be the role of the professional nurse to assess a community or aggregate's need for knowledge about the cost, quality, and access to health care services and to teach consumers accordingly (Maraldo, 1990). Different communities will have different needs. An example of an aggregate within a community is pregnant women who use drugs. However, there are many other aggregates within communities that are in need of intensified health education, such as those presented by AIDS-affected clients, cancer patients, gerontological clients, and so on. The nurse managing care for these clients will require a greater understanding of the sociocultural and political aspects of the community as the emphasis in health care reform shifts to health promotion and health protection in these under-researched populations (AACN, 1992; NLN, 1992). Whatever the future holds for health care, nurses utilizing the Neuman Systems Model to guide care for a variety of clients can improve the quality, access, and cost of health care service. This chapter can serve as a template for how that care can be delivered more effectively through utilizing the client, nursing, and health care systems as subsystems of the larger comprehensive social system.

REFERENCES

Abel, E. L., and Sokol, R. J. 1991. A revised conservative estimate of the incidence of FAS and its economic impact. *Alcoholism: Clinical and Experimental Research* 15:514–524.

An Agenda for Nursing Education Reform: In Support of Nursing's Agenda for Health Care Reform. 1992. New York: National League for Nursing.

Chasnoff, I. J. 1991. Cocaine and pregnancy: Clinical and methodologic issues. *Clinical Perinatology,* 18(1):113–123.

Flandermeyer, A. 1987. A comparison of the effects of heroin and cocaine abuse upon the neonate. *Neonatal Network* 6(4):42–48.

Gaffney, T., and Mikulencak, M. 1993. Restructuring health care includes discussing options. *American Nurse* 25(2):18, 24.

Hadeed, A., and Seigel, S. 1989. Maternal cocaine use during pregnancy: Effect on the newborn infant. *Pediatrics* 84:205–210.

Health Care Reform: The Clinton Plan, Assessing the Implications. 1992. Dallas: Ernest and Young.

Janke, J. 1990. Prenatal cocaine use: Effects on perinatal outcome. *Journal of Nurse Midwifery,* 35(2):74–77.

Jones, K. 1991. Developmental pathogensis of defects associated with prenatal cocaine exposure: Fetal vascular disruption. *Clinical Perinatology* 18(1):139–145.

Klerman, L. V., Brown, S. S., and Poole, V. L. 1993. The role of family planning in promoting healthy child development. Paper prepared for Task Force on Meeting the Needs of Young Children, Carnegie Corporation of New York, February.

Maraldo, P. J. 1990. The nineties: A decade in search of meaning. *Nursing & Health Care* 11(1):11–14.

Mays, L. C., Granger, R. H., Bornstein, M. H., and Zuckerman, B. 1992. The problem of prenatal cocaine exposure: A rush to judgment. *JAMA* 267:406–408.

National Institute on Alcohol Abuse and Alcoholism. 1990. Seventh Special Report to the U.S. Congress on Alcohol and Health From the Secretary of Health and Human Services. Rockville, Md.

Phibbs, C. S., Bateman, D. A., and Schwartz, R. M. 1991. The neonatal costs of maternal cocaine use. *JAMA* 266:1521–1526.

Position statement for addressing nursing education's agenda for the 21st century. 1992. Washington, D.C.: American Association of Colleges of Nursing.

Torrence, C., and Horns, K. 1989. Appraisal and caregiving for the drug addicted infant. *Neonatal Network* 8(3):49–59.

Webb, K. 1992. "Dr. Clinton" proposes a remedy for America's health ills. *UAMS Journal* 1:22–27.

Zuckerman, B., and Frank, D. A. 1992. Crack kids: Not broken. *Pediatrics* 89:337–339.

26

IMPLEMENTING THE NEUMAN MODEL IN A PSYCHIATRIC HOSPITAL

Betty Scicchitani

Julie G. Cox

Loretta J. Heyduk

Patricia A. Maglicco

Nancy A. Sargent

BACKGROUND INFORMATION

Friends Hospital, the first private not-for-profit psychiatric hospital in the United States, was founded in 1813 by members of the Religious Society of Friends (Quakers). It was established to provide human care for persons "deprived of the use of their reason." In the early 1800s Friends Hospital was a leader in the "moral revolution." The Quakers emphasized humane treatment of clients, that is, care with respect and kindness no matter what degree of mental illness was manifested.

Although many changes have taken place in psychiatric care, the philosophy of Friends Hospital has remained consistent. The nursing philosophy was based on a wholistic stance and emphasized the assessment of clients' strengths. this supported the Quaker belief of "that of God in everyone." Another key belief of the Quakers is decision making by consensus. Thus a participatory management style was the mode of operation of the nursing department.

Nursing department leaders at Friends have always looked for what was current, innovative, and future-oriented in nursing practice. In the late 1980s and early 1990s it became clear that the new economics of health care was going to have a major impact on delivery of nursing care. Financial reimbursement agencies presented providers with increasing demands. These included shorter lengths of stay, outcome studies, and justification for specific modalities of care. Adapting to these demands required creativity in overall systems of care delivery. These efforts had to be balanced in ways that would not compromise the care of clients. It was paramount that nurses not lose their commitment to the client. As change began in response to some of these demands, the department determined the need to implement a nursing model.

It was hoped that the model selected would:

• Define the practice of nursing at Friends
• Provide a unifying framework for nursing practice
• Promote efficiency of communication
• Promote ease of data collection
• Promote accountability
• Guide in-service and daily practice
• Provide a basis for outcome studies
• Lend itself to quality improvement
• Provide a basis for professional growth and greater autonomy.

SELECTION OF THE MODEL

Having identified what was needed from a nursing model, the department designed a selection process that acknowledged change theory and the department's commitment to participatory management. For this reason the department valued maintaining the broadest possible involvement of nursing staff. Also important in the selection process was finding a model that would recognize and reframe existing strenghths in the department while at the same time facilitate a sorting out of the concepts. With these goals in mind, the process of selecting a model was designed with two main components. These were a self-study, similar to those conducted in academic settings, and an examination of several models suggested for a psychiatric treatment setting.

The self-study employed a two-pronged approach. It facilitated examination of the department as a whole—its philosophy, valued concepts, history, and ideals—as well as its place in the larger hospital system. In addition, the personal beliefs and philosophies of the professional nursing staff were assessed and described. A task force was established with representation from all levels, shifts, and services in the department. A consultant familiar with a variety of models worked with this group and its co-chairs. With her help a questionnaire for all nurses was used to collect data regarding the staff's views of the four paradigms—*person, environment, health,* and *nursing.* Also assessed was the staff's familiarity or allegiance to any particular model and exposure to the use of nursing models in general.

The task force collected and examined the various written statements of hospital mission and philosophy, nursing department philosophy, and the statements of philosophy of the various units of service. Policies and procedures were examined to identify implied statements of belief. The hospital was a long-established institution of the Society of Friends, so the history and myths regarding the hospital's founding and development also offered clues that demanded attention. For example, the founder and early directors of the hospital had followed the Friends' ideal, seeking "that of God" in "those temporarily deprived of the use of their reason." In addition, the use of the external environment had long been emphasized in the care of clients. These ideas contributed to an understanding of the four paradigms.

Upon recommendation of the consultant, four models were identified, and study groups were established to examine each of them. Opportunities for involvement of all nurses were facilitated by establishing study groups on each shift. Each group was given its task in the form of materials about a specific model, suggestions for studying the materials, and a set of questions to which the group would provide written answers. These questions were designed to assess the degree to which the model met criteria for selection. Criteria included the fit with current practice in the hospital; social utility, social congruence, and social significance of the model; and pragmatic concerns regarding the model's ease of implementation. The questions further encouraged and assessed the study group's understanding of the model by identifying the four paradigms and the underlying assumptions of the model.

Each of the groups worked diligently to complete the task within a two-month period, and considerable interest developed in the models studied during the process. In addition to the written report, each group was invited to make a brief videotape sharing impressions of the model and the experience of working in the study group in a more informal way. These videotapes and written reports were made available to all nurses. Strong enthusiasm for both Neuman's model and one other model brought the task force members to a temporary impasse in making the final recommendation. A survey of all nurses, both management and staff, did little to bring about a decision.

In making the choice, nursing management found a major conflict between pragmatic concerns and a more long-term view. A site visit was made to two hospitals, each using one of the models. The visits provided the task force with ideas regarding implementation of the models but were less helpful in resolving the conflict. The model supported by many staff nurses employed language that seemed readily understood and concepts that suggested immediate application, particularly in the geriatric service. Many of the management staff, on the other hand, saw the general system base of the Neuman Model as having much broader application and utility. The stress base was a familiar concept to many, and the three levels of prevention as intervention offered support for expansion of nursing roles and services into new settings. Ultimately, the management group chose the Neuman model based on a more long-term view of practice and the setting in which it occurs. This decision was announced to the hospital in a poster session and tea, which is a formal tradition in the hospital.

IMPLEMENTATION OF THE MODEL

An introductory poster session was held to familiarize all nursing staff with aspects of the Neuman conceptual model and application of the model to client case studies.

A decision was made by the nurse managers that the model be implemented across all hospital units at the same time. This pattern of implementation provided an opportunity to build on the nurses' growing enthusiasm for the project. A new task force was established to guide in the implementation process. Again by design, this new task force included a broad range of membership. Individuals from nursing administration and in-service education, and an individual from each nursing unit in the hospital including the partial hospital program were assigned to participate. Initial goals of the task force were as follows:

1. To study the model in more depth and become familiar enough with it to assist in teaching the model to other nurses
2. To develop an education plan
3. To design nursing assessment tools consistent with the model

The educational process started when the task force began work on the first goal through reading assignments, videotape reviews, lectures, and discussion. The plan included presentations about the model at regularly scheduled workshops for staff nurses and nursing management and at the seminar for the nursing community. The plan so included a periodic newsletter devoted to definitions and explanations of the model as well as updates on the task force work. the revised nursing assessment tool was a radical change from the previous tool. It was based on the one developed by Betty Neuman and emphasized client and staff perceptions related to stressors, coping devices, and so on. In addition, supplemental assessment tools were created to structure exploration of target complaints, as needed (for example; sleep disturbance, appetite disturbance, spirituality, and psychosis). Nurse managers piloted the forms, and staff nurses were then encouraged to use the tools and adapt them to their individual style of practice prior to formal in-service education. In retrospect, this sequence was not helpful in decreasing staff anxiety about their lack of a knowledge base in the Neuman Model.

To generate enthusiasm and to answer specific questions about the model, Betty Neuman was invited to consult with the nursing department. In addition, a workshop was held in which Neuman provided an overview of the model. A panel of nurses from other institutions in the area that were also using the Neuman Model discussed their experiences in implementing the model. All Friends Hospital nurses and guests from the surrounding community were included in the workshop.

The Annual Nursing Management Workshop, which includes all nursing management staff, was also devoted to the study of the Neuman Model. The emphasis of this workshop was a review of systems theory and stress theory as the theoretical underpinnings of the model. The department of nursing Annual Seminar for the Nursing Community presented the Neuman Model. Finally, The Annual Nursing Workshop for Staff Nurses, which followed the seminar, summarized much of the content that had been explored throughout the year. Concerns related to the use of the assessment tool were addressed, and the results of audits of the supplemental assessment tools were discussed. In addition, a simulation game (Duke, 1986) was designed and used to enhance an understanding of the model (see Appendix A).

On the basis of the outcome of the staff nurse workshop, a second revision of the nursing assessment tool was planned, and nurses were asked to submit proposals for revised forms to the task force for review. Changes in the original form were made and approved.

The task force then focused on interdisciplinary education regarding the nursing department's use of the model. A presentation to all disciplines was made at an interdisciplinary literature seminar, and the Neuman Model was viewed positively.

The task force then turned to continuing integration of the model into nursing practice. Integration of the Neuman Model into the nursing department's practice standards and philosophy was established. The nurse internship program and the orientation program for new nurses were revised to include the Neuman Model. The nursing tool used to assess clients at risk of suicide was examined for congruence with the model. The task force looked at client records on various nursing units to examine how the model was used by the nurse in his or her care of the client. Nurse members of the task force were encouraged to review the findings with their unit staff.

The department of nursing views integration of the model as an ongoing process; therefore, the task force, which guided initial implementation, became a standing committee of the department. As changes occur more rapidly in response to external pressures such as managed care, the committee faces many challenges. These include redesigning the assessment tool and accommodation to vast reorganization in the department and the hospital.

OUTCOME

The use of models and theoretical constructs was not new to this nursing staff. In a survey conducted prior to the selection of the model, 68 percent of the nurses had identified one or more constructs that they frequently used in nursing care. The attribution of change based on the Neuman Model therefore awaits research. It is, however, possible to describe behaviors that show the influence of the Neuman Systems Model. The most prominent behaviors in each of the four paradigms of person, health, environment, and nursing, as identified by the authors, will be described.

Person

There has been a fairly dramatic increase in the attention focused on client perceptions. In an institution that has always considered the uniqueness of each individual, the magnitude of the change came as somewhat of a surprise. It may be that the idea of "that of God in every person" that exists as part of Friends Hospital's heritage found its modern expression most clearly in the clients' statements about themselves, their current situation, and their aspirations for the future. It seems as though the nurses' natural concern for sensitivity to individual needs was enhanced by an assessment tool structured to document client perception, nurse perception, and the degree of congruence between them. The department has long subscribed to the concept that what a person perceives is happening to him or her is more influential in determining behavior than what is actually happening. It was the Neuman Model, however, that so clearly showed the interplay of client and nurse perception, with all of its implications for accurate and individualized interventions. A logical extension would be greater individuality and specificity of care, an ideal subject for future nursing research.

Health/Wellness and Environment

Neuman defines wellness as "the condition in which all system parts and subparts are in harmony with the whole system of the client" (Neuman, 1989). She defines environment as consisting of "both internal and external forces surrounding the client, influencing and being influenced by the client, at any point in time, as an open system" (Neuman, 1989). Acceptance of these definitions results in the commitment to assess the client's relationships to five variables: physiological, psychological, sociocultural, developmental, and spiritual. The most prominent nurse behavior identified by the authors is the continued commitment to assessment of all five variables, even in the face of pressure to focus on the "most significant reason" for hospitalization. While supporting the need for early focus, nurses are aware that many risk factors that potentially jeopardize movement toward wellness are identified only by assessment of all five variables. Similarly, strengths that could be used to facilitate movement toward wellness may go unrecognized and untapped unless all five variables are assessed.

The pull between lengthy assessment and early focus was apparent in the process of revision of the nursing assessment tools described earlier. Many of the decisions revolved around how "comprehensive" and how "focused" to be in the initial assessment tool. The nurses' choice of the more lengthy version of the assessment tool indicated their continued insistence that wholeness is essential to the practice of nursing. It remains for the organization's nursing leadership to continually assist staff nurses to interpret and use data in the most meaningful and practical way. To this end, future studies in the clinical decision-making process will be important.

Nursing

As one would expect from a systems model, the relationship among variables has attained greater clarity. Ideas appear more fluid and less compartmentalized. This is most apparent in nurses' understanding of primary, secondary, and tertiary interventions. They have moved away from the tendency to categorize interventions as "before, during, and after hospitalization," to the more complex concept of "retaining, regaining, and maintaining" wellness independent of the location of the intervention or of the tasks necessary. The more fluid conceptualization has allowed a corresponding fluidity in nursing interventions. For example, client education now occurs whenever and however it is needed, and is much less likely to be seen as "discharge teaching." there has also been an increase in the scope of teaching and in the creativity with which it is accomplished.

FUTURE IMPLICATIONS FOR THE USE OF THE NEUMAN SYSTEMS MODEL

Simultaneously with the selection and implementation of the Neuman Systems Model, nurses, as part of the larger hospital organization, participated in three major changes: the complete restructuring of the interdisciplinary treatment plan and treatment planning process; the beginning implementation of the philosophy and techniques of continuous quality improvement; and the beginning decentralization of clinical services via formation of service unit teams. As a system the nursing department responded to each of these changes by engaging in internal reorganization, with increasing depth of practice. The reciprocity between the Neuman Systems Model and each of the changes supports the wisdom of the original choice of the Neuman Model. However, it is imperative that this be substantiated by research. The most likely sequence would be research on the impact of the model on the clinical decision-making process of the nurses, followed by a second research study of client outcomes in relation to nursing decisions. Only then can we say that we have met the goals for implementation of a nursing model *and* the utility of this model has been fully proved.

REFERENCES

Neuman, B., ed. 1989. *The Neuman Systems Model,* 2d ed. Norwalk, Conn.: Appleton & Lange.

APPENDIX A

Game Simulation "Neuman: It's in the Bag"

"Neuman: It's in the Bag" was designed to help nurses integrate the Neuman Systems Model into practice. Game simulation was one technique used during the implementation phase of the Neuman Model. At the Annual Department Workshop for Nurses, nurses were divided into small groups of six to eight participants. Each group was given a large manila envelope representing the fictitious Mrs. Mertz. In addition to an attractive magazine picture representing Mrs. Mertz, a typed definition of the Neuman client system was pasted onto the envelope. Mrs. Mertz's case study was then read aloud to the groups. The case study content was selected to be representative of a typical psychiatric client the nurse might expect to encounter.

Within the larger envelope were additional smaller envelopes labeled with various aspects of the Neuman Model and the corresponding definitions (flexible line of defense, normal line of defense, internal lines of resistance, basic structure, stressors). Small strips of paper were distributed to the groups. These papers contained brief statements about the client (e.g., "plays bridge for leisure." "good marital relationship," "complains of frequent headaches," "poor appetite," "white female," "65 years old," "mother died at age 67," etc.). The statements were taken from Mrs. Mertz's nursing assessment. The groups were given a 30-minute time limit and asked to discuss the placement of each statement into the appropriate envelope (aspect of the model). No specific roles were assigned to group members. Each group was free to approach the task in its own way.

At the end of the 30 minutes, a representative of each group was asked to present the contents of one of the small envelopes. In addition, the group was asked, based on its understanding of the Neuman Model, to defend its placement of the nursing assessment statements into that particular aspect of the model. This assignment invariably led to a discussion of the use of the model in organizing client information into a workable framework (the translation of theory into practice). The instructional objective was not that the groups agreed on their placement of the statements but rather that each group, based on its understanding of Neuman's model, reached a consensus about the relationship of the model to the case study content presented (i.e., group members could discuss the outcome in terms of where they were going and how they got there). The workshop participants' evaluations of the tool were generally favorable. Participants indicated that they thought the game simulation enhanced their appreciation of how the model is a useful way to organize their nursing practice.

REFERENCES

Duke, B., 1986. A taxonomy of games and simulations for nursing education. *Journal of Nursing Education* 25, (5): 197–206.

27

NEUMAN IMPLEMENTATION IN A CANADIAN PSYCHIATRIC FACILITY

Dorothy M. Craig
Corinne Morris-Coulter

The Whitby Psychiatric Hospital (WPH) is an accredited mental health facility in Ontario funded by the Ontario Ministry of Health. The hospital first opened its doors in 1919 and is one of 10 tertiary care psychiatric institutions in the province. With a catchment area of two million people, who are both rural and urban dwellers, the hospital serves seriously and persistently mentally ill individuals. Comprehensive mental health services are provided to individuals, families, and groups with an inpatient capacity of 325 beds.

The hospital employs 341 nursing staff, including both registered nurses and registered nursing assistants. The nurses have preparation at the diploma, bachelor's, and master's level of nursing, and many have worked in diverse clinical settings.

A range of multidisciplinary programs is provided at the hospital. Adolescents and adults suffering from schizophrenia, affective disorders, major psychoses (including psychoses with developmental handicaps), personality disorders, dementia, and acquired brain damage are served. Each clinical program is housed in a separate building on the spacious hospital grounds.

The goal of the hospital is to provide comprehensive treatment and rehabilitation programs to individuals with mental illness and to assist clients to reintegrate into the community at their most independent levels. The mission statement of the hospital includes the belief that each individual has physical, psychosocial, economic, and spiritual needs and that care for persons should be governed by the principles of availability, accountability, continuity, coordination, and community involvement (Ontario Ministry of Health, 1993).

The philosophy of the nursing department at the hospital is based on the premise that nurses endeavor to maintain and enhance the strengths and coping skills of clients. In-hospital treatment is seen as temporary, goal-directed, and only a part of the total client care continuum that exists between WPH and the community it serves, Durham Region.

SELECTION OF A CONCEPTUAL MODEL

The College of Nurses of Ontario (CNO) is the regulatory body for nurses practicing in the province. The mandate of the CNO is to protect the public, and each practicing nurse is required to hold a current Certificate of Competence. In 1990 the CNO released the Standards of Nursing Practice, which stated: "Four universal concepts—nursing, person, health, and environment—form the foundation for a variety of conceptual frameworks, or ways of organizing knowledge and beliefs about nursing. All relationships within the nursing context can be seen as combinations of or interactions among these basic elements" (College of Nurses of Ontario, 1990).

These standards acted as a catalyst for theory-based practice. The assistant administrator of patient services and the director of nursing at WPH recognized the merits of integrating theory-based practice and supported choosing a nursing model to guide nursing practice at the facility. Nursing administration believed that a conceptual model would assist nurses to carry out complete client assessments and organize the data to ensure that care plans met individual needs and built on client strengths and past effective coping patterns. Also, it was felt that clients would become more involved in their care plans, working with nurses toward realistic independent living. Truly a new partnership with the client was envisioned, with nurses able to clearly articulate their roles in the health care delivery system to clients and other health professionals.

A core group of nurses representing the nursing department under the leadership of the director of nursing critically examined several nursing models. Input from both management and front-line nurses was sought by the core group, and the Neuman Systems Model was selected as the model to guide nursing practice the WPH. It was agreed that the model was congruent with the philosophy of the nursing department. The model was viewed as a framework for psychiatric nurses in the practice setting to promote optimal levels of health by creating partnerships with seriously and persistently mentally ill clients (Morris-Coulter, Adler, Allan, MacDermaid, McMullan, Peterson, and Pritchard, 1993; Neuman, 1989).

IMPLEMENTATION OF THE NEUMAN SYSTEMS MODEL

In December 1991 an implementation project was developed to introduce the model to all nursing staff. The project followed the initiatves taken by the Middlesex London District Health Unit in London, Ontario, to introduce the model in the practice setting (Drew, Craig, and Beynon, 1989).

The introduction of theory-based nursing practice at WPH was also guided by the diffusion of innovations theory (Rogers, 1983). The diffusion of innovations theory focuses on social systems and explains the process by which an innovative idea gains acceptance within a community. According to the theory, when many people are involved in decision making, the adoption of new ideas is slowed, and particular efforts must be make to help members of the social system become aware of the new idea and its attributes. The use of peer networks to encourage acceptance of the ideas will speed the rate of adoption. Individuals in the social system are categorized according to their rate of adoption of the innovation as innovators, early adopters, early majority, late majority, and laggards (Rogers, 1983). This classification system can be used not only to guide research into the process of innovation but also to assist in the identification of potential key players in the early stages of an innovative project. Hence, the diffusion of innovations theory was a valuable framework to consider when encouraging nurses to adopt the innovative Neuman Systems Model in practice.

First, a steering committee was formed to develop a strategic plan. The committee was composed of 10 nurses, including the director of nursing as the chairperson. The remaining nine members represented front-line nursing, nursing management, nursing quality assurance, hospital education services, nursing education, and nursing research. Membership was voluntary and was open to any interested nurses working within the hospital. The purposes of the committee were (1) to plan, implement, and evaluate the use of the Neuman Systems Model at WPH; (2) to facilitate the use of the model by providing educational programs; and (3) to promote communication about the use of the model with all service areas at the hospital (Drew, Craig, and Beynon, 1989).

The steering committee recruited nurses from each of the 15 clinical settings to act as Neuman representatives. Two or, at some sites, three nurses agreed to represent each clinical setting, and they met monthly or bi-monthly with the steering committee to share ideas and generate practical approaches to assist nurses to use the model in their respective clinical settings. The Neuman representatives were asked to (1) function as the link between the steering committee and the nursing staff, (2) generate interest in learning about and using the model, and (3) share their knowledge and experience with the staff in the clinical areas (Drew, Craig, and Beynon, 1989). The Neuman representatives were free to call on individual steering committee members if they required guidance. According to the diffusion of innovations theory (Rogers, 1983), the initial members of the steering committee would be classified as innovators, and the Neuman representatives would be identified as early adopters.

The steering committee recognized the importance of establishing collaborative relationships among all levels of nursing, including practice, education, research, and administration. The committee was sensitive to the fact that implementation of the Neuman Systems Model would represent significant change for all members of the WPH culture. It was anticipated that individuals engaged in the implementation project needed to experience gradual stages of change before adopting the model so that they would not feel overwhelmed. Therefore, the committee members felt strongly that developing strong collaborative and participatory relationships would encourage the adoption of new ideas, foster model use, and ultimately enhance the quality of client care (Figure 27–1).

ACTIVITIES DESIGNED TO PROMOTE USE OF THE MODEL

Front-line nurses represented the largest group of players integral to the implementation project at WPH. The nursing cohort presented unique learning needs in relation to using the Neuman Systems Model in the mental health practice setting. The challenge of introducing the model to nursing staff from different treatment programs was heightened by the variation in nursing educational preparation, clinical experience, shift schedules, type of nursing care delivery system, and the geographical isolation of the practice site. A dymanic program of learning activities was established to target in a coordinated manner the diverse educational variables of the large nursing complement.

The diffusion of innovations theory states that individuals are more likely to engage in innovations that are simple, compatible with values and beliefs, advantageous, and cost-efficient (Rogers, 1983, 233). Based on this premise, the steering committee introduced a range of learning opportunities aimed at effectively introducing the Neuman Systems Model to practicing nurses. Educational events were designed to meet three generalized objectives: (1) to develop a sense of enthusiasm for learning about the Neuman Systems Model, (2) to begin to promote an understanding of the theoretical components of the model, and (3) to provide opportunities for application of the model in mental health nursing practice (Drew, Craig, and Beynon, 1989). It was expected that meeting these objectives would encourage the nurses to adopt the model as quickly as possible.

The steering committee categorized learning activities into three broad areas of focus, including promotion, resource, and evaluation (Figure 27–1). Hence, three subcommittees comprised of steering committee members and Neuman representatives were formed to define the focus and introduce activities related to the focus area at both the nursing and hospital level.

Promotion

The general purpose of this focus was to promote awareness and generate interest among participants in the Neuman Systems Model implementation project.

The promotion subcommittee initiated a host of strategies to raise the consciousness of nurses and hospital personnel about the project. Promotion activities were geared to the individual nurse, nursing team, multidisciplinary team, and general hospital.

Congruent with the diffusion of innovations theory, the promotion sub-

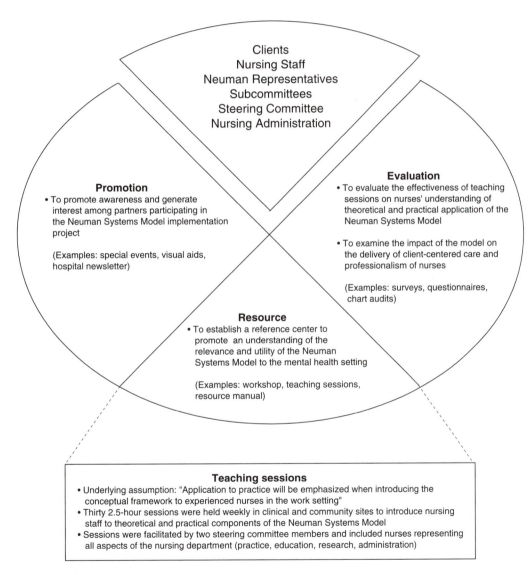

Figure 27–1. Nurse–client partnerships—activities designed to promote collaboration in the Neuman Systems Model implementation project.

committee planned activites that communicated in familiar, simple, and non-threatening terms the benefits of implementing the Neuman Systems Model (Rogers, 1983). The subcommittee conveyed positive messages about the model in an effort to alleviate nurses' anxiety, uncertainty, and resistance to learning about the theoretical framework.

The promotion subcommittee initiatives seemed to have considerable impact on the target population at WPH. The visual symbol of an apple was chosen to represent the implementation project and as an aid to interpret theoretical components of the model. The subcommittee capitalized on the use of apple images/themes to promote the project in an eye-catching and innovative manner. Various mediums were accessed to attractively market the model. Several examples of formal and informal activities included regular releases of written material to highlight the project, a monthly column entitled "Neuman's Nook" in the hospital newsletter, and Neuman bulletin boards located on all clinical sites and outside the staff of client libraries. The presence of visually attractive Neuman material effectively communicated particular components of the model and the large-scale implementation project. Staff contests were regularly scheduled, including cryptograms and crossword puzzles to familiarize nursing and hospital staff with Neuman terminology. The nursing department promoted special events to celebrate the implementation project at WPH, specifically during the annual Canadian Nurses Week and on project anniversary dates. Sanctioned/endorsed opportunities to commemorate theory-based practice served as a venue for key players to share experiences with the model, receive recognition for participating in the innovation, and promote the professional image of mental health nurses in the facility.

Resource

The resource focus was designed to impart information regarding theoretical and practical components of the Neuman Systems Model in the mental health setting. An underlying assumption of this focus was the belief that introduction of the model would build on nurses' existing knowledge and that application to practice would be emphasized with experienced nurses in the work setting (Drew, Craig, and Beynon, 1989).

The diffusion of innovations framework guided resource learning activities (Rogers, 1983). Efforts were made to describe the Neuman Systems Model in a way that was compatible with how the mental health nurses were already practicing, making it "triable" or user-friendly. Therefore, implementation activities focused on using the model congruent with the nursing process, and nurses were encouraged to shift toward creating collaborative partnerships with clients and setting mutual goals in the plan of care. The innovation of the Neuman Systems Model was evident as nurses were challenged to explore realistic optimal wellness with seriously and persistently mentally ill clients. The model prompted nurses to consider all levels of intervention, including health promotion initiatives, when working with clients in a tertiary care psychiatric facility.

The shift toward client-centered care was a good fit with the nursing care delivery system and the multidisciplinary approach at WPH.

The general purpose of this focus was to establish resources to promote an understanding of the relevance and utility of the Neuman Systems Model to mental health nursing. In response to nurses' requests for evidence of model implementation in other practice settings, an extensive literature review was conducted, and a binder of reference material was prepared for each clinical and community area.

The resource subcommittee established a network of nursing professionals interested in sharing experiences about the Neuman Systems Model. Collegial links were formed with clinical facilities and community agencies using the model in the practice setting. Academic liaison with graduate nursing faculty at the University of Toronto in Ontariao further promoted an understanding of the relevance of theory-based practice. Ongoing correspondence with Dr. Betty Neuman and members of the Neuman Trustee Group served to focus and energize the implementation project.

Prior to introducing the model to front-line nurses, the steering committee and Neuman representatives participated in an intensive full-day workshop to become familiar with the model. Two delegates from the Neuman Trustees Group facilitated a comprehensive and dynamic in-service for key players in the implementation project. The learning experience seemed to validate plans to use the model at WPH, formalized the role of key players, and provided nurses with an opportunity to share perceptions of theory-based practice and dialogue with experts in the use of the Neuman Systems Model.

Under the scope of the resource focus, the steering committee designed a comprehensive teaching package to formally introduce the model to a population of 341 nurses. Partners of committee members presented in total thirty 2.5-hour teaching sessions biweekly over a six-month period to introduce all nursing staff to the model. The sessions were purposly held in 12 different clinical and community sites to ensure continuity of client care, to promote staff attendance, and to ground the learning experience in the psychiatric practice setting. Staff from all areas of the hospital were welcome to attend any of the scheduled sessions. The teaching sessions were well attended by nurses, including those in practice, education, research, and administration.

The purpose of the teaching sessions was to provide nurses with a preliminary opportunity to learn about the Neuman Systems Model in a familiar setting. The sessions were divided into two parts presented in seminar format with group discussion. The first half of the sessions was devoted to general comments regarding use of conceptual frameworks, selection of the Neuman Systems Model at WPH, and basic theoretical components of the model itself. The second half of the teaching session focused on application of the model to practice, specifically mental health nursing. Prior to the sessions, Neuman representatives from each hosting clinical area were asked to formulate a mock client case study that personified the profile of a mental health client from their practice area.

Representatives were asked not to use actual client case studies at this point in the project, as the aim of the introductory session was to learn about the model and to ensure that nurses visiting from other clinical areas had the same data base from which to apply the model. The intent was to gradually shift toward using the Neuman Systems Model when working with actual clients.

Practical application of the model at WPH was assisted by the "Neuman Assessment Flowsheet," created by the steering committee and revised by nurses from all areas of the hospital. While the data sheet was initially designed as a learning tool for the teaching sessions, positive feedback from practicing nurses has led to plans to incorporate the instrument into the nursing documentation system. Key players in the implementation project unanimously agreed that inclusion of a written form on the client's chart visually reinforced the use of the Neuman Systems Model at WPH.

Evaluation

The general intent of this focus was to introduce a systematic way of evaluating the impact of planned change, specifically the innovation of implementing the Neuman Systems Model in a mental health facility. In relation to the diffusion of innovations framework, the evaluation subcommittee was interested in determining whether implementation of the Model was advantageous and cost-effficient (Rogers, 1983). This focus was interested in exploring whether use of the model was perceived as beneficial to the clients, nurses, and other members of the multidisciplinary team. In keeping with the constraints of the economic climate and diminishing resources, the subcommittee prudently considered the "cost" of the project, examining time, energy, and money spent in relation to perceived benefits of theory implementation.

The identified purposes of the evaluation focus were to evaluate the effectiveness of teaching sessions of nurses' understanding of theoretical and practical application of the Neuman Systems Model, and to examine the impact of the model on the delivery of client-centered care and on the professionalism of nurses. Several mechanisms designed by the evaluation subcommittee were used to examine the effectiveness of ongoing learning activities, including surveys, evaluation/comment sheets, and nursing chart audits. The subcommittee developed a formal linkage with the nursing quality management committee at WPH for the purpose of facilitating methods of evaluation.

PROJECT IMPLEMENTATION TIME LINE

The Neuman Systems Model implementation project was based on the stages proposed in the strategic path of the Middlesex-London Health Unit (Drew, Craig, and Beynon, 1989). The time frame for the venture was tailored to meet the learning needs and interests of the unique nursing culture at WPH. An extensive and valuable period of time was taken in the selection of a conceptual model by the nursing department and in preparing nursing staff to move toward theory-based practice. Phase 1 of the implementation project was completed in six months, during which time the entire nursing complement was introduced to the Neuman Systems Model via promotion, resource, and evaluation learning activities. In addition, approximately 90 percent of the nursing department participated in teaching sessions offered by the steering committee.

Phase 2 of the implementation project is currently in place and will cover the span of one year. During this stage, steering committee members are serving as a resource to Neuman representatives, who are facilitating practical application of the model in the clinical and community setting. The thrust of Phase 2 includes using the conceptual framework in the assessment, planning, implementation, and evaluation stages of working with actual clients in the psychiatric practice setting.

The Neuman Systems Model has challenged nurses at WPH to begin to work collaboratively with seriously and persistently mentally ill clients in the pursuit of optimal wellness. The conceptual framework enables nurses to deliver levels of wholistic care to clients in a tertiary psychiatric care facility.

Phase 3 learning activities are currently being planned by key players in the project in response to nursing staff feedback and ongoing evaluation. The exact time frame for Phase 3 is yet to be determined. Examples of future challenges to be addressed in the final stage of the implementation project at WPH include such initiatives as ongoing process and outcome evaluation of theory implementation, nursing research activities testing use of model in mental health care, expanded application of the model to include families and groups, and communication of the impact of implementing the Neuman Systems Model to all members of the multidisciplinary team.

REFLECTIONS TO DATE

The introduction of the Neuman Model at WPH has been an exciting and challenging process. The innovators and early adopters have been a dynamic force in marketing the model concepts and acting as role models for their peers. Their efforts have not only made the projects a success to date but also have paved the way to meet the challenges of Phase 3 with enthusiasm and commitment.

REFERENCES

College of Nurses of Ontario. 1990. *Standards of Nursing Practice for Registered Nurses and Registered Nursing Assistants.* Toronto, Ontario.

Drew, L., Craig, D., and Beynon, C. 1989. The Neuman Systems Model for community health administration and practice. In *The Neuman Systems Model: Application to Nursing Education and Practice,* edited by B. Neuman. East Norwalk, Conn.: Appleton & Lange.

Morris-Coulter, C., Alder, L., Allan, L., MacDermaid, L., McMullan, J., Peterson, C., and Pritchard, H. 1993. Partnerships in theory: Implementation of the Neuman Systems Model at an Ontario psychiatric facility. Poster presented at the Fourth 1993 Biennial International Neuman Systems Model Symposium, Rochester, N.Y.

Neuman, B., ed. 1989. *The Neuman Systems Model: Application to Nursing Education and Practice.* East Norwalk, Conn: Appleton & Lange.

Ontario Ministry of Health. 1993. *Whitby Psychiatric Hospital Operational Plan 1992— 114.* Oshawa, Ontario: OMH.

Rogers, E. M. 1983. *Diffusion of Innovations,* 3d ed. New York; Free Press.

OKLAHOMA STATE PUBLIC HEALTH NURSING
Neuman-Based

Toni D. Frioux
Anita Gayle Roberts
Sandra J. Butler

Health care is changing and evolving at an ever increasing rate as to type and quality of care demanded by the population. This phenomenon prevails in all areas of health care. The public health setting is no exception. Thus the need becomes increasingly evident for a structure in which to frame nursing service delivery. This structure provides a "system for observing, ordering, clarifying and analyzing events" (Bush, 1979, 13). Nursing in the community health setting requires a unique blend of public health and nursing concepts. The Neuman conceptual model provides a comprehensive and flexible framework that integrates both the knowledge and the skills necessary for nursing intervention in a community health setting. The public health nursing staff, with varied educational and work experiences, provides care for a diverse population. Selection of a broad practice framework such as the Neuman Model is especially applicable for public health nursing service delivery in Oklahoma.

Reviewed by Dorothy Craig, Eleanor Stittich, and Patricia Chadwick.

OKLAHOMA PUBLIC HEALTH ORGANIZATIONAL STRUCTURE

The Oklahoma State Department of Health, overseen by the state board of health, has statutory responsibility for the public health of all Oklahoma residents. This responsibility is serviced through local county health department sites, with public health nurses providing the majority of all direct client services. Advanced registered nurse practitioners account for approximately 15 percent of the total public health nursing population, and they provide expanded services, including primary care in maternity, family planning, and child health services.

At the state level, client service delivery is grouped into two divisions: Personal Health Services, organized primarily around public health programs; and Local Health Services, focusing on direct service provision. Each Personal Health Services program is responsible for financial management and development of a specific program, such as family planning or immunizations. The public health nurse is responsible for providing direct public health nursing interventions to local population groups. These interventions may be program specific, such as immunizations, or may address nonprogrammatic health care needs, such as community education activities. Nursing Service provides the structure for the delivery of effective nursing care to individuals, families, and communities under the direction of a nurse executive. Nursing Service plays a pivotal role, bridging the gap between state Personal Health Program personnel and public health nurses housed within the local county health department sites.

Service delivery is planned locally and implemented by the District Nursing Supervisor (DNS), Public Health Nurse (PHN), and the Public Health Administrator. Each DNS is assigned to a specific geographic area and is responsible for program planning, implementation, monitoring, and evaluation. Programs at the local county health departments are implemented according to staff availability, community needs for each program, and physical plant availability. DNSs are the liaison between the Oklahoma State Department of Health Nursing Service, the programs, and the PHNs at the local sites. This system results in a complex set of varying and sometimes conflicting program standards and outcome criteria. Nursing Service's role is to assure delivery of efficient and cost-effective services to local county health departments clients, families, and aggregates. The supervisor assumes primary responsibility in directing implementation of nursing theory into local programs.

CULTURAL DIVERSITY

Though varied as to beliefs and values, Oklahoma public health nurses are historically attuned to cultural diversity. With over 30 tribes in the state, Oklahoma has the largest American Indian population in the United States. Assessing clients using methods that produce culture-specific information is essential. Languages, tribal governments, economic status, health beliefs, and approaches to health care needs vary from tribe to tribe. The PHN is an essential component in the delivery of health care to the American Indian population. He or she must collaborate with the individual, the individual's family, tribal health providers, United States Public Health Service, and many other entities that influence health care in order to provide comprehensive care. The PHN must be cognizant of each tribal belief regarding health care. The flexibility of the Neuman Systems Model provides a conceptual approach to addressing the problems of cultural differences. Hispanic, African Americans, and Asian American populations present cultural challenges to the primarily female Caucasian public health nurses as well. The wholistic nature of the Neuman Model requires that assessmentt data be collected on physical, psychological, cultural, developmental, and spiritual variables. The model is especially successful when applied in the cross-cultural context of the diverse population by the primarily female Caucasian public health nurse. Neuman describes this "unique feature" of the model, stating that "the kinds of data obtained from the client's own perception of his/her condition influence the overall goals of care" (Neuman, 1982, 16). The use of a standardized protocol, made possible through use of a nursing model, provides a comprehensive structure within which to base a coherent nursing practice—one focused on preventive health modalities and in keeping with emerging health care reform issues.

PUBLIC HEALTH NURSING AND THE NEUMAN SYSTEMS MODEL

Oklahoma's public health nursing is well grounded in the American Nurses' Association's Conceptual Model of Community Health Nursing. As ANA states,

> Community health nursing is a synthesis of nursing and public health practice applied to promoting and preserving the health of populations. The practice is general and comprehensive. It is not limited to a particular age group or diagnosis, and is continuing, not episodic. The overall reponsibility is to the population as a whole; nursing directed to individuals, families, or groups contributes to the health of the total population. (American Nurses' Association, 1980; 1).

Neuman's primary goal of nursing is to retain, attain, and maintain client system stability. This compatibility with the ANA model allows the Neuman Systems Model (1989) to be utilized within the larger health system to promote healthy populations.

Neuman sees nursing as a unique profession concerned with all client system variables that affect an individual's response to environmental stressors. Community health nursing has traditionally utilized a wholistic approach to care. Assessment identifies those factors within a broader context that affect a client's response to stressors. The Neuman Model compares to the goal of public health in that both dictate the philosophic premise of a comprehensive, dynamic view of individuals, groups, and communities subject to environmental stressors. These stressors can occur anywhere within and among the various societal subsystems and can be categorized within the five broad Neuman Model variables: physiological, psychological, sociocultural, developmental, and spiritual.

For use within community settings, the Neuman Model provides a systematic and logically related set of concepts incorporating the essential components of nursing practice and the scientific theories on which practice is based. Stanhope and Lancaster (1984) note various types of subsystems found in communities. These areas include economic, educational, religious, health care, political, welfare, law enforcement, energy, and recreational systems. Where the stability of one subsystem is affected, the stability of another is usually also affected. The Neuman Systems Model is an appropriate conceptual model for community health nursing because it emphasizes a wholistic practice approach in which any system part, or subparts, can be organized into an interrelating whole that ideally functions as a total system (Neuman, 1989).

The authors recognize that the concept of community health nursing is related to a care philosophy rather than a practice setting; however, for purposes of this chapter, community health and public health nursing terms are used interchangeably. The goal-directed approach, evident in the Neuman Model, focuses on primary, secondary, and tertiary preventions as interventions. These interventions are compatible with the overall philosophy of the State of Oklahoma Nursing Service. In fact, many of the Neuman concepts, such as primary, secondary, and tertiary preventions as interventions, are already used in community health nursing. Therefore implementation of the model did not involve a shift in focus. Dever's (1980) epidemiologic approach for assessing communities is familiar to public health nursing and interfaces well with application of the Neuman Model.

Familiarity with primary, secondary, and tertiary preventions as interventions allows the public health nurse to utilize Neuman intervention modalities in any client situation or setting. These care modalities give clear distinction and direction for retaining, attaining, and maintaining system stability at each of the intervention levels, wherever and however the client is defined within the health care system. The following scenario is a typical example of the application of different levels of interventions involving a county that has experienced major flooding. The primary level of preventive intervention includes working with a designee to prepare media coverage regarding the high risk for spread of disease; assisting organization of efforts to bring in bottled water for drinking; and providing tetanus immunizations. The secondary level of prevention focuses on educational interventions. For example, area-wide media coverage should be arranged to announce and educate the community as to the need for an order to water boil, along with signs and symptoms of disease. The tertiary level of prevention includes interventions to maintain community optimal health or stability in order to enhance or return the community to its former health level.

Participation in community disaster planning, assistance in grant writing for funds for flood control measures, and organization of early case-finding strategies are examples of the tertiary level of preventions.

IMPLEMENTATIONS OF THE NEUMAN SYSTEMS MODEL

The need for a nursing model was identified while revising job descriptions and developing a job performance tool for documenting differentiated practice areas. A risk management committee was activated to both describe and quantify the needs for future state nursing practice. Staffing plans and compensation proposals were developed as well. Another committee developed standardized care plans with community health-related nursing diagnoses. Each of these diverse activities identified the need for an organizing framework for nursing practice. The Neuman Model's systematic perspective is flexible enough to meet changing program demands, while providing a reliable framework for quality nursing practice. Neuman Model application is relevant for all levels of nursing practice within the Oklahoma State Department of Health system, thus accommodating and facilitating extended roles of the PHNs in service delivery as part of the larger system.

As new community needs are identified and programs developed, greater organizational structuring is required. For example, the growing complexity of public health service delivery created the need to integrate all service program standards under an umbrella or unifying framework. Examples of such standards include record keeping, epidemiological data collection, and documentation of care provided. The Neuman Systems Model was chosen as the base or structure for practice. In the culturally diverse state population, where priorities and program care focuses change dynamically, the model provides flexibility and stability.

Because the Oklahoma State Health Department Nursing Service values collaborative decision making and participatory management in its relationships with public health nurses, a strategic plan was developed for introducing the Neuman Systems Model to local public health nurses. A two-day orientation education session developed for key PHNs and supervisors was conducted. Dr. Raphella Sohier, a Neuman trustee, was recruited to present an introduction to the use of nursing theories and specifically the Neuman Systems Model.

Dr. Sohier used an innovative approach in introducing the model and its application. A segment of *My Fair Lady* was used as an example to which she applied the Neuman Systems Model. Evaluations of the orientation session were positive; however, some questioned the value of using a nursing model. Most PHNs have either associate degree or diploma preparation with no prior formal education experience with practice models. After the session was held, however, situational problems such as staff turnover and changing workload priorities reduced continuity in the overall learning and implementation of the Neuman Model.

In retrospect, the orientation training may have been conducted prematurely. Prior to Dr. Sohier's training session, it would have been advantageous to provide a knowledge foundation of systems theory to clarify the value of adopting a nursing model. Confusion resulted in resistance to early acceptance of the model. If this process is to be repeated in the future, the approach would be to adapt the existing nursing tools (such as public health nursing practice guidelines, approved orders, forms, and nursing standards) to the Neuman Systems Model *prior* to formalized model presentations. It would be important to conduct a thorough analysis of PHN learning readiness, followed by development of specific learning tools based on this analysis. Pre- and posttesting would indicate further learning needs.

Nursing Service could benefit from having nursing consultants who focus specifically on model implementation; however, without this support, model implementation became everyone's responsibility. Each director of nursing service was required to become familiar with the Neuman Model for nursing practice. The initial implementation plan required the supervisors to cooperatively study the Neuman Model with the PHNs and together develop specific "tools" for model implementation in their community health practice. This has had an important unifying effect as nursing leaders shared the development of Neuman Model expertise, which continues to motivate staff creativity at all levels of involvement.

MODEL EDUCATION PROTOCOL

An effective and positive approach to educating public health nursing personnel is "Roberts' Five-Minute SPOT" (Short Period of Teaching). To explain the Neuman Model efficiently and effectively, Gayle Roberts developed an innovative teaching technique utilizing adult learning principles. Brevity and flexible delivery modalities of the SPOT retain attention as it focuses on teaching one aspect of the model within a brief five-minute summary. That is, presentation of new information in concise terms facilitates long-term change. (Kouzes and Posner, 1991). Familiarity with the nursing model by all nursing personnel facilitates a common language and organizational structure. The first SPOT focuses on the system core, or basic structure energy resources. Examples of system cores or basic structure facts are applied to the individual, family/group, and community. Second, the lines of defense are reviewed. The model presentation is complete within a total of 10 sessions. The SPOT has been an effective strategy for combining both technical and conceptual data. Sessions were formatted in a self-paced learning packet for use in conjunction with our orientation program. This enables new employees to quickly become knowledgeable in using the model early in their community health nursing practice. Other teaching tools such as overheads, laminated posters, and handouts are also effective. All public health nurses will use common client case situations as learning strategies to share and confirm model application.

FUTURE IMPLICATIONS

Despite problems that were encountered early, Nursing Service remains committed to Neuman Model implementation. Concepts from the model provide a conceptual base for developing standards for community health nursing practice. Nursing standards for the care of children with special health care needs are being developed. These children often require a transdisciplinary approach that enables other disciplines to become familiar with Neuman concepts in the public health setting. Nursing practice guidelines are changing to reflect Neuman assessmant variables and to incorporate the prevention levels as intervention care modalities. Also, the Adult Health Record uses the Neuman assessment variables for a baseline health history.

The state's Nursing Service is cognizant of the need to incorporate Neuman Model concepts into all future public health nursing activities. The self-paced, competency-based orientation plan, which has been implemented, provides a basic introduction to the Neuman Model. Development of model implementation tools and examples of model application will continue to be a priority. Each model application brings Nursing Service closer to full model implementation; however, much work still remains. Nursing Service needs nursing consultants who can focus specifically on model application in order to expedite the implementation.

CONCLUSION

The model's goal-directed approach, which focuses on primary, secondary, and tertiary prevention interventions, is compatible with the overall philosophy of health care reform. With increased emphasis on health promotion and disease prevention, public health nursing is in a unique and timely position to respond to this national trend. By utilizing a comprehensive, flexible approach such as the Neuman Model, nursing becomes an active participant in health care service provision as the paradigm shifts from an acute care to the more efficient and cost-effective prevention intervention delivery system.

The Oklahoma State Department of Health Nursing Service is confident that the Neuman Model provides a flexible, broad practice framework that structures the nursing care for our culturally diverse population. The model allows for a comprehensive, wholistic, systematic client care approach while providing efficient, cost-effective, and high-quality client care. Utilization of the Neuman Model is particularly germane given this time of rapidly changing health care demands.

REFERENCES

American Nurses' Association: 1980. *A Conceptual Model of Community Health Nursing.* Kansas City, Mo.: ANA.

Bush, H. A. 1979. Models in nursing. *Advanced Nursing Science* 1:13–21.

Dever, G. E. A. 1980. *Community Health Analysis.* Germantown, Md.: Aspen.

Kouzes, J. M., and Posner, B. Z. 1991. *The Leadership Challenge.* San Fancisco: Jossey-Bass.

Neuman, B., ed. 1982. *The Neuman Systems Model: Application to Nursing Education and Practice.* East Norwalk, Conn.: Appleton-Century-Crofts.

Neuman, B. 1989. *The Neuman Systems Model.* Norwalk Conn.: Appleton & Lange.

Stanhope, M., and Lancaster, J. 1984. *Community Health Nursing,* 2d ed. St. Louis: C. V. Mosby.

29

NEUMAN-BASED EDUCATION, PRACTICE, AND RESEARCH IN A COMMUNITY NURSING CENTER

Patricia Hinton Walker

"Nurse-organized and nurse-managed health services have a long and distinguished history" (ANA, 1987). From the late 1800s up to the present, nursing centers (frequently called community nursing centers in the literature) have consistently attempted to provide professional nursing services to the nation's underserved populations with a nursing model of care. These alternative care delivery systems have historically provided direct access to professional nursing services; today, nurse-managed care is reemerging, in community nursing centers. This chapter presents a brief history of nursing centers and discusses the development of the Community Nursing Center at the Univeristy of Rochester School of Nursing. Using the Neuman System Model as part of its organizing framework, this innovative community nursing center provides opportunities for student learning, faculty practice in a revenue-generating business model, and future directions for nursing research.

New opportunitites for clinical and health services research in nursing centers provide a pathway to the future as the nursing profession struggles to demonstrate the value of direct nursing services. As nursing models of care and access to direct nursing service are promoted as part of the answer to America's health care dilemma, it is important for members of the profession to provide explanantion, justification, and research data that support the use of nursing models of care nationally. In this chapter, the rationale for selecting the Neuman Systems Model for interdisciplinary practice will be presented, along with some new perspectives about the use and evaluation of the model related to the delivery of cost-effective, quality care.

DEFINITION AND HISTORICAL PERSPECTIVE

An official definition of nursing centers is provided in the ANA publication *The Nursing Center Concept and Design* (1987): "Nursing centers—sometimes referred to as community nursing centers, nurse-managed centers, and nursing clinics—are organizations that give the client direct access to professional nursing services." Additionally, care in nursing centers is described as professional nurses using nursing models of care to "diagnose and treat human responses to potential and actual health problems, and promote health and optimal functioning among target populations and communities" (ANA, 1987). Nursing services provided by these centers are wholistic and client-centered and require some form of reimbursement. A review of the nursing literature indicates that clinical services of nursing centers are primarily in two broad categories—care for the chronically ill and wellness care. Historically and today, in most community nursing centers in the United States these services are targeted toward the care of underserved populations, and the majority of these centers are connected in some way to an academic institution such as a school of nursing.

Nursing centers have been in existence since 1893, when the Henry Street Settlement was established by Lillian Wald in New York City. Since then, many outstanding leaders—individuals whose names are recognized as contributing significantly to nursing's history—can be found amidst the history of nursing centers. Names such as Margaret Sanger, Mary Breckinridge, Lydia Hall, and M. Lucille Kinlein stand out—all with efforts to shape new directions for care (ANA, 1987). Common to the development of professional nursing practices for all these famous leaders was a nursing model of care that included prevention and health promotion, a wholistic, client-centered approach, direct access to professional nursing services, and autonomy over administration and delivery of professional nursing practice.

A brief summary of the history of nursing centers by Aydelotte and Gregory in the NLN publication *Nursing Centers: Meeting the Demand for Quality Health Care* (1989) describes the following names, places, and events:

1. Lillian Wald's Henry Street Settlement, established in 1893, provided care to the sick and impoverished.

2. In 1916 Margaret Sanger opened the first birth control clinic to provide contraception and family planning information to the poor.

3. Mary Breckinridge, a certified nurse-midwife, established the Frontier Nursing Service in 1920 to serve mothers and babies in remote eastern Kentucky.

4. In 1961 Lydia Hall established the Loeb Center at Montefiore Hospital in New York, where professional nurses were the only individuals to provide care in a unique setting between hospital and home.

5. In 1965 the nurse practitioner role was established to provide primary care for a client's first contact in an illness-related health care system.

6. In 1971 M. Lucille Kinlein established an autonomous independent nursing practice.

7. The 1970's marked the beginning of many academic-based nursing centers designed to provide direct services, student experiences, and faculty practice sites.

8. O. Marie Henry urged the profession to establish nursing centers in institutional, community, and primary care settings to provide direct access to nursing care, promote student learning, and foster research.

9. In the 1980s nursing centers proliferated, and approximately 150 nursing centers were recorded as in existence. (NLN, 1989)

BACKGROUND

The Community Nursing Center (CNC) of the University of Rochester School of Nursing was established as an organizational response to both internal and external identified needs of the school. This CNC, unlike other nurse-managed centers in the country, was designed in the beginning to provide a variety of services in both urban and rural areas—as a center without walls. Cornerstones of this CNC include (1) development of innovative practice models in urban and rural communities; (2) the analysis and development of health policies that will improve access, quality, and cost-effectiveness of care, particularly to underserved populations; and (3) building community partnerships with existing agencies and providers rather than duplicating already existing services. The CNC, developed in the context of "unification," provides nursing practice, education, and research opportunities for nurse practitioner and nonnurse practitioner faculty. Students at all levels (undergraduate, master's, doctoral) have opportunities for learning experiences in primary care, community health, and the development of autonomous practice roles for professional nurses consistent with the directions of health care reform.

Although most other nursing centers in the United States were developed at one site with selected populations, this CNC was developed as a "center without walls." Opportunities for diverse and autonomous practices in the community were determined necessary for the following reasons:

1. The University of Rochester faculty have a rich history with faculty practice.

2. Strong nurse practitioner programs with varying populations of interest were part of this history as well.
3. Community needs for underserved popluations were diverse—in urban and rural areas.
4. The philosophy was to improve access to care by linking nurse-managed care to community agencies in close proximity to clients' home, work, or school.
5. Consistent with goals of Health People 2000, elderly, chronically ill adults and children, adolescents, and women will be priorities for care.

This CNC was designed as a comprehensive model to foster group practice among faculty while providing new role models and learning experiences for students. Four "service clusters" were developed as follow:

> (1) Services for Life Transitions and Developmental Changes related to birthing, parenting, puberty and adolescence, midlife changes, aging, divorce and death, the final transition; (2) Service for Longer-Term Continuity of Care, designed to enhance quality of life for individuals and families experiencing chronic illness, physical and/or developmental disabilities, and the challenges associated with aging; (3) Services for Organizations, Businesses and Health Care Providers, including expert consultation, clinical case management services, staff development and health education programs and employee wellness programs; and (4) Services for Life-Altering Crises, designed for informal care-givers, such as families of Alzheimer's patients and survivors of trauma such as spouse and child abuse victims. (Hinton Walker, 1991)

These service clusters reflect what Toffler (1990) calls "flex firms" in his book *Power Shift*. Clusters of services suggest a constellation of smaller organizations that can be responsive and trade ideas, data, strategies, and resources to achieve a common goal. Figure 29–1 reflects this concept. As the CNC grows, each service cluster will develop its own internal organizational stucture. Consistent with this concept of flex firms, design of data bases and information systems must be flexible enough to support innovative practice delivery models, student learning experiences, and clinical and health services research.

Lange (1983) discussed important issues of survival of nursing centers in an economic environment that has not traditionally supported reimbursement for preventive services or for direct nursing care. Higgs (1988) further identified concerns related to financial support for nursing centers. Lundeen (1988) also described challenges of obtaining funding and financial support. In order to address these concerns, remain viable, and make a significant contribution to the nursing profession, the University of Rochester CNC maintains a three-pronged approach to CNC stability. The three elements believed necessary for survival are (1) a nursing model of care, (2) impact on health policy, and (3) use of sound business principles (see Figure 29–2). The nursing model of care chosen for this innovative CCNC was the Neuman Systems Model.

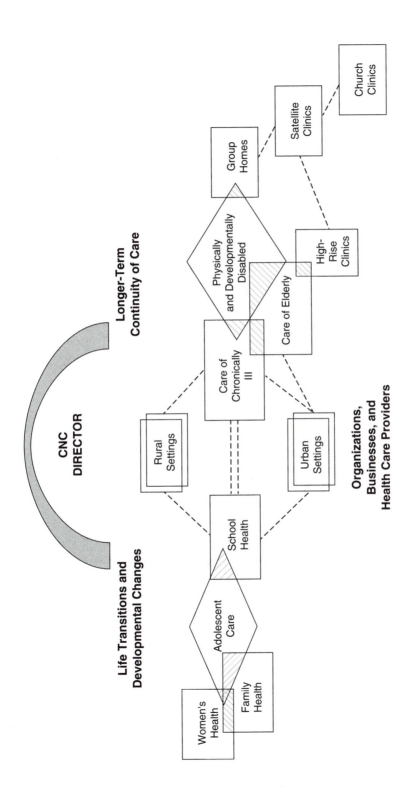

Figure 29–1. *(Copyright 1991, University of Rochester.)*

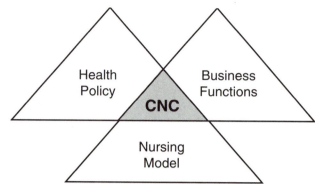

Figure 29–2. *(Copyright 1991, University of Rochester.)*

THEORETICAL FRAMEWORK

The Neuman Systems Model was the nursing model of choice for a number of reasons. Since the CNC was designed as a "center without walls" with a variety of practices and services offered, it was imperative that the nursing model chosen would view the individual as client, the family or group as client, and the organization or community as client (see Figure 29–3). Neuman writes that the

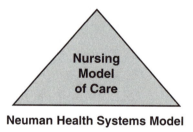

Neuman Health Systems Model

Mutual goal setting between client and provider

Focus of care consistent with community-based practice

Primary and tertiary prevention as intervention

Wholistic approach with attention to:

Stressors	*Variables*
Intrapersonal	Physiological
Interpersonal	Developmental
Extrapersonal	Psychological
	Spiritual
	Sociocultural

Figure 29–3. *(Copyright 1991, University of Rochester.)*

client system may be narrowly defined as an individual or person, or broadly defined as situations dictate from one client as a system to the global community as a system. What is defined or included within the boundary of the system must have relevance to nursing and represent the reality of its domain of concern (Neuman, 1989).

The Neuman Systems Model also provides a wholistic framework for nursing and is considered predominantly wellness-oriented. One of the critical reasons for choosing the Neuman Systems Model was the view of the client from a wholistic framework. All five variables—physiological, psychological, sociocultural, developmental, and spiritual—are integral to the wide variety of CNC services and the many underserved populations needing nures-managed care. Many nursing models are wholistic and focus on the physiological, psychological, and sociocultural factors in the client or patient. However, the Neuman Systems Model considers the client as a composite of these variables "functioning harmoniously or stable in relation to both internal and external stressors." This prevents possible fragmentation and failure to interrelate various aspects of the client system.

The CNC faculty have identified points of developmental transitions as significant times for professional nurses to positively influence change toward wellness. The inclusion of the "developmental" variable was a key component in describing and marketing services to populations of all ages who need direct access to professional nursing services. Consequently, one of the service clusters is identified as "life transitions and developmental changes." In addition, this service cluster emphasizes the primary prevention strategies discussed in the Neuman Systems Model (see Figure 29–4).

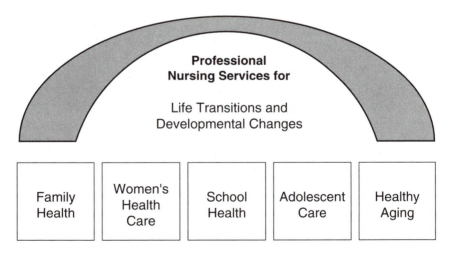

Figure 29–4. *(Copyright 1991, University of Rochester.)*

Since the CNC was designed as a futuristic organization, the addition of the spiritual variable was a very important factor. Naisbitt's *Megatrends* predicted a spiritual revival in the 1990s. Toffler also writes of a spiritual revival that will influence decision making and values of aggregate populations in the future. Explanation of the spiritual variable as innate, influencing other variables, and positively or negatively affecting the impact of stressors on the client system is consistent with the philosophy and values of those practicing in the Univerity of Rochester Community Nursing Center.

The Neuman Systems Model view of clients is also consistent with the philosophical approach of the CNC to care. "The model and the CNC both emphasize a partnership with the client—or client-centered care. . . . The Community Nursing Center's approach to care incorporates Neuman's mutual decision-making and assists the client to make healthy choices—weighing quality of life issues with feasibility/desire for lifestyle pattern change for healthy living" (Hinton Walker, 1992). The concept of overall goals for the client system is also consistent with the Neuman Systems Model. In community-centered care, the nurse can neither change the fact that the client is experiencing a life transition/developmental change nor cure a chronic condition. However, through mutually determined interventions between the client and the nurse, prevention of further breakdown form intra-, inter-, and extrapersonal stressors can be accomplished. The goal of care in the nursing center is not to "cure" but to provide caring by assisting the client toward attaining and maintaining wellness. Therefore the outcomes of CNC care for the client system include (1) informed decision making, (2) healthy choices, and (3) a quality improvement in well being (see Figure 29–5). This is consistent with Neuman's main nursing goal, which is to facilitate optimal wellness. This is accomplished through nursing actions initiated to "retain, attain, and maintain optimal client health or wellness, using the three preventions as interventions to keep the system stable" (Neuman, 1989).

Prevention as intervention as a format for care is relevant to the needs of clients in the community, especially in light of health care reform. The Neuman Model's "focus on primary prevention as a mode of nursing intervention is consistent with a community care organization in a setting like the University of Rochester School of Nursing that features primary care practice and education of nurse pracitioners" (Hinton Walker, 1992). Secondary and tertiary prevention as intervention is also especially relevant to care of the chronically ill populations of all ages in community settings. Prevention, maintenance of function, and mutual goal setting and decision making are necessary for successful care of the chronically ill. Nurse practitioners are uniquely prepared to identify medical and nursing problems, evaluate changes, and manage the patient and family in a collaborative way during the chronic illness trajectory. "New practice environments such as community nursing centers offer opportunities for both collaborative and consultative models of practice with physicians" (Hinton Walker, 1993).

The Neuman Systems Model "presents a comprehensive systems-based conceptual framework for nursing. It represents the client within the systems perspective wholistically and multidimensionally. It is considered a wellness model . . . and wellness attainment, and maintenance are major considerations in its use" (Neuman, 1989). The CNC is also a comprehensive systems-based approach to delivery of nursing services to populations needing wholistic care. The model's focus on wellness, with significant attention to health maintenance for chronically ill individuals and groups, is also consistent with the philosophy and values of the CNC. Finally, the structure of the delivery of professional nursing services across the wellness—illness continuum in the Neuman Systems Model (primary, secondary, and tertiary prevention interventions) provides a framework for integrated care required in the future for cost-effective, quality care.

CLINICAL SITES AND STUDENT EDUCATION

The University of Rochester is a private institution of higher learning and serves as a national research institution offering undergraduate, graduate, and profes-

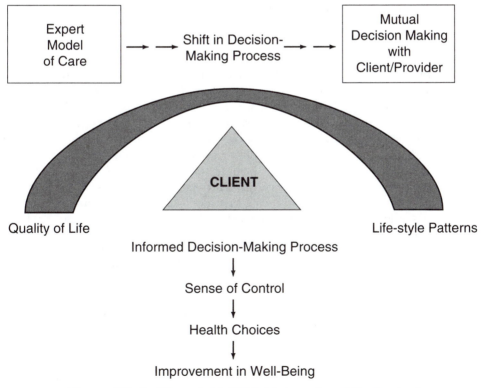

Figure 29–5. *(Copyright 1991, University of Rochester.)*

sional instructional programs of excellence. The School of Nursing offers an upper-division undergraduate program leading to the BS degree for both generic and registered nurse students. The school also offers graduate study in seven clinical components leading to the master's degree as well as a research-focused PhD program and a postdoctoral research program. At the master's level, specialization concentrations offered include Nursing Administration, The Care of Children and Families, Medical-Surgical Nursing, Primary Care Nursing (Adult and Family Nurse Practitioner), Community Health Nursing, Psychiatric-Mental Health Nursing, and Women's Health Care. At the graduate level students work closely with preceptors in skill building, experiencing new roles, and learning about new health care delivery systems throught the CNC. Using their own practice populations and administrative roles as a framework for learning, CNC advanced-practice nurses as clinical faculty serve as mentors during students' clinical experiences.

A variety of CNC service sites that function through the CCNC provide faculty practice, student learning experiences, and future research opportunities. Through innovative arrangements and joint ventures with community agencies, the CNC director had arranged nurse-managed practices with varied populations consistent with the goals of Health People 2000. These CNC practice sites and clinical learning experiences for students in both urban and rural sites are described below.

There are three practices in rural settings. These include the Women's Health Centers in Livingston County; an innovative practice in a country jail along with a mobile van in Wyoming County; and a developing adolescent practice in Ontario County. These three practices are approximately one hour from Rochester.

The Women's Health Centers, a division of the Livingston County Health Department in rural New York, provide health care by nurse practitioners for women and their partners. Primary prevention is the major nursing intervention provided by the CNC nurse practitioner to these predominantly female clients. Wholistic care is provided with special attention to physiological, developmental, and sociocultural variables. External environmental stressors (lack of transportation, distance from health care providers, and poverty) impact the ability to access primary care and preventive health care services in these rural areas. Nurse practitioner students in the women's health care program at the master's level are working with the CNC clinical faculty member for enhanced learning experiences in a rural setting. There are future plans to include opportunities for selected undergraduate students as well.

Practices in the Wyoming County Hospital constitute a full-time rural practice for one of the CNC's experienced nurse practitioners. Students in the family nurse practitioner program use this seasoned CNC clinical faculty member as a preceptor for new and different learning experiences. The Wyoming County Jail, which is located in the county seat of Warsaw, New York, has the capacity for 64 inmates, both male and female. The jail houses county inmates (sentenced from local courts) as well as state and federal inmates. The state and federal inmates are held on a temporary basis while they are to be tried or are in transition from one facility to another. This practice site was traditionally a physician-staffed site with episodic care as its main focus. Attention to the impact of stressors on physiological variables in the population continues to be a dominant focus of the practice; however, since June of 1992 the CNC clinical faculty member has initiated several improvements using a nursing model of care. The practitioner interventions include attention to documentation of care, case management during referrals and transfers, and attention to the psychological variable through structured referral to psychiatric services and a significant reduction in the use of controlled substances. With the constant ebb and flow of federal inmates, many cultural groups are represented. This diversity requires the nurse practitioner to pay special attention to the sociocultural variable and requires additional primary prevention as an intermediary between inmates and guards. Other primary prevention interventions such as health education had not been a priority in the past. This has been integrated into the prisoner visits since the CNC nurse practitioner arrived. Future plans include structured health education classes and limited opportunities for undergraduate clinical experiences.

The second practice for this seasoned CNC practitioner and educator is the Wyoming County Rural Mobile Clinic, in the same rural area as the Wyoming County Jail. This practice is implemented through a Mobile Health Van (MHV), and outreach effort of the Wyoming County Hospital and the CNC that was initiated in September 1993. A 28-foot-long converted recreational vehicle reaches into communities where no primary care providers have been consistently available to underserved populations. In this practice, primary prevention interventions comprise a large part of the practice; however, secondary and tertiary prevention interventions are also a focus of care with chronically ill and elderly populations reached by the van. In addition to care coordinated through community agencies, the MHV assists the small industrial businesses of the county to provide primary prevention intervention, including primary care services, educational programs, and screening initiatives to employees and employers.

A third rural practice is in Canandaigua, New York, about 45 minutes from Rochester. This is a collaborative practice with pediatricians of the Canandaigua Medical Group. The practice consits of comprehensive primary care of children from birth to 18 years of age. Although other providers (physicians) see adolescents, referrals and consultations regarding care are a very important part of this CNC clinical faculty practice role. In addition to comprehensive primary care services provided to both well and ill children and adolescents, the practice is strongly focused on prevention and health promotion activities. Adolescents are often seen for wellness care (e.g., school physical). Other frequent problems are associated with developmental changes such as irregular menses, at-risk behaviors noted by parents, and headaches/stomach problems associated with stress.

A wholistic care approach includes consideration of developmental, sociocultural, psycho-emotional, and spiritual factors. Intrapersonal, interpersonal, and extrapersonal stressors are addressed with interventions such as health counseling and teaching about self-esteem, decision making regarding risk behaviors, communication with parents, and need for support systems. At this time, these interventions are primarily with individuals and occasionally with families. Contraception and sexually transmitted diseases are discussed with all adolescents globally, with specific counseling as appropriate for individuals and families. Future plans are to develop this practice into a structured adolescent program that would formalize many of the individual intervention strategies and offer them to groups of teens and/or parents in evening or after-school classes. The CNC faculty member currently provides clinical experiences as a preceptor for students in the pediatric nurse practitioner program.

Under the service cluster "services to organizations and businesses," consultation services in organizational development are also provided to rural hospitals in the Fingerlakes area outside Rochester. The Neuman Systems Model is used in these consultations, focusing on the organization/community as client. Attention is focused on assessment of the five variables in the Neuman Model, with prevention intervention strategies to address intra-, inter-, and extrapersonal stressors as appropriate in these varied settings. Examples of interventions include attention to interpersonal stressors damaging relationships between nurses and administration in one setting, development of a proactive staffing plan in another consultation, and development of a strategic plan to address significant changes in hospital roles and services in the context of health care reform. This latter consultation was designed as a primary prevention intervention to increase flexible lines of defense and reduce future external environmental stressors. Opportunities for students in the nursing administration master's program are facilitated through preceptor experiences in the consultation and management arena of the CNC.

In addition to CNC outreach efforts in rural areas, practices are also functioning in the urban Rochester area that provide faculty practice and student learning experiences. One practice is at the hillside Children's Center, which serves troubled and emotionally disturbed children and families. This facility provides residential treatment, a campus school, day treatment, emergency shelter/crisis counseling, and therapeutic foster family care. Services in this setting include care for seriously mentally ill children and hearing impaired mentally ill children; care for seriously emotionally disturbed children requiring a therapeutic living environment; emergency housing, crisis counseling, diagnostic assessment, and after-care services to children and families in crisis situations; and prevention of permanent placement outside families by providing services to strengthen the family whenever possible. The CNC practitioners provide primary health care nursing services to at-risk female clients, group health education programs, and individual health counseling. In this practice attention is paid to all five variables in the Neuman Model and significant intra-, inter-, and extrapersonal stresses. Students from the women's health and pediatric practitioner programs have utilized this site and CNC clinical faculty as preceptors during the years this practice has been in existence.

Another significant practice is the Senior Health Service, a new practice developed at the Regional Council on Aging for elderly patients. These services include physical examinations, mental health assessments, functional assessments, consultation, health education, and referrals. There is a growing practice involving "house calls" for seniors who are physiologically and/or psychologically unable to leave their homes for health care. The wholistic nursing model approach in this practice consistently addresses all five variables, and interventions include primary, secondary, and tertiary prevention as intervention. Students in the adult and family nurse practitioner programs have used this CNC practice site for clinical experiences.

School health services are also a component of the services offered in the urban area by the CNC clinical faculty. Primary prevention interventions are offered, including school, sports, and camp physicals done by nurse practitioners; a puberty education class conducted as a joint venture with the department of medicine; and selected consultations as many communities consider school-based or school-linked clinics. Students primarily in the pediatric nurse practitioner program participate in these practice opportunities. The Neuman developmental variable and environmental stressors are addressed in this CNC practice.

FUTURE DIRECTIONS AND EVALUATION

The systematic evaluation plan for this new and innovative CNC is consistent with the philosophy and intent to impact health policy, implement a nursing model of care, and monitor and determine costs through the application of sound business principles. This three-pronged approach is critical if nursing centers are to impact and support health policy reform. Both the Neuman Systems Model and David Gil's model for social policy reform are being explored by nurses as organizing frameworks for evaluation and health policy analysis.

In David Gil's model for health policy analysis, he identifies five institutional processes involved in the implementation of policy that directly impact outcomes. These are: development, management, and conservation of resources; organization of work and production; exchange and distrubution of goods, services, rights, and responsibilities; governance and legitimation; and reproduction, socialization, and social control (Gil, 1990). For the purposes of evaluating CNC contributions and impact, institutional systems and processes directly impacting the *development, management, and conservation of resources* exist in the creative joint ventures and collaboration of the CNC with community agencies to decrease demand for space and equipment resources. CNC *organization of work and production* relates in this model to the use of nurse practitioners as providers rather than traditional physician care models. Since the primary mission of most community nursing centers is to provide services to underserved populations who have rights to care but little access, this addresses the process of *exchange and distribution of goods, services, rights, and responsibilities.* The goal of community-centered practice in this community nursing center is to impact governmental policy and funding of health care provided by nurse practitioners under *governance and legitimation.* Lastly, informing the consumers, other providers, and legislators about the quality and cost-effectiveness of nurse-managed care addresses *reproduction, socialization, and social control.*

Perhaps the most important contribution of Gil's work and model is that he identifies outcomes that will measure the effectiveness of health care policy. These outcomes involve improvement in: circumstances of living of individuals, groups, and classes; power of individuals, groups, and classes; nature and quality of human relations among individuals, groups, and classes; and overall quality of life. Outcome measures discussed here become part of the systematic plan for measurement of quality of nursing interventions in CNC sites. CNC faculty have begun identifying instruments that relate to these outcomes, such as health status measurement tools, healthy life-styles, and quality of life instruments. Using selected instruments developed for specific populations receiving care through CNC practice sites, students and faculty will have opportunities to participate in the evaluation of nurse-managed care with frequently served populations—the elderly, chronically ill, adolescent, and children and families.

The nursing interventions defined in the Neuman Systems Model will be used as a framework for categorizing interventions into *primary, secondary, and tertiary prevention interventions.* These intervention groupings will be used to clarify and define services, but more importantly as a framework for tracking costs and case management across sites and through episodes of care over time. The most significant goal of managed care for the future will be to reduce costs of "secondary interventions" (such as emergency room visits, acute care length of stay, medications, and diagnostic tests) by providing effective primary and tertiary interventions as defined by the model. Assessment instruments will be implemented that incorporate Neuman's five factors—*developmental, physiological, psychological, spiritual, and sociocultural.* In addition, barriers and problems with access to care for underserved populations will be explored and grouped in categories of *intrapersonal, interpersonal, and extrapersonal stressors.* In these ways, the model will be used both as methodology and as evaluation in future research and special projects.

The Neuman Systems Model and Gil's Policy Analysis Model have been integrated into a systematic plan for data organization, monitoring, evaluation, and research for the Univeristy of Rochester Community Nursing Center (see Figure 29–6). The blending of these conceptual models will serve the dual purposes of providing care and measuring cost-effectiveness and quality outcomes of care. These evaluation measures will be critical to support changes in health policy and continuation of the focus of preventive care in the future. Health policy analysis and use of sound business principles will also play a vital role for survival of this nursing center and other community nursing centers as they attempt to address the needs of underserved and vulnerable populations. Since

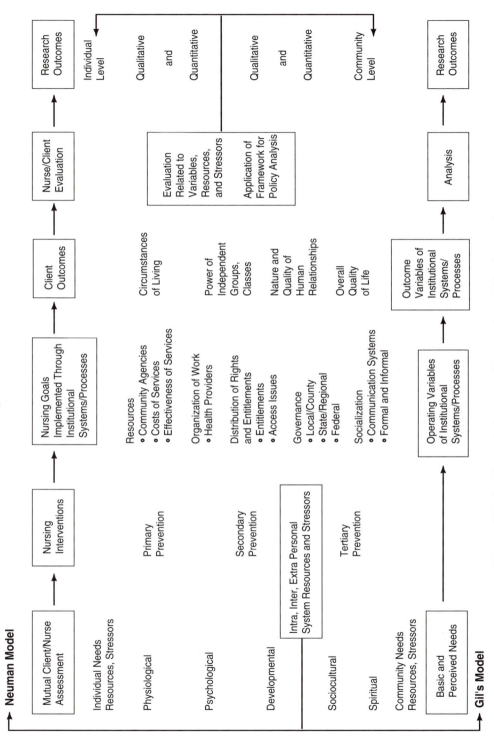

Figure 29–6. *(Copyright 1991, University of Rochester.)*

primary care and preventive services are the basis of practice in most nursing centers, the Neuman Systems Model should be considered as one of the key nursing models for nursing centers.

CONCLUSION

The integration of Neuman's and Gil's models provides a sound conceptual framework with potential to shape the future direction for faculty practice, student learning experiences, and research that will contribute to the advancement of the nursing profession. The Neuman Model emphasizes a partnership with the client and categorizes primary care, prevention, and health promotion as "primary prevention interventions." When managing care over time, nurse practitioners provide health maintenance care, reeducation, and monitoring of conditions after discharge from acute care institutions. Neuman defines these as "tertiary interventions." For the purposes of costing out care for future CNC managed care contracts, services such as emergency room visits, number of hospitalizations,and inpatient days will be categorized under "secondary prevention interventions." The Neuman Model consequently serves as both a framework for providing wholistics care and an evaluation of the cost-effectiveness of care by using Neuman's prevention categories of services for managed care. In the context of health care reform in the future, the Neuman wholistic approach to care and Gil's quality outcomes will provide significant contrubutions to a new health care system that hopefully emphasizes comprehensive care and prevention services.

REFERENCES

Gil, D. G. 1990. *Unravelling Social Policy*. Rochester: Schenkman Books, Inc.

Lang, N. M. 1983. Nurse managed centers—will they thrive? *American Journal of Nursing* September: 1290–1298.

Neuman, B. 1989. *The Neuman Systems Model*. Norwalk: Appleton & Lange, 22, 25, 34.

The Nursing Center: Concept & Design 1987. Kansas City: American Nurses' Association.

Nursing Centers: Meeting the Demand for Quality Health Care 1989. New York: National League for Nursing.

Toffler, A. 1990. *Power Shift*. New York: Bantam Books.

Walker, P. H. 1991. The community nursing center for nurse practitioners, an opportunity to develop entrepreneurial skills. *Rochesier Nursing* Fall: 18–19.

Walker, P. H. 1992. Neuman Systems Model: Right choice for community nursing center. *Neuman News* March: 1–2.

Walker, P. H. 1993. Care of the chronically ill: Paradigm shifts and directions for the future. *Holistic Nursing Practice* 8:1.

30

THE NEUMAN SYSTEMS MODEL ADAPTED TO A CONTINUING CARE RETIREMENT COMMUNITY

Marion L. Rodriguez

INTRODUCTION: APPLYING THE NEUMAN SYSTEMS MODEL TO CLINIC NURSING

This chapter focuses on the application of the Neuman Systems Model to clinic nursing practice of a continuing care retirement community (CCRC). The Neuman Systems Model was adapted to the clinic of the Collington Episcopal Life Care Community, Incorporated, a CCRC in Mitchellville, Maryland, on the periphery of Washington, District of Columbia. There are 370 residents at Collington.

The community has a health center (dedicated in October 1988) that includes a clinic for the independent-living residents and a 70-bed in-patient unit. The clinic is under the direction of the clinic coordinator (the author). The health services department is managed by the director of health services.

Today there is much emphasis on using a theoretical basis for nursing research, nursing curricula, and nursing practice to increase nursing professionalism. In recent years there has been an increase in the number of clinicians predicating their practice on a specific theoretical model. Nurses in long-term care settings must now join the cadre of practitioners adapting nursing models to their practice. A section of this chapter, devoted to a literature search, addresses the rationale for applying theory to practice.

THE NEED FOR THEORY-BASED PRACTICE IN LONG-TERM CARE

The population of elderly persons is escalating, and the number of CCRCs is increasing proportionately. Care of the residents in these communities is of importance to health care professionals involved in the practice of gerontological nursing. That care can no longer be predicated on "gut feelings" or the philosophy of "this is the way we have always done it." Approaches to gerontological nursing practice *must* have a theoretical basis to justify all nursing actions. Tollett (1982) succinctly states that the Neuman Systems Model's simplicity and universality promote its use among various nursing specialties, as well as among the various health care professionals.

With this statement in mind, it becomes apparent that the author must begin to formulate a theoretical basis for both the organizational structure and the care/interventions of the Collington CCRC clinic. It was imperative that the author review the literature for identification of the rationale for theory-based nursing practice and then study the various models to find one that could best be adapted to the Collington clinic.

NURSING MODEL APPLICATION TO PRACTICE: LITERATURE REVIEW

Theorists and researchers in nursing have long stressed the importance of having a theoretical basis for nursing practice. Therefore a literature search was initiated to examine ideas, comments, and theories that would underscore the value of having a theoretical basis for the daily practice of nursing, at all levels and in the various specialties.

Parse (1990) states that theory-based practice is the challenge for nurses of the '90s:

> Theory-based practice is necessitated by the times. Nurses need to be more knowledgeable and expectations, of their employers and the public, are greater. Nursing care is becoming more concentrated in community-settings and family homes, and health promotion and quality of life are becoming a major focus of practice in all settings. What grows more important then is the use of nursing models to guide this focus of practice. (p. 53)

Fitzpatrick, Whall, Johnson, and Floyd (1982) note:

> As nursing continues to develop its own approaches to person, environment, and health, a distinctive theoretical base of nursing becomes more evident. (p. vi)

Nurses in clinical settings may ponder how they can apply theory to practice. Fawcett (1988) discusses several approaches that may be used to identify theories that researchers and clinicians can use to explain and describe nursing practice. The author recommends that nurses search the literature for information relevant to their practice then conduct a study to ascertain whether a selected theory is applicable to that aspect of nursing practice. Observations of actual clinical practice can be formalized to serve as theories.

Christmeyer, Catanzareti, Langford, and Reitz (1988) indicate that a conceptual framework provides a foundation for nursing practice and forms the structure for organizing its systems, methods, and tools. Nurses at their facility have found that using a conceptual framework to guide practice, education, and research facilitates nursing professionalism and serves as the link between nursing theory and practice. This approach was used by Reitz at Johns Hopkins to formulate the framework of a concept for nursing practice, which eventually became the foundation for a Nursing Intensity Index. The Framework for Nursing Practice (FFNP) incorporates concepts such as health, the nature of nursing, and the correlation between the two. It is an ideal clinical model.

Hanchett (1990) discusses the use of nursing frameworks and theories to guide community nursing practice for clients. This is in compliance with the American Public Health Association (1980) and the American Nurses' Association's (1980) "call" for a synthesis of public health and nursing knowledge. In Hanchett's article, four nursing models are presented: Orem's (Self-Care), Roy's (Adaptive), King's (Human Systems), and Rogers's (Unitary Man). Community nurses will base their practice on the model that is most useful to them. Knowledge of the four models can provide direction to the public health nurse/community nurse practitioners and researchers. The Neuman Systems Model, though not mentioned in this article, was found to be easily adaptable and particularly useful in public health nursing worldwide.

Application of the Neuman Systems Model to Nursing Practice

Select applications of the Neuman Systems Model to practice are presented in this chapter. Some applications are particularly relevant to the Collington CCRC clinic.

Neuman (1989) has included many authors who have demonstrated the model's applicability to nursing practice, in areas such as:

1. Community health administration and practice
2. Joint use—community health practice and student teaching
3. Assessment of the community-as-client
4. Community psychiatric nursing
5. Family theory
6. Intervention modality for the renal patient
7. Application to perinatal nursing
8. Application to the hospital setting
9. Uses in other countries

There are applications of the model to a gerontological curriculum; however, there are no examples of the model's application to long-term care (nursing home of CCRC) in either the 1982 or 1989 editions of *The Neuman Systems Model*.

Community Health Administration in Canada's Manitoba and Ontario Provinces

The Neuman Systems Model provided a systematic approach for examining three different issues pertaining to the efficient, effective delivery of health services in the provinces of Manitoba and Ontario. Drew, Craig, and Beynon (1989) discuss the application of the Neuman Model for analysis of an organizational matrix that integrates community health programs into the global framework of the province of the Manitoba health care delivery system. Select concepts of the Neuman Systems Model provided the conceptual basis for developing provincial standards for community health nursing practice and also introduced a theoretical framework for public health nursing. The Neuman Systems Model became the theoretical framework for providing care to clients and families. The model was appropriate because of:

1. Its emphasis on a wholistic approach to nursing
2. Its goal-directed approach
3. The easy interpretation of concepts across departments

This laid the foundation for community nursing practice in Manitoba and Ontario and provided future direction for the delivery of quality community services in these Canadian provinces.

The Community as Client

Beddone (1989) applied the Neuman Systems Model to the assessment of the community as client. The rationale for community assessment is the provision of guidelines for program planning. Data can be collected about client needs from the prospective clients and caregivers. In this application, an assessment guide was developed to allow a large suburban health department to assess the health care needs of aggregate postnatal parents and to identify any probable barriers to satisfying those needs. The assessment tool provides the direction necessary for community health nurses to assess the system using a flexible and comprehensive nursing framework. Since community health nursing already embraces the concepts of primary, secondary, and tertiary prevention, the use of the Neuman Systems Model does not involve a major shift in focus.

Family Theory

Reed (1989) applied the Neuman Systems Model to family theory and stated that since the model is predicated on systems theory, it lends itself well to the incorporation of family theories. It provides a theoretically valid and consistent means to assess families and then offers methods to intervene appropriately. The Neuman Systems Model includes the individual, the family, or the community as a client system. Intervention is effected when assisting individuals, families, and groups to retain, attain, and maintain an optimal level of wellness by intervening to reduce stressors and adverse conditions that affect or could affect client functioning.

Implications in Long-Term Care

These analogies were helpful during the formulation of this application of the Neuman Systems Model to a CCRC clinic. The aforementioned nursing scholars have stated that using many perspectives emphasizes the importance of applying theory to practice. Other nurses have presented their applications of the Neuman Systems Model to their area of practice. It is now time for practitioners in long-term care settings to apply theory to practice and then share these theoretical applications with others.

ADAPTING THE NEUMAN SYSTEMS MODEL TO THE COLLINGTON CLINIC

Rationale for Selecting the Neuman Systems Model

The Neuman Systems Model, which is based on systems theory, seemed to be adaptable to the problems of the Collington clinic as well as the stressors experienced by the residents relocating to this retirement setting.

Application of the Neuman Systems Model to the Clinic

After much deliberation about approaches to adapting the Neuman Systems Model to the Collington clinic, it seemed practical to present two applications. These applications are presented in Figure 30–1, which depicts the clinic as the client, and Figure 30–3, which depicts the resident as the client. The "clinic as the client" pertains to the clinic system and its organizational components (i.e., "what makes it tick"), the stressors that constantly bombard the system, and the interventions implemented to resolve them.

The *basic core* of the clinic is the staff, which includes the coordinator, a registered nurse, licensed practical nurses, and certified nursing assistants. Their philosophy, past education, and experiences are integral parts of the basic core. The basic core is surrounded by the service implemented by the staff. These services are included in the clinic logo (see Figure 30–2).

Use of Neuman Model: The Lines of Defense, the Lines of Resistance, and the Five Variables

The flexible line of defense is represented by policies and procedures that are the framework of the department. Failure to have them formulated and imple-

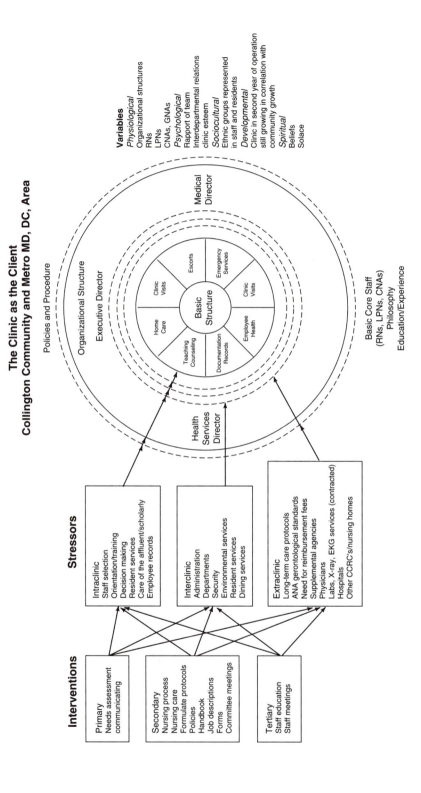

Figure 30–1. The Neuman Systems Model adapted to the Collington clinic.

mented would result in the clinic's functioning haphazardly, without direction or protocol. Policies and procedures are used to orient new staff and are used as reference points during the daily operation of the clinic.

The normal line of defense is the organizational structure of hierarchy of the clinic staff. Information about departmental structure is shared during orientation. Team cohesiveness and cooperation are stressed. It the team is intact and functioning as a unit, this line will be difficult to penetrate.

The lines of resistance are represented by the director of health services, the medical director, and the executive director of the Collington community. At this level, these persons preserve the integrity of the clinic systems when stressors threaten the flexible or normal lines of defense. When these lines are penetrated and the interventions are not effective, the results could include instability, disruption of services, and departmental collapse.

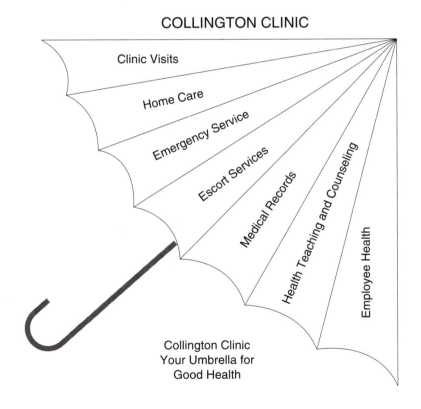

HELP WHEN YOU NEED IT

Figure 30-2. The Collington clinic logo.

There are five variables ever present in the clinic system. They are defined as follows:

- Physiological—individual or group physical structure
- Psychological—staff support, esteem
- Sociocultural—interdepartmental relations, ethnicity
- Developmental—clinic growth correlated with community growth
- Spiritual—beliefs of the group that assist staff to cope with population morbidity and mortality

Stressors

Stressors are intraclinic, interclinic, and extraclinic.

Intraclinic stressors include staff selection, orientation training, employee health records, appropriate decision making, providing resident services, and caring for the affluent, scholarly, formerly high-level professionals who are often demanding and intolerant.

Interclinic stressors are those activities that involve coordinating services with other departments. These interdepartmental interactions are usually implemented without discord. However, when a problem arises in the interaction between departments, stress ensues and the issue must be resolved as amicably as possible.

Extraclinic stressors encompass such areas as long-term care protocols, the American Nursing Association Standards, establishing fees for services, working with supplemental nursing agencies, physician schedules and requests, timely diagnostic testing and reporting, hospital discharges back to the Collington community, and communication with other CCRCs and nursing homes.

Interventions to resolve stressors are primary, secondary, and tertiary, as depicted in Figure 30–1. the interventions are currently in progress and ongoing.

APPLICATION OF THE NEUMAN SYSTEMS MODEL TO THE RESIDENT

Use of Neuman Model: The Five Variables

The basic structure of the resident encompasses the needs of any organism, including food, warmth, shelter, coping patterns, love, and care. The elderly client often has difficulty maintaining the integrity of the basic structure due to problems within the five variables shown in Figure 30–3:

- Physiological—deterioration of body systems
- Psychological—cognitive changes
- Sociocultural—retirement, family/friend separation, death of spouse
- Developmental—experiencing the last developmental stage, which is traumatic for many
- Spiritual—seeking comfort in spiritual beliefs during stressful times

The basic structure is surrounded by the clinic services provided to the residents.

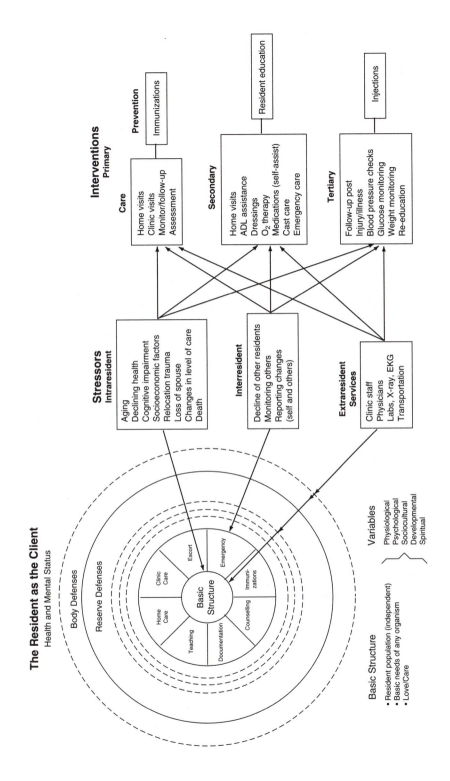

Figure 30–3. The Neuman Systems Model adapted to the Collington residents.

Lines of Defense and Resistance

The flexible line of defense represents the health and mental status of the resident. If health and mental status are in excellent condition, stressors will have negligible effect; if not, penetration will occur.

The normal line of defense is represented by the body's defenses. Neuman (1989) states it is what the client has become over time and represents the usual wellness status. Illness results when this line is penetrated.

Lines of resistance serve to defend the client when the lines of defense are penetrated. When coping is ineffective, there will be draining of reserves, leading to incapacities and possibly death. If the system copes effectively, the system reconstitutes and recuperates. The clinic staff intervenes during these bouts of stressor bombardment and client coping efforts.

Stressors

Stressors are intraresident, interresident, and extraresident.

Intraresident stressors include declining health, possible cognitive impairment, socioeconomic factors (e.g., reduced income, retirement), relocation trauma, selling of a home, changes in level of care (necessitating a move to the health center or hospital), death of a spouse, and thoughts of one's own death.

Interresident stressors include, but are not limited to, seeing the decline and death of other residents, monitoring a neighbor who shows signs of early cognitive impairment, and reporting changes in oneself and others.

Extraresident stressors are often services such as physician consultation, diagnostic laboratory tests, transportation to the Metro (subway), shopping trips, and other medical-related appointments. Anxiety ensues and increases when procedures and appointments are not on schedule or a diagnosis is not favorable.

Primary care includes home visits by staff to assess problems, clinic visits by residents to report their concerns, monitoring, follow-up, and assessment. Prevention at this stage can include immunizations for influenza, diphtheria, and pneumonia.

Secondary care involves home visits by staff to provide care for postoperative conditions, assisting with activities of daily living (ADLs), medication assistance, cast care, emergency assessment, and transfers to the health center or a hospital. Prevention at this level addresses education relevant to the current problem.

Tertiary care is initiated after illness or injury, during glucose monitoring of the diabetic resident, and during weight assessment. This is the maintenance phase. Prevention includes administering injections such as B-12, interferon, liver extract, calcimar, insulin, and allergy medications.

The nursing process and nursing diagnosis are used to further assess, diagnose, plan, intervene, and evaluate management care strategies applicable to the Collington CCRC clinic. Plans are being implemented to revise the current assessment tool to include all parameters of the Neuman Systems Model.

CONCLUSION

The adaptation of the Neuman Systems Model has been well received at Collington, both by staff and the independent-living residents. Staff plans include coordinating the theoretical model with the Minimum Data Set (MDS), the Maryland Minimum Data Set (MMDS), and the Care Plan process. It has been an exciting venture to have interdisciplinary involvement in a theory-based effort.

As a continuing consultant, the author is currently adding another dimension to the model that reflects the nursing unit as the client. This adaptation will depict those specific stressors that impact the basic core of a nursing unit as well as nursinng interventions and lines of defense that impede their progress.

The adapted model is presented during orientation to the clinic and the inpatient unit, and is included in the policy manuals and resident handbooks. Continuing evaluation of the efficiency of the model will be assessed during review of the admission process, MDS, MMDS, Care Plan, and quality improvement modalities. This evaluative process will be presented during the quarterly meetings.

The adaptation/application of the Neuman Systems Model to the Collington clinic and residents will significantly enhance interdisciplinary team approaches to care planning and continuous quality improvement.

REFERENCES

American Nurses' Association. 1989. Standards for Gerontological Nursing.

Beddone, G. 1989. Application of the Neuman Systems Model to the assessment of the community-as-client. In *The Neuman Systems Model,* edited by B. Neuman, 363–370. Norwalk, Conn.: Appleton & Lange.

Christmeyer, C., Catanzareti, M., Langford, A., and Reitz, J. 1989. Bridging the gap: Theory to practice—part I: clinical applications. *Nursing Management,* 19(5):42–50.

Drew, L., Craig, D., and Beynon, C. 1989. The Neuman Systems Model for community health administration and practice: Provinces Manitoba and Ontario Canada. In *The Neuman Systems Model,* edited by B. Neuman, 315–341. Norwalk, Conn.: Appleton and Lange.

Fawcett, J. 1989. Conceptual models and theory development. *JOGN 17*(4): 400–403.

Fitzpatrick, J., Whall, A., Johnson, R., and Floyd, J. 1982. *Nursing models and Their Psychiatric Mental Health Applications.* Bowie, Md.: Robert J. Brady.

Hanchett, E. 1990. Nursing models and communitiy as the client. *Nursing Science Quarterly* 3(2): 67–72.

Neuman, B. 1990. Health as a continuum based on the Neuman Systems Model. *Nursing Science Quarterly* (3): 129–135.

Neuman, B. 1989. *The Neuman Systems Model.* East Norwalk, Conn.: Appleton & Lange.

Parse, R. 1990. Nursing theory based practice: A challenge for the 90s. *Nursing Science Quarterly* 3(3): 52.

Reed, K. 1989. Family theory related to the Neuman Systems Model. In *The Neuman Systems Model,* edited by B. Neuman, 385–395. East Norwalk, Conn.: Appleton & Lange.

Reed, K. 1982. The Neuman systems Model: A basis for family psychosocial assessment and intervention. In *The Neuman Systems Model: Application to Nursing Education and Practice,* edited by B. Neuman, 188–195. East Norwalk, Conn.: Appleton & Lange.

Tollett, S. 1982. Teaching geriatrics and gerontology: Use of the Neuman Systems Model. In *The Neuman Systems Model: Application to Nursing Education and Practice,* edited by B. Neuman. East Norwalk, Conn.: Appleton-Century-Crofts.

Section V

Nursing Research and the Neuman Systems Model

Introduction

Theory development and testing are cyclical and essential components in the development and progress of knowledge. One cannot exist without the other, and both require complementary and integrated processes. Progress in the discipline is contingent on the dialectical development of both and on careful attention to the integral relationship between them. An effective section on research should ground the reader in the current state of the art related to a theory or topic, propose future directions, support a blueprint for action, and challenge the reader to transcend existing ideas and frameworks. Research using the Neuman Systems Model and a conceptual model is presented in this section; different authors address different aspects of theory testing and theory development. Together they give the reader an overview of what has been done and what could be done to further the development of the Neuman Systems Model.

In the first chapter Meleis calls for a post–theory testing era. She challenges the existing use of the concept of theory testing and proposes a transformative world view from a mechanistic view of testing to a more holistic and integrative approach to theory support. The proposed view, she argues, is more congruent with some principles essential in nursing as a human and caring science. She addresses the significance of considering gender, culture, and more sensitivity to consumer involvement in theory development and testing.

Using theory to guide research is sometimes constrained by the need to have researchers' thorough understanding of a theory as an imperative requirement to meaningful and authentic utilization of theory—not always an easy task with the many esoteric concepts that tend to be used in nursing. Although attempts are always made to operationalize the abstract concepts in a theory and to utilize the theory in research, such attempts are sometimes authentic and congruent with the theory and at other times are incongruent. Therefore questions arise as to the meaning of theory research utilization, and when research can be classified as being based on a particular theory, and whether or not a theory concept should be used in all parts of the research to be classified as theory-based research. Anticipating all these questions, Fawcett facilitates this complex process for theory users by providing the reader with six rules for research, based on conceptual models. Furthermore, she translates these rules and relates them more specifically to the Neuman Systems Model.

Readers will find that this section is a valuable resource for intiating or building on existing research; that is, the abstracts provided by Louis provide examples of ways in which Neuman's model has been used in research. The references provided by each author in this section represent the state of the art in research related to Neuman. The list of areas of suggested research intended to develop a middle range theory is another tangible resource for researchers and clinicians who are interested in using Neuman's model.

The Neuman Systems Model has been used extensively in master's theses and doctoral dissertations. Recently, Louis demonstrated that between 1989 and 1993 the utility of Neuman's model was demonstrated in 40 clinical reports and in 100 research studies. Louis proposes that one of the driving forces of the phenomenal increase in the use of Neuman's model in both practice and research can be attributed to the international symposia that bring nurses from different parts of the world together to discuss her model and work related to it.

Theory students as well as expert researchers will find the chapter by Breckenridge a useful demonstration of how a middle range theory may evolve from practice within the Neuman Systems Model. A typology of clients' decision making related to dialyses was proposed, demonstrating how the major concept in the Neuman model, as perceived optimal wellness, can lead to the further development and refinement of the systems model.

Developing this point further, Smith and Edgil advocate the creation of a center or an institute that nurtures collaborative, interdisciplinary, and multisite efforts to formulate and test practice theories within the Neuman Systems Model. Such a center would also be built on the principle of diversity of philosophical and methodological stances. There is ample evidence in nursing that centers and institutes of research invariably enhance scholarly productivity, particularly of tangible support through resources provided. The proposed center would provide mechanisms for immediate retrieval of the most current research using the model as well as offer the potential for developing collaborative efforts between novice and expert model users. Equally important, researchers can find others who may be interested in the same phenomenon early on in their research.

Several conclusions can be drawn from the following section as a whole. First and foremost, the Neuman Systems Model is gaining momentum in research inasmuch as it has already demonstrated its utility in practice and in master's theses and doctoral dissertations. Second, organized theory-based structures in the form of symposia meetings, treatises, and presentations help promote the use and implementation of theories to carry this conclusion further. Therefore, the development of a center may further enhance the utilization of theory. Third, the utility of theory in research is a complex phenomenon that involves considering the different components of utilization. While traditionally theory utilization in research was equated with theory testing, it is apparent now that theories could also be used in selection of nursing phenomenon for developing appropriate research methodologies, data analyses, and interpretation. There is an increasing flexibility in operationalizing theories in research as evidenced from the many examples provided in this section. Fourth, a number of authors are proposing that the next steps in further developing Neuman's Model is to focus on the construction of middle range theory, particularly in the area of predicting the outcomes of preventive interventions.

Future consideration of the theory research dialectic could include the ways by which research findings have changed the assumptions or the propositions advanced by Neuman. When this happens, the research practice theory circle would be completed.

Afaf Ibrahim Meleis

31

THEORY TESTING AND THEORY SUPPORT
Principles, Challenges, and a Sojourn into the Future

Afaf Ibrahim Meleis

There is a general agreement among theoreticians, clinicians, and researchers that nursing is both a human science and a practice-oriented science, and that nursing deals with human beings who are embedded in a context. That context ranges from the immediate environment to a society at large to a world that is interconnected. To test theories considering the environment without the larger context is like trying to understand the responses of fish without understanding the nature of the water that determines their very existence. This reconceptualization of the discipline drives a reconsideration of the whole notion of theory testing. Therefore, the purpose of this chapter is to analyze some of the trends that may influence theory testing and to propose a framework that is more concurrent with these trends.

More specifically, this chapter has three objectives. First, I will argue that there are some principles that are imperative for any theory validation. Any theory testing process that does not address these principles is inadequate, lacks vigor, and more importantly lacks social consciousness. It would be a theory devoid of critical thinking about our moral obligations as a discipline. Second, I will argue that a rigid notion of theory testing is limiting and incongruent with the properties of the discipline of nursing. I will further demonstrate that the nature and meaning of validation may have to undergo some major changes.

This chapter is based on a keynote address given at the Fourth International Neuman Symposium, University of Rochester, New York, April 23, 1993.

These changes in the process of validation and testing of theory may be a response to contextual changes and a reflection of the nature of nursing as a human science and its practice orientation. This view of theory validation is empowering to nurses. Third, I will propose several approaches to be used as a flexible framework for theory validation. These principles and approaches may be used to develop a futuristic agenda to validate Betty Neuman's systems theory.

PRINCIPLES

Our world is going through some major transitions, and globalization is becoming a way of life. I believe these transitions create some very necessary but not sufficient principles that need to be considered for any form of theory testing and/or validation. These principles could become guidelines for the substance and process of theory testing.

I propose six principles. These are: gender sensitivity, diversity, vulnerability, internationalization, culturally competent care, primary health care, and consumer involvement. I will elaborate on each principle briefly. The intent of the articulation of these principles is to stimulate and challenge the reader to consider how each of these principles may influence the processes and context of the current and future work in theory validation.

1. Principle of Gender Sensitivity

Theory testing that is confined to only men or only women has been demonstrated to be sexist and biased. Similarly, theory testing using the experiences of one sex as the norm for the other has proven futile. An assertion could be made that there is more heightened awareness of the fallacy of normative universalization based on one gender. For example, assuming that what stresses one gender is also stressful to the other has limited the careful attention to potential differences based on qualitatively and historically different lived experiences. Therefore, because the work role has proved to be a source of stress for men, it was then assumed to create similar situational stresses for women. Recent research has helped in questioning the relationships between the work role and stress for women and uncovered the significance of the spousal and maternal role in women's health outcomes. These findings illustrate how imperative it is to consider gendered experiences in testing of theories.

2. Principle of Diversity

Transitions create movements, and there have been extensive population shifts that have affected the sociocultural make-up of the health care system. The US, for example, is a notion that has citizens representing Hispanic, African, Portuguese, Middle Eastern, German, Slavic, Chinese, and Japanese cultures, to name a few. Large cities in many countries are microcosms of this diversity. There are millions of migrants and immigrants who are opting or being forced to leave their countries of birth and establish residence and new identities in another city or another country.

Immigrants and migrants from different cultural heritages and different rural areas bring with them their own health beliefs, values, healing modalities (Leininger, 1977), and forms of defense against stress that have not been well understood by mental health care professionals. Their stress is buffered by their own cultural values and exacerbated by extended family, racism, and stereotypes. When they come into a health care system, they baffle health care providers because their customs are different from the prevailing cultural norms. Some like to shop for health professionals. Others prefer the old, distinguished-looking male health providers over the young and seemingly inexperienced. Some will only undress in front of female providers but are not able to express their need and thus are diagnosed as difficult patients or noncompliant. Others are not able to use verbal communication to reveal their interpersonal or intrapersonal stressors.

Diversity also creates a challenge for health workers who represent different countries and for administrators who manage multicultural and multinational workforces. Diversity has created the need for models to help in ensuring a healthy multicultural working situation and for careful attention to assumptions and the premises of theories that are based on individuals and on the ability to communicate freely and openly. This need requires some careful attention to the development of models that are sensitive to the special needs of minorities and to their own cultural assumptions. Similarly, testing models that are sensitive to diversity are lacking (Davis et al., 1992). **Theory testing that does not honor diversity is limited and prejudicial.** It also continues to support the supremacy of one group, and the generalization based on one.

3. Principle of Vulnerability

The third major principle to guide theory testing is related to the emergence and visibility of new vulnerable populations and the lack of reassurances that support and tend to their needs. For example, either the size of the frail elderly population is increasing in some parts of the world, or the problem is highlighted because the extended family's resources are depleted and the environment and the resources to support them are nonexistent or inadequate in most of the world. In addition to lack of resources, access of the elderly to resources is constrained by other factors as well, such as economics, transportation, and lack of experience in caring for the elderly.

Other emerging vulnerable populations are created by an increasing tendency to care for patients outside hospitals and in their own communities. Although populations in developing countries have always demonstrated a preference for home deliveries, early discharge, home care, and dying at home, this pattern is more recently observed in more developed countries, where economic and insurance company constraints are sending people out of the hospital and to their homes early. Other vulnerable and at-risk populations are also emerging because people are living longer with chronicities and requiring different supportive care.

The meaning of vulnerability is also mandating some conceptual changes in how vulnerable populations are defined. There is a need for an expanded definition of vulnerability to encompass sociopolitical and cultural barriers and not only biomedical risks. Vulnerability, therefore, can be better understood when we consider the daily lived experiences of populations as they themselves see it. To use Neuman's theory, do these vulnerable groups have qualitatively different normal lines of defense? The emergence of these vulnerable populations creates the need to question assumptions about clients' defenses, resistance, and health and the definitions used to guide research related to nursing theories. It also raises questions about the congruency of current approaches for theory testing that were designed to reflect primarily biomedical concerns.

4. Principle of Culturally Competent Care

With increasing diversity and the change in the definition of vulnerable populations, health care professionals are looking for ways to increase cultural sensitivity and cultural competence in health care.

Similarly, acknowledging diversity and vulnerability as principles for theory validation necessitates considering culturally competent care as another principle. Assistance in developing lines of defense, buffers to stress, and modifiers of adaptation that are limited to one culture may create more stress and may weaken lines of defense in other cultures. Our challenge here is to develop tests for theory within a context of cultural sensitivity and with consideration to culturally competent care as an outcome variable.

The effects of the nurse and client socioeconomic status and cultural heritage on health practices, patterns of illness, and style of intervention need to be integrated in theory testing. Knowledge that evolves from sociocultural and economic context, representing different societies, will empower nurses to provide needed care and can more realistically influence health care policies.

5. Principle of Internationalization

Understanding and interpreting the responses of minority immigrants or migrants to health and illness in the United States (understanding and interpreting responses is the essence of what nursing is about) is enhanced by understanding these responses within the context of the minority immigrants' own cultures. While some understanding of responses can be developed by studying health care needs and responses of minorities in North America, scientists who have a working systematic knowledge of immigrant minorities in their own countries produce much richer understanding of explanatory frameworks that can influence the way nurses manage the health care needs of these immigrants.

Becoming knowledgeable about health care in other countries has the bonus of making clinicians and scientists (who have worked abroad) more sensitive and more interested in recruiting and considering underserved populations in the work related to theory validation. It forces us to examine our own biases and prejudices.

Through increasing internationalization, nurses in many regions of the world can learn about the different culturally appropriate nursing therapeutics, to decrease stress, mobilize energy, or bolster lines of defense. Examples of culturally appropriate nursing therapeutics include music from India, herbs from China, meditation from Japan, social support from Colombia, and music and dance rituals from Egypt. Internationalization in theory testing also helps in considering what is within socioeconomic constraints in different societies. It is a humbling experience to witness what nurses in some countries have been able to do to help their patients create supportive environments, mobilize energy, and boost the level of integrity of human systems in spite of the constraints of limited economic and modernization resources. They have utilized local healers, indigenous practices, and common local practices. If these strategies are not considered in testing theories, theories may be limited in scope and potential. Sharing and reciprocating such practices can increase nurses' repertoires of nursing therapeutics, which would in turn enhance their effectiveness in caring for diverse populations.

International theory testing may be enhanced through exchange programs and through international networking. Examples are networks provided by specialty organizations or national organizations in nursing or in other disciplines and sister country programs (AAN, 1992). The Neuman Systems Model Trustees Group, Inc., could develop a commitment to internationalization and mobilize some resources for it.

6. Principle of Primary Health Care

Theory testing needs to be put into the context of health care reform management nationally and internationally. In 1978 a jointly planned meeting of WHO, UNICEF was convened in Alma Ata in the USSR (WHO, 1978). It included 134 member countries and a number of informal and formal organizations. These representatives participated in signing an international declaration pledging to bring health to all populations by the year 2000. The declaration was based on the strong conviction that such goals will not be attained without a refocus of health care on primary health care (PHC). PHC must be considered in any form of knowledge development and testing. During the meeting it was reaffirmed that progress in science and the development of new technology are not the answer for assuring quality care.

PHC is defined as a way of thinking, a way of acting, a movement, a process, a strategy, and a goal. It is essential health care, based on practical scientific and social acceptability. The goal is to enable people to lead socially and economically proactive lives.

Theory testing may presume a just and equitable system and may promote the maintenance of a status quo. Social consciousness and responsibility make it imperative that we consider testing of status quo, and creating an environment that is more congruent with addressing global concerns. Doing that may promote more fundamental changes in the theories proposed for testing.

7. Principle of Consumer Involvements

The process of theory development and testing has been conceptualized as expert-driven. An expert-driven approach presupposes that it is the experts who best know the clients' experiences, situation, and outcomes. With many well-informed consumers in the United States and with an increasing desire and demand for total involvement in all aspects of health care, we can no longer assume that theory validation is the prerogative only of scientists or professionals. If we have accepted consumer involvement in the health–illness process, then we need to consider consumers' essential role in participation in the development of approaches to validate theories.

CHALLENGES

If nurse scholars consider the importance of these principles in their theory validation work, then we must face the challenges that result from this approach to theory validation. I have selected four challenges to review. These are marginalized experiences, criteria to ensure rigor and enhance credibility, how to enhance theory validation for theory-based practice and practice-based theories, and how to promote the role of clinicians as resources for theory validation.

1. Marginalized Experiences

Theories provide us with frameworks that help us to make sense of our world in a systematic way. Theories have tended to normalize deviant experiences and trivialize marginalized views. This normalization and trivialization are a product of an attempt to address majority experiences and those that have some universal properties and potential. When we consider the seven principles as essential to guiding theory testing and validation, then the challenge that scholars confront is how and in what form the experiences of vulnerable, stigmatized, and disenfranchised populations will be reflected in the process and product of theory validation. Which populations are included, and how do the results of their experiences get reflected in the theory?

2. Rigor and Credibility

If generalization cannot be used, what other criteria *can* be used to judge the usefulness of a theory? And what criteria can be used to ensure rigor and enhance credibility within the context of the seven principles addressed above?

How can networking that is based on diversity and internationalization be developed within the constraints of limited resources to ensure culturally competent validation? What determines the credibility and rigor in narratives based on personal experiences?

3. Theory-Based Practice and Practice-Based Theory

Another important challenge facing theory validation is predicated on increasing the link among practice, theory, and research. Some clinicians ask, why bother? We now have theories that provide nurses with guidelines to help them in establishing trusting relationships, enhancing self-care, supporting adaptation, speeding recovery, increasing the potential of wounds to heal, developing primary, secondary, and tertiary prevention as intervention, and decreasing confusion. The stages that nurses have gone through to achieve a scholarly and a scientific role have some universal features. The first stage has been clinical practice; the second stage has been functional, including teaching, education, and administration; the third stage has been research; and the fourth has been theory. Our challenge now is to consider how these stages may influence clinical practice and in turn influence theory validation. However, we also need to uncover other models that may emerge from our practice. How do we practice within a theory but maintain the openness to uncover other phenomena that may not lend themselves to explanation with that theory?

4. Clinicians as a Resource for Theory Validation

A final challenge for us is how to integrate theory validation and development in the role of nurses who are in advanced nursing practice. Nurses are interested in how patients are living, the experience of being hospital patients, how the hospital environment and the home environment may influence this experience, and what nurses can do to make the experience as comfortable as possible for the patients and their significant others. Clinicians are in the best possible position to develop knowledge based on their practice. The question that challenges nursing practice and nurse administrators is what strategies are most effective in increasing nurses' participation in the development and validation of theories?

To consider this question we have to consider our assumptions about nursing and nurses. *Clinical nurses are not merely reservoirs for theory use; they are also resources for theory development.* The assumption of this duality is essential because theory development and validation are dialectically related; one cannot contribute to knowledge development effectively without the other. The nature of nursing practice, the intensity of nurses' association with their clients, and the wisdom they gain from the clinical work could be the genesis for theory development. Acknowledging and valuing the rich potential nurses have to contribute to the growth of nursing knowledge and theory may help them articulate and share their insights and ideas with others. Such an opportunity for exchange is the essence of theory development (Meleis and Jennings, 1989).

THEORY SUPPORT: AN ALTERNATIVE TO THEORY TESTING

The whole notion of theory testing and validation is problematic because it tends to presume that a theory can be subjected to a single validation test and that such a validation test renders the theory credible or noncredible. How many of us have heard colleagues and students say, "We do not want to or cannot use nursing theories because they have not been validated," to which I always respond, "Give me examples of theories you think have been validated and tested." Upon further discussion, it becomes apparent that the notions of testing and validation are quite complex and are not easily translatable to psychoanalytic theories, Erickson's theory of development, of Maslow's hierarchy, all of which have been used extensively.

Nursing literature is rich with clinicians' experiences and narrative analyses demonstrating either the utility of nursing theories or the goodness of fit between a theory and a clinical situation. What is the use of these critical narratives, and what do they demonstrate? Several previous discussions of this subject of validation affirm the emerging pattern of support instead of validation.

In 1985 I discussed three different theories of truth that were proposed by Armour (1969), Kaplan (1964), and Meleis (1985). The rationale behind this discussion was to demonstrate that one theory of truth was insufficient for nursing as a human science. The first, the correspondence theory of truth, is based on the principle that a statement or a theory is reported to be true when there is a fit between the theoretical view and objective data. The principle of this theory of truth places the focus on research as the only way to validate the theory. The second theory, coherence, is driven by a principle of logic that is checked through tests of consistency, integration of relatedness, and simplicity of form. Tests of validation for coherence are not based on research as much as they are based on theoretical and conceptual analyses. The third theory is that of pragmaticism, which focuses on the utility of a theory and on its utilizers.

These theories were used as a framework for theory validation. One type of discussion addressed the changing nature of the consideration of truth as objective and as a reflection of reality. This discussion added to an understanding of the complexity of truth and the inappropriateness of a single approach to it. Silva and Sorrell added to this discussion by expanding validation of theory to include a host of criteria. They asserted that testing to verify nursing theory could be done through critical reasoning, description of personal experiences, and application to nursing practice (Silva and Sorrell, 1992). They went even further and developed a number of criteria to be used to judge the credibility of the validation tests.

I would like to propose that what we are after for theory validation could be better served if we consider the concept of *theory support*. I am proposing "theory support" to substitute theory validation and testing for the reasons that I have discussed. Theory support is a broader concept, more friendly to alternative ways of theory validation, and more congruent with the nature of the discipline. It is not validation of a theory that we are looking for; we need to think of support and affirmation of parts of theories, and we need to think of components of theories. Even though we cannot say that *all* individuals experience their health and illness situation in certain ways, it is still extremely useful to understand the experience of the few who experience it in certain unique ways, particularly for members of sciences that deal with human experiences and with practice-oriented issues. What other criteria can affirm or support a theory?

These accounts, exemplars, stories, and relationships adhere to credibility criteria, and that provides them with the strength to hold up the theory. *Theory support* includes increased advocacy of central statements, appropriateness with some central problem in the discipline, and new insights about nursing phenomena. Theory support can also be obtained through networks formed to evaluate the theory's potential and capability. Other criteria can affirm or support theory scholars in the discipline of nursing, and I mean by scholars, both scientists and clinicians, can provide support for theories through a number of approaches. These approaches are not proposed here as new and different (Meleis, 1985; Meleis 1991; Silva and Sorrell, 1992). Rather, I am proposing legitimizing the work that has been used in supporting theories that may not qualify as testing or validation because of the limited definitions of these concepts.

I therefore propose the following approach in theory support:

1. Supporting nursing theory through philosophical analyses
2. Supporting nursing theory through conceptual analyses
3. Supporting nursing theory through existing data, through the analytical synthesis of single utilization studies, through component-based meta-analyses, and through the utilization of national and regional data bases
4. Supporting nursing theory through new data and through the use of narrative studies based on clinicians' experiences and the assessment of clients' situation and the therapeutics used. Interpretive studies based on clients' experiences could be used to provide theory support, as well as studies that support the utility of nursing therapeutics and further development of predictive theory studies.

CONCLUSION

There is a dialectic relationship between theory development and theory validation. Focusing on one without the other limits the potential of progress in knowledge development in nursing. The nature and meaning of validation may have to undergo some major changes similar to those that have accompanied theory development. Changes in the processes to validation and testing of theory may be a response to contextual changes, to the nature of nursing as a human science, and/or to its practice orientation. There is a momentum for quality health care that is accessible to all populations as manifested in national and international health care debates and initiatives. There is an urgent need to consider theory validation within this framework.

In this chapter, seven principles that I believe are essential for any work related to theory support were discussed. I have also challenged the reader to think of what is needed to consider on the sojourn into the future of theory validation. To base validation on these principles will require that we discuss and resolve some pressing challenges. Four of these challenges are (1) ways by which theory validation may reflect responses of marginalized experiences, (2) identification of criteria for rigor and credibility appropriate for theory support, (3) ways by which the balance between validation of theory through theory-driven practice and practive-based theory can be maintained, and (4) how to utilize clinicians as resources for theory support.

I have also proposed that theory support may have been dominated inappropriately (though metatheorists continued to promote these approaches to theory development exclusively until the late 1980s) by positivist and mechanistic criteria. Theory development has escaped this route and followed a course that respected the nature of nursing as a human science. Theory development has been based on insights from clinical practice, personal experiences, and conceptual analyses. We have had visionary theorists such as Dr. Neuman who conceptualized human beings as having a core and lines of resistance and defense to protect that core. A client as a human being was also vividly conceptualized as having flexible, accordion-like outer shields to ward off stressors, with loops linking the core to the environment. These are innovative ideas in theory development that were not bound by positivist or mechanistic philosophical thoughts. Yet theory validation continues to be based on more traditional and borrowed approaches from the natural and physical sciences.

Theory testing has been based predominantly on research reports and equated with research. Research was limited to investigations based on analytical designs to the exclusion of interpretive designs. While theory development may have been more congruent with the nature of nursing, it is only recently that theory testing is undergoing some fundamental changes, making it more congruent with the nature of nursing as a discipline and a profession.

Educators have demonstrated the utility of theories in curricula, and clinicians have described their experiences in using nursing theories as frameworks for their practice and have explained patient response and outcomes using theories. Some clinicians presented clinical evidence that the outcomes were related to the assessment and actions of nurses. Administrators presented narrative descriptions of processes of implementing a nursing theory and reflected on how the process of defining outcomes has become more systematic, orderly, and convincing. These narratives may not meet the criteria for theory testing; however, they may be considered as validation of theories if *theory support* rather than *criteria for theory testing* is used as a framework for validation.

The new philosophical era, that of postmodernism, may also be an era of post-theory testing, allowing deconstruction of theory validation and a reconstruction of a more congruent concept of theory support.

Language is powerful. there is a very significant metaphoric symbolism attached to concepts. A change from *testing* to *support* for theory validation is more than a semantic change. It is empowering to all those who have made a significant contribution to interpreting, using, refining, and developing theories. They may not make a difference in theory testing, but they would make a great difference in theory support.

REFERENCES

American Academy of Nursing. 1992. *The International Role of the American Nurses Association and American Academy of Nursing: A White Paper.* Washington, D.C.: American Academy of Nursing.

Armour, L. 1969. *The Concept of Truth.* Assem: Van Gorcum and Co.

Davis, L. H., Dumas, R., Ferketich, S., Flaherty, M. J., Isenberg, M., Koerner, J. E., Lacey, B., Stern, P., Valente, S., and Meleis, A. I. 1992. The AAN Expert Panel Report: Culturally competent health care. *Nursing Outlook 40(6): 277–283.*

Kaplan, A. 1964. *The Conduct of Inquiry: Methodology of Behavioral Sciences.* San Francisco: Chandler Publishing Co.

Leininger, M. 1977. Cultural diversities of health and nursing care. In *Nursing Clinics of North America,* edited by H. Dietz, Philadelphia, W. B. Saunders Co. 5–18.

Meleis, A. I. 1985. *Theoretical Nursing: Development and Progress.* Philadelphia: Lippincott Co.

Meleis, A. I. 1991. *Theoretical Nursing: Development and Progress,* 2d ed. Philadelphia: Lippincott.

Meleis, A. I., and Jennings, B. 1989. Theoretical nursing administration: Today's challenges, tomorrow's bridges. In *Dimensions and Issues in Nursing Administration,* edited by B. Henry, C. Arndt, M. DiVincenti, and A. Marriner, 7–18. Boston: Blackwell Scientific Publication.

Silva, M., and Sorrell, J. 1992. Testing of nursing theory: Critique and philosophical expansion. *Advances in Nursing Science* 14(4): 12–23.

World Health Organization. 1978. *Primary Health Care Report of the International Conference on Primary Health Care.* Alma Ata, USSR, September 6–12. Health for All Series, No. 1. Geneva: WHO.

32

CONSTRUCTING CONCEPTUAL-THEORETICAL-EMPIRICAL STRUCTURES FOR RESEARCH
Future Implications for Use of the Neuman Systems Model

Jacqueline Fawcett

The purpose of this chapter is to identify strategies for constructing logically consistent conceptual-theoretical-empirical structures for research based on the Neuman Systems Model. The chapter opens with a discussion of the components of conceptual-theoretical-empirical structures and progresses to the identification of general rules for conceptual model-based research and the specific rules for Neuman Systems Model-based studies. The chapter concludes with a presentation of guidelines for designing studies that reflect the rules for Neuman Systems Model-based research.

Reviewed by Patricia Hinton Walker.

COMPONENTS OF CONCEPTUAL-THEORETICAL-EMPIRICAL STRUCTURES

Conceptual models, such as the Neuman Systems Model, guide middle-range theory development and the selection of research methods. Three levels of abstraction are evident in both theory-generating and theory-testing research: conceptual models, middle-range theories, and empirical indicators (Figure 32–1).

Conceptual Models

Conceptual models are the most abstract component of conceptual-theoretical-empirical structures. A conceptual model is defined as a set of abstract and general concepts and the propositions that state something about the concepts (Fawcett, 1989). The Neuman Systems Model is one example of a conceptual

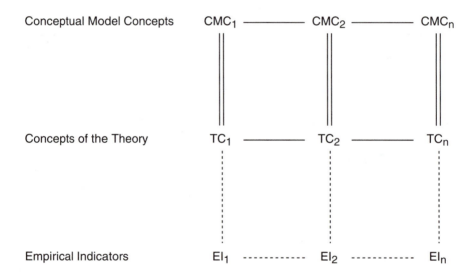

Conceptual Model Concepts   CMC$_1$ ————— CMC$_2$ ————— CMC$_n$

Concepts of the Theory   TC$_1$ ————— TC$_2$ ————— TC$_n$

Empirical Indicators   EI$_1$ ----------- EI$_2$ ----------- EI$_n$

Legend:

═════ Propositions linking conceptual model and theory concepts
------- Operational definitions
——— Relational propositions linking conceptual model concepts and theory concepts

Figure 32–1. General form of a conceptual-theoretical-empirical structure. (From Fawcett, J., and Downs, F. S. 1992. *The Relationship of Theory and Research,* 2d ed. Philadelphia: F. A. Davis, p. 106, with permission.)

model of nursing. The Neuman Model concepts of *primary prevention* and *client system stability* are examples of conceptual model concepts. An example of a conceptual model proposition from the Neuman Model is the statement that *primary prevention promotes client system stability.*

The function of a conceptual model of nursing is to provide a global frame of reference for observing and understanding people and their environments, and a context for the nursing process. Given the abstract nature of conceptual models, their concepts are not directly observed in the real world nor are their propositions amenable to direct empirical testing.

Middle-Range Theories

Middle-range theories are at the intermediate level of abstraction in conceptual-theoretical, empirical structures. They are less abstract than conceptual models but more abstract than empirical indicators. A middle-range theory may be defined as a set of relatively specific and concrete concepts and propositions that account for or characterize a phenomenon (Barnum, 1990). Examples of middle-range theory concepts are *preoperative information* and *physiological coping behaviors.* These concepts are linked by the proposition stating that *provision of preoperative information is associated with use of physiological coping behaviors postoperatively* (Ziemer, 1983).

The function of a middle-range theory is to describe, explain, or predict responses of specific people experiencing specific situations and events within the context of specific environments. The specificity of these theories means that their concepts can be observed and their propositions can be empirically tested in a direct manner.

Empirical Indicators

Empirical indicators are the most concrete component of conceptual-theoretical-empirical structures. Empirical indicators are the real-world representatives of middle-range theory concepts. More specifically, they are the actual instruments, experimental conditions, and research procedures that are used to observe or measure the concepts of a middle-range theory. An example of an empirical indicator that is an instrument is the Physical Coping Behavior Scale (Ziemer, 1983). An example of an empirical indicator that is an experimental condition is an audiotape of preoperative information. An example of an empirical indicator that is a research procedure is the stipulation that data are to be collected three days after surgery.

RULES FOR CONCEPTUAL MODEL-BASED RESEARCH

Conceptual models guide research by stating what phenomena make up the domain of inquiry and specifying methodological directives about how the domain is to be investigated, how theories are to be generated and tested, how data are to be collected, and how those data are to be analyzed (Laudan, 1981; Schlotfeldt, 1975). More specifically, a fully developed conceptual model reflects a particular research tradition that is made up of the six rules for inquiry that are listed in Table 32–1.

Rules for research based on the Neuman Systems Model are beginning to be formulated. The rules listed in Table 32–2 were extracted from the content of the Neuman Systems Model and the literature based on this model, including a recent article by Grant, Kinney, and Davis (1993) and discussion with the Neuman Systems Model Trustees Group (personal communications, April 24, 1993).

GUIDELINES FOR CONSTRUCTING NEUMAN SYSTEMS MODEL-BASED STUDIES

The general rules for research (Table 32–1) and the rules for Neuman Systems Models-based research (Table 32–2) can be restated in the form of guidelines for designing and reporting the results of studies based on the Neuman Systems Model. These guidelines are listed in Table 32–3.

The first and second guidelines highlight the need to explicate the fact that the study is guided by the Neuman Systems Model and to provide an overview of the modes that clarifies the relationship between the content of the model and the study purpose. An example of the first guideline is drawn from a study of the impact of cancer on long-term survivors (Loescher, Clark, Atwood, Leigh, and Lamb, 1990):

> The conceptual framework for this study was adapted from the three major components of Betty Neuman's total person framework: stress, reaction, and reconstitution. (p. 223)

TABLE 32–1. RULES FOR CONCEPTUAL MODEL-BASED RESEARCH

- The first rule identifies the phenomena that are to be studied.
- The second rule identifies the distinctive nature of the problems to be studied and the purposes to be fulfilled by the research.
- The third rule identifies the subjects who are to provide the data and the settings in which data are to be gathered.
- The fourth rule identifies the research designs, instruments, and procedures that are to be employed.
- The fifth rule identifies the methods to be employed in reducing and analyzing the data.
- The sixth rule identifies the nature of contributions that the research will make to the advancement of knowledge.

TABLE 32–2. RULES FOR NEUMAN SYSTEMS MODEL-BASED RESEARCH

- The first rule of Neuman's Systems Model states that the phenomena to be studied encompass (1) physiological, psychological, sociocultural, developmental, and spiritual variables; (2) properties of the central core of the client system; (3) properties of the flexible and normal lines of defense as well as of the lines of resistance; (4) characteristics of the internal, external, and created environments; (5) characteristics of intrapersonal, interpersonal, and extrapersonal stressors; and (6) elements of primary, secondary, and tertiary prevention interventions.
- The second rule states that the clinical problems to be studied are those that deal with the impact of stressors on client system stability with regard to physiological, psychological, sociocultural, developmental, and spiritual variables, as well as the lines of defense and resistance. One purpose of Neuman Systems Model-based research is to predict the effects of primary, secondary, and tertiary prevention interventions on retention, attainment, and maintenance of client system stability. Another purpose is to determine the cost, benefit, and utility of prevention interventions.
- The third rule stated that subjects can be the client systems of individuals, families, groups, communities, organizations, or collaborative relationships between two or more individuals. Data encompass both client system and investigator perceptions and strategies for negotiated goal setting, and may be collected in inpatient, ambulatory, home, and community settings.
- The fourth rule states that this nursing model is an appropriate base for inductive and deductive research using both qualitative and quantitative research designs and associated instrumentation.
- The fifth rule states that data analysis techniques associated with both qualitative and quantitative research designs are appropriate.
- The sixth rule states that research will advance understanding of the influence of prevention interventions on the relationship between stressors and client system stability.

The second guideline is exemplified by the following quotation from a study of patient perceptions of mechanical ventilation conducted by Gries and Fernsler (1988):

> The purpose of this study was to ascertain patient perceptions of the mechanical ventilation experience in a critical care unit. Neuman's model of nursing represents a total person approach to promoting and understanding of people, their environment, and the relationship of variables in the person and environment that may affect individual function. People are viewed as open systems who interact with the environment by adjusting themselves to it, or it to themselves. By this interaction the individual maintains a steady state of balance when confronted with a stressor. . . . Individual perception of the stressor is mediated by the time of occurrence, past and present conditions, the nature and intensity of the stressor, and the amount of energy required to adapt. . . . Because the meaning of the stressor to the patient is of primary importance in the Neuman model, nursing intervention cannot be planned without an understanding of the meaning of the experience for the person. (pp. 52–53)

The third guideline requires an explicit statement of the linkage between concepts of the Neuman Systems Model and the middle-range theory concepts that constitute the study variable. It is important to note here that few studies require the use of *all* of the Neuman Systems Model concepts. Rather, most studies are guided by just a few of the conceptual model concepts. The linkages

TABLE 32–3. GUIDELINES FOR CONSTRUCTING NEUMAN SYSTEMS MODEL-BASED STUDIES

1. Explain that the Neuman Systems Model is the underlying guide of the study.
2. Discuss the Neuman Systems Model in sufficient breadth and depth so that the relationship between the model and the purpose of the study is clear.
3. State the linkages between the relevant Neuman Systems Model concepts and the study variables.
4. State the linkages between the relevant Neuman Systems Model propositions and the study aims and/or hypotheses.
5. Ensure that the methodology reflects the Neuman Systems Model:
   • Select study subjects from a population that is appropriate for the focus of the Neuman Systems Model.
   • Select instruments that are appropriate measures of Neuman Systems Model concepts.
   • Select statistical techniques that are in keeping with the focus of the Neuman Systems Model.
6. Include conclusions regarding the empirical adequacy of the theory and the credibility of the Neuman Systems Model in the discussion of the study findings.

between Neuman Systems Model concepts and middle-range theory concepts typically are phrased as "Neuman Systems Model concept$_n$ is represented (or indicated) by study variable$_n$." An example is taken form Leja's (1989) study of the effect of guided imagery on postsurgical depression:

> The person's flexible lines of defense are defined by Neuman as "a dynamic, rapidly changing protective buffer." This is represented in the study by a measurement of depression level prior to the person's confrontation with home discharge. The primary prevention is guided imagery discharge teaching. The impact of the primary prevention is indicated by the measurement of depression after the discharge teaching. (p. 8)

The fourth guideline extends the explanation of the association between the conceptual model and the research by requiring an explicit statement of the linkage between relevant Neuman Systems Model propositions and the study aims, purposes, or hypotheses. That linkage is evident in the following quotation from the report of a study of the effect of turning on postoperative outcomes for coronary artery bypass graft (CABG) patients (Gavigan, Kline-O'Sullivan, and Klumpp-Lybrand, 1990):

> The Betty Neuman Systems Model . . . suggests that nursing interventions involving primary prevention will strengthen an individual's defenses and reduce the possibility of a person's encounter with a stressor. . . . Primary prevention in this study refers to regular turning of individuals in an experimental group. Immobility is the indicator of a stressor, and the impact of stressors is examined by documenting the incidence of pulmonary complications in both the control and the experimental group and noting each study participant's length of hospital stay. This study postulates that because immobility is a postoperative stressor, primary prevention through the provision of regular turning

procedures in the immediate postoperative period has the potential to build an individual's defenses and decrease the likelihood of the patient's encounter with a stressor. This will be indicated by decreased incidence of pulmonary complications and shorter length of hospital stay for CABG individuals in the experimental group. (p. 70)

The fifth guideline requires a study design that clearly reflcts the focus of the Neuman Systems Model. Consequently, the study sample should be drawn from a population that is a legitimate client system, including "individuals, groups, families, communities and collaborative relationships between 2 or more individuals" (Grant et al., 1993, 55). Moreover, the instruments should operationalize the relevant Neuman Systems Model concepts. Inasmuch as no particular methodology is required by the Neuman Systems Model, the data analysis plan should be appropriate for the type of research—qualitative or quantitative—undertaken.

In qualitative studies, the Neuman Systems Model influences the research design by facilitating the selection of methods for the discovery of new middle-range theories. Thus, as can be seen in Figure 32–2, theory generation proceeds from the Neuman Systems Model directly to the empirical indicators. The data obtained from the empirical indicators are then analyzed, and a new middle-range theory emerges. Figure 32–2 illustrates that linkages are forged directly from the Neuman Systems Model concepts and propositions to the empirical indicators and then from the empirical indicators to the concepts and propositions that make up the newly discovered middle-range theory.

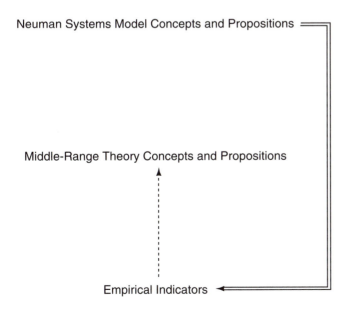

Neuman Systems Model Concepts and Propositions

Middle-Range Theory Concepts and Propositions

Empirical Indicators

Figure 32–2. Theory generation from the Neuman Systems Model.

Blank, Clark, Longman, and Atwood's (1989) research report exemplifies the influence of the Neuman Systems Model on the design of a qualitative study. With regard to study subjects, they explained:

> Neuman indicates that stressors experienced by the patient and stressors experienced by the caregiver are not always compatible. Therefore, for [the] purposes of this study, stressors in both patients and caregivers were assessed to develop a more accurate representation of their home care needs. . . . The subjects were outpatients in a tertiary care center receiving high-technology therapy on an outpatient basis, with most of their day spent at their own home or a temporary one, usually an apartment near the cancer center. (pp. 81–82)

Blank and her colleagues (1989) also explicated a link between the Neuman Systems Model and study instruments. They stated:

> Two interview guides developed by Newman to assess patient and caregiver stressors were used for [the] purposes of this study. The Neuman Stressors Inductive Interviews were conducted to provide qualitative data regarding patient and caregiver needs. (p. 81)

Finally, the data analysis plan used by Blank, Clark, Longman, and Atwood (1989) reflects the Neuman Systems Model. As can be seen in the following quotation, they used Neuman's concept of three types of stressors to establish a priori categories for content analysis of qualitative data. More specifically, as Blank et al. explained:

> Data from interviews were tape-recorded and transcribed for content analysis. Consistent with the underlying [conceptual] model, the data were analyzed in relation to: intrapersonal stressors, . . . interpersonal stressors, . . . and extrapersonal stressors. . . . Stressors identified by the subjects were categorized according to the definitions offered by Neuman. Construct validity of the categories has been built in through the coding process and is consistent with the Neuman [Systems Model]. Definitions from the Neuman model were used to categorize the stressors identified by the patients and caregivers. The individual stressors identified by the subjects were then placed in the categories offered by Neuman. Data placement in categories [was] validated by two of the researchers. (p. 82)

A descriptive classification theory of patient and caregiver needs emerged from the data analysis. Needs were induced from each category of stressors. The conceptual-theoretical-empirical structure for the study conducted by Blank et al. (1989) is illustrated in Figure 32–3.

In quantitative studies, the Neuman Systems Model influences the research design by again facilitating the selection of the methods required to test a middle-range theory that has been derived from the model. As illustrated in Figure

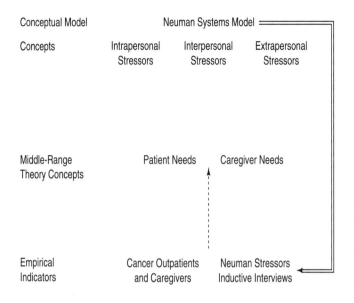

Figure 32–3. Example of theory generation from the Neuman Systems Model. (Diagram constructed from Blank, Clark, Longman, and Atwood, 1989.)

32–4, theory testing proceeds from the relevant Neuman Systems Model concepts and propositions to the middle-range theory and then to the empirical indicators. The data obtained from the empirical indicators are analyzed by following the methodological guidelines of the conceptual model, and in middle-range theory is supported or refuted.

The study conducted by Courchene, Patalski, and Martin (1991) exemplifies the influence of the Neuman Systems Model on the design of a quantitative study. The purpose of their study was to compare the health status of nurses who frequently administer Cyclosporine A (CyA) with that of nurses who have no exposure to CyA. The investigators proposed that "CyA may represent an environmental stressor capable of penetrating the individual nurse's health-protective lines of defense or resistance and consequently altering the state of wellness of that individual" (p. 498). They went on to explain that "The normal line of defense represents adaptation over time, that is, usual coping patterns, life style factors, or (for this study) work habits that protect the individual form environmental stressors" (p. 498).

The study subjects were nurses who administered CyA and those who did not. Courchene, Patalski, and Martin (1991) explained:

> The study group consisted of 22 nurses in an urban teaching hospital who regularly handled CyA and administered the medication to the pediatric transplant patients. This group of nurses was selected because the CyA contamination of the skin of nurses who work with pediatric transplant patients with CyA is a

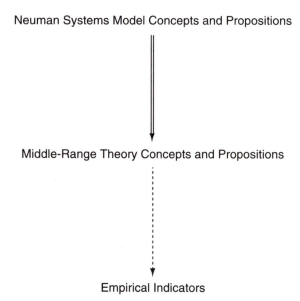

Neuman Systems Model Concepts and Propositions

Middle-Range Theory Concepts and Propositions

Figure 32–4. Theory testing
and the Neuman Systems

Empirical Indicators

> common occurrence. The control group consisted of 31 medical-surgical nurs-
> es employed on inpatient units at another large urban teaching hospital. The
> control group primarily cared for adults and had no exposure to CyA. (p. 498)

The influence of the Neuman Systems Model on the selection of the study
instrument is also evident. Courchene et al. (1991) commented:

> A self-report Health Status Questionnaire was used consisting of 122 items. It
> requested information regarding specific diseases, identification of symptoms
> and assessment of gynecological history, life style factors, protective work prac-
> tice habits, exposure to antineoplastic drugs, and exposure to CyA. (p. 498)

The Neuman Systems Model had no direct influence on the method of data
analysis employed in the study. However, the chi-square statistic used by
Courchene and her colleagues (1991) is an appropriate statistical technique for
analyzing the data they obtained. The conceptual-theoretical-empirical structure
for the study conducted by Courchene et al. is illustrated in Figure 32–5.

The final guideline listed in Table 32–3 requires attention to the empirical
adequacy of the middle-range theory and the credibility of the Neuman Systems
Model. The abstract and general nature of the Neuman Systems Model precludes
direct empirical testing. The propositions of the Neuman Systems Model are
instead tested indirectly through the empirical testing of the theories that are
derived from or linked with the model. If the findings of theory-testing research

support the theory, it is likely that the Neuman Systems Model is credible. If, however, the research findings do not support the theory, both the empirical adequacy of the theory and the credibility of the Neuman Systems Model must be questioned. If the credibility of the Neuman Systems Model is questioned, then serious consideration must be given to modifying its concepts and/or propositions. The willingness to consider modifying conceptual models on the basis of empirical evidence prevents their treatment as "the truth" or ideologies that should never be questioned. Indeed, Grant and her colleagues (1993) pointed out that "Investigators must identify the strengths and weaknesses of a . . . model and interpret data around a consistent frame of reference" (p. 55).

Examples of the contribution on research findings to the credibility of the Neuman Systems Model are drawn from two studies. Ali and Khalil (1989), who studied the effect of psychoeducational intervention on anxiety among Egyptian bladder cancer patients, claimed that their findings supported the Neuman Model. They stated, "Results of the study support the Betty Neuman Health-Care Systems Model, which suggests that nursing intervention (psychoeducational

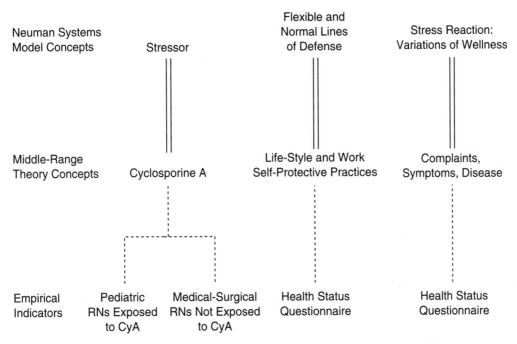

Figure 32–5. Example of theory testing and the Neuman Systems Model. (Diagram constructed from Courchene, Patalski, and Martin, 1991.)

preparation) increases resistance to stressors and strengthens the flexible line of defense as exhibited by a marked decrease in state anxiety postoperatively and before discharge" (p. 241).

In contrast, findings from the study conducted by Gavigan and her colleagues (1990) did not support the Neuman Systems Model proposition that primary prevention (regular turning) builds client system defenses and decreases the likelihood of encounters with stressors (pulmonary complications, length of hospital stay). The investigators reported no statistically significant differences in pulmonary complications and length of stay in both the surgical coronary care unit and the hospital between CABG patients who were turned every two hours for the first 24 hours and those who remained in a supine position during that time.

CONCLUSION

Application of the guidelines for constructing Neuman Systems Model-based studies should result in the development and reporting of logically consistent conceptual-theoretical-empirical structures. The results of such studies should advance nursing knowledge by enhancing our understanding of the effects of using the Neuman Systems Model on client system stability.

REFERENCES

Ali, N. S., and Khalil, H. Z. 1989. Effect of psychoeducational intervention on anxiety among Egyptian bladder cancer patients. *Cancer Nursing* 12:236–242.

Barnum, B. J. S. 1990. *Nursing Theory: Analysis, Application, Evaluation,* 3d ed. Glenview, Ill.: Scott Foresman/Little Brown Higher Education.

Blank, J. J., Clark, L., Longman, A. J., and Atwood, J. R. 1989. Perceived home care needs of cancer patients and their caregivers. *Cancer Nursing* 12:78–84.

Brown, M. W. 1988. Neuman's Systems Model in risk factor reduction. *Cardivascular Nursing* 24(6):43.

Courchene, V. S., Patalski, E., and Martin, J. 1991. A study of the health of pediatric nurses administering Cyclosporine A. *Pediatric Nursing* 17:497–500.

Fawcett, J. 1989. *Analysis and Evaluation of Conceptual Models of Nursing,* 2d ed. Philadelphia: F. A. Davis.

Gavigan, M., Kline-O'Sullivan, C., and Klumpp-Lybrand, B. 1990. The effect of regular turning on CABG patients. *Critical Care Nursing Quarterly* 12(4):69–76.

Grant, J. S., Kinney, M. R., and Davis, L. L. 1993. Using conceptual frameworks of models to guide nursing research. *Journal of Neuroscience Nursing* 25:52–56.

Gries, M., and Fernsler, J. 1988. Patient perceptions of the mechanical ventilation experience. *Focus on Critical Care* 15:52–59.

Laudan, L. 1981. A problem-solving approach to scientific progress. In *Scientific Revolutions,* edited by I. Hacking, 144–155. Fair Lawn, N.J.: Oxford University Press.

Leja, A. M. 1989. Using guided imagery to combat postsurgical depression. *Journal of Gerontological Nursing* 15(4):6–11.

Loescher, L. J., Clark, L., Atwood, J. R., Leigh,S., and Lamb, G. 1990. The impact of the cancer experience on long-term survivors. *Oncology Nursing Forum* 17:223–229.

Louis, M., and Koertvelyessy, A. 1989. The Neuman Model in nursing research. In *The Neuman Systems Model,* 2d ed., edited by B. Neuman, 93–113. Norwalk, Conn.: Appleton & Lange.

Schlotfeldt, R. M. 1975. The need for a conceptual framework. In *Nursing Research I,* edited by P. J. Verhonick, 1–24. Boston: Little, Brown.

Ziemer, M. M. 1983. Effects of information on postsurgical coping. *Nursing Research* 32:282–287.

33

THE NEUMAN MODEL IN NURSING RESEARCH
An Update

Margaret Louis

Conceptual models and conceptual frameworks have been identified as synonymous terms (Fawcett, 1989; Johnson, 1968). It is generally agreed that conceptual models and frameworks represent less formal and less well-developed attempts at organizing phenomena than do other more developed entities, such as theory statements (Silva, 1981). However, in nursing the distinction between theories and models or frameworks is often unclear. This may best be attributed to the range of the phenomena as well as the degree of specificity of the concepts and hypotheses formulated.

A conceptual model or framework is generally perceived as loosely conceived and providing a broad outline for the organization of the phenomena being studied. The organizing scheme is based on the relevance of the phenomena under study, even though developed propositions stating the relationship among the concepts are generally missing at this level of knowledge development. The lack of conceptual relationships is significant because without them there is no basis for explanation and prediction of phenomena. Explanation and prediction are two important aims of science. Conceptual frameworks are seen by some as the precursors of theory (Silva, 1981).

Conceptual frameworks characteristically are not empirically testable by a direct method; rather, they provide a perspective from which specific theories or hypotheses are developed and evaluated (Fawcett and Downs, 1992; Suppe and Jacox, 1985). Few would debate the need for conceptual models and frameworks in nursing research. A conceptual model or framework provides focus

Reviewed by Cynthia Capers. Editorial comments by Cynthia Capers.

for the inquiry as well as a coherent guide to observations, and as such is a scheme for interpreting and organizing knowledge or to refine theory. As Schlotfeldt noted (1975), the conduct of research without the presence of such a scheme is indeed research in a vacuum. For some nurses the use of conceptual models and frameworks has become a sine qua non in both master's theses and doctoral dissertations. Published nursing research also includes conceptual frameworks or theories.

All disciplines possess a knowledge base that is distinctive and individualized in its perspective. The responsibility for the development of the knowedge base falls primarily on the community of scholars from within each discipline. Disciplined inquiry, or research concerning the phenomena of the discipline, is the vehicle leading toward accomplishment of that endeavor. The body of knowledge characterizing each discipline undergoes continuous change due to advancements and synthesis of knowledge; thus the research process is a dynamic one. While these statements apply to all disciplines, they are especially true and appropriate in nursing, as evidenced by the increasing number of refereed research journals, conferences sponsored by societies focusing on research efforts, the increasing number of nursing doctoral programs, and the vigorous debates over nursing theory development and testing.

While much agreement is found on the need to use conceptual models and frameworks in nursing research, more rigorous examination of the logical relationships between these and the components of the research is needed. For example, it is not unusual to read a study in which a conceptual model or framework is described in the introduction but reference is never again made to the conceptual framework. In addition, Hayman (1987) observed that great conceptual leaps are often made between theoretical formation and explanation of clinical phenomena. The results obtained in experimental intervention studies are frequently attributed to the intervention, with no further mention of the theoretical structure or even a hint that any relationship might exist.

Conceptual models and frameworks represent a stage in theory development, and so the time and effort in selecting a conceptual model are well spent. When the conceptual model or framework can be readily linked to the research problem, then the design, selection of data collection strategies, analysis, and especially interpretation of the data can flow from that conceptualization. Identifying this link is a concern that frequently arises related to the selection of a particular conceptual model or framework to be used in conducting research. Many (Fawcett and Downs, 1992; Laudan, 1977; Schlotfeldt, 1975; Silva, 1981) have formalized the steps used when selecting a conceptual model or framework in empirical research. The *Guide for Selection and Use of a Conceptual Model or Framework in Research* (Louis and Koertvelyessy, 1989) was developed to incorporate these various works into one tool. The *Guide* was used to assess inclusion of Neuman Model phenomena in the reviewed studies (Neuman, 1989).

As noted by Laudan (1993), theories and models are modified or changed more readily than the criteria used to assess their value. For example, in 1989 Dr. Neuman added the concepts of "spirituality" and "created environment" to the Neuman Systems Model. However, the criteria for science have remained essentially the same (Laudan, 1993). The *Guide* is used again to determine the depth and breadth of the use of the Neuman Model in the reported research literature and to offer updated continuity from the previous review (1989) (see Appendix A).

RESEARCH USE OF THE NEUMAN SYSTEMS MODEL

The purpose of the remainder of this chapter is to discuss the use of the Neuman Systems Model in nursing research and provide an update from previous citations of research studies identified as being based on the model. Over the years Dr. Neuman has been aware that the Neuman Systems Model was being used in master's theses and doctoral dissertations due to the extensive number of graduate students who have made personal contacts. To assess how these and other studies were applying the model in the research process, a survey was made of Dr. Neuman's personal contact list as well as an extensive search of published literature through CINAL and MEDLINE. The result identified a marked increase in use of the model and in the number of published studies using the model. Over 40 publications, between 1989 and 1993, were identified in which the Neuman Systems Model was reported as guiding nursing practice with clients in various settings (Appendix B). Use of the model as a teaching aide was also identified in these publications.

In relation to research-based publications for the five years between 1989 and 1993, nearly 100 research studies were identified in which the Neuman Systems Model served as the organizing framework. A summary of the identified research based on the Neuman Systems Model follows. In addition, to facilitate networking and collaboration of nurses interested in and conducting research using the Neuman Systems Model, Appendix A includes an annotated bibliography of selected studies, and Appendix B includes citations of research studies (either in process or completed).

Summary of Use of the Model in the Research Process

The phenomena of the model used in reviewing the studies are those identified by Neuman (in Fawcett and Downs, 1992) and include:

1. The physiological, psychological, sociocultural, developmental, and spiritual variables
2. Properties of the central or basic core structure of the client system
3. Properties of the flexible and normal lines of defense as well as the lines of resistance
4. Characteristics of the internal, external, and created environments
5. Characteristics of intra-, inter-, and extrapersonal stressors

6. Elements of primary, secondary, and tertiary prevention as intervention modalities

When complete study reports could be assessed, they were reviewed for use of the model based on the above phenomena and the five criteria identified in the *Guide for Selection and Use of a Conceptual Model or Framework in Research*. A brief description of the five criteria follows.

Criterion 1: Provide an Outline of the Phenomena to Be Investigated.
All six categories of the phenomena for the Neuman Systems Model were found in the studies reviewed. The five variables—physiological, psychological, sociocultural, developmental, and spiritual—were all used in varying degrees. Several studies included all five variables (Barrow, 1992; Vujakovich, 1993; Decker and Young, 1991). The psychological and sociocultural were the most frequently included. The physiological variable was found in Therrien's (1993) work with weight gain and breast cancer treatments, Heffline's (1991) study of postanesthesia shivering, and Speck's (1990) work with nursing students and injection skill. Interestingly, the spiritual variable, added recently, was found more frequently than the developmental variable, which was included in Neuman's first writings of the model. Use of the spirituality concept was found in work by Decker and Young (1991), Fulton (1993), Ivey (1993), and Klimek (1993). The developmental variable was specifically included in Speck's (1990) study of use of guided imagery by nursing students.

The system properties of the central core also varied in the studies reviewed and included cancer patients, families and their caregivers, nurses as caregivers, or nursing as a career. Several studies used children or the elderly as the system.

The lines of defense, both flexible and normal, and lines of resistance were studied by Barrow (1992) and Courchene, Patalski, and Martin (1991). Several studies used interventions of guided imagery (Leja, 1989; Speck, 1990) to strengthen flexible lines of defense. The distinction between strengthening a line of defense and reducing a stressor is not clearly distinguished in the studies. This is an important area for further research clarification.

Characteristics of the environment (internal, external, and created) were studied by Barrow (1992). Courchene, Patalski, and Martin (1991) identified the environment as the client system core in their study of the health of nurses administering cyclosporine A. Hinds (1990) used environemnt as a predictor of quality of life. Environment as a concept was infrequently included.

Study of a stressor in relation to nursing practice seems to be the key component in almost all of the studies. The stressor concept may be a major reason the Neuman Systems Model is chosen to guide a study. One can readily see the relationship between the various stressors and the client or study problems. Consequently, the researcher can easily envision how to use the Neuman Systems Model to guide a study of how, why, and what to do when encountering stressors.

All three levels of prevention as interventions were used in the studies. Some studies investigated all three (Loescher et al., 1990; Robin, 1991), and others investigated only one or two levels as the researcher deemed appropriate (Hinds, 1990; Leja, 1989; Puetz, 1990). There is great variation as to how the model has been used. For example, the client system is usually identified as individuals, two groups such as client and nurse or client and family, and caregivers or nurses.

Criterion 2: Direct the Method to Be Used in the Investigation. This

step includes identifying the nature of the problem and purposes of the research project. Neuman (1985, 1989) has identified the clinical problem as being of interest in relating the impact of the stressor on the stability of the client and the ability to predict the prevention as intervention mode required to retain, attain, or maintain client system stability. More specifically, she sees a relationship of harmony to wellness and perceptions to wellness, and a congruence of client and caregiver perceptions.

Many studies used a design level that does not allow prediction to be made about the efficacy of the prevention as intervention concept. This is not a negative but simply reflects the type of design that the researcher used in testing the model. Approximately one-third of the designs used were of an experimental type, and of these only about five were identified as experimental with randomization, control group, and manipulation of subjects. Another six were identified as having used intact groups in the study, thus decreasing the generalizability of the findings.

Criterion 3: Guide Data Collection and Analysis. Neuman has identi-

fied the model as being appropriate for use with individuals, families, and communities. The studies used children with injection pain (Maron, in process), adults with postoperative shivering (Heffline, 1991), and perceptions of the patient and nurse (Puetz, 1990). Anxiety was a variable studied by many as a response to stressors.

Families were studied in their role as caregiver, and in their response to a family member's illness, including head trauma and cancer. Homogeneous community groups such as clerical workers, nursing students, community and acute care nurses, and nonnurse professional women were also studied. Other groups under study included those whose basic core structure was described as coronary artery bypass graft (CABG) clients, and older adults postoperatively. Cancer-related groups comprised about one-fourth of the subject groups and data sets.

Analysis techniques varied, with most of the studies using quantitative analysis as appropriate to the design and data collected. Researchers were able to use the model with a variety of designs, including methodological studies (Ivey, 1993; Robin, 1991).

Criterion 4: Guide the Interpretation of the Findings. Findings were related back to the model in most instances, and the model was used to focus findings and identify future research needs.

Overall the studies did advance understanding of the relationship between prevention as intervention and client system stability. Some studies found no significant relationships. Others indicated decisive results. Before making value judgments of this contradiction, one needs to carefully examine each study individually to assess the rigor of the study. Another area for assessment is whether the prevention as intervention used in studies with nonsignificant findings was truly strong enough to make the predicted impact on the stressor and response to it to retain, maintain, or attain client stability. In some studies the prevention as intervention that was used seemed to be either too weak or not applied for a sufficient time period to logically expect a reduction of the stressor or a strengthening of the lines of defense and resistance. Puetz (1990) discussed a need for greater or stronger intervention and over a longer period of time to achieve the predicted outcome for future study related to coronary artery bypass graft clients.

The studies that were reviewed do indicate support that the model can be successfully used in empirical research that incorporates the phenomena of the model (Neuman, 1992) and meets the five research process criteria. The ability to make predictions based on the model is less conclusive. The mixed findings suggest the need for continued rigorous studies using the model.

Criterion 5: Direct the Use of Findings for Future Studies and Nursing Practice. Findings from studies using the model did identify future study and practice impact. The studies suggesting the next research direction were the clearest and easiest to follow. Barrow (1992) proposed further study related to the internal lines of resistance and the CCRN credential, and Filmore (1992) recommended further study of preventions as interventions in relation to educational interventions for preoperative clients. Others proposed interventions for practice situations were based on their findings, such as Courchene et al.'s (1991) proposal of primary prevention interventions for the pediatric nurse to reduce the impact of the stressor (exposure to CyA). If all researchers would complete this final recommended step following the analysis of their work, it would enhance the overall knowledge base of nursing and future use of the model. It is the researcher who is best prepared to make these recommendations because of his or her intimate knowledge of the total study.

SUMMARY

In summary, the Neuman Systems Model has been successfully used to guide research studies to include all six categories of phenomena of the model (Neuman, 1992). Research reports indicate use of the model for all stages or steps of the research process. The model has been used with experimental and nonexperimental types of research. The model seems to be most useful when stress and responses to it are being considered in almost any grouping of study subjects.

The increase over the last five years in articles and studies using the model may be attributed in part to the Biennial Neuman Systems Model International Symposia, where nurses from around the world present and discuss their use of the model. For these nurses the symposia provide a vehicle for discussion and resolution of the questions they may have. My own experience has been that these symposia are a very fertile environment for researchers in particular to gain insights into research questions and the dilemmas encountered when attempting to conduct research using a nursing model.

Overall the findings from this review support the position that the model has definite value in guiding nursing research and that the model can be tested using the scientific method.

FUTURE IMPLICATIONS FOR USE OF THE NEUMAN SYSTEMS MODEL IN NURSING RESEARCH

The Neuman Systems Model is used widely in research, and the research supports the view that the model is being successfully applied in directing nursing practice (over 100 published articles were found). Review of research studies suggests more testing is needed to clarify questions related to the Neuman Systems Model. Additional questions include: What is the relationship between prevention as intervention and the stressor or the response to the stressor? To what extent can the applied preventions as interventions retain, attain, or maintain desired client system stability? Are the interventions of sufficient strength or vigor? Is there a distinction between strengthening a line of defense and reducing a stressor?

Review of the research using the Neuman Systems Model supports the continuing need for rigorous examination of the relationships between components of the model and the prediction of outcomes for the client. Studies are also needed to determine the impact of nursing interventions in relation to projected changes in health care delivery systems. Future refinement of professional nursing practice and desired outcomes will require scientific data to support the need for preventions as interventions provided by nurses to retain, attain, and maintain the health of their clients.

To facilitate networking and collaborating of nurses who are interested in the Neuman Systems Model or are conducting research using the model, Appendix A includes citations and an annotated bibliography of the use of the model, and Appendix B includes citations of studies that are in process as well as completed research studies.

REFERENCES

Fawcett, J. 1989. *Analysis and Evaluation of Conceptual Models of Nursing,* 2d ed. Philadelphia: F. A. Davis Company.

Fawcett, J., and Downs, F. S. 1992. *The Relationship of Theory and Research,* 2d ed. Philadelphia: F. A. Davis Company.

Hayman, L. L. 1987. Fatal flaws. *Nursing Research* 56(5):267.

Johnson, D. 1968. Theory in nursing: Borrowed and unique. *Nursing Research* 17(3): 206–209.

Laudan, L. 1977. *Progress and Its Problems: Towards a Theory of Scientific Growth.* Berkeley: University of California Press.

Laudan, L. 1993. How scientific controversies end. Colloquium, Philosophy Department, University of Nevada, Las Vegas, March 30.

Louis, M., and Koertvelyessy, A. 1989. The Neuman Model in nursing research. In *The Neuman Systems Model,* 2d ed., edited by B. Neuman. San Mateo, Calif.: Appleton & Lange.

Schlotfeldt, R. M. 1975. The need for a conceptual framework. In *Nursing Research 1,* edited by P. J. Verhonick, 1–24. Boston: Little, Brown.

Silva, M. C. 1981. Selection of a theoretical framework. In *Readings in Nursing Research,* edited by S. D. Krampitz and N. Pevlovich. St. Louis: Mosby.

Suppe, F., and Jacox, A. 1985. Philosophy of science and the development of nursing theory. In *Annual Review of Nursing Research,* Vol. 3, edited by H. Werley and J. J. Fitzpatrick. New York: Springer.

Stevens-Barnum, B. J. 1990. *Nursing Theory Analysis, Application, Evaluation,* 3rd ed. Glenview, Ill.: Scott, Foresman/Little, Brown Higher Education.

APPENDIX A ————————————

Annotated Bibliography of Selected Completed Studies Applying the *Guide for Selection and Use of a Conceptual Model or Framework in Research*

Barrow, J. M. 1992. Type A behavior, job stress, social support, and job satisfaction in critical care nurses. Unpublished thesis, Northwestern State University of Louisiana, Shreveport, Louisiana.

1. *Provide an outline of phenomena to be investigated.* The Neuman Systems Model was used with critical care nurses (CCRN) as the client. Leaving critical care nursing was identified as analogous to their system core being penetrated. The line of resistance was the social support CCRNs receive, the normal line of defense was the inherent behavior type of the CCRN (type A or B), the flexible line of defense was their degree of job satisfaction, and job stress was the stressor that could cause a reaction.

2. *Direct the method to be used in the investigation.* The descriptive correlational design study tested six hypotheses developed from the model. Data were collected using tools designed to measure the variables as defined from the model.

3. *Guide data collection and analysis.* The subjects and population were CCRNs and were the identified client. Analysis tested the hypotheses developed from the model.

4. *Guide the interpretation of the findings.* The stressors were found to be related to the lines of resistance and flexible line of defense as identified in the study. However, the normal line of defense was not supported as being related to the lines of resistance, flexible line of defense, or stressor.

5. *Direct the use of findings for future studies and nursing practice.* Barrow proposed that the CCRN credential acts as a secondary or tertiary prevention as intervention. Further study was suggested related to the internal lines of resistance and the CCRN credential.

Courchene, V. S., Patalski, E., and Martin, J. 1991. A study of the health of pediatric nurses administering cyclosporine A. *Pediatric Nursing* 17(5):497–500.

1. *Provide an outline of phenomena to be investigated.* Pediatric nurses were identified as the client and CyA as environmental stressor.

2. *Direct the method to be used in the investigation.* They tested if the exposure of pediatric nurses' skin to CyA, an immunosuppressant, was related to their health status. The flexible line of defense was identified as being penetrated when the nurse had complaints, symptoms, or disease.

3. *Guide data collection and analysis.* The subjects and setting used by the researchers were congruent with the model. They did not measure serous fluids for contamination even though their literature suggested such from rat studies.

4. *Guide the interpretation of the findings.* The findings were consistent with the model.

5. *Direct the use of findings for future studies and nursing practice.* They proposed primary prevention actions for the pediatric nurse to reduce the impact of the stressor (exposure to CyA).

Decker, S. D., and Young, E. 1991. Self-perceived needs of primary caregivers of home-hospice clients. *Journal of Community Health Nursing* 8(30):147–154.

1. *Provide an outline of phenomena to be investigated.* The Neuman Systems Model provided the interview guide for the qualitative and quantitative data collected in this study.

2. *Direct the method to be used in the investigation.* Twenty-one primary caregivers for hospice patients were interviewed. The patient and family were both identified as client system cores.

3. *Guide data collection and analysis.* An instrument was designed to elicit information about intra-, inter-, and extrapersonal stressors in regard to physiological, psychological, sociocultural, developmental, and spiritual aspects of the caregivers' life situation.

4. *Guide the interpretation of the findings.* Decker and Young identified needs that were translated into five diagnoses.
5. *Direct the use of findings for future studies and nursing practice.* Primary preventive interventions such as ongoing assessment, teaching, and provision of adequate respite were proposed as ways the nurse can assist the caregivers to withstand the stressors impinging upon them.

Fillmore, J. A. 1992. The effects of preoperative teaching on anxiety levels of hysterectomy patients. Unpublished thesis, University of Nevada, Las Vegas.

1. *Provide an outline of phenomena to be investigated.* The Neuman Systems Model guided this study of the effects of preoperative teaching on anxiety levels of hysterectomy patients.
2. *Direct the method to be used in the investigation.* The experimental study included 40 women, divided at random to either preoperative teaching for hysterectomy surgery or routine preparation for the same surgery. The model was used to guide the content for the preoperative teaching intervention (teaching or primary prevention).
3. *Guide data collection and analysis.* Primary intervention was identified as preoperative teaching aimed at strengthening the flexible line of defense to prevent hazard from occurring or to decrease the impact of the stressor (surgery). Surgery, a stressor, was identified as both physical and psychological. It was proposed that as the client's knowledge of surgical experience increases, there is a strengthening of the normal line of defense, which increases the ability to cope more successfully with the stress of surgery.
4. *Guide the interpretation of the findings.* The findings were interpreted using the Neuman Systems Model. The findings showed the anxiety levels of the experimental group were lower, suggesting support of the Neuman Systems Model even though the anxiety levels were not statistically significant.
5. *Direct the use of findings for future studies and nursing practice.* Recommendations included further study of prevention as intervention strategies in relation to educational intervention.

Hinds, C. 1990. Personal and contextual factors predicting patients' reported quality of life: Exploring congruency with Betty Neuman's assumptions. *Journal of Advanced Nursing* 15:456–462.

1. *Provide an outline of phenomena to be investigated.* The study applied seven variables of interest to the Neuman Systems Model.
2. *Direct the method to be used in the investigation.* The congruency of seven quality of life predictor variables with the Neuman Systems Model for lung cancer patients was assessed.
3. *Guide data collection and analysis.* Person/client, environment

(including created environment), health, nursing, and intervention were compared to seven quality of life measures.

4. *Guide the interpretation of the findings.* Hinds found congruence between Neuman Systems Model concepts and the quality of life measures.

5. *Direct the use of findings for future studies and nursing practice.* Goals for nursing were proposed through use of the Neuman Systems Model.

Ivey, B. 1993. Evaluation of social support tools for women with diagnosed breast cancer. Unpublished thesis, University of Nevada, Las Vegas.

1. *Provide an outline of phenomena to be investigated.* Ivey used the Neuman Systems Model to guide a methodological study of the use of previously developed social support tools with women diagnosed with breast cancer.

2. *Direct the method to be used in the investigation.* Over eighty women with breast cancer were included in the survey study assessing their social support. Neuman Systems Model concepts were assessed with the questionnaires under study.

3. *Guide data collection and analysis.* Tests to measure the Neuman Systems Model's spiritual variable were used.

4. *Guide the interpretation of the findings.* The tools were found to have support in measuring sociocultural variables as defined by the model. It was also identified that intra-, inter-, and extrapersonal stressors can be assessed with the PRQ.

5. *Direct the use of findings for future studies and nursing practice.* Ivey identified that the PRQ has support for reliability, concurrent validity, and construct validity in assessing the sociocultural concept in women with breast cancer.

Leja, A. M. 1989. Using guided imagery to combat postsurgical depression. *Journal of Gerontological Nursing* 15(4):6–11.

1. *Provide an outline of phenomena to be investigated.* The Neuman Systems Model was used to a guide study of the impact of guided imagery (primary prevention) for elder postoperative persons about to be discharged (stressors) and the subsequent strengthening of the line of defense.

2. *Direct the method to be used in the investigation.* The client groups and the two hypotheses tested were congruent with the Neuman Systems Model.

3. *Guide data collection and analysis.* The independent variable was guided imagery (GIDT) of the home environment, including care of wound, ADL, etc. The dependent variable, psychological response, was measured using the Beck Depression Scale.

4. *Guide the interpretation of the findings.* Findings suggest GIDT used as primary prevention did strengthen older persons' line of defense, thus supporting the Neuman Systems Model's theory relative to primary prevention. The findings did not support that this was significantly different from routine discharge planning, however.

5. *Direct the use of findings for future studies and nursing practice.* Leja suggested further study, such as increasing the sample size over 10 and assessing areas other than just depression in relation to the psychological variable.

Loescher, L. J., Clark, L., Attwood, J. R., Leigh, S., and Lamb, G. (1990). The impact of cancer experience on long-term survivors. *Oncology Nursing Forum* 17(20):223–229.

1. *Provide an outline of phenomena to be investigated.* The Neuman Systems Model was used to guide the exploratory study of needs of adult survivors of cancers.

2. *Direct the method to be used in the investigation.* It was proposed that the cancer as stressor was capable of invoking physiological, psychological, or socioeconomic system instability based on the Neuman Systems Model. A wholistic approach was proposed to better assess the open system of intra- and extrapersonal environmental factors' interaction by adjusting to the situation.

3. *Guide data collection and analysis.* The Cancer Survivor Questionnaire (22 short open-ended items) of changes, problems/concerns, and needs was used. It was worded to elicit emic (subject's own words) answers.

4. *Guide the interpretation of the findings.* Both qualitative and quantitative analyses were used. Deductive findings were analyzed in relation to physiological, psychological, and socioeconomic changes, problem/concern, and needs. The findings were consistent with the Neuman Systems Model in relation to intra- and interpersonal relationships.

5. *Direct the use of findings for future studies and nursing practice.* Conclusions and recommendations were made in primary, secondary, and tertiary prevention modes. Use of the model enhanced the study and allows for projection of the findings beyond the 17 subjects.

Mendez, D. 1990. College students' image of nursing as a career choice. Unpublished thesis, University of Nevada, Las Vegas.

1. *Provide an outline of phenomena to be investigated.* The Neuman Systems Model guided the comparative survey of college students—161 nonnursing and 93 nursing students—in relation to their image of nursing as a career and ideal profession.

2. *Direct the method to be used in the investigation.* She tested five hypotheses of factors related to a nursing career and an ideal career.

3. *Guide data collection and analysis.* Mendez took the position that nursing's image is a stressor impinging on nursing's flexible lines of defense. Her tools measured perception of an ideal career and of nursing as a career. Her core groups were college students, those enrolled in a nursing major, and those not enrolled in a nursing major.

4. *Guide the interpretation of the findings.* The findings were presented in relation to secondary prevention, with the public and nurses' own image being the stressor that needs intervention. The study dealt with stressors being intra-, inter-, and extrapersonal to nursing. The flexible and normal lines of defense were identified.

5. *Direct the use of findings for future studies and nursing practice.* It was noted that nursing needs to deal with its stressor (image) for recruitment and retention of professional nurses.

Pardee, C. J. 1992. Evaluating family caregivers' ability to select appropriate care techniques following discharge instructions on post traumatic brain injury symptoms. Unpublished thesis, Grand Valley State University, Michigan.

1. *Provides an outline of phenomena to be investigated.* The Neuman Systems Model was identified as appropriate for use when developing an educational plan for family members of brain-injured individuals. The family caregiver was the client, a system composed of physiological, psychological, developmental, sociocultural, and spiritual variables. The family members were identified as having had their flexible and normal lines of defense penetrated by the stressor of brain injury to a family member. Nursing interventions under study were actions to support the family in responding to the stressor.

2. *Direct the method to be used in the investigation.* Subjects and setting were congruent with the model. The hypothesis derived from the model was "family caregivers will increase their ability to select appropriate action for posttraumatic brain injury symptoms when provided with information on cognitive dysfunction and behavioral changes compared to families who do not receive instruction."

3. *Guide data collection and analysis.* In the experimental design the independent variable was the education program and the dependent variable the caregivers' posttest score on action related to brain injury symptoms.

4. *Guide the interpretation of the findings.* The research hypothesis was supported.

5. *Direct the use of findings for future studies and nursing practice.* Pardee did not specifically include the model in discussion of the findings as related to future study or practice.

Puetz, R. 1990. Nurse and patient perception of stressors associated with coronary artery bypass surgery. Unpublished thesis, University of Nevada, Las Vegas.

1. *Provide an outline of phenomena to be investigated.* In a study of nurse and patient perceptions of stressors associated with coronary artery bypass surgery (CABG), the Neuman Systems Model was applied using two system cores: the patient with CABG and the nurse.

2. *Direct the method to be used in the investigation.* The prevention as intervention was the alliance between patient and nurse to identify the patient needs. Incongruence between nurse and patient can become a stressor to the patient.

3. *Guide data collection and analysis.* Three hypotheses related to the congruence of the nurse and patient perceptions of stressors related to CABG were tested. Intrapersonal stress was determined to be the conditioned responses to life events, loss, grief, developmental changes, and conformity to social norms as measured by CSSS. Interpersonal responses to the interaction between patient and spouse, significant others, nurse, physicians, and other patients were measured by CSSS. Extrapersonal responses to financial concerns, visiting hour restrictions, hospital environment, and hospital equipment were also measured by CSSS.

4. *Guide the interpretation of the findings.* Puetz found incongruencies between patient and nurse perception of stressors. Self-perception was reflected by how one integrates stimuli from the psychological, social, emotional, and physical aspects of the environment. Incongruencies found were identified as being due to the nurse not assessing "individual" patient needs and not assessing the patient's ability to meet those needs.

5. *Direct the use of findings for future studies and nursing practice.* It was proposed that the duration of the intervention needs to be greater (longer than one 12-hour shift), or perhaps the skill of the nurse needs to be increased to be effective in identifying the patient's view of his or her stressors and needs.

Robin, N. S. 1991. Clinical evaluation of the ectopic pregnancy risk assessment screening tool: A retrospective study. Unpublished thesis, University of Texas Health Science Center at Houston.

1. *Provide an outline of phenomena to be investigated.* The Neuman Systems Model was used to guide a validation study of a tool to diagnose ectopic pregnancy and use of the information obtained from the tool in primary, secondary, and tertiary prevention. Patient education and maintenance of health to sustain a safe and viable pregnancy was seen as primary prevention. Secondary prevention dealt with screening and case finding. Tertiary prevention included

education of pregnant women with signs and symptoms of ectopic pregnancy, as identified with the tool, to strengthen the lines of defense to keep the stressor from penetration.

2. *Direct the method to be used in the investigation.* The hypothesis tested was "Does the Ectopic Pregnancy Risk Assessment Screening Tool differentiate women who subsequently are diagnosed as having ectopic from intrauterine pregnancy?"

3. *Guide data collection and analysis.* The pregnant woman was identified as the client.

4. *Guide the interpretation of the findings.* Robin discussed the findings in relation to the Neuman Systems Model, seeing it as a valuable tool for screening. These findings can then be used in client education to strengthen the lines of defense and protect the central core structure of the client as a system.

5. *Direct the use of findings for future studies and nursing practice.* Implications for practice and recommendations for further research were congruent with the use of the model in the study.

Therrien, S. 1993. Weight gain in women with stage I and stage II breast cancer. Unpublished thesis, University of Nevada, Las Vegas.

1. *Provide an outline of phenomena to be investigated.* Weight gain in 213 women with stage I and stage II breast cancer over a 12- and 24-month period was studied.

2. *Direct the method to be used in the investigation.* The Neuman Systems Model was used to guide study, with the main focus being limited to physiological factors. Other Neuman Systems Model concepts were assessed to describe the sample.

3 *Guide data collection and analysis.* Data collection was related to the four hypotheses and the physical concepts of weight gain, stage of disease, and use of chemotherapy or a Tamoxifan-only treatment.

4. *Guide the interpretation of the findings.* It was found that both groups, stage I and stage II, gain weight over 12 and 24 months, regardless of treatment type (chemotherapy or Tamoxifan only). Weight gain was not statistically different between the groups.

5. *Direct the use of findings for future studies and nursing practice.* Future studies were identified as well as the need to include other Neuman Systems Model concepts to be wholistic in further determining the full impact or relationship of factors to weight gain in breast cancer women.

Wilkey, S. F. 1990. The effects of an eight-hour continuing education course on the death anxiety levels of registered nurses. Unpublished thesis, University of Nevada, Las Vegas.

1. *Provide an outline of phenomena to be investigated.* Two theories were combined for a framework to study the effects of an eight-hour continuing education course on the death anxiety levels of registered nurses. The primary prevention mode of intervention of the Neuman Systems Model identified the purpose, hypothesis, significance, and interventions tested. The belief-oriented approach used was the social learning theory of Bandura.

2. *Direct the method to be used in the investigation.* Primary prevention as a treatment modality focused on need determination, objective and goal identification, education, and other supportive interventions that augment the existing strengths related to the nurse's flexible line of defense. The process of dying and the event of death are major stress-producing forces, whether intra-, inter-, or extrapersonally. As environmental stressors, dying and death can create significant anxieties and fears to threaten the stability and equilibrium of an individual, family, or community. Certain attitudes, abhorrence, shame surrounding the dying process, and the event of death are also used with the model. Intrapersonal stressors were identified as primordial anxieties of nonexistence, fears regarding "afterlife," lack of experience in confronting death as an inevitable life occurrence, and lack of knowledge of the dying and death process.

3. *Guide data collection and analysis.* The intervention of information was aimed at increasing the strength of the nurse's flexible line of defense as it relates to death anxiety to better prepare the nurse for more effective confrontation in situations of dying and death.

4. *Guide the interpretation of the findings.* The two hypotheses tested found anxiety as measured did decrease but not significantly and that differences between the groups of nurses with and without education program were not significant.

5. *Direct the use of findings for future studies and nursing practice.* Future study suggested use of the model for enhancing the use of primary prevention as intervention.

APPENDIX B ─────────────

Research Studies Using the Neuman Systems Model (1989–1993)

Adams, D. In process. Focus on concept of hope within the spiritual variable in care of AIDS clients. Dissertation study, Wayne State University, Michigan.

Agcaoili, R. M. In process. Stressor reduction effectiveness for parents and children of pre and post operative telephone contact with parents of pediatric day surgery clients. Thesis study, D'Youville College, Buffalo, New York.

Ali, N. S., and Khalil, H. A. 1989. Effect of psychoeducational intervention on anxiety among Egyptian bladder cancer patients. *Cancer Nursing* 12(4):236–42.

Anderson, B., and Lowry, L. W. 1990. Do clients incorporate the ventilator into their created environment? Paper presented at the Third Biennial Neuman Systems Model International Symposium, Dayton, Ohio, November 14–16.

Barnes, K. M. 1993. The relationship between mistreatment of the elderly, quality of care and demographic characteristics. Paper presented at the Fourth Biennial Neuman Systems Model International Symposium, Rochester, New York, April 22–24.

Barrow, J. M. 1992. Type A behavior, job stress, social support, and job satisfaction in critical care nurses. Unpublished thesis, Northwestern State University of Louisiana, Shreveport, Louisiana.

Blank, J. J., Clark, L., Longman, A. J., and Atwood, J. R. 1989. Perceived home care needs of cancer patients and their care givers. *Cancer Nursing* 12(2):78–84.

Bolen, S. 1990. The relationship between spiritual well-being and life satisfaction in the elderly. Paper presented at the Third Biennial Neuman Systems Model International Symposium, Dayton, Ohio, November 14–16.

Bowdler, J. E., and Barrell, L. M. 1987. Health needs of homeless persons. *Public Health Nursing* 5(3):135–140.

Cammuso, B. S. 1993. Caring and accountability in nursing practice in Ireland and the United States: Helping Irish nurses bridge the gap when they choose to practice in the United States. Paper presented at the Fourth Biennial Neuman Systems Model International Symposium, Rochester, New York, April 22–24.

Cantin, B., and Mitchell, M. 1989. Nurses' smoking behavior. *Canadian Nurse* 85(1):20–21.

Carroll, T. L. 1989. Role deprivation in baccalaureate nursing students pre and post curriculum revision. *Journal of Nursing Education* 28(3):134–139.

Case, S. C. 1992. The immediate perceived needs of family members of trauma patients and how they differ from the nurses perceptions of needs. Unpublished thesis, University of Nevada, Las Vegas.

Clark, C., Cross, J. R., Deane, D. M., and Lowry, L. W. 1991. Spirituality: Integral to quality care. *Holistic Nursing Practice* 5(3):67–76.

Clark, C. A., Cross, J., Deane, D., and Lowry, L. W. 1990. Operationalizing the spiritual variable of Neuman Systems Model: An interdisciplinary inquiry. Paper presented at the Third Biennial Neuman Systems Model International Symposium, Dayton, Ohio, November 14–16.

Collins, A. S. 1993. Effects of positional changes on selected physiological and psychological measurements in clients with atrial fibrillation. Paper presented at the Fourth Biennial Neuman Systems Model International Symposium, Rochester, New York, April 22–24.

Courchene, V. S., Patalski, E., and Martin, J. 1991. A study of the health of pediatric nurses administering cyclosporine A. *Pediatric Nursing* 17(5):497–500.

Craig, D. 1993. Older adults' use of nursing services, life stress, ways of coping and health, mood and energy for life. Paper presented at the Fourth Biennial Neuman Systems Model International Symposium, Rochester, New York, April 22–24.

Cross, J., and Deane, D. 1990. Evolution of spiritual inquiry at Wright State University–Miami Valley. Paper presented at the Third Biennial Neuman Systems Model International Symposium, Dayton, Ohio, November 14–16.

Davis, A. In process. Social support and fear of recurrence in women who have had breast cancer ten years post-diagnosis. Dissertation study, University of Alabama, Birmingham.

Deane, D., Cross, J. R., and Barber, S. 1990. Spiritual well-being and role attitudes of student nurses. Paper presented at the Third Biennial Neuman Systems Model International Symposium, Dayton, Ohio, November 14–16.

Decker, S. D., and Young, E. 1991. Self-perceived needs of primary caregivers of home-hospice clients. *Journal of Community Health Nursing* 8(30):147–154.

Dombeck, M-T. B. 1993. Bifurcation and self-organization as a consequence of spiritual disequilibrium. Paper presented at the Fourth Biennial Neuman Systems Model International Symposium, Rochester, New York, April 22–24.

Fillmore, J. A. 1992. The effects of preoperative teaching on anxiety levels of hysterectomy patients. Unpublished thesis, University of Nevada, Las Vegas.

Fulton, R. A. 1990. Concept analysis of spirituality. Paper presented at the Third Biennial Neuman Systems Model International Symposium, Dayton, Ohio, November 14–16.

Fulton, R. A. B. 1993. Spiritual well-being of baccalaureate nursing students and nursing faculty and their responses about spiritual well-being of persons. Paper presented at the Fourth Biennial Neuman Systems Model International Symposium, Rochester, New York, April 22–24.

Gavigan, M., Kline-O'Sullivan, C., and Klumpp-Lybrand, B. 1990. The effect of regular turning on CABG patients. *Critical Care Nursing Quarterly* March:69–76.

Gibson, D. E. 1990. A Q-Analysis of interpersonal trust in the nurse–client relationship. Paper presented at the Third Biennial Neuman Systems Model International Symposium, Dayton, Ohio, November 14–16.

Girts, D., and Agostinelli, M. 1990. What do intubated patients perceive as effective nursing interventions to minimize stress? Paper presented at the Third Biennial Neuman Systems Model International Symposium, Dayton, Ohio, November 14–16.

Gloss, E. F., and Crowe, R. L. 1993. Coronary artery disease: Post menopausal women, power and anxiety. Paper presented at the Fourth Biennial Neuman Systems Model International Symposium, Rochester, New York, April 22–24.

Goedecke, D., and Jones, E. 1993. A comparison of personal factors in pregnant and non-pregnant adolescent girls. Paper presented at the Fourth Biennial Neuman Systems Model International Symposium, Rochester, New York, April 22–24.

Grant, J. 1992. Needs and resources of head injured adults being cared for in the home. Unpublished dissertation, University of Alabama, Birmingham.

Hainsworth, D., and Grimes, G. 1993. Use of the Neuman Model as a framework for research and educational interaction for nurses who care for terminally-ill patients and their families. Paper presented at the Fourth Biennial Neuman Systems Model International Symposium, Rochester, New York, April 22–24.

Hayes, K. 1990. The relationship between informal support and learned helplessness on the informal caregiver of the person with AIDS. Paper presented at the Third Biennial Neuman Systems Model International Symposium, Dayton, Ohio, November 14–16.

Heffline, M. S. 1991. A comparative study of pharmacological versus nursing interventions in the treatment of post anesthesia shivering. *Journal of Post Anesthesia Nursing* 6(50): 311–320.

Heiber, K. 1990. Nurses' spiritual well-being and attitudes regarding spiritual care. Paper presented at the Third Biennial Neuman Systems Model International Symposium, Dayton, Ohio, November 14–16.

Herrick, C. 1990. Neuman Systems Model for nursing practice as a conceptual framework for a family assessment. Paper presented at the Third Biennial Neuman Systems Model International Symposium, Dayton, Ohio, November 14–16.

Hinds, C. 1990. Personal and contextual factors predicting patients' reported quality of life: Exploring congruency with Betty Neuman's assumptions. *Journal of Advanced Nursing* 15:456–462.

Hobbs, B. B. 1990. The nurse manager's role in relation to the chemically impaired hospital nurse. Paper presented at the Third Biennial Neuman Systems Model International Symposium, Dayton, Ohio, November 14–16.

Huffstutler, S. In process. Changes in registered nurses on completion of their baccalaureate degree in nursing. Dissertation study, Auburn University.

Hui-Tseng, T. 1993. Cognition and anxiety level of pre-cardiac catheterization patients before and after education program. Paper presented at the Fourth Biennial Neuman Systems Model International Symposium, Rochester, New York, April 22–24.

Ivey, B. 1993. Evaluation of social support tools with women with diagnosed breast cancer. Unpublished thesis, University of Nevada, Las Vegas.

Kahn, E. C. 1990. Comparative study of perceived needs of family members of critically ill patients and family members of "Do Not Resuscitate" patients in the intensive care unit. Paper presented at the Third Biennial Neuman Systems Model International Symposium, Dayton, Ohio, November 14–16.

Klimek, S. 1993. Comparison of breast self examination practices of professional nurses and professional women not in health care. Unpublished thesis, University of Nevada, Las Vegas.

Laschinger, H. K., and Duff, V. 1991. Attitudes of practicing nurses towards theory-based nursing practice. *Canadian Journal of Nursing Administration* March/April:6–10.

Leja, A. M. 1989. Using guided imagery to combat postsurgical depression. *Journal of Gerontological Nursing* 15(4):6–11.

Lin, C. In process. Health belief knowledge related to cardiology of the elderly Tai population. Dissertation study, University of Alabama, Birmingham.

Lindell, M., and Olsson, H. 1991. Can combined oral contraceptives be made more effective by means of a nursing care model? *Journal of Advanced Nursing* 16:475–479.

Loescher, L. J., Clark, L., Atwood, J. R., Leigh, S., and Lamb, G. 1990. The impact of cancer experience on long-term survivors. *Oncology Nursing Forum* 17(20):223–229.

Louis, M. A. 1990. Refining preferred other network of elder widows using NSM with matrix analysis. Paper presented at the Third Biennial Neuman Systems Model International Symposium, Dayton, Ohio, November 14–16.

Lowry, L. W. 1990. Perceptions of newly graduated RNs concerning internalizations and application of NSM: A longitudinal study. Paper presented at the Third Biennial Neuman Systems Model International Symposium, Dayton, Ohio, November 14–16.

McDaniel, G. S. 1990. The effects of two methods of dangling on heart rate and blood pressure in postoperative abdominal hysterectomy patients. Paper presented at the Third Biennial Neuman Systems Model International Symposium, Dayton, Ohio, November 14–16.

Maron, S. K. In process. The effect of a cognitive intervention strategy on the preschool age child's perception of pain. Thesis study, Wright State University.

Mead-Bennett, E. 1990. An investigation of sleep loss in pregnancy using concepts from the Neuman Health Care Systems Model. Paper presented at the Third Biennial Neuman Systems Model International Symposium, Dayton, Ohio, November 14–16.

Mendez, D. 1990. College students' image of nursing as a career choice. Unpublished thesis, University of Nevada, Las Vegas.

Mirenda, R. M. 1990. Environment: A concept analysis. Paper presented at the Third Biennial Neuman Systems Model International Symposium, Dayton, Ohio, November 14–16.

Moseley, C. A. In process. Energy as related to the Neuman Model basic structure. Thesis study, Texas Woman's University, Denton, Texas.

Norris, B. W. 1990. Physiologic response to exercise in client with mitral valve prolapse syndrome. Paper presented at the Third Biennial Neuman Systems Model International Symposium, Dayton, Ohio, November 14–16.

Pardee, C. J. 1992. Evaluating family caregivers' ability to select appropriate care techniques following discharge instructions on post traumatic brain injury symptoms. Unpublished thesis, Grand Valley State University, Michigan.

Paul, P. In process. Pre and post discharge needs of clients 55 years of age or older. Dissertation study, University of Alabama, Birmingham.

Peske, G. W. 1990. The effectiveness of a learning activity package (L.A.P.) used in discharge teaching of the patient with chronic obstructive pulmonary disease. Paper presented at the Third Biennial Neuman Systems Model International Symposium, Dayton, Ohio, November 14–16.

Polomeno, V. In process. Family stress and high-risk pregnancy in newly immigrated families. Dissertation study, University of Montreal, Canada.

Poole, V. 1993. Pregnancy wantedness, attitude toward pregnancy and use of alcohol, tobacco, and street drugs during pregnancy. Paper presented at the Fourth Biennial Neuman Systems Model International Symposium, Rochester, New York, April 22–24.

Price, J. In process. Correlation between nurse employee work attendance and job stress. Thesis study, Barry University, Florida.

Puetz, R. 1990. Nurse and patient perception of stressors associated with coronary artery bypass surgery. Unpublished thesis, University of Nevada, Las Vegas.

Robin, N. S. 1991. Clinical evaluation of the ectopic pregnancy risk assessment screening tool: A retrospective study. Unpublished thesis, University of Texas Health Science Center at Houston.

Rose, B. S. In process. Bringing nursing theory to the front line of the acutely ill congestive heart failure client. Thesis study, Catholic University.

Rowles, C. J. 1993. The relationship between selected personal and organizational variables and the tenure of directors of nursing in nursing homes. Paper presented at the Fourth Biennial Neuman Systems Model International Symposium, Rochester, New York, April 22–24.

Shackleford, C. M. In process. Evaluation of intrapersonal and interpersonal stressors in the emergency department related to high burnout and turnover rates. Thesis study, University of Michigan.

Shambaugh, B. F. 1992. Evaluation of the effectiveness of the Neuman Systems Model as a theoretical framework for baccalaureate nursing programs. Unpublished dissertation, University of Massachusetts, Amherst.

Sipple, J. A. 1990. Curriculum change based on Neuman Model: Australian update. Paper presented at the Third Biennial Neuman Systems Model International Symposium, Dayton, Ohio, November 14–16.

Skipworth, D. In process. Intervention study for test effectiveness of a stress management support program for caregivers of frail elders. Dissertation study, University of Alabama, Birmingham.

South, L. In process. Self concept of children with cancer and their need for social support. Dissertation study, University of Alabama, Birmingham.

Speck, B. J. 1990. The effect of guided imagery upon first semester nursing students performing their first injections. *Journal of Nursing Education* 29(8):346–350.

Suttmiller, J. 1990. NSM and stressors, social support, coping responses and effectiveness in daughters with institutionalized mothers. Paper presented at the Third Biennial Neuman Systems Model International Symposium, Dayton, Ohio, November 14–16.

Therrien, S. 1993. Weight gain in women with stage I and stage II breast cancer. Unpublished thesis, University of Nevada, Las Vegas.

Vaughn, M., Cheatwood, S., Sirles, A. T., and Brown, K. C. 1989. The effect of progressive muscle relaxation on stress among clerical workers. *AAOHN Journal* 37(8): 302–306.

Virgin, S. In process. Hardiness in deans of schools of nursing. Dissertation study, Auburn University.

Vujakovich, M. A. In process. Relationship between family stress and coping behaviors in families of head injured individuals (Neuman). Thesis study, D'Youville College.

Waker, C. D. 1990. Professional nurses' levels of spiritual well-being and attitudes toward providing spiritual care. Paper presented at the Third Biennial Neuman Systems Model International Symposium, Dayton, Ohio, November 14–16.

Wilder, B. In process. Hardiness in older women age 65 and above. Dissertation study, Auburn University.

Wilkey, S. F. 1990. The effects of an eight-hour continuing education course on the death anxiety levels of registered nurses. Unpublished thesis, University of Nevada, Las Vegas.

Williamson, J. W. 1990. The influence of self-selected monotonous sounds on the night sleep patterns of post operative open heart patients. Paper presented at the Third Biennial Neuman Systems Model International Symposium, Dayton, Ohio, November 14–16.

Woodruff, D. 1990. Nevada nurses attitudes toward mandatory continuing education. Unpublished thesis, University of Nevada, Las Vegas.

Editorial Comments

Cynthia Flynn Capers

The following editorial comments connect Louis's chapter entitled "The Neuman Model in Nursing Research: An Update" to the development of middle range theories.

Nursing conceptual models are a rich source for the development of middle range theories. From Louis's analysis of research studies using the Neuman Systems Model, it is evident that theories pertaining to several of Neuman-based concepts could emerge. The following six areas of potential mid-range theory development are noted.

1. *Variables:* Descriptions and interrelatedness of the five variables of the person as relevant to assessment and diagnosis of health problems, and management of client care.
2. *Central core:* Description of the central/basic core of client systems and how the integrity of the core is related to overall levels of wellness of client systems.
3. *Lines of resistance:* Description and differentiation of the lines of defense, including the flexible and normal lines of defense and the internal lines of resistance.
4. *Created environment:* Description of the created environment and predictions about how this type of environment serves as a stressor and/or resource for client systems.
5. *Stressors:* Examination of the interrelatedness of intrapersonal, interpersonal, and extrapersonal stressors and the relevance that this interrelatedness has to levels of wellness.
6. *Prevention as intervention:* Further specification pertaining to the prescriptive value of primary, secondary, and tertiary prevention as intervention modalities.

Reconstitution and *client stability* are two additional concepts of the Neuman Systems Model that provide a base for mid-range theories. Reconstitution could be specified with identifiable behaviors and descriptors associated with the process of reconstituting. These behaviors could then be related to specific clinical situations. Finally, secondary preventions that promote reconstitution could be delineated.

Client stability could be developed to further specify clients stabilizing at levels below, the same, or above levels of wellness that were evident prior to interacting with stressors. Pertinent questions for theory development include: What are the factors that are related to each level of client stability? How do these attained levels of stability relate to the lines of defense and subsequent interactions with stressors? What are the nursing implications associated with client stability and varying levels of wellness?

From the proposed topics it is clear that the Neuman Systems Model is useful for the development of mid-range theories. Practice-based research programs can be developed with concepts of the Neuman Systems Model serving as the basis for research and selected clinical situations as the "operations" of the model's concepts. Through the development and implementation of several related studies, propositions derived from the Neuman Systems Model can be tested. In a heuristic manner, then, mid-range theories can emerge. These theories will be grounded in research and have specific applications to nursing practice.

The Neuman Systems Model has been useful for the development of individual research studies. It is now time for the model to be used as a base for establishing research programs for the purpose of developing and testing mid-range theories.

34

NEPHROLOGY PRACTICE AND DIRECTIONS FOR NURSING RESEARCH

Diane M. Breckenridge

This chapter focuses on how the author has used the Neuman Systems Model to develop middle range theory based on practice. The Health Care Focus for Renal Clients (Figure 34–1) and the Framework for Nephrology Nursing Practice (Figure 34–2) were developed and revised for practice (Breckenridge, 1982, 1989). Working with the Neuman Systems Model since the mid-1970s, the author more recently is finding that the philosophical underpinnings, concepts, and assumptions of the Neuman Systems Model have given directions for timely research of renal clients and nephrology practice decisions. The author will explain how the Neuman Systems Model gives direction for research based on practice.

THE NEED FOR PRACTICE-BASED RESEARCH

Nurses and other health care providers need to be aware of the current health care reform proposals, health policies, and regulations that specifically apply to their clinical practice area. This is particularly pertinent in the area of nephrology nursing since the end-stage renal disease (ESRD) program is the only national catastrophic health care reimbursement program in the United States. The Medicare ESRD program was implemented in 1973, providing dialysis to all clients in need regardless of age, medical condition, and/or ability to pay. Evans (1981) found that prior to this program the typical dialysis client was white, under 55 years of age, middle income, and male. Since the program's imple-

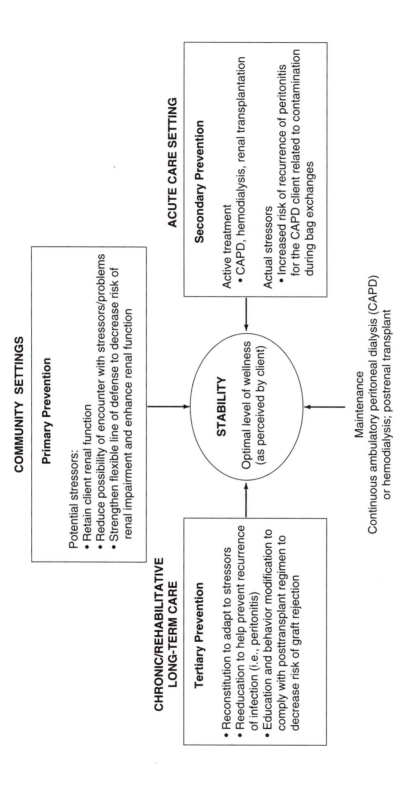

COMMUNITY SETTINGS

Primary Prevention

Potential stressors:
• Retain client renal function
• Reduce possibility of encounter with stressors/problems
• Strengthen flexible line of defense to decrease risk of renal impairment and enhance renal function

ACUTE CARE SETTING

Secondary Prevention

Active treatment
• CAPD, hemodialysis, renal transplantation

Actual stressors
• Increased risk of recurrence of peritonitis for the CAPD client related to contamination during bag exchanges

CHRONIC/REHABILITATIVE LONG-TERM CARE

Tertiary Prevention

• Reconstitution to adapt to stressors
• Reeducation to help prevent recurrence of infection (i.e., peritonitis)
• Education and behavior modification to comply with posttransplant regimen to decrease risk of graft rejection

STABILITY

Optimal level of wellness (as perceived by client)

Maintenance
Continuous ambulatory peritoneal dialysis (CAPD) or hemodialysis; postrenal transplant

Figure 34–1. Neuman-based health care focus for renal clients.

Nursing Process Format

I. Establish nursing diagnoses
- Assessment of potential and actual stressors (client's and caregiver's perceptions)

II. Formation of nursing goals (negotiated with client)
- Establish expected outcomes (client goals)
- Plan of care
  – Primary   Prevention interventions
              Retain existing renal functions
              Strengthen client's resistance to infection
  – Secondary CAPD; hemodialysis; transplantation; (renal replacement treatments)
              Posttreatment interventions
  – Tertiary Reeducate to prevent recurrence of infection (i.e., peritonitis)

III. Nursing outcomes
- Implementation–include: nurse consultation with other health care providers to direct total client care
- Evaluation
  – Measure expected outcomes
  – Reassess client stressors (problems)
  – Revise client problems and nursing goals
- Nephrology health care team
  – Nurse
  – Physician
  – Nutritionist
  – Clergy

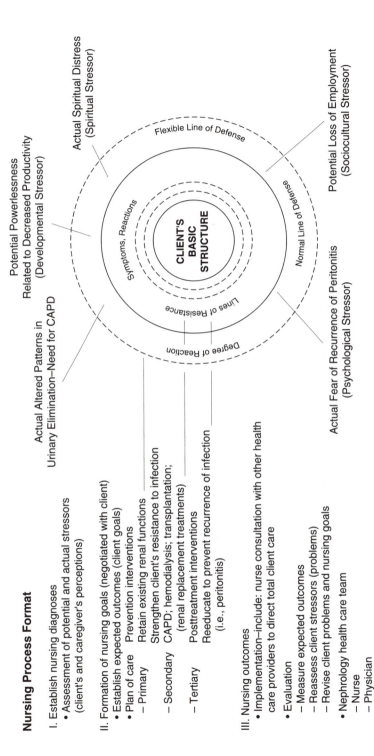

Figure 34–2. Neuman-based framework for nephrology nursing practice.

501

mentation there has been rapid growth both in the ESRD population and subsequently in program costs.

In 1974, 16,000 ESRD clients were covered under the program for $250 million as compared to only 1,000 clients in 1969, prior to the passing of the ESRD Medicare legislation. The latest number of clients is more than 140,000, at a cost exceeding $4 billion (Evans, Blagg, and Bryan, 1981; National Kidney Foundation, 1987, 1992).

Since 1982 the United States federal government's position has been to lower the amount of money reimbursed for treatment. This is being done by encouraging the less expensive forms of treatment modalities such as transplantation, home hemodialysis, self-care hemodialysis, and the home treatment of continuous ambulatory peritoneal dialysis (CAPD) (Richard, 1986). In fact, the cost of CAPD is approximately $10,000 per year as compared to $23,000 per client for in-center hemodialysis. Only 16,969 clients in the United States received CAPD in 1990, while 106,523 clients received in-center hemodialysis.

Moreover, research indicates that those clients undergoing the home treatment of CAPD have the highest quality of life when compared to in-center hemodialysis clients (Evans, Manninen, Garrison, Hart, Blagg, Gutman, Hull, and Lowrie, 1985; Bremer, McCauley, Wrona, and Johnson, 1989). Therefore, why are so many more clients on hemodialysis when the cost factor of CAPD is less than half that of hemodialysis and when the quality of life is higher? Is this because clients in the United States are counseled about all the treatment modalities and have a voice in which type they prefer? Research to gain more understanding of this phenomenon is being conducted by this author.

THE NEED FOR RESEARCH-BASED PRACTICE FOCUSED ON PREVENTIVE INTERVENTIONS

Since the cost to treat ESRD is so high, there needs to be an increased emphasis on the prevention of renal disease and continuing research to develop the most cost-efficient methods to treat clients with ESRD with the goal of reconstitution to an optimal level of functioning. Klingenstein (1986) states that the ultimate goal in the care of a client with renal disease, whether the person is newly diagnosed with renal hypertension or has progressed to ESRD, is to prevent further deterioration in functioning and to restore the client to a maximum level of satisfaction with life.

QUANTITATIVE RESEARCH APPROACH TO DEVELOP MIDDLE RANGE THEORY

Quantitative research is the paradigm used to investigate research hypotheses based on questions derived from a thorough literature search. To guide quantitative research based on the Neuman Systems Model, the three-level conceptual-theoretical-empirical structure, proposed by Fawcett and Downs (1992), and exemplified by Ziemer (1983) based on the model, was used for the renal client on the home dialysis modality of CAPD (Table 34–1). Since there is an identified need, based on the literature, to increase the area of primary prevention for renal clients, the Neuman Systems Model concept of primary prevention was explicated. This concept is based on the Neuman Systems Model's assumption that primary prevention is circular in nature and tends to lead back from tertiary prevention implemented after the initial secondary intervention of maintenance CAPD.

This conceptual-theoretical-empirical structure focuses on the effects of teaching aseptic technique for maintenance CAPD clients as a primary prevention as intervention to prevent or decrease the incidence of peritonitis. This adapted structure was conceptualized after the development and utilization of the Systematic Nursing Assessment Tool for the CAPD Client (Breckenridge, Cupit, and Raimondo, 1982, 1983) with research conducted to determine the major problem areas (stressors) for CAPD clients. The conceptual-theoretical-empirical structure is a formalization, for research purposes, of the Health care Focus for Renal Clients and a Framework for Nephrology Nursing Practice (Breckenridge, 1982, 1989).

One of the identified stressors/problems, peritonitis, was selected as the outcome because it is a major complication of CAPD (Zappacosta and Perras, 1984). Middle range theory that could be generated from this research focuses on the effects of teaching aseptic technique for the bag exchanges necessary for maintenance CAPD to prevent or decrease the incidence of peritonitis.

TABLE 34–1. CONCEPTUAL/THEORETICAL/EMPIRICAL STRUCTURE FOR STUDY OF THE EFFECT OF TEACHING STERILE TECHNIQUE ON CAPD COMPLICATIONS

Neuman Systems Model Concepts	Stressors	Primary Prevention	Lines of Defense	Impact of Stressors
Concepts of the theory	Renal Failure	Teaching	Compliance with strict sterile technique of bag exchanges	Complications: peritonitis
Empirical Indicators	CAPD 4 bag exchanges daily	CAPD booklet; audiotapes with information	Assessment tool to evaluate if patient is complying with strict sterile technique	Complications: "Systematic Assessment Tool"

QUALITATIVE RESEARCH APPROACH TO DEVELOP MIDDLE RANGE THEORY

Another research approach could be done from a qualitative paradigm. The broad question of asking the client his or her perception of the major stress area or areas of health concern is a premise of the Neuman Systems Model. It is the first question of the Neuman Systems Model generic Assessment and Intervention Tool (see page 59).

Research related to quality of life of ESRD clients on dialysis modalities reflects that past trends in determining quality of life have been based on the health care provider's perspective (Evans et al., 1985; Deniston et al., 1986). There is a great need for specific tools to measure the quality of life from the client's perspective (Wu, 1993). Therefore the contribution of a conceptual model that has as the phenomenon of study the client's perspective is both timely and necessary. The Neuman Systems Model assumes that when there is client system stability, then optimal wellness, as perceived by the client, has been achieved.

To conduct qualitative research, an interview guide (Table 34–2) was developed (Breckenridge 1992, 1993) to elicit perceptions of clients as to why their dialysis treatment modality was chosen. For the preliminary data, obtained from a pilot study, a grounded approach was used to analyze the data as articulated by Fox and Swazey (1974, 1978), O'Brien (1983), and Artinian (1987) based on Glaser and Strauss (1967) for the discovery of grounded theory and the emergence of themes. As data from focused interviews and observations were analyzed, more and different themes emerged. A typology of the clients' themes reflected why the decision was made. These themes were:

- *Self-decision:* Client's own decision.
- *Access-rationing decision:* Based on factors of availability of space at a center.
- *To live decision:* Client states dialysis is necessary to live.
- *Physiologically dictated decision:* Client's physiological limitations dictate the modality.
- *Expert decision:* Health care provider (i.e., physician, nurse) made the decision.

TABLE 34–2. INTERVIEW SCHEDULE FOR PRELIMINARY DATA OF PILOT STUDY FOR CLIENT PERCEPTIONS OF WHY DIALYSIS TREATMENT WAS CHOSEN

---

1. In your opinion or with your story, can you tell me what are the reasons you are on the dialysis modality that you are on?
2. Prior to being on this present dialysis modality, have you been on another type of dialysis?
   If yes, for how long?
3. What caused you to switch from one to the other?
4. Which modality do you prefer and for what reasons?

- *Significant other decision:* Significant other (i.e., family member) made the decision.
- *To be cared for decision:* Client states he or she is cared for by another.
- *No client choice in making decision:* Client states he or she had no choice in modality.

This typology of client themes is the generation of a beginning middle range theory. The Neuman Systems Model categories of intrapersonal, interpersonal, and extrapersonal stressors to classify the emergent themes of why the decision was made could be done in a further content analysis of this qualitative data. This was the approach used by Blank, Clark, Longman, and Atwood (1989) in their qualitative study and constructed into a conceptual-theoretical-empirical structure (Figure 34–3). The validation of these themes from the pilot study data will need to be determined by carrying out a qualitative grounded approach study in which the number of clients is determined when saturation of themes is reached.

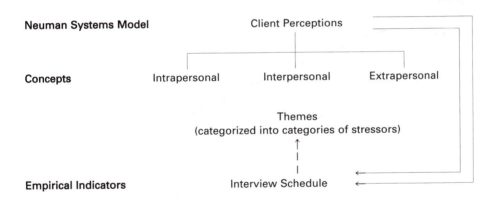

Neuman Systems Model   Client Perceptions

Concepts   Intrapersonal   Interpersonal   Extrapersonal

Themes
(categorized into categories of stressors)

Empirical Indicators   Interview Schedule

Themes Categorized into Categories of Stressors[a]

Intrapersonal:	Self-decision
	Physiologically dictated decision
	To live decision
Interpersonal:	Expert decision
	Significant other decision
	To be cared for decision
Extrapersonal:	Access-rationing decision
	No client choice in making decision

[a]Breckenridge, D. M. 1992. Unpublished raw data. University of Maryland at Baltimore.

Figure 34–3. Conceptual/Theoretical/Empirical Structure for Study of Dialysis Modality Decisions.

FUTURE DIRECTIONS FOR PRACTICE-BASED RESEARCH TO VALIDATE AND SUPPORT THE NEUMAN SYSTEMS MODEL

Meleis (1993) has underscored the importance of conducting research with vulnerable populations. Clients with ESRD certainly represent one such population. Meleis (1993) advocates that even if a theory cannot be validated because nurses cannot determine if all individuals experience their situation in a certain way, it is still useful to understand the lived experience of a few. This qualitative perspective is one of the approaches of Meleis's (1993) definition of theory support.

Directions into the 21st Century

The primary purpose of this chapter is to increase awareness of how the Neuman Systems Model gives direction for the phenomenon to be studied for specific client populations and in specific practice settings. The research approach—qualitative or quantitative—will be selected based on the existing knowledge about the phenomenon of concern. Development of middle range theory will be validated well into the 21st century through theory testing and supportive approaches. These approaches will increase the body of research-based knowledge for practice with specific client populations and in specific clinical settings.

REFERENCES

Artinian, B. 1986. The research process in grounded theory. In *From Practice to Grounded Theory: Qualitative Research in Nursing,* by C. Chenitz and J. M. Swanson. Redding, Massachusetts: Addison-Wesley Publishing Co.

Blank, J. J., Clark, L., Longman, A. J., and Atwood, J. R. 1989. Perceived home care needs of cancer patients and their caregivers. *Cancer Nursing* 12:78–84.

Breckenridge, D. M. 1989. Primary prevention as an intervention modality for the renal client. In *The Neuman Systems Model: Application to Nursing Education and Practice,* 2d ed. East Norwalk, Conn.: Appleton & Lange, Inc.

Breckenridge, D. M. 1982. Adaptation of Neuman health-care systems model for the renal client. In *The Neuman Systems Model: Application to Nursing Education and Practice.* East Norwalk, Conn.: Appleton-Century-Crofts.

Breckenridge, D. M., Cupit, M. C., Raimondo, J. 1982. Systematic nursing assessment tool for the CAPD client. *Nephrology Nurse* January/February:24–31.

Breckenridge, D.M. 1992. *Pilot study.* Unpublished. University of Maryland at Baltimore.

Breckenridge, D. M. 1993. Patient perceptions of why dialysis treatment was chosen. Proposal submitted to National Institute of Health.

Bremer, B. A., McCauley, C. R., Wrona, R. M., and Johnson, J. P. 1989. Quality of life in end-stage renal disease: A reexamination. *American Journal of Kidney Diseases* 13 (3):200–209.

Deniston, O. L. Carpentier-Alting, P., Kneisley, J., Hawthorne, V. M., and Port, F. K. 1989. Assessment of quality of life in end-stage renal disease. *Health Services Research* 24(4):555–578.

Evans, R. W., Blagg, C. R., and Bryan, F. 1981. Implications for health care policy: A social and demographic profile of hemodialysis patients in the United States. *Journal of the American Medical Association* 245(5):487–491.

Evans, R. W., Manninen, D. L., Garrison, L. P., Hart, G., Blatt, C. R., Gutman, R. A., Hull, A. R., and Lowrie, E. G. 1985. The quality of life of patients with end-stage renal disease. *The New England Journal of Medicine* 312(9):553–559.

Fawcett, J., and Downs, F. S. 1992. *The Relationship of Theory and Research,* 2d ed. Philadelphia: F. A. Davis Company.

Fawcett, J. 1990. The Neuman Systems Model: Directions for Research. Paper presented at the Third Biennial Neuman Systems Model International Symposium.

Fox, R. C., and Swazey, J. P. 1974, 1978. *The Courage to Fail: A Social View of Organ Transplants and Dialysis.* Chicago: The University of Chicago Press.

Glaser, B., and Strauss, A. L. 1967. *The Discovery of Grounded Theory: Strategies for Qualitative Research.* New York: Aldine Publishing Company.

Klingenstein, J. A. 1986. Successful rehabilitation of the renal client. In *Comprehensive Nephrology Nursing,* edited by C. J. Richard. Boston: Little, Brown.

Meleis, A. I. 1993. Theory testing and theory support: Principles, challenges and a sojourn into the future. Papre presented at the Fourth International Neuman Symposium, University of Rochester, New York, April.

National Kidney Foundation. (1987, 1992). Telephone communication. New York, New York.

O'Brien, M. E. 1983. *The Courage to Survive: The Life Career of a Dialysis Patient.* New York: Grune & Stratton, Inc.

Richard, C. J., ed. 1986. *Comprehensive Nephrology Nursing.* Boston: Little, Brown.

Wu, A. 1993. Quality of life. Paper presented at the University of Maryland at Baltimore and Johns Hopkins University Research Symposium, March.

Zappacosta, A. R., and Perras, S. T. 1984, 1990. *Continuous Ambulatory Peritoneal Dialysis.* Philadelphia: J. B. Lippincott.

Ziemer, M. M. 1983. Effects of information on postsurgical coping. *Nursing Research* 32:282–287.

35

FUTURE DIRECTIONS FOR RESEARCH WITH THE NEUMAN SYSTEMS MODEL

Mary Colette Smith
Ann Estes Edgil

The purpose of this chapter is to propose a plan for testing middle range theories within the Neuman Systems Model. A view of research as consisting of conceptual, substantive, and methodological domains, and as occurring in prestudy, central, and follow-up stages (Brinberg and McGrath, 1985) is used to organize the plan. The plan involves creation of an Institute for the Study of the Neuman Systems Model to formulate and test practice theories through collaborative, interdisciplinary, and multisite efforts. The chapter includes guiding directions for the work to be done, an organizational structure specifying personnel requirements, and a task analysis of what and who would be appropriate to participate in task completion. The direction for research with the model can be stated as:

1. Identifying and assembling resources
2. Formulating principles/presuppositions
3. Identifying concepts and interrelationships
4. Synthesizing existing research based on the concept
5. Generating research questions/hypotheses
6. Conducting the research
7. Developing structural models for testing

8. Refining the theories
9. Generating new theories

It is only through a cohesive program of research involving collaboration of persons with a wide range of expertise that the implicit theories within the Neuman Systems Model can be recast into propositions for investigation. Coordinating the efforts, monitoring progress, and housing resources in a central place would seem to be indispensable to moving forward with the theory development essential for use of the model.

GUIDING DIRECTIONS

Future directions for research with the Neuman Systems Model originate in an assumption that philosophy of science is the transcending system within which inquiries reside and with which they should correspond. Scholarly inquiry is assumed to embody distinct but interlocking domains of expertise relevant to the study of the phenomena under consideration. Adherence to the rubrics of the embedding systems of philosophy of science and scholarly inquiry is essential to the validity, replicability, and credibility of research endeavors.

Philosophy of Science

Investigators studying phenomena of the model will need to take a posture on the nature of scientific knowledge and on what kind of evidence is required as explanation in a practice discipline. Issues such as the structure of theories, the relationship between theory and evidence, the role of observation, and the processes by which science changes or develops have long been debated in the philosophy of science community. Although absolute finality has not been reached on many of the issues, within the last decade a new understanding of the logic of science has been forged (Phillips, 1987). For example, Karl Popper's critical rationality insight marked the boundary between science and nonscience. Specifically, Popper (1968) reached the conclusion that the essence of science is testability, or more precisely the openness to refutation. According to this position, knowledge grows by the process of error elimination rather than by the process of proving items to be true.

Scholarly Inquiry

Because of the enormous complexity of human beings, the abstract nature of conceptual frameworks, and theory testing that requires concrete real-world phenomena and analysis of events, a perspective of distinct but interlocking domains is proposed. Brinberg and McGrath (1985) refer to aspects of research as conceptual, substantive, and methodological. The conceptual domain consists of ideas, concepts, relationships, and underlying assumptions (p. 25). The substantive domain consists of the focal topic, phenomena, and processes of interest

(p. 25). The methodological domain consists of designs, methods, and strategies of research for examination of the concepts and phenomena (p. 26). Brinberg and McGrath suggest that different types of expertise are required for each of the domains and that not all persons are equally qualified or interested in all domains. Additionally, they describe research as occurring in stages of prestudy (definition and refinement of elements), central (conduct of the study), and follow-up (generalization). The underlying concern in this perspective is validity, which has different meanings in each of the domains and the stages. (The reader is referred to the Brinberg and McGrath [1985] text for details of the Validity Network Schema.) The concern about conceptualization and measurement in the social sciences described by Blalock (1982) serves as yet another source for the perspective adopted here. Conceptualization involves processes by which ideas are moved to research operations, while measurement serves as the linking process between operations and mathematical language (Blalock, 1982, 11–12).

Embedding Systems

The Neuman Systems Model is based in general systems theory and wholism, with a view of nursing as being concerned with action in stress-related situations (Neuman, 1989, 11). These foundations serve as transcending and embedding systems for a conceptual domain with which topical phenomena and methodological treatment must be consistent. Neuman (1989, 17–22) has made explicit a set of assumptions upon which any exploration would be based, constituting a foundational system for all inquiry related to the model. Also serving as embedding systems are national health and nursing priorities, with which model research can easily be articulated.

SUMMARY

Using a philosophy of science perspective, a view of research based in scholarly inquiry, and consolidation of resources, the following plan for testing middle-range theories of the model is proposed as a support system for researchers, practitioners, and educators using the model. The institute will provide a planned and coordinated effort to enhance use, confirm authenticity, and maintain integrity of the model. Conceptual, substantive, and methodological orientations operating throughout prestudy, central, and follow-up stages of research were proposed. The future of research is one that is characterized as collaborative, interdisciplinary, funded, and articulated with the national priorities in this country and in other countries. As we move toward the 21st century, the future for use of the Neuman Systems Model demands a cohesive and conceptually, methodologically, and substantively sound foundation. Through the institute, the existing spirit and resources can be mobilized into greater realization for the long-term agenda for action.

ORGANIZATIONAL STRUCTURE

An organizational structure for the Institute for the Study of the Neuman Systems Model is presented in Figure 35–1. The structure consists of the Neuman Systems Model Trustees Group, a coordinating council, consultant panel, two core groups, four concept panels, and support staff. Based on the anticipated work that needs to be done as we move toward the 21st century, sets of expertise have been identified and clustered. The organization is not unlike those of other institutes and is modeled from an Agency for Health Care Policy Research and Patient Outcomes Research Team project (Goldenberg, 1992), on which the first author served as an investigator.

The Trustees Group, as responsible for ensuring the integrity of the model, is the body to which all research endeavors are accountable. Conceivably, the trustees could serve in an advisory capacity, but at this stage of conceptualizing the institute, they seem to be the logical choice for accountability. The trustor, Betty M. Neuman, RN, PhD, FAAN could retain or delegate administrative and/or scientific aspects of the institute. The trustees would seem to be operating in the conceptual domain, yet they would be accountable for ensuring the appropriate correspondence of substantive phenomena for study and methodological strategies as consistent with assumptions of the model. They will advise the coordinating council of potential panel and core members. A coordinating council is proposed to serve as a type of steering committee for the operations of the institute. The council should consist of persons with conceptual, substantive, and methodological orientations. Because of the administrative aspect of coordination of panel and core activities, one member should possess this type of expertise. This person will be assisted by the project manager from the support staff. The council, with advice from the trustees and assistance from the support staff, is responsible for identifying and assembling personnel and resources. With the number and variety of personnel involved in the institute, one of the primary functions of the council is communication. Monthly meetings or conference calls would be mandatory to monitor progress toward ultimate goals. Table 35–1 depicts a list of activities required to realize the plan proposed in this chapter.

The consultant panel, to be named early in the planning, should be comprised of persons reknowned for their insights in embedding systems of the model. The panel will include experts in the areas of philosophy of science, stress, systems, and research designs. Discussing research directions for theory development, Suppe and Jacox (1985) recommended being adequately informed of contemporary philosophy of science literature. Because of the essential foundations of the model in stress and systems theory, persons in these domains would be indispensable to the work of the institute. Also recommended by Suppe and Jacox (1985) is the use of multiple approaches and attention to methodological and evaluation developments as applicable to theory development and evaluation. Persons flexible and amenable to diversity in research designs will be sought as consultants on this panel.

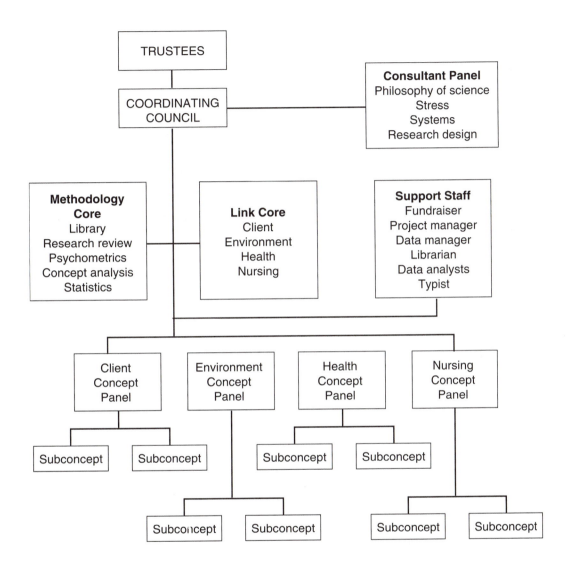

Figure 35–1. Organizational Structure for the Institute for the Study of the Neuman Systems Model. *(Copyright © 1993 by Mary Colette Smith, Ann Edgil, and Betty Neuman. Structure adapted with permission from Goldenberg, R. L. 1992.* Patient Outcomes Research Team (PORT): Low birthweight in minority and high-risk women *(Tech. Rep.). Birmingham, AL: University of Alabama at Birmingham (p. III-2). All rights reserved. No part of this document may be reproduced, quoted, or cited without prior permission of the authors.)*

TABLE 35–1 TASK ANALYSIS

Prestudy tasks

Tasks to be done	Trustees	Coordinating Council	Consultant Panels	Methodology Core	Link Core	Support Staff	Concept Panels	Subconcept Groups
Prestudy								
1.0 Identify and assemble resources	•							
1.1 Consultants	•		•					
Philosophy								
Stress								
Systems								
Design								
1.2 Coordinating council	•	•	•					
Conceptual								
Substantive								
Methodological								
Administration								
1.3 Methodology core		•	•	•				
Library								
Research review								
Psychometrics								
Concept analysis								
Statistics								
1.4 Link core		•	•		•			
Client								
Environment								
Health								
Nursing								
1.5 Support staff		•				•		
Project manager								
Data manager								
Librarian								
Data analysts								
Fund raising								
1.6 Concept panels		•	•				•	
Client								
Environment								
Health								
Nursing								

Tasks 2.0–9.2

Tasks to be done	Trustees	Coordinating Council	Consultant Panels	Methodology Core	Link Core	Support Staff	Concept Panels	Subconcept Groups
2.0 Formulate presuppositions	•		•					
2.1 Philosophy								
2.2 Inquiry research								
2.3 The model								
3.0 Identify concepts and subconcepts			•		•		•	•
4.0 Conduct integrative research review	•		•	•	•	•	•	•
4.1 Questions								
4.2 Criteria								
4.3 Evidence table								
5.0 Conduct concept analyses		•						
6.0 Construct interrelationships		•						
6.1 Maps								
6.2 Models								
7.0 Assess instrument status			•	•	•		•	•
7.1 Construct validity								
8.0 Design studies								
8.1 Question								
8.2 Terms								
8.3 Literature review								
8.4 Instrument development								
8.5 Design/method								
8.6 Subjects/settings								
8.7 Research team								
8.8 Data presentation				•		•	•	•
8.9 Data analysis								
Central Stage								
9.0 Conduct study								
9.1 Collect data								
9.2 Analyze data								

Tasks 9.3–Dissemination

Tasks to be done	Trustees	Coordinating Council	Consultant Panels	Methodology Core	Link Core	Support Staff	Concept Panels	Subconcept Groups
9.3 Present								
9.4 Interpret								
9.5 Findings								
9.6 Conclusions								
9.7 Discussion								
9.8 Recommendations								
9.9 Articulation with other concept projects			•	•			•	•
9.10 New research questions								
Follow-up Stage								
10.0 Robustness				•			•	•
10.1 Replication	•						•	•
Dissemination								

Smith, M. C., Edgil, A., and Neuman, B. (1993, April). Nursing research and the Neuman Model: Directions for the future. The Neuman Model in Research, Practice and Education. The Fourth Biennial International Neuman Systems Model Symposium, Rochester, NY. Reprinted with permission.

514

The methodology core, serving all concept panels, provides the expertise to conduct the literature searches, develop new instruments, refine existing instruments, coordinate concept analyses, and oversee any statistical analyses. One of the primary functions of the library and research review core personnel would be to identify and classify all research, published and unpublished, based on the Neuman Systems Model. The result of the research review is anticipated to be a litany of concepts, phenomena, subjects, variables, and model focus reported to date in the literature.

The "link" core functions as a concept, intervention, and variable coordinating group. This unbiased body is commissioned to formulate the linkages among concepts and subconcepts, with a view to conceptual mapping leading to the development of structural equation modeling. This group is concerned with primary, secondary, and tertiary intervention, and the interacting physiological, psychological, sociocultural, developmental, and spiritual variables.

The support staff serve to facilitate the day-to-day operations of the institute. Positioned in this group is a fund raiser, whose role it is to keep the institute financially afloat. The project manager is responsible for personnel acquisition, management, paper movement, schedules, and so forth. The data manager maintains all data, stores them, keeps them in retrievable fashion, keeps them current, and retains all data records. The project librarian sets up a functional library of sources, reprints, and other appropriate documents for project personnel usage. The data analysts carry out statistical treatments, construct visual displays, and in the case of qualitative data, execute the necessary steps for analysis.

The concept panels are the most critical parts of the institute. They will consist of persons with conceptual orientations, and those with substantive orientations so that the abstract concept can be appropriately made concrete and feasible for study. It is expected that the concepts, after the concept analyses, will be comprised of subconcepts, at which time additional subpanels may be formed.

This institute is proposed for the specific purpose of promoting the study of the Neuman Systems Model as the paradigm for nursing research. At this time, it is conceivable that work on the "theory of prevention as intervention" (Koertvelyessy cited in Neuman, 1989, 38) could be a point of departure for discussion in each of the concept panels and in the link core as well. Selected substantive phenomena for study might include practice theories related to breast cancer in high-risk females, immunizations in special groups of children, and high-risk behaviors in sexually active adolescents.

TASK ANALYSIS

A set of activities viewed as essential to launching the institute is organized around Brinberg and McGrath's (1985) research stages—prestudy, central, and follow-up. The task analysis of what needs to be done, and by whom, is depicted in Table 35–1.

The prestudy stage encompasses identifying and assembling persons identified in the organizational structure and conducting the work preliminary to theory exploration and testing. One of the most important aspects of the prestudy stage is the identification of funds to support the efforts of the institute. The trustees will need to pool knowledge and available financial resources to bear on this problem. Without funding, the consultants charged with assistance in making explicit the embedding systems and formulating the fundamental presuppositions will not be available. A person skilled in fund identification and fund raising needs to be hired at the earliest possible time. Already in place, the trustees can begin discussion on concepts and subconcepts and identify potential members of the concept and link panels. The integrative research review could be conducted on a multisite and continuing basis, organized by the trustees in the absence of a coordinating council. A time frame should be formulated to ensure that tasks are achieved in a reasonable period. It should be recognized that the prestudy stage will require considerable time. While some may be anxious to move on to the central stage for conduct of studies, it will be important to value and appreciate the preliminary work that must precede the research of testing. Dillon (1984) classified research questions as ranging from whether or not a phenomenon exists, to once establishing that it does, what it looks like. The next step is the question of relationships, and finally, after answering the prior questions, moving on to questions of explanation, prediction, and control.

It is during the prestudy stage that the conceptual domain will be operationalized through substantive phenomena identification. Conceptual maps can be constructed and propositions formulated for investigation. The integrative review will make explicit the concepts, subjects, methods, instruments, and results. Examination of instruments used and assessment of needed instruments will be an outcome of this activity. From the research review, new questions for study will emerge.

Concluding the prestudy stage is the design of the new studies by the concept panels. The usual steps of the research process are carried out through the data analysis phase.

The central stage consists of the activities associated with conduct of a study. Critical to this stage will be the articulation of results across studies with the unbiased perspective of the link core. From their deliberations, further questions for investigation should arise.

The follow-up stage is the time to test robustness of findings by identifying replications for study and establishing the boundaries of the findings (where they do and do not apply). Findings from a single study are viewed as insufficient for change in practice or policy.

Throughout the process, dissemination can occur without violation of scientific integrity rules of premature reporting. Of value to the scientific community in nursing would be communicating the presuppositions, concept analysis results, and research review.

REFERENCES

Blalock, H. M., Jr. 1982. *Conceptualization and Measurement in the Social Sciences.* Beverly Hills: Sage.

Brinberg, D., and McGrath, J.E. 1985. *Validity and the Research Process.* Newbury Park: Sage.

Dillon, J. T., 1984. The classification of research questions. *Review of Educational Research,* 54:327–361.

Goldenberg, R. M. 1992. Patient Outcomes Research Team (PORT): Low birthweight in minority and high-risk women. Technical proposal, University of Alabama at Birmingham, Birmingham, Alabama.

Neuman, B. 1989. *The Neuman Systems Model,* 2d ed. Norwalk: Conn.: Appleton & Lange.

Phillips, D. C. 1987. *Philosophy, Science, and Social Inquiry.* Oxford: Pergamon Press.

Popper, K. 1968. *Conjectures and Refutations.* New York: Harper Torchbooks.

Suppe, F., and Jacox, A. K. 1985. Philosophy of science and the development of nursing theory. *Annual Review of Nursing Research* 3:241–267.

Section VI

International Use of the Neuman Systems Model

36

THE NEUMAN MODEL
Examples of its Use in Canadian Educational Programs

Dorothy M. Craig

The Neuman Model is currently being used as the basis for curriculum content in a number of educational institutions in Canada. The experience of 12 of these institutions, representing six Canadian provinces, will provide insights into how the model is used and the model's strengths. For some nursing programs the Neuman Model forms the basis for the whole curriculum, but for others the model is used as a framework to guide specific courses. Aspects of the model that Canadian teachers have found difficult to work with will also be noted. Information about the nursing programs was provided by a contact person from each educational institution.

THE CURRICULUM BASE

In 1990 the faculty in the College of Nursing at the University of Saskatchewan implemented a revised curriculum based on the Neuman Systems Model. The first students in this revised program are currently completing their third year.

The Neuman Systems Model was used to select program and specific course content and to structure course sequence (Dyck, Innes, Rae, and Sawatzky, 1989). The Neuman concept of levels of prevention form the focus for specific years of the program, starting with primary prevention in year one, secondary in year two, tertiary in year three, and integration of all three levels in year four. In similar fashion various client systems are emphasized in given years, starting with individual systems in year one, family systems in year two, and community systems in year three, with an integration of all systems in the final year.

Examples of how the model determined course selection are as follows: Normal human physiology (primary prevention) is taught in year one, and pathophysiology (secondary prevention) is taught in year two; interpersonal relationships (individual client system) is taught in year one, and family dynamics (family client system) is taught in year two. The human variables, as identified in the model, guided specific course selection such as growth and development, transcultural nursing, and ethics. (*Contact: S. Dyck, RN, BScN, MContEd, Professor, College of Nursing, University of Saskatchewan, Saskatoon, Saskatchewan.*)

The Neuman Model was selected as the basis for the first year of a new baccalaureate program in Prince Edward Island (PEI). Since its initial class of students were enrolled in September 1992, first-year courses have just been completed for the first time. Detailed planning for the second-year curriculum is beginning. The curriculum is designed to prepare beginning practitioners to practice nursing based on the philosophy of primary health care (WHO, 1978). Basic to this design are the beliefs that the client is the primary decision maker in his or her own health care activities and that the nurse functions with a wholistic concept of that client and an awareness of the role of collaborator in achieving desired health goals.

After considering a variety of conceptual frameworks for nursing, the faculty at PEI chose the Neuman Model to guide their first-year students in developing their knowledge and skills as nurses. The model's major concepts of health, nursing, and person (client or patient) are compatible with those held by the faculty and intrinsic to their stated philosophy of health care and nursing as outlined above.

Student experience included interacting with healthy individual senior citizens in their own homes to conduct introductory level health history and assessment, and contributing to the assessment and care of hospitalized adults in an acute care setting. In both instances, the Neuman Model provided a process for completing a client-driven nursing assessment and enhanced the students' client-centered versus illness-centered approach to the nursing role. (*Contact: M. F. Munro, RN, PhD, Associate Professor and Founding Dean of Nursing, School of Nursing, University of Prince Edward Island, PEI.*)

THE CLINICAL SETTING

The Neuman Systems Model has been used by the University of Calgary, Faculty of Nursing since 1990. This model was chosen because it fit well with the faculty's philosophy of nursing.

Students apply the model in the clinical setting. The Neuman assessment format is a useful organizing framework for beginning students as they start to collect data about individual clients. Senior students use the same framework when critically analyzing their data to ensure that they have been wholistic in their assessment and in their understanding of the relationships that are important to their clients.

Neuman's inclusion of strengths and stressors in her model reminds faculty and students to focus on client activities that promote and maintain health as well as on those that may create problems. Students more readily focus on health concerns. Neuman's model also prompts them to remember a client's strengths. (*Contact: C. Rogers, RN, MHSc, Associate Dean, Undergraduate Program, Faculty of Nursing, The University of Calgary, Calgary, Alberta.*)

The Neuman Systems Model is used at Brandon University in the practicum courses—Nursing in the Community and Long-Term, Rehabilitative, and Palliative Care Nursing. In these courses, postdiploma nursing students make a transition from institutionally based to community-based care, and from an individual client to a family and community as client perspective. These paradigm shifts can be difficult, and experience reveals that realization is facilitated in several ways by the Neuman Model.

First, the model is a comprehensive and wholistic vision of a client system and its relationship with the environment. The model's flexible and broad definition of person transfers readily from individual client to family and community as client. Accordingly, the opportunity to appraise each client group with a single conceptual framework expedites the students' struggles with the paradigm shift. Second, the students find the emphasis on stressors and reactions in the model fits with their previously acquired experience and knowledge and eases the institution to community shift. In addition, the course on long-term care incorporates the concept of chronicity and its impact on families. Conceptualization of this impact from a systems perspective enables students to make a quick recognition of multiple stressors and actual and potential reactions experienced by families coping with chronic illness. The transfer from institution to community is also facilitated by the model's incorporation of environment as a key concept. (*Contact: R. Will, BN, MBA, Assistant Professor, Department of Nursing and Health Sciences, Brandon University, Brandon, Manitoba.*)

The practice component of the primary health course in the post-BN/RN program at the University of New Brunswick engages students in conducting a community assessment in order to determine the health challenges of a select community. The identified health challenges subsequently guide the students in selecting interventions that are responsive to the needs of the community. Students select a nursing model to direct the assessment phase and ensure implementation and evaluation.

A prevalent choice among these students is the Neuman Systems Model. Although students experience some difficulty grasping the language of the model, they embrace the theoretical underpinnings of systems theory and are familiar with the levels of intervention espoused by this model. These factors facilitate the acceptance of this model by students who have several years of nursing experience but have not previously been involved in theory-driven nursing practice. (*Contact: D. McCormack BN, MScN, Assistant Professor, Faculty of Nursing, University of New Brunswick, Fredericton, New Brunswick.*)

COMBINED CURRICULUM AND PRACTICE SETTINGS

At the University of Moncton students learn about the Neuman Systems Model during the second year of the program. First they study the model in the Nursing Principles and Theory course. Then during the same year, they learn to apply the model in a community setting.

During the third year of the program, students are expected to demonstrate a more in-depth comprehension of the model. Again, the model is used during home visits to convalescent patients and their families. Students evaluate patient and family health, prepare a care plan, and implement care. They explain their findings and their interventions using the conceptual framework of the model. Fourth-year students often choose the Neuman Model as a basis for nursing practice during their independent study course. (*Contact: V. Wade, MS [Nursing], Professor, Faculty of Nursing, Universite de Moncton, Moncton, New Brunswick.*)

COMMUNITY HEALTH

At the University of Western Ontario, the Neuman Systems Model was selected because of its consistency with the community health nursing course in year four of the undergraduate nursing program, when the community as the client is the focus. The model has been well documented in terms of fit and utility for this client group. Congruent with the goals and concepts of this course were Neuman's (1) total person approach to client care in order to help individuals, families, and groups attain and maintain a maximum level of wellness by purposeful intervention; (2) aim of nursing as the reduction of stress factors and adverse conditions that potentially or actually impact on client functions, and (3) view of prevention at three levels—primary, secondary, and tertiary—which correspond to the tenets of community and public health nursing. (*Contact: D. Goldenberg, RN, PhD, Associate Professor, Faculty of Nursing, University of Western Ontario, London, Ontario.*)

At the University of Windsor the study of conceptual frameworks in nursing, including the Neuman Systems Model, is an integral part of the four-year baccalaureate program curriculum at the School of Nursing. Neuman's model is the first nursing model that is introduced to third-level students in the Family and Community Health Nursing courses. These students use the model to guide their assessment and intervention when caring for children, postpartum women, adults, elderly, and their families in a community setting. In the fourth level, students have the option of applying various nursing models in their independent study and the senior Family and Community Health Nursing course. Many students continue to use the Neuman Model as a guide to study health needs and behaviors of families, aggregates, organizations, and community. (*Contact: L. Matuk, BA, BSc, RN, MScN, Assistant Professor, School of Nursing, University of Windsor, Windsor, Ontario.*)

THEORETICAL PLURALISM

Where theoretical pluralism is the approach of the nursing program, students often choose the Neuman Systems Model. Postbasic RN students enrolled at the University of Victoria (where both distance and campus courses are offered) or at one of the collaborative partner sites at Okanagan University College, University College of the Cariboo, or Malaspina College take three core clinical courses and two options of advanced clinical courses. The core clinical courses focus on family, population, and geographical community as client. Students in the BSN program at all sites are introduced to a variety of nursing models and frameworks in all clinical courses that they can use to guide their practice. Many students in both the population and community as client courses choose to use the Neuman Systems Model. (*Contact: G. Beddome, RN, MSN, College Professor, Okanagan College, Kelowna, British Columbia.*)

At the University of Toronto it is felt that Neuman's model makes a valuable contribution to the discipline and practice of nursing. The model is based on systems theory; hence it is "wholistic" (Neuman, 1992, 177). The value of the model is seen in its comprehensiveness and thus its usefulness in structuring nursing knowledge development and practice activities across a wide variety of situations. Because the model focuses on understanding the intricate relationship between persons and their environment with the goal of bringing/keeping the two in balance, it offers a powerful tool to assist students to focus on promoting wellness. Nurses find the model relevant and useful across health care settings and in their work with individuals, family groups, and communities. In fact, graduate nursing students, who study Neuman's model in a required course, have identified these strengths of the model repeatedly.

The ongoing challenge, of course, lies in the development of practice content that derives from the Neuman Systems Model so that it is more than a theoretical guide to practice. Nursing's substantive and distinctive contribution to society can then be better articulated, alongside the role that Neuman herself has played in this direction (D. Wells, MHSc, PhD candidate, personal communication, April 15, 1993). (*Contact: D. Craig, MScN, Associate Professor, Faculty of Nursing, University of Toronto, Toronto, Ontario.*)

The Neuman Systems Model has been incorporated into the curriculum of the four-year nursing baccalaureate program at Ryerson within a perspective of theoretical pluralism. The nursing theories and models of Roy, Orem, and Neuman were identified as most accurately representing the values and beliefs of the faculty and were selected to guide the curriculum. Students are introduced to nursing theory as a basis for practice in the first semester of the program; specific nursing theories and models are introduced throughout the course of the program to direct both the clinical practice courses and the choice of content within specified nursing classroom courses.

At this point in the program, the clinical field officially expands to incorporate the community, and the Neuman Systems Model provides the theoretical focus for clinical practice and course content in semesters six and seven. The selection of the Neuman Model for these experiences is congruent with the Neuman-based *Standards of Nursing Practice for Community Health Nurses in Ontario* (RNAO, 1985). The Neuman Model is perceived as being less structured than the other models used in the curriculum and more compatible with student learning at an advanced level.

The Neuman Model underpins the Community Health Nursing course offered in semester six. In this course students are introduced to the nurse's role in health promotion and disease prevention for families, groups, and communities. Neuman's model provides the framework for assessment of family, group, and community as client and for investigation of primary, secondary, and tertiary prevention as intervention. Students use the Neuman Model to guide their investigation of current issues in community health and present their findings throughout the latter half of the course. (*Contact: J. Pearce, RN, BN, EdD [candidate], Professor and Associate Director, Ryerson Polytechnical Institute Toronto, Ontario.*)

At the University of Ottawa students of the generic program are exposed to a variety of practice theories and conceptual frameworks in nursing throughout their studies. The Neuman Systems Model has been selected to provide the structure for the majority of the nursing courses in the third and fourth year of the basic program: Health Assessment; Family Nursing in the Community; Community Mental Health Nursing; Community Health Nursing; and Nursing Management of Multiple Stressors in Acute Care.

In the baccalaureate program for registered nurses, the Neuman Systems Model is the framework of choice for two of the most important concentrations: community/occupational health nursing and perinatal nursing. The courses for which it serves as the basic structure are Community Health Nursing; Occupational Health Nursing; Nursing Management of the At Risk Gravida, during Antipartum; During Intrapartum; Nursing Management of the Neonate at Risk. (*Contact: M. A. Loyer, RN, PhD, Asociate Professor, Faculty of Health Sciences, University of Ottawa, Ottawa, Ontario.*)

SUMMARY

Nurses working with the Neuman Model in educational programs in Canada reported a number of model strengths. The focus of the model on a wholistic approach addressing levels of prevention guides students to focus on the health of the client in the context of his or her unique environment. The model also assists students in clinical settings to carry out in-depth assessments and to categorize the data obtained in a meaningful way so that specific interventions can be planned with the client.

Students reported some difficulties understanding the complexity of the model and the developmental and spiritual variables. Also it was not always easy to differentiate between the lines of defense and resistance or to assess the degree of stressor penetration.

Further explanations about these areas and a simpler illustration of the model's concepts would assist educators and students in their use of the model. In spite of these concerns, educators reported that the Neuman Model was very often chosen by students for its ability to guide them in providing excellent client care, particularly in the community setting.

REFERENCES

Dyck, S. M., Innes, J. E., Rae, D. I., and Sawatzky, J. E. 1989. The Neuman Systems Model in curriculum revision: A baccalaureate program, University of Saskatchewan. In *The Neuman Systems Model,* 2d ed., edited by B. Neuman, 225. East Norwalk, Conn.: Appleton & Lange.

Neuman, B., ed. 1989. *The Neuman Systems Model,* 2d ed. East Norwalk, Conn.: Appleton & Lange.

Registered Nurses' Association of Ontario. 1985. *Standards of Nursing Practice for Community Health Nurses in Ontario.* Toronto: RNAO.

WHO. 1978. *Primary Health Care: Report of the International Conference on Primary Health Care.* Geneva, Switzerland: WHO.

37

COMMUNITY/PUBLIC HEALTH NURSING IN CANADA
Use of the Neuman Systems Model in a New Paradigm

Dorothy M. Craig

In Canada, community health/public health nursing has been going through major changes in organizational structure, service delivery methods, and roles for nurses. Two documents—one on program and service guidelines (Ontario Ministry of Health, 1989) and the other on the preparation and practice of community health/public health nurses in Canada (Canadian Public Health Association, 1990)—have challenged nurses to examine the scope and mandate of community/public health nursing. With an increasing awareness of the role played by the broad determinants of health, these documents have identified the need for a wide range of approaches: from a focus on the individual to broad population-based strategies.

In Ontario the program and service guidelines have precipitated a shift from the nurse as generalist to specialty or focused nursing practice. In many health units nurses now work as members of program teams, some of which are interdisciplinary. Thus a nurse may work on a team, for example, that addresses the older population or one that addresses maternal and child health. In other Canadian provinces similar changes in service delivery are occurring.

Teaching Health Units have also been initiated in Ontario. Agreements have been signed by a number of public health units with local universities to work in partnership in education, research, and practice. The benefits of these joint ventures will include more effective learning opportunities for students and more opportunities for service providers and researchers to work together on clinically relevant research.

Three nurses who are working in community/public health nursing have provided some examples of how these changes are affecting nurses and clients in their agencies and how the Neuman Systems Model has been used to ensure that the client system integrity is maintained and enhanced.

THE ELGIN–ST. THOMAS HEALTH UNIT

The Public Health Nursing Division (PHND) of the Elgin–St. Thomas Health Unit, St. Thomas, Ontario, used a professional model of practice for over 10 years. Staff used the nursing process, identified nursing diagnoses, and documented their nursing interventions using a problem-oriented record. During an extensive revision of the PHND's philosophy a need for a more effective practice model was identified. Nurses felt that the current model was too broad and open to a number of interpretations. Provincial community health nursing standards also stipulated the use of a nursing theoretical model for practice.

There was complete agreement among PHND staff and administrators to use the Neuman Systems Model (NSM) as the model for nursing practice in the agency. The NSM was seen as the best fit with public health nursing practice, and it was felt that the flexibility of the model would guide the move from individual and family work to the changing paradigm of nursing practice as work with aggregates and communities.

An action plan was developed to introduce the NSM to staff and to implement the model into practice. A series of in-service sessions were held using both internal resources and external experts on the use of the NSM. A series of fact sheets were developed, and copies of Neuman's books were made easily accessible to staff. As the implementation plan progressed, staff evaluation indicated that nursing records should be adapted to reflect the language and concepts of the NSM. Staff felt that this move would assist with the integration of the concepts in their practice.

To ensure that staff had ownership of the record revision project, a committee was formed of staff members and one supervisor. Revision of the record became an orderly and efficient cycle of development, analysis, and evaluation until the work was completed. The nursing supervisor, who worked with the committee, analyzed the process of the record development and found it an effective exercise in planned change.

The NSM was particularly helpful in establishing the parameters for the area of client assessment in the record. It is well known that the record can set expectations for practice as it defines the types of information that are to be documented. For example, in the new record nurses were to document strengths and limitations of the client system and stressors on which to base nursing diagnoses. These expectations support the use of the six assessment questions developed by Neuman to assist nurses in their assessments of clients' needs for nursing intervention (Neuman, 1989, 62–63).

The move to work with aggregates and communities necessitated the development of an appropriate assessment form that differed significantly from the one used for individuals and families. For example, when the school was identified as the client, the functional patterns of the school required assessment. Also in keeping with the NSM, the strengths and limitations of the school to cope with its health problems needed to be assessed in order to determine the best role for the nurse in the resolution of health problems. Since a model of community development was accepted for practice, the six NSM assessment questions were revised so that their meaning was not lost but the wording was appropriate for the community as client. The use of the NSM with the community as client has only been in place for one year and has not been fully evaluated.

Working with the NSM has been an exciting and challenging experience for nurses and has expanded horizons on the possibilities for new and innovative nursing responses to client needs. Further work with the model will continue. A need has been identified by nursing staff to capture more of the wholistic view of the client on the nursing record. The record will also be used to determine the quality of nursing care to communities and aggregates, so it will be a vital document in the quality assurance program. (*Contact: Geraldine Craddock, Elgin–St. Thomas Health Unit, St. Thomas, Ontario.*)

THE MIDDLESEX–LONDON HEALTH UNIT

The Public Health Nursing Division of the Middlesex–London Health Unit (MLHU), an official health agency located in London, Ontario, Canada, has been working with the Neuman Systems Model since 1985. Initial use of the model was with individuals, families, and small groups such as prenatal and parenting classes. The division's documentation system, including an audit tool, was revised to support the use of the model. In addition, a tool was developed to assist nursing managers to use the model in their supervisory practice. Since the introduction of the model the division has been restructured from nurses working as generalists in district teams to nurses working in more specialized teams. The Neuman Systems Model continues to be used as the framework for nursing practice.

As a result of the move from individual and small group focus and the need to include population-based health promotion strategies, recent work within the nursing division is focusing on the development of skill in model use at the aggregate and population level. The phrase "community as partner" is currently being used as a reminder that current efforts to enhance the health of the population are through community participation, coalition building, and intersectoral collaboration.

A formalized agreement among the MLHU, the University of Western Ontario, and the provincial Ministry of Health has designated the MLHU as a Teaching Health Unit. This program allows health unit staff to work closely with students and faculty. Such a collaborative program will not only provide relevant student placements but also opportunities for staff members of the MLHU to engage in collaborative research with faculty members. To date, the dialogue resulting from this arrangement has identified particular benefits for students. One of these benefits relates to the collaborative efforts that could enhance student learning about the Neuman Systems Model. The Neuman Systems Model is taught in the undergraduate nursing program, and health unit staff act as a resource regarding the model and its application to practice for both faculty and students. Students also receive guidance in using the model during their field placements in the MLHU. The possibility of fourth-year undergraduate students using the model during their practicums offers opportunities for the model to be tested and refined for the practice of public health nursing.

These are times of change and times of opportunity for nurses to reexamine their roles and demonstrate the uniqueness of their contribution to the health care system. The NSM continues to offer a flexible yet comprehensive, meaningful framework to guide the practice of community/public health nursing at the individual and population level. (*Contact: Charlene Beynon, Middlesex–London Health Unit, London, Ontario.*)

AN ADOLESCENT PROJECT IN CALGARY, ALBERTA: THE NURSE AS ENABLER

Traditionally, adults have decided what adolescent problems are and have developed programs to address those adult-perceived needs. These programs have had a minimal impact on enhancing the positive life-style behaviors of adolescents. For example, one author, after an extensive review of school-based alcohol programs, suggested that all school-based preventive programs need to have their conceptual bases and their strategies reconsidered (Mauss, Hopkins, Weisheit, and Kearney, 1988).

This report will describe a project with adolescents aimed at ensuring that adolescents defined their own needs and the strategies that would be used to meet these needs. Ultimately, it was expected that the project would have a positive impact on the students' health.

The NSM was used as the conceptual framework for the project, and Social Marketing Theory (SMT) (Kotler and Roberto, 1989) was integrated into this framework. The decision to use the NSM was based on two important concepts in the model: the wholistic approach to the client and the view of nurses in a collaborative, facilitative role. Thus in this project the adolescents were the experts, and the nurse's role was that of enabler. Nursing expert roles can create rifts between professionals and communities, with resultant services that rob people of power (Labonte, 1989). Enabler roles empower people by providing them with means or opportunities (Meriam-Webster, 1986). SMT is a strategy for convincing individuals to make behavior changes. SMT advocates that the likelihood of an individual's responding to new information increases with the audience's interest or involvement in the issue. Thus it was important to ensure that any student project capture the students' interest and involvement.

The NSM defined the environment that should be explored before implementation of the project. For example, data were acquired about the client system (the adolescent population of the school) by interviewing the counseling and teaching staff and the school nurse. An environmental survey was also completed, and this revealed important information about the school's lines of resistance, the flexible and normal lines of defense, and the extrapersonal stressors. During the assessment phase support was enlisted for the project from school personnel and students. Some of the findings from the assessment were as follows:

1. *Physiological variable:* Students went to see the nurse with a variety of complaints (including headaches, stomach aches, and fatigue) and for immunization. Many students were overweight, and food choices often included "junk food."

2. *Developmental variable:* The students were viewed as concrete learners, and the school's goal was to provide them with trade skills. Some of the students had experienced failures in regular academic school settings.

3. *Psychological variable:* Students' relationship problems with their parents were of concern to school staff. Many of the adolescents were identified as suspicious of adults and very slow to trust others. Concern existed about the adolescents' self-esteem, related to nonachievement in an academic school setting.

4. *Sociocultural variable:* Students' high-risk life-style behaviors of smoking, use of alcohol and other drugs, and poor nutrition were identified by school staff. Gang violence was identified by some students.

5. *Spiritual variable:* A noon-hour worship group met regularly. This group was led by a teacher.

6. *Lines of resistance:* The school provided a safe atmosphere in which to learn work skills. The school tried to provide a learning environment that encouraged students to set up and meet short-term goals, thus enhancing their self-esteem and protecting their client integrity.

7. *Normal lines of defense:* The usual wellness level of students was reported as suboptimal, since there were high rates of absenteeism and high usage of the two holding beds in the nurse's room.

8. *Flexible lines of defense:* The flexible lines of defense were weak-

ened for the client system due to unhealthy life-style practices as mentioned above.

9. The *extrapersonal environment* included a fast food outlet and a convenience store close to the school, giving students ready access to food, candy, and cigarettes.

Using the Neuman Model to complete the client (the school) assessment identified how complex the stressors were for the students. It was evident that any new project that had the goal of impacting on student health must work in partnership with students to be effective.

Initially, 13 students from grades 10 to 12 agreed to meet in a focus group to discuss their health problems and to take an active part in their own health care. The group met twice weekly for 45 minutes, with an average attendance of seven students.

The Nominal Group Process (Van de Ven and Delbecq, 1972) was used to assist students to identify their stressors. After two meetings and much discussion the students identified the issue of child abuse as a topic they would like to learn more about. They also felt that once they had learned more about child abuse they would be able to help their peers by sharing this information with them. Subsequently, the group members prepared questions and invited a guest speaker to the group to discuss the topic with them and to answer their questions.

After the information session the students decided to complete a pamphlet and posters to inform other students about child abuse. The students worked on their own ideas for the pamphlet and posters, and the nurse was present for support and guidance. Student ownership of the project was very evident as students automatically accepted roles of chairperson and recorder at group meetings.

The finished products were very impressive, and students were proud of their accomplishments. School staff were also impressed with the pamphlet and posters. The pamphlet was published in the Board of Education's *Educational and Health Newsletter;* as a result of this, requests for the pamphlet came from health teachers, counseling departments, and an Educational Leadership Administration Centre. At an interagency level, the Canadian Red Cross Society requested that the students develop a pamphlet on child abuse as a permanent resource for their child abuse prevention program. The Red Cross program is targeted to all grade eight classrooms in Calgary, Alberta; thus the potential reach of the program is large.

The media were also involved in the dissemination of the results of this project as students were interviewed by a weekly community newspaper with a circulation of over 202,000. Also, one student and the nurse were interviewed by a local radio station.

Although school staff reported an increase in disclosure of child abuse, no direct association can be made between this reported increase and the school project. However, the students who worked on the project gained new skills and felt a sense of pride in their work, which will undoubtedly add to their sense of self-esteem and increase their normal and flexible lines of defense. The paradigm shift in nursing roles from "expert" to "enabler" may be difficult for nurses, but from the experience of this project it has the potential for the most lasting outcomes. (*Contact: Candace Lind, Wood's Homes, Calgary, Alberta.*)

REFERENCES

Canadian Public Health Association. 1990. *Community Health–Public Health Nursing: Preparation and Practice.* Ottawa: CPHA.

Kotler, P., and Roberto, E. 1989. *Social Marketing: Strategies for Changing Public Behavior.* New York: The Free Press.

Labonte, R. 1989. Community and professional empowerment. *The Canadian Nurse* 85(3):23–26.

Mauss, A. L., Hopkins, R. H., Weisheit, R. A., and Kearney, K. A. 1988. The problematic prospects for prevention in the classroom: Should alcohol education programs be expected to reduce drinking in youth? *Journal of Studies on Post Anesthesia Nursing* 5(1):54–55.

Merriam-Webster, Inc. 1986. *Webster's Ninth New Collegiate Dictionary.* Markham: Thomas Allen & Son.

Ministry of Health. 1989. *Mandatory Health Programs and Service Guidelines.* Toronto: Author.

Neuman, B. 1989. *The Neuman Systems Model,* 2d ed. East Norwalk, Conn.: Appleton & Lange.

Neuman, B. 1982. *The Neuman Systems Model: Appliation to Nursing Education and Practice.* East Norwalk, Conn.: Appleton-Century-Crofts.

Van de Ven, A. H. and Delbecq, A. L. 1972. The nominal group as a research instrument for exploratory health studies. *American Journal of Public Health* 62:337–342.

38

NEUMAN-BASED EXPERIENCES OF THE MIDDLESEX–LONDON HEALTH UNIT

Charlene E. Beynon

In 1985 the Public Health Nursing Division of the Middlesex–London Health Unit (MLHU), located in Central Canada, initiated a three-year project to implement the Neuman Systems Model as the division's theoretical framework for nursing practice. For a complete discussion of the structure and process used to facilitate this project see Drew, Craig, and Beynon (1989).

This chapter describes subsequent experiences, including those following the completion of the implementation phase. Recommendations developed from the project are presented, as well as staff comments about the model's utility and its continuing ability to direct the practice of public health nursing in an ever-changing environment. Beginning work in applying the model to the community as client is included.

OVERVIEW OF THE PROJECT

The introduction of *Standards of Nursing Practice for Community Health Nurses in Ontario* (RNAO, 1985) promoted the concept of theory-based practice throughout the province. The availability of such standards, which were based on the Neuman Systems Model, affirmed the decision to implement this particular model in the Public Health Nursing Division. Principles that directed the project were extensive staff and management participation, formative and sum-mative evaluation, and ongoing dialogue about the model and its utility to the practice of public health nursing. A variety of activities were developed to fos-ter understanding and to accommodate different learning styles. It was expect-ed that new knowledge derived from the learning activities would be applied to day-to-day practice. Application of the Neuman Systems Model was discussed at team meetings and during individual meetings with the team supervisor.

EXPERIENCES FOLLOWING THE PROJECT

In 1989 the first theory-based record was introduced. Since that time, all nursing records have been based on the Neuman Systems Model, and the audit tool has been revised to reflect this change. Since the division's existing problem-orient-ed record was compatible with the Neuman Systems Model, a decision was made to learn the model during the three-year implementation phase, rather than learning how to complete a "Neumanized" record. Staff were encouraged to refer to model definitions often and to start assessing, making diagnoses, iden-tifying nursing outcomes, and evaluating interventions in terms of the model. The goal was to think and act using the new system rather than continuing to translate from the old.

The Neuman Systems Model has been incorporated into the division's orga-nizational culture. For example, the division's philosophy of nursing was revised to incorporate theory-based practice, and the performance appraisal tool for public health nurses was modified to include application of the model to prac-tice. Furthermore, staff have used the model as an organizing framework to develop a staff education program on aging, and public health nurses use the model's language when talking with colleagues. The Neuman Systems Model also has been used as the foundation to develop a specific model for public health nursing in schools.

Anecdotal comments from staff and management and review of records reflect that practice has been strengthened by the use of the Neuman Systems Model. Historically, practice expectations assumed client involvement, but the use of the Neuman Systems Model legitimized actively inviting the client's per-ception and participation in identifying both concerns and possible solutions. Family assessments are more comprehensive, and the inclusion of the spiritual variable has added a new dimension to practice beyond an inquiry of religious practices. Inclusion of the sociocultural variable has increased the cultural sen-sitivity of practitioners' interactions with clients and groups in a community with a rapidly changing ethnic profile.

Two committees, the Neuman Steering Committee and the Neuman Repre-sentatives (Drew et al., 1989), which were instrumental in guiding and mon-itoring the implementation project, were maintained for 15 months and nine months, respectively, following completion of the project. These committees required both staff and management participation. The decision to maintain the committees was significant in that it facilitated monitoring the model's use following the official end of the three-year project, and the retention of both committees helped to maintain the progress that had been achieved during that time.

The Neuman Bulletin Board and *Neuman Notes,* a division newsletter, continue to be used as strategies to reinforce practice expectations and to update staff regarding further developments as the model is used in other settings and countries including the United States, Australia, Sweden, and other European nations. Future plans include periodic refresher days, encouraging research projects and student placements that support use of the Neuman Systems Model, and inviting staff to share experiences and new learning gained from using the model in practice.

STAFF COMMENTS AND EXPERIENCES

Staff were surveyed annually during the project years. At the end of the second year, staff affirmed the same benefits of using the Neuman Systems Model in their practice as had been identified at the end of the first year. Staff observed that the model:

- Identifies and recognizes the importance of the client's perception
- Incorporates a wholistic approach
- Includes all levels of prevention
- Promotes a comprehensive and goal-directed approach
- Helps organize data
- Provides guidance in determining intervention (Drew et al., 1989)

At the end of the second year, staff also reported that the model's terminology was a continuing source of concern. The difficulty of documenting use of the model on the problem-oriented record was identified as a critical issue. As the model's terminology was internalized during the project years and became more meaningful in the practice setting, the model's language became less of a concern. The introduction of the theory-based record in 1989 reinforced the expectation that the Neuman Systems Model be used as the division's framework for nursing practice and required that practitioners be familiar with the model in order to accurately document nursing actions.

At the end of the third year, survey results indicated that there was a definite shift from "sometimes use" to "usually use" the model when assessing individuals, families, and groups; when formulating nursing diagnoses, expected outcomes, and nursing interventions; in recording; and in case consultations with supervisors. Staff identified remaining learning needs, such as using the model with special populations. They were now able to acknowledge and demonstrate personal responsibility in meeting these needs. The most frequently cited reinforcers for using the model were discussions at team meetings, case discussions with supervisors, and reading circulated articles.

Although initially somewhat skeptical of the Neuman Assessment/Intervention Tool (Neuman, 1989), public health nurses have found the tool helpful in focusing visits and interventions. Staff were encouraged to modify the questions to reflect their own interviewing styles and clients' developmental stages and situations, while maintaining the tool's intent. Following use of the tool in practice, it was recommended that an additional question of "What are you not able or willing to do regarding the identified concern?" be added to the tool (K. Mepham, personal communication, 1988).

The following comments from public health nurses are reflective of the range of experiences in learning and using the model within the division:

> At first the model is intimidating—once the words become familiar it is a friendlier model to use. It does permit an efficient organization of data. It has improved my assessments to include previously overlooked areas such as spiritual. It has assisted me to identify why nursing strategies are or haven't been effective with the inclusion of both the client's and the nurse's perception. I think I am discharging more efficiently . . . and with less guilt.

The following comments came from a practitioner new to the division:

> Using the Neuman Systems Model focuses my approach on the client as a whole with all factors that may be affecting functioning. . . . The model focuses on the client and the client's perception . . . thus encouraging active involvement in the learning/change process.

An experienced nurse writes:

> It is clearer to me what strengths and weaknesses individuals have and hence it makes our mutual plan . . . easier to negotiate and evaluation of outcomes is simpler to do.

Another experienced nurse responded:

> I feel mighty good when I see it all together. . . . The model definitely provides for a thorough assessment of the individual and family. This valuable data collection helps in planning interventions realistically. I feel that the model helps make us better interviewers and counsellors. . . . I have had to "de-program" and change my attitude regarding the model, but it is coming. I feel much more positive.

One nurse spoke about the decision to learn the model:

> When change is imminent, you have a choice. You can resist or go with the

flow. I decided to go with the flow by getting involved. . . . It helped me to understand the (Neuman) framework and it gave me a forum in which to answer my questions. Best of all, it gave me a sense of owning the framework, a feeling I would have lost, had I stayed "on the outside" looking in.

And as a final comment, one nurse stated:

For the past year, I have felt increasingly comfortable with the model. I have totally incorporated it into my thinking during the assessment, intervention, evaluation and documentation phase of all contacts with individuals and families. *Finally,* it is a *natural* process now after many months of trying to work through it step by step and *WORK* it was! It seems to be the perfect model for us to use in Community Health Nursing. . . . It truly seems feasible to use it with population based programs just as easily as with individuals and families. I am personally looking forward to applying it there.

RECOMMENDATIONS: LESSONS LEARNED

For a project such as this to be successful and to sustain momentum over a period of time, it is critical to have a clear vision and organizational commitment as well as staff who are supported and willing to accept a challenge to modify the way nursing is practiced in their agency. The probability of achieving the desired outcomes is increased by specifying a reasonable time frame for the implementation phase with a specific completion date identified at the outset. Formative evaluations during the implementation phase are critical.

In this organization, the Director of Public Health Nursing assumed the role of project sponsor (Bryson, 1991), thereby ensuring that the project was sanctioned and received sufficient support and resources to survive despite numerous other challenges. A supervisor (designated as the project coordinator), a steering committee, and a staff representative and supervisor in each of the nursing teams assumed the responsibility of ensuring that the momentum was maintained. Staff and management involvement in introducing the project and sustaining progress is essential in promoting individual ownership and survival of such a project.

When a change in practice is launched, it is imperative to recognize current strengths and expertise and yet be clear that a change in practice is intended. Otherwise the response may be "we already do this," and the full potential of using a nursing model will not be realized. A focus on enhancing quality of care and perceived benefits to the individual practitioner is a useful approach to promoting a change in practice.

It is also important to acknowledge the limits of using any model. It was necessary to clarify that the model should not be viewed as a programmed tool that automatically provides answers but rather as a framework that has the capability of clarifying and strengthening nursing actions. Throughout the project it was emphasized that using the model did not lessen the need for a solid knowledge base and clinical judgment. Likewise it was acknowledged that using the model did not replace the need for incorporation of other tools and theories, which still would be required according to the client's need and situation.

In addition to the identified "Critical Elements to Promote Success" (Drew et al., 1989) that were identified early in the project, the use of humor and opportunities to celebrate accomplishments were sought. A "raffle" was held using the parts of the model as tickets. The prize was a T-shirt with the slogan "Neuman to the Core." This same slogan was printed on pens that were distributed to staff to complete the survey at the end of the third year. During a staff meeting the official end of the project was celebrated complete with balloons, sparklers, and a cake decorated with the model. One of the nursing teams prepared a skit and composed a song to commemorate the division's experiences. This time of celebration was a way of congratulating the staff for a job well done and providing yet another opportunity to review and reinforce expectations. This event was enjoyed by staff, and the feedback received was "Why didn't we do this when we started?"

As a time-saving measure, it is recommended that a historical record of project events be maintained as they occur. Such accounts are useful to share with other agencies who are considering implementation of theory-based practice. The development of resource binders that include learning activities, articles, and samples of recording using the model are convenient for periodic review by individuals and groups of staff. Such references are also helpful in providing new staff with a consistent orientation to the project and practice expectations.

Ongoing consultation and networking with other model users are extremely beneficial during the project years and after the implementation phase has been completed. Contact from other users has functioned as the "external conscience" in identifying issues that require follow-up within the division, for example, development of a standardized aggregate record. Planning specific strategies to reinforce and enhance continuing model usage following the project is highly recommended.

THE NEUMAN SYSTEMS MODEL'S FIT WITH A CHANGING PRACTICE ENVIRONMENT

Since the decision was made to implement the Neuman Systems Model as the Public Health Nursing Division's framework for practice, many stressors have occurred within the internal and external environment. The recession and changing societal expectations are demanding that practitioners recognize and respond to the broad determinants of health, demonstrate interdisciplinary and intersectoral collaboration, and reallocate already scarce resources to health promotion and disease prevention. It is increasingly expected that the consumer will be included in problem identification and decision making in a manner that empowers and acknowledges cultural, linguistic, and racial diversity.

Since 1989 there has been a heightened emphasis on disease prevention, health promotion, and health protection within the Province of Ontario's public health system. This shift in focus has resulted in the development of programs that emphasize population-based approaches and require interdisciplinary practice and broad community participation and support.

Concurrent with the changes in practice resulting from the above programs and in preparation for the 21st century, the scope and mandate of public health nursing have and continue to be critically examined across the country (CPHA, 1991). From these discussions the unique goal of public health nursing has been defined as "to promote and preserve the health of populations" (CPHA, 1991, 3). Such a definition, with its emphasis on population-based approaches and view of the community as the client, is necessitating changes in the practice of public health nursing. There is now a greater emphasis on groups and aggregates and an acknowledged need for different strategies and modes of intervention. Examples of such strategies are community development, social marketing, and healthy public policy.

In view of the aforementioned stressors, it has become evident that a model is needed to guide public health nursing practice in these times of change. Furthermore, such a model must be broad in scope—one that is wellness focused; incorporates a broad definition of health; is empowering; promotes ownership of concerns, involvement, participation, and partnership with others; is consistent with the science and principles of public health; accommodates interdisciplinary practice; and may be used with individuals, families, groups, communities, and entire populations. The Neuman Systems Model offers the Public Health Nursing Division such a model, and the model has withstood the challenges presented by these and other stressors in the internal and external environment.

Staff experience with the model has provided evidence that the Neuman Systems Model can be used with individuals, families, groups, or the community and is compatible with population-based approaches. The Neuman Assessment/Intervention Tool (Neuman, 1989) is used effectively as a community development tool with focus groups to assist communities in identifying areas of concern and determining possible solutions. In using the model, the "consumer's" perception and participation are actively sought in identifying such concerns and possible solutions. Inclusion of the five variables—physiological, psychological, developmental, sociocultural, and spiritual—recognizes the need for a broad definition of health, recognizes the many determinants of health, and acknowledges the impact of societal and environmental factors on health. Although the Neuman Systems Model has been used primarily by nurses, its terminology and foundation in systems theory make it appropriate to be used by other disciplines. Potential use of the model by other disciplines makes the selection of the Neuman Systems Model as the theoretical framework for the practice of public health nursing especially pertinent.

If a model that focused primarily on the care of individuals and families had been selected, it would have been difficult to continue to consistently use one model in the face of the shift to health promotion and population-based approaches, and the view of the community as the client. The need to change models or to introduce additional models during times of significant change would have severely threatened the commitment to theory-based practice. The adoption of the Neuman Systems Model as the division's framework has made such transitions less difficult.

REMAINING CHALLENGES

Despite the Neuman Systems Model's ability to be used with the community as client, additional work is needed to develop skill in this area of practice. The model does offer a comprehensive framework to work with a community in identifying what data are needed, organizing the data in a systematic and meaningful manner (Figure 38–1), and prioritizing and selecting interventions.

Used in conjunction with other resources (such as morbidity and mortality reports, census data, economic indicators, and other techniques, including windshield surveys and interviews with key informants and community members), a comprehensive community assessment and profile can be generated using the model. The Neuman Assessment/Intervention Tool (Neuman, 1989) offers a way to organize interviews with community members and provides a means of validating information collected from other sources. The five variables assist in making a truly wholistic assessment and in identifying actual or potential issues within the community that the community may wish to address, such as:

- Physiological: burden of illness
- Psychological: sense of well-being, economic base
- Sociocultural: recreational, cultural opportunities; ethnic profile
- Developmental: length of time as a community
- Spiritual: sense of hope

Similarly, by classifying stressors using the model's intra-, inter-, and extra-environmental terminology, actual or potential stressors can be identified in consultation with the community, such as:

- Intraenvironmental: conflict *within* the community, for example, NIMBY ("not in my backyard") conflict over the location of a group home, federal penitentiary for women, or needle exchange program
- Interenvironmental: issues *between* neighboring communities, for example, debate over annexation
- Extraenvironmental: issues *distal* to the community, for example, pollution, cross-border shopping, free trade agreements

In addition to developing expertise in using the model with the community as client, a continuing challenge is to remain attentive to model issues. Practi-

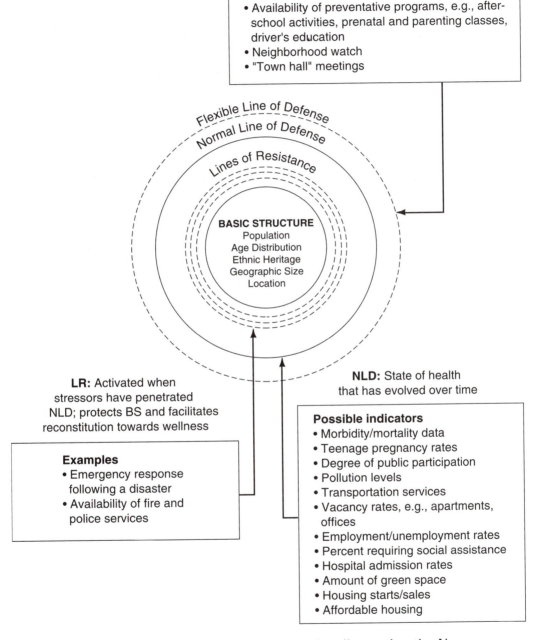

FLD: Protective accordion-like buffer that protects the NLD from invasion by stressors

Possible indicators
- Availability of preventative programs, e.g., after-school activities, prenatal and parenting classes, driver's education
- Neighborhood watch
- "Town hall" meetings

Flexible Line of Defense
Normal Line of Defense
Lines of Resistance

BASIC STRUCTURE
Population
Age Distribution
Ethnic Heritage
Geographic Size
Location

LR: Activated when stressors have penetrated NLD; protects BS and facilitates reconstitution towards wellness

Examples
- Emergency response following a disaster
- Availability of fire and police services

NLD: State of health that has evolved over time

Possible indicators
- Morbidity/mortality data
- Teenage pregnancy rates
- Degree of public participation
- Pollution levels
- Transportation services
- Vacancy rates, e.g., apartments, offices
- Employment/unemployment rates
- Percent requiring social assistance
- Hospital admission rates
- Amount of green space
- Housing starts/sales
- Affordable housing

Figure 38–1. Viewing the community as the client using the Neuman Systems Model.

tioners new to the division and experienced staff need to remain current about the model as it evolves and is further developed in practice settings around the world. This task needs to be shared by staff and management and is likely to be most successful if periodic "checkups" are included in operational plans and annual review of programs. Networking with model users in other settings is a valuable motivator and reinforcer. Consistent use of opportunities to incorporate the model into in-service programs, case consultations, and discussions at staff meetings; circulation of relevant articles; and distribution of newsletters that provide model updates and address practice issues are all effective strategies in ensuring that the commitment to theory-based practice and the chosen model is maintained.

FUTURE IMPLICATIONS FOR USE OF THE NEUMAN SYSTEMS MODEL IN THE 21ST CENTURY

With the coming of the next century, all practitioners will be challenged by a changing practice environment. Current events suggest that public health nursing will continue to increase its emphasis on health promotion, community participation, and population-based approaches and, as a result, will demand of its practitioners new skills and interventions. In addition, this environment probably will become increasingly culturally diverse and will offer diminishing resources. Most likely, differing patterns of health needs related to life-style and chronic illnesses, poverty, environmental stressors, and a changing demographic profile will emerge. This environment will demand heightened accountability and excellence in practice. The ability to make difficult practice decisions and to use nursing interventions that are research-based and known to be effective will be paramount.

The Neuman Systems Model offers a framework to guide the practice of nursing in a changing environment. As previously stated, no model will replace the need for a credible knowledge base or strong clinical judgment, but because the Neuman Systems Model "provides structure, organization, and direction for nursing action, yet is flexible enough to deal adequately with infinite complexity" (Neuman, 1989, 16), the Neuman Systems Model can guide and direct the practice of public health nursing in meeting the challenges and expectations of the next century.

SUMMARY

The process of implementing a nursing framework has been energizing and challenging for our Public Health Nursing Division. The structures and strategies implemented during the project were effective in managing the project and sustaining achievements postimplementation.

Following the implementation phase the model continues to be used in daily practice and incorporated into the division's culture. The selection of the Neuman Systems Model as the framework for practice has and continues to be an excellent choice despite changes in practice expectations. The staff are now planning to use the model in new areas of practice as the scope and mandate of public health nursing continue to evolve.

REFERENCES

Bryson, J. M. 1991. *Strategic Planning for Public and Nonprofit Organizations.* San Francisco: Jossey-Bass.

Canadian Public Health Association. 1990. *Community Health—Public Health Nursing in Canada: Preparation and Practice.* Ottawa: CPHA.

Drew, L. L., Craig, D. M., and Beynon, C. E. 1989. The Neuman Systems Model for community health administration and practice: Provinces of Manitoba and Ontario, Canada. In *The Neuman Systems Model,* edited by B. Neuman, 315–341. Norwalk, Conn.: Appleton & Lange.

Neuman, B., ed. 1989. *The Neuman Systems Model,* 2d ed. Norwalk, Conn.: Appleton & Lange.

Registered Nurses' Association of Ontario. 1985. *Standards of Nursing Practice for Community Health Nurses in Ontario.* Toronto: RNAO.

39

THE NEUMAN SYSTEMS MODEL IN A CHRONIC CARE FACILITY: A CANADIAN EXPERIENCE

Margot Felix
Cora Hinds
Sister Carmen Wolfe
Antoinette Martin

> "Professional activities can be best controlled by a group which belongs to that profession with the view to understanding the functions, determining the needs and examining the alternatives."
>
> (*The Division of Labor in Society*, Durkheim, 1893)

> "Nursing professionalism is dependent upon the development of a scientific nursing theory base."
>
> (Neuman, 1985)

This chapter describes the implementation of a Project Management Plan incorporating the Neuman Model to guide practice in a tertiary care institution. This chapter will:

1. Describe the context within which the Neuman Systems Model was selected to guide practice.
2. Utilize the model to demonstrate the progression of client care along the continuum through graduate care.
3. Discuss the implementation of the model on a chronic care unit.
4. Present feedback of nurses' utilization of the model in practice.

The Project Management Plan and graduate care are defined as follows:

- The *Project Management Plan* is a dynamic working document conceived to guide the implementation process of the Neuman Systems Model at Elisabeth Bruyère Health Centre.
- *Graduate Care* is care along a continuum from partially independent functioning in the community to full chronic and palliative inpatient care.

There is widespread concern among health care professionals about the growing number of elderly people in Canadian society and the rising cost of providing medical care and supportive services to those who need them (Angus, 1990). By 2010 in Ontario alone, the number of people 65 years of age and older will have grown by 18 percent (Ministry of Health, 1991). The health and activity limitation survey (Statistics Canada, 1990), conducted in 1986 and 1987, revealed that 45.5 percent of people aged 65 and over experience some form of disability and that disability increases sharply with age. In addition, an estimated 40,000 nonelderly people with physical disabilities and chronic illnesses will require publicly funded long-term care support and services (Ministry of Health, 1991).

The complexity and different etiologies associated with chronic illnesses require a multidisciplinary team approach to enhance or palliate the health status and the quality of life of chronically ill individuals. Nurses who are key members of the team have an important contribution to make to the well-being of the chronically ill. However, role clarification for each discipline is a prerequisite to practice within multidisciplinary teams for efficient and effective interventions and outcomes. The nursing profession, as a subcomponent of the health care system and a full team member, should be able to articulate and clarify its contribution to the health status of society. "In defining its parameters, not only can the nursing profession underline its independence, but underscore the fact that multidisciplinary interdependence can be realized only if a minimum of independence has been achieved by each of the professions involved" (Coutu-Wakulczyw and Beckingham, 1993, 83). The Neuman Systems Model, which uses a multidisciplinary approach, provides a mechanism for communicating more effectively about nursing practice with both nurses and other disciplines.

Nursing practice based on a theoretical framework is well recognized by the College of Nurses of Ontario. Frameworks provide a road map for practice. They tell the clinician what to look for when interacting with clients and how to interpret observations. It also tells the practitioner how to plan interventions in a general manner and provides beginning criteria for evaluation of intervention outcomes (Fawcett, 1984). In short, practice based on a model is essential to the complex decision making required of nurses when caring for clients, such as the chronically ill.

CONCEPTION OF THE PROJECT MANAGEMENT PLAN

The project was conducted at the Elisabeth Bruyère Health Centre (EBHC), a 324-bed chronic care facility serving an essentially geriatric population, with an average age of 80 years, in the Ottawa-Carleton region. The philosophy of the nursing department is premised on the worth, dignity, respect, and wholeness of individuals. The provision of high-quality wholistic care within an interdisciplinary framework is a goal that is prominently reflected in the philosophy of the nursing department.

This project utilizing the Neuman framework is a three-year undertaking that has been financed within the nursing services' global budget. The plan has been operationalized using a committee structure drawn from nursing services. An ad hoc committee, called the "Neuman Working Group," was formed comprised of individuals from nursing research and education. By consensus, members committed themselves to implementing the project. A schematic representation of the project is shown in Figure 39–1. The activities of the Neuman Working Group are listed in this diagram.

THE MODEL SELECTION

In the process of selecting a model for the project, seven commonly used nursing frameworks were considered. The Neuman Systems Model was finally chosen because of its congruency with the client care goals of EBHC, which are based on a total person approach and encourage the involvement of families in the care process. The Neuman Model is derived from Gestalt and field theories of the interaction between person and environment, theoretical formulations of stress and adaptation, general systems theory of the nature of living open systems, and formulation of levels of prevention. Thus both inductive and deductive strategies were used (Neuman, 1982).

Elements of the Neuman Systems Model, which uses a systems approach, are congruent with both the graduate care concept and the multidisciplinary approach used at EBHC. Clients benefit from a comprehensive range of services, which include health promotion, functional rehabilitation, maintenance, and palliation. The importance of a client's family and friends is recognized, and their involvement in the individual's overall plan of care is encouraged. The model's comprehensiveness is an added dimension in terms of its adaptability. It takes into account the roles of all nursing personnel and their contribution, the provision of nursing care, and the range of services offered in a chronic care facility.

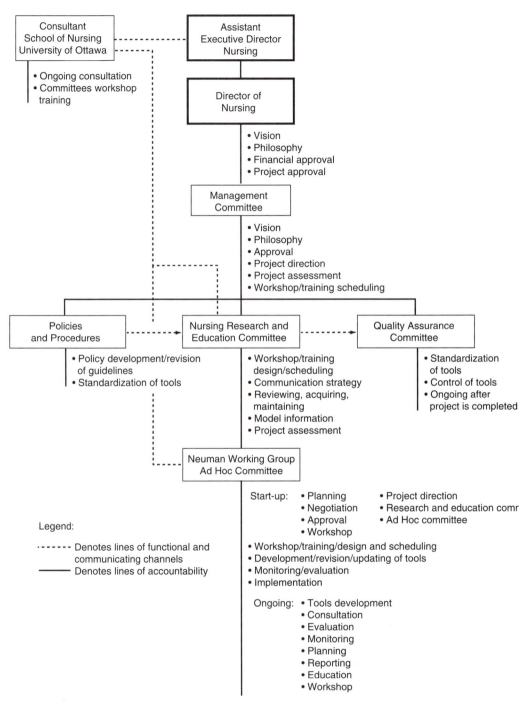

Figure 39–1. A schematic representation of the organization and structure of the project.

OPERATIONALIZATION OF THE PROJECT

The process of moving toward theory-based practice began with the adoption of a Project Management Plan by nursing administration. The plan provided a mechanism that facilitated the development of standards for effective and efficient delivery of care and, at the same time, allowed nurses to further develop their professional autonomy.

The implementation strategy included a six-month start-up period. The initial activity consisted of a half-day session by one of the authors (C. Hinds) to introduce the model to senior and middle management personnel and the Nursing Research and Education Committee. It was followed three months later by a two-day workshop by Betty Neuman and Rosalie Mirenda. These activities served as a catalyst for creating interest in the model and motivating nursing personnel. They also informed other disciplines within the institution and the larger nursing community of the move to theory-based practice at EBHC. Furthermore, through participation of university personnel, these teaching sessions established the linkage between education and practice.

TOOLS DEVELOPMENT

The EBHC Neuman Systems Model nursing health assessment tool and the nursing care plan were developed by the Neuman Working Group. These two tools were developed in accordance with the assessment format utilized by Neuman. In order to simplify and encourage the use of the tool by nurses, lists of possible patient symptoms that are commonly found to alter the functional pattern of patients were included under each of the five variables and three environmental stressor categories identified by Neuman. A sample of the assessment impressions and nursing care plan is shown in Figure 39–2. These instruments were first tested in a workshop session utilizing a case study. A second testing of the instruments was conducted using as a control group registered nurses from a nondemonstration unit who had no prior knowledge or instruction in the use of the Neuman Model. Comments received from this testing served as the basis for modifying the assessment tool and nursing care plan. It also provided direction for the development of the in-service educational program on the use of the model prior to its implementation on the demonstration unit. These tools continue to be tested and refined. The authors will share complete assessment tool upon request.

IMPLEMENTATION OF THE MODEL

Testing on a Demonstration Unit

A 53-bed unit consisting of both male and female patients with multiple chronic health problems and an average stay of two years was selected for testing the newly designed tools. The process began with an in-service educational program consisting of four modules, each lasting 45 minutes. The sessions were conducted on the unit and were made available to each shift and offered at a time suggested by the nurses. Nursing staff included registered nurses, registered nursing assistants, and nurse's aides. This ensured maximum attendance at these educational sessions. Principles of adult education and learning were incorporated in the education program design, thus fostering flexibility and allowing

List	Resident/Family/Other Perception	Nurse Perception
Nutrition		
Respiratory status		
Circulatory status		
Bowel function		
Bladder function		
Skin integrity		
Sleep pattern		
Mobility		
Sensory function		
Motor function		
Hygiene		
Eating		
Others		

Figure 39–2. A sample of summary of impressions following client assessment.

Service de sante' des
Soeurs de la Charite' d' Ottawa/Sisters of Charity of Ottawa
Health Service

NURSING CARE PLAN
Neuman Systems Model

Allergy □	Sex: Male □ Female □ Age ( )	Admission Date:

Discharge Plan: Yes □ No □	Rehabilitation □	Respite Care □

Diagnosis	Code Status	Dentiers/Dentures
	#_____	□Upper/supérieur Lower/inférieur □ □Partial upper Partial lower □

I. Physical (Lifestyle)

Personal Habits:

Smoking: Yes □ No □
Alcohol: Yes □ No □

Diet:

Collation: Yes □ No □
Food Allergies: Yes □ No □

Sleep/Rest Patterns:

Rest during day: Yes □ No □

Functional Patterns (A.D.L.)
Eating:

Feeds self   Yes □ No □
Feeds self with
assistance   Yes □ No □
Partial assistance   Yes □ No □
Total feed   Yes □ No □
Difficult total feed   Yes □ No □
Tube feeding   Yes □ No □

Elimination:

Continent   Yes □ No □
Incontinent: Bowel □ Bladder □
Ostomy □   Brief (M) □ (L) □
Bladder training   Yes □ No □
Times: _____
Catheter □ Size: _____
Condom □ Size: _____
Toiletting:
Independent   Yes □ No □
With assistance   Yes □ No □
With constant presence Yes □ No □

Bathing:

Bathes self with supervision   □
Washes face and hands only   □
Promotes self care/Bathes
   with assistance   □
Complete bath in bed, tub,shower   □
Dress/Undress   □
Grooms self   □
Needs total grooming care   □
Tub bath—day _____

Ambulation/ Mobility:

Type:_____
Walks—supervision with or without
   mechanical aids   □
Walks—with staff constant presence   □
Propels self in wheelchair within
   institution   □
Circulates in wheelchair with
   assistance   □
Turn position/skin care   □
Special position skin care   □
Passive exercises _____
_____   □

Transfer Picto:

1. 2. 3. 4.
5. 6. 7. 8.
9. 10. 11. 12.

Instrumental Activities of Daily
Living (I.A.D.L.)

Uses facial tissue   Yes □ No □
Uses telephone   Yes □ No □
Uses bedside bell   Yes □ No □
Operates radio   Yes □ No □
Operates television   Yes □ No □
Handles own cigarette   Yes □ No □
Communication board   Yes □ No □

II. Psychological (Mental Status)
Memory Attention Span:

Confusion   □
Recent Memory Loss   □
Confabulation   □
Remote Memory Loss   □

Mood:

Appropriate   □   Inappropriate □
No response   □   Depressed □
Agitated   □   Irritable □
Anxious   □   Other: ____
_____
_____

Speech:

Unable to speak   □
Clear   □
Dsyphasia   □
Expressive aphasia   □
Aphasia   □

Chambre/Room: _____   Nom/Name: _____

Figure 39–2. (cont.)

NURSING CARE PLAN
Neuman Systems Model

Palliative Care ☐	Chronic Care ☐	Coroner: Yes ☐ No ☐
Dentition naturelle/ Natural Teeth ☐ Upper/supérieure ☐ Lower/inférieure	Hearing aid/Prothèse auditive ☐ Right/droit ☐ Left/gauche	Eye glasses/Lunettes Reading glasses Yes ☐ No ☐ Regular Yes ☐ No ☐

Thought Process/Thought Content:

Coherent ☐	Incoherent ☐
Evasive ☐	Slow to respond ☐
Logic ☐	Illogic ☐
Delusions ☐	Hallucinations ☐

Cognitive Function: Consciousness:

Alert ☐	Lethargic ☐
Semiconscious ☐	Comatose ☐

Orientation:
Oriented to:
Person ☐   Place ☐   Time ☐
Wanders on unit   Yes ☐ No ☐
Tends to go outside   Yes ☐ No ☐
Relationship to Person:

Cooperative ☐	Defensive ☐
Hostile ☐	Aggressive ☐
Abusive ☐	Disturbs others ☐

III. Sociocultural
Support systems
available   Yes ☐ No ☐
Languages spoken: _____
_____
LOA's: _____
Frequency of family visits:
_____
_____
Level of family support
required: _____
_____

Next of Kin:
1. Name: _____
Relationship: _____
Tele (H): _____
    (W): _____

III. Sociocultural (cont'd)
Next of Kin
2. Name: _____
Relationship: _____
Tel: (H): _____
    (W): _____

IV. Developmental:
Marital status: _____
Educational level: _____
Past occupation: _____

V. Spiritual:
Religious preference: _____
Important religious practice: _____
_____
Seeks spiritual assistance: _____
_____
Ministry Consultant   Yes ☐ No ☐
Date: _____
Questions moral and ethical
implication of therapeutic regimen:
_____
_____
Sacrament of the sick: Yes ☐ No ☐
Date: _____

Health & Safety:
Smoking Hazard: Robot ☐
    Smoking apron ☐
Supervision   Yes ☐ No ☐
Constant Presence: Yes ☐ No ☐
History of self injury: Yes ☐ No ☐
History of fall: Yes ☐ No ☐
Seat belt: Yes ☐ No ☐
Choking: Yes ☐ No ☐

Health & Safety (cont'd)
Laptable: Yes ☐ No ☐
Restraint: Yes ☐ No ☐

Wanderer:
Green Dot: Yes ☐ No ☐
Electronic Device: Yes ☐ No ☐
Bedside Rails: Up—Yes ☐ No ☐
    Down—Yes ☐ No ☐

Behavior Modification:
Plan: Yes ☐ No ☐

Treatments:
Vital signs: _____

Médicin/Physician: _____

Figure 39–2.

learning to occur at a pace suited to individual nurses. The change was introduced with minimum disruption of the ward routine and produced little resistance from nurses.

Content of the Modules

Module 1. Material covered in this module included the scope of nursing, the concept of autonomy in nursing, and developmental, traumatic, and planned change. Principles of change used by Lewin (1951) and theories of attitude change (Insko, 1967) (Figure 39–3) were incorporated in the material presented to the nurses. The work of these two authors was also integrated to provide a mechanism for feedback and follow-up as the implementation progressed.

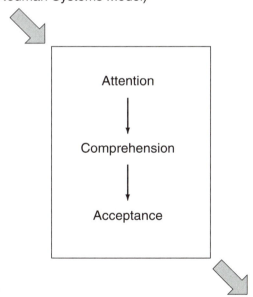

Underlying Theories:
Stimulus, response, and reinforcement theories of attitude change

Stimulus (the Neuman Systems Model)

Attention

Comprehension

Acceptance

Response
(attitude change)

Figure 39–3. Theories of attitude change. (Adapted by permission from Insko, C. A. 1967. *Theories of Attitude Change.* Englewood Cliffs, N.J.: Prentice Hall, pp. 13, 14.) (See also Hovland, Janis, and Kelley [1953])

Module 2. The second module dealt with the process of choosing a model, the pros and cons of using models in nursing, and how various models differ from each other. The final segment focused the question, why the Neuman Systems Model?

Module 3. The third module covered elements of the Neuman Model, which were presented in two sessions one week apart. Before the second session a quiz was administered to the nurses to assess their knowledge of the content offered to this point. The quiz included some scenarios for practical application of the model (for example, "After assessing Mrs. Peters using the Neuman Systems Model Health Assessment tool, one of the nursing diagnoses was potential alteration in skin integrity related to immobility. At what level of prevention should the nurse base his or her intervention?"). Similar types of questions were asked at the end of the educational program to test participants' knowledge and understanding of the model.

Module 4. The fourth module dealt with interviewing techniques, explanation, and use of the Neuman Assessment Tool, which was developed specially for use in the chronic care setting. The end of this session was seen as the beginning of an ongoing learning process that would eventually result in internalization of the model through practice. This was facilitated through twice weekly team meetings led by RNs where staff members discussed their practice using the model to assess client health status. This process served to increase staff confidence and comfort in using the model. Ongoing support and consultation were provided to the unit staff by the nurse educator and the unit manager.

Following each of the four educational sessions, feedback about the content was obtained from participants.

THE NEUMAN SYSTEMS MODEL: *A FRAMEWORK FOR ASSESSING THE CARE NEEDS OF THE CHRONICALLY ILL*

Neuman (1989) describes her multidimensional framework as based on two major components: stress and the reaction to stress. The total person (client system) is an open system in interaction and total interface with the environment. "Man" is a composite of *physiological, psychological, sociocultural, developmental, and spiritual variables* (Neuman, 1989, 29). This view is congruent with the basic principle of the proposed reform of the long-term care system in Ontario (Ministry of Health, 1990). Neuman's model can be used to assess either an individual, a group or family, or a community. Our view is that Neuman's model has utility for assessing, enhancing, and palliating the health status of chronically ill individuals in chronic care institutions.

In Figure 39–4, a system (either an individual or a group of chronic care users) is depicted as having a *basic structure or central core,* which is composed of factors basic to all organisms or to all systems, and to survival (Neuman, 1989). Although the chronically ill suffer irreversible changes to the system, there is the potential for them to achieve a maximum level of functioning; hence emphasis must be placed on wellness rather than illness. Stressors may impair the core of some composite variables within individuals, but through systematic interventions they can be assisted to attain an optimal level of functioning and well-being. Surrounding this basic structure are the *lines of resistance,* which protect the central core against stressors to decrease the degree of reaction to it. The *normal line of defense* is the normal adaptational state the person has developed over time, and is considered a normal state of wellness for that individual (Neuman, 1982, 1989). In this case of chronically ill clients with reduced normal lines of defense, they will adapt to their new state of health or optimum potential. The *flexible line of defense,* which surrounds the normal line of defense, is the dynamic state of wellness that may be particularly susceptible to situational circumstances. It can be thought of as an accordion-like structure that functions to prevent stressors from penetrating the normal line of defense (Neuman, 1982). The newly acquired health status or optimum functional level of chronically ill clients in chronic care institutions must be maintained.

Stressors can be subsumed under three categories: *intrapersonal, interpersonal,* and *extrapersonal factors.* A reaction occurs in response to a stressor. The nature and the degree of the reaction is determined by the interrelationship of the five variables. Health is defined on a wellness–illness continuum (Neuman, 1982). This definition fits well with the philosophy of care at EBHC, which embraces the notion of a continuum and the graduate care concept. Here the role of nursing is to promote system stability through the use of purposeful interventions. The level of intervention will be determined by the actual or potential penetration of the normal line of defense and is developed at three modes or levels of prevention: primary, secondary, and tertiary (Neuman, 1982). This thinking is in line with the proposed legislation of the Ontario Ministry of Health, Regulated Health Professions Act (RHPA), and promoted by the College of Nurses of Ontario. It states that "the practice of Nursing is the promotion of health and the assessment of the provision of care and the treatment of health conditions by supportive, preventive, therapeutic, palliative and rehabilitative means in order to attain or maintain optimal function."

INTERVENTIONS IN CHRONIC CARE

Caring for the chronically ill in chronic care institutions represents an intervention on behalf of persons with chronic conditions in order to offset the func-

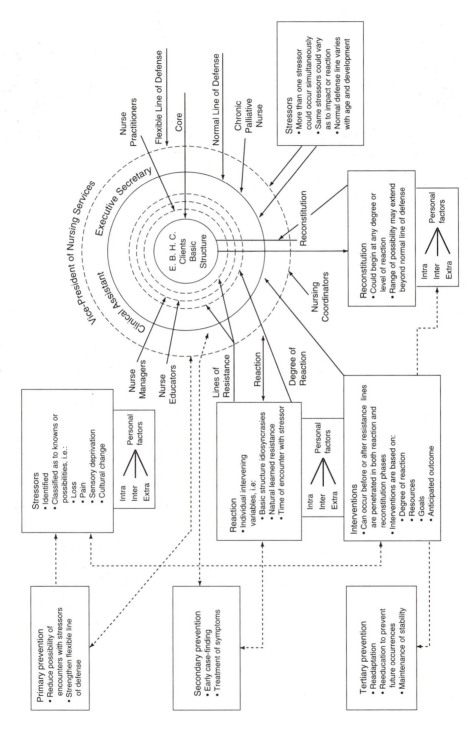

Figure 39-4. The Neuman Systems Model: Adapted to chronic care units at Elisabeth Bruyère Health Centre (EBHC).

tional losses that have resulted from illness or injury. The intervention may be introduced to prevent an impairment, to avoid a disability, or to offset the consequences of a handicap (Lubkin, 1986). Some interventions may be advocated prior to the existence of an anticipated illness in an effort to maintain wellness; such interventions should be considered an appropriate part of chronic care (Lubkin, 1986). Congruent with the Neuman Systems Model, intervention can begin at any point at which a stressor is either suspected or identified in the trajectory of a chronic condition or in the care continuum. One would carry out the intervention of primary prevention when a reaction had not yet occurred, although the degree of risk or hazard was known or present. The intervener would perhaps attempt to reduce the possibility of the individual's encounter with the stressor or in some way attempt to strengthen the individual's flexible line of defense to decrease the possibility of a reaction (Neuman, 1982). For example, a person with a cardiovascular accident (CVA) and residual hemiplegia may be immunized against influenza. This primary prevention intervention is an anticipatory strategy to offset a debilitating illness that could lead to complications and exacerbation of an existing condition.

Assuming either that the above intervention was not possible or that it failed and a reaction occurred, intervention at the level of secondary prevention would be offered in terms of prompt treatment of existing symptomatology. Treatment could begin at any point following the occurrence of symptoms. Optimum use would be made of individuals' resources—both external and internal—in an attempt to stabilize their condition or help strengthen their internal lines of resistance to reduce the reaction (Neuman, 1989). Assessing both the internal and external resources of the ill person gets at the total meaning of the experience for the individual (Neuman, 1982; Rubenstein, 1983). This assessment permits appropriate ranking of patient needs. Should the individual fail to reconstitute, death occurs as a result of the failure of the basic core structure to support the intervention (Neuman, 1982, 1989). Reconstitution can be thought of as beginning at any point following interventions. It should be kept in mind that reconstitution may progress beyond, or stabilize somewhat below, the individual's previous normal line of defense or usual level of wellness (Neuman, 1989).

Tertiary prevention begins following the active treatment or secondary prevention stage where some degree of reconstitution or stability has occurred (Neuman, 1982, 1989). The emphasis on tertiary prevention is therefore aimed at maintaining a reasonable degree of adaptation. This implies proper mobilization and utilization of the individual's existing energy resources. When applied to persons in chronic care facilities, tertiary prevention can be considered rehabilitation in the global sense of the term where the primary goal would be to strengthen clients' resistance to stressors through reeducation and readaptation in order to limit or prevent recurrences of reaction or regression. Here reconstitution is seen as a dynamic state of adaptation to stressors in the internal and external environment, integrating all factors for optimum use of total patient resources. This dynamic view of tertiary prevention moves the patient back ideally to optimum system stability.

OPTIMIZING CARE AND CONSERVING RESOURCES

Rubenstein (1983, 1984) suggests that assessment can circumvent inappropriate use of health care services, prevent waste of scarce resources, and contribute to avoidance of imposed disability resulting from inappropriate diagnosis and labeling of old persons. Successful assessment leads to improved nursing diagnostic accuracy, more appropriate intervention outcomes for persons with chronic care needs, and improved functional status of the elderly. Neuman (1982) identifies three basic principles in developing an assessment tool related to the total person model:

1. Good assessment requires knowledge of all the factors influencing a patient's perceptual field.
2. The meaning that a stressor has to the patient is validated by the patient as well as by the caregiver, thus the notion of choice.
3. Factors in caregivers' perceptual field that influence their assessment of the patient's situation should be made clear (Neuman, 1982).

Critical to assessment in chronic care is the paradigm that examines what Katz and Akpom (1976) refer to as activities of daily living. This is the assessment of an individual's functional capacities that typically include bathing, dressing, transferring, toileting, and feeding. In fact, these are performance measures that determine capacity for independence and identify areas of dependency, which if appropriately ameliorated, will increase independent functioning. In addition, the individual's cognitive capacities, social interactions and family supports, eating practices, resources in the physical environment, and mental health functioning are generally included in the assessment process and are captured within the elements of the model.

Assessment becomes a tool for encouraging maintenance of wellness and identifying resources within the individual, the family, and the environment that can contribute to and enhance the wellness of the individual. Wellness is not only the absence of pathology but also maintenance or improvement of one's functioning (Robertson, 1986). In contrast to acute care, chronic care shifts from a focus on disease or pathology to a focus on function, and then to maintaining function through appropriate intervention. Appropriately targeted interventions that are based on accurate assessments not only benefit patients but also encourage judicious use of scarce resources. The Neuman Systems Model provides a mechanism whereby these objectives can be met, while at the same time allowing nurses in chronic care facilities to fulfill their mandate of total patient care and articulate their unique contribution along the chronic care continuum.

NURSING: A SUBSYSTEM OF THE CHRONIC CARE CONTINUUM

When viewed as a system, chronic care facilities have a reciprocal relationship with the environment of the larger health care system and the larger social system surrounding it, while at the same time sharing with the parts and subparts of its own smaller system. For example, a chronic care facility as a subsystem of the health care system is related to other parts of the larger system, which also shares the goal of maintaining the integrity of chronically ill clients at an optimal level of wellness or health status. Nursing, a subpart of the system, can affect the entire health care system and in turn be affected by it. As front-line providers, nurses, who fall within the subsystem of nursing administration, can in Neuman's terminology be conceptualized as the lines of resistance surrounding the core, that is, the chronically ill individual (Figure 39–4). These sharing relationships of parts and subparts of the health care system represent a type of interdependency requisite for optimal functioning and, in fact, the eventual survival of the entire system. Thus the larger system can be described as a pervasive order that holds together the parts (Neuman, 1982).

NURSES' PERCEPTION OF THE USEFULNESS OF THE MODEL

Following the completion of the demonstration project, nurses in the project were asked to respond to a questionnaire that assessed their perceptions of the usefulness of the model and their concerns about applying the model in practice. The questionnaire also allowed nurses to provide feedback that would assist in refining the implementation process on other units. Responses were made to a Likert scale that ranged from 1 (not useful) to 5 (very useful). Twenty-nine (98 percent) of nurses responded to the questionnaire. Overall, nurses found the model to be very useful (75 percent), neutral (21 percent), and not useful (4 percent). With respect to planning patient care, 63 percent of the nurses felt that using the model increased their understanding of the needs of residents/patients and assisted them in approaching patient care wholistically. These verbatim quotes reflect the nurses' perceptions:

> "The assessment tool helps us to see the resident as a whole person."
> "Good patient assessment, good knowledge of the patient thereby impacting on a better quality of care."
> "A new interest in documenting the monthly patient review."

These quotes clearly reflect benefits nurses perceived in utilizing the Neuman Systems Model in practice. Thirty-seven percent of nurses were neutral in their view to this question. There were a few negative comments made by nurses, and these were generally in relation to the length of time it took to complete the assessment tool (for example, "It takes a long time to complete the assessment form because of the detailed needs of the residents"). A more detailed account of the nurses' responses to this questionnaire will be reported elsewhere.

NEUMAN SYSTEMS MODEL: A DETERMINANT FOR CHANGE

The Neuman Systems Model offers a new approach for thinking about the care of the institutionalized chronically ill. The framework provides a meaningful index to assess the health status of the chronically ill. Utilizing this model, impairments of the five variables—physiological, psychological, sociocultural, developmental, and spiritual—find their clinical expression in signs and symptoms of organ system dysfunction and in disability. Prompt intervention at the appropriate level of prevention will prevent further deterioration of the individual. The Canadian health care system relies heavily on inpatient institutional care to meet the needs of chronically ill and dependent elders. However, the changing demographics of an aging society in a climate of limited resources is demanding reassessment and critical examination of the way in which the needs of institutionalized chronically ill and dependent elderly are met.

The Neuman Systems Model emphasizes identification of actual and potential problems in the functioning of the system and the delineation of intervention strategies that maximize efficient and effective system operation (Coutu-Wakulczyk and Beckingham, 1993). Rubenstein (1983) makes the observation that unless assessment results in improved comprehensive services, it is legitimate to ask whether assessment has any impact on the provision of services. In addition to being important to the individual being assessed, assessment contributes in a significant way to the accumulation of data that are essential when planning resource allocation that can influence the availability of chronic care services and access to them (Rubenstein, 1984).

At the present time, nursing services are in the process of expanding the use of the model. A framework has been developed for quality assurance based on the Neuman Quality Improvement Process (Hinton Walker, in press). In addition, a nursing research informatics committee is involved in application development of a computerized nursing care plan utilizing the Neuman framework and the nursing process. These will provide a data base that can be used for clinical nursing research in the field of chronic illness.

CONCLUSION

In conclusion, the Neuman Systems Model, with its underpinning in general systems theory, provides a useful framework for interpreting current trends within the health care system and, at a micro level, offers direction for use in a chronic care institution. The model provides a way of thinking about the care for institutionalized chronically ill populations. It offers a systematic approach to care and provides an analytical tool for explaining the way in which stressors interact within a system. The model also provides a problem-solving approach using the three levels of prevention. Thus this model has the capacity to meet the needs of the target population at any stage in the wellness–illness continuum.

REFERENCES

Angus, D. 1990. A great Canadian prescription: Take two commission studies and call me in the morning. In *Restructuring Canada's Health Services System: How Do We Get There from Here,* edited by R. B. Deber and G. G. Thompson. Toronto: University Press.

Coutu-Wakulczyw and Beckingham. 1993. Selected nursing models applicable to gerontological practice. In *Promoting Healthy Aging: A Nursing Community Perspective,* edited by Beckingham-Dugas. Toronto: Mosby Year Book Inc.

Durkheim, E. 1893. *De la Division Sociale du Travail.* Presse Universitaire de France, 9e édition, 1973.

Fawcett, J. 1984. *Analysis and Evaluations of Conceptual Models of Nursing.* Philadelphia: F. A. Davis Co.

Hinton Walker, P. In press. *Neuman Quality Improvement Process.*

Hovland, C., Janis, I., and Kelley, H. H. 1953. *Communication and Persuasion.* New Haven, Conn.: Yale University Press.

Insko, C. A. 1967. *Theories of Attitude Change.* Englewood Cliffs, N.J.: Prentice Hall, 13, 14.

Katz, S., and Akpom, A. 1976. A measure of primary biological and social functioning. *International Journal of Health Services* 6(3):494.

Lewin, K. 1951. *Field Theory in Social Sciences.* New York: Harper.

Lubkin, I. M. 1986. *Chronic Illness: Impact and Interventions.* Boston: Jones and Bartlett.

Ministry of Health. 1990. *Strategies for Change: Comprehensive Reform of Ontario's Long-Term Care Services.* Toronto: Queen's Printer for Ontario.

Neuman, B. 1982. *The Neuman Systems Model: Application to Nursing Education and Practice.* East Norwalk, Conn.: Appleton-Century-Crofts.

Neuman, B. 1989. *The Neuman Systems Model.* East Norwalk, Conn.: Appleton-Century-Crofts.

Regulated Health Professions Act, RHPA Tour Information Session. 1992. College of Nurses of Ontario.

Robertson, D. 1986. Alternative mode for health care delivery. In *Aging with Limited Health Resources,* Ministry of Supply and Services Canada.

Rubenstein, L. Z. 1983. The clinical effectiveness of multidimensional geriatric assessment. *Journal of the American Geriatric Society* 31(12):758–762.

Rubenstein, L. Z. 1984. Geriatric imperatives: Geriatric assessment programs. *Journal of the Medical Society of New Jersey* 81(8):651–654.

Statistics Canada. 1990. Barriers Confronting Seniors with Disabilities in Canada, Special Topic Series, The Health and Activity Limitation Survey.

40

COMMUNITY-AS-CLIENT ASSESSMENT
A Neuman-Based Guide for Education and Practice

Gail Beddome

The focus of this chapter is on the use of the Community-as-Client Assessment Guide (Beddome, 1989) by registered nurses enrolled in a bachelor of science of nursing (BSN) program in British Columbia. A review of the assessment guide and suggested modifications are discussed. Use of the assessment guide by BSN students with aggregate and community clients, as well as selected examples of data analysis, nursing diagnosis, and primary, secondary, and tertiary levels of preventive interventions are described with future implications for the guide's use as based on the Neuman Systems Model.

Health care reform has become a theme for the '90s as governments around the world are struggling to contain escalating illness care costs. Canada has embraced a changing health paradigm by adopting primary health care principles (WHO, 1978) and community development (Green and Kreuter, 1991) approaches to shift the focus from illness care to health care delivery. Evidence of health care reform in Canada includes an emphasis on health promotion (Epp, 1986; CPHA, 1986), individual and community empowerment (Labonte, 1990), a shift of secondary care from hospital to community, hospital bed closures, and more community programs (Seaton et al., 1991). At regional levels, health care reform has resulted in creative options for cost containment while also ensuring quality health services. Some examples of new programs include hospital–community partnerships, hospitals without walls, and nurse-managed

Reviewed by Jean Kelley and Charlene Beynon.

clinics. Another outcome of health care reform is that nurses are increasingly working in community and nontraditional programs and ideally will integrate primary health care principles and community development approaches with a health promotion focus into their practice (Clouthier Laffrey and Page, 1989; Doucette, 1989).

While nurses in both hospital and community settings recognize the need for new health care approaches (Beddome, Clarke, and Whyte, 1993)—for example, a beginning shift to health promotion-focused practice (Berland and Whyte, 1991)—many recognize that they lack the knowledge and/or skill required to practice within the new paradigm, motivating their return to the university setting for a BSN education. Students enrolled in the BSN program at the University of Victoria, or one of its partner sites, are exposed to a variety of nursing models, including the Neuman Systems Model (Neuman, 1982).

COMMUNITY-AS-CLIENT ASSESSMENT GUIDE

The Community-as-Client Assessment Guide (Beddome, 1989), an adaptation of the Neuman Systems Model, provides an organizational framework allowing for collection of data about geopolitical and aggregate needs from the perspectives of both clients and caregivers (Neuman, 1982). The assessment must also take into consideration community resources and resource utilization patterns. Methods of data collection for community assessment include observational surveys, key informant interviews, participant observation, and secondary analysis of existing data (Goeppinger, 1985).

The Community-as-Client Assessment Guide is based on the Neuman Systems Model, which deals with system parts as well as the whole. This model provides "structure, organization, and direction for nursing action, and is flexible enough to deal adequately with infinite complexity" (Neuman, 1982, 11). Furthermore, a systems approach is neither in competition with nor exclusive of other nursing assessment approaches (Beddome, 1989). The guide's broad application makes it suitable for both geopolitical communities (Aroskar, 1982) and aggregates (Williams, 1982).

Confusion about whether the client is a geopolitical or aggregate client can be reduced by a clear definition of the client system that is the target of data collection and nursing intervention (Beddome, 1989). Once the decision is made concerning the focus of data collection, the client system can be classified as community as client or aggregate as client. The community as client is defined by visible geographical separations, such as rivers, roads, and institutional walls, or invisible political separations, such as state, provincial, or national boundaries. The aggregate as client is defined by demographic characteristics such as socioeconomic status, culture, age, values, or policies (for example, inner-city street people or preschool children).

The intra-, inter-, and extrasystem environmental concepts of the Neuman Systems Model can be applied to both the geopolitical and aggregate clients as illustrated in Figure 40–1. The intrasystem in both client systems is the people. In the geopolitical client it is all the people living within an identified geopolitical boundary (Aroskar, 1982), such as the citizens of a particular city. The aggregate intrasystem is a group of individuals who have in common one or more personal or environmental characteristics (Williams, 1982), such as people with AIDS within a particular hospital or city. The assessment of any intrasystem population reflects the physiological, psychological, developmental, sociocultural, and spiritual characteristics of the Neuman Model. These five variables interact with the intersystem and extrasystem. For example, a geopolitical or an aggregate community client with the core sociocultural variable of a diverse mix of cultures and high unemployment will have distinctly different needs from a community that is more homogeneous.

The five variables—physiological, psychological, developmental, sociocultural, and spiritual—of the Neuman Systems Model work well when applied to people but are less easily defined when applied to environmental inanimate objects such as buildings, roadways, and communication systems within a community (Beddome, 1989). Therefore, when the community system as a whole is assessed, subsystems must be addressed as one of the interdependent units of complicated social relationships and biophysical influences (Stewart, 1985).

The inter- and extrasystems of both geopolitical and aggregate clients are assessed according to eight subsystems: health and safety, sociocultural, education, communication and transportation, recreation, economics, law and politics, and religion (Anderson and McFarlane, 1988; Stewart, 1985). Guided by the purpose and focus of the assessment, nurses must make clinical judgments about whether they need general or specific information. For example, if the nurse wants to know what recreation resources are available for an aggregate of elders living in a particular city, the data collection would be much more specific than if the nurse wants to know what recreation resources are available for all people of a geopolitical community living in the same city.

The aggregate intersystem is confined to the immediate caregiving system, for example, volunteer organizations, hospital, or health department. The assessment of the aggregate intersystem would include relevant data of the immediate caregiver subsystems; for example, the nurse might want to assess the number and educational background of staff at a women's center. A geopolitical community intersystem assessment would include relevant data from each of the eight subsystems, for example, the media resources that are available to advertise support group activities.

The geopolitical community client extrasystem includes areas of influence, such as beliefs, laws, and resources from neighboring and greater communities (Stewart, 1985). A geopolitical extrasystem assessment would include the influence of a larger area, such as the reduction of transfer payments from the federal government to the Canadian provinces for health care, considered according to the eight subsystems. The aggregate extrasystem includes the eight subsystems of the geopolitical intersystem. The aggregate extrasystem assessment, like the intersystem assessment, includes relevant data from each of the eight sub-

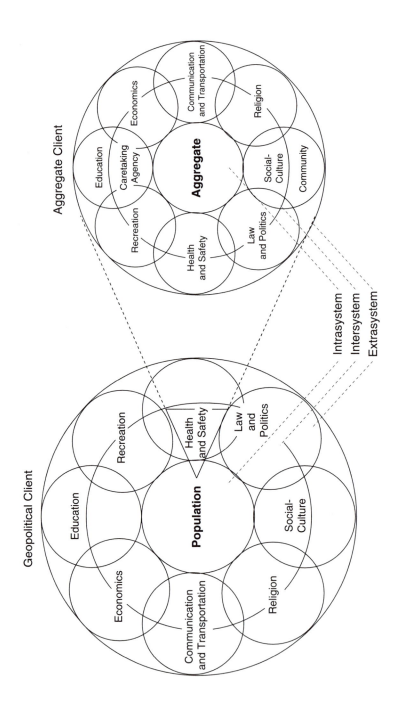

Figure 40–1. Schematic illustration of the Neuman Systems Model applied to a geopolitical client and an aggregate community as client.

systems of the geopolitical intersystem; for example, a reduction in funding may result in a reduction of programs at the aggregate intersystem level. This is illustrated more fully in the Community-as-Client Assessment Guide in Appendix A.

Analysis of intra-, inter-, and extrasystem environmental data is done to determine the impact of intra-, inter-, and extrasystem stressors upon the client system, as well as the strength of the client system lines of resistance to protect from stressors and reconstitute when necessary. Consistent with systems theory, a threat or stressor in one part of the system has implications for instability of all other parts. The flexible line of defense acts as the system boundary and controls exchanges of material, energy, or information through such things as laws, policies, conflict resolution, and decision making. For example, cost containment and reduced federal funding for health care is an extrasystem stressor that may penetrate both the geopolitical community and aggregate clients' flexible lines of defense. Stressor penetration would then result in the client system's normal line of defense being challenged, causing periods of instability until the system could reconstitute by using available resources (lines of resistance), both internal and external. The normal line of defense is the system's state of health developed over time and is reflected in health indicators and social determinants such as life-style, immunization rates, available housing, employment, and crime rates. The flexible line of defense includes activities and programs such as "Neighborhood Watch" and "Buckle-Up" that reflect the system's basic beliefs and values about health care. Client stability takes place through primary, secondary, and tertiary prevention (Neuman, 1982). An example of community-as-client reconstitution using tertiary prevention is health care reform by rethinking health policy and writing new health legislation at many levels of government.

Nursing diagnoses are statements using model language of actual or potential problems related to intra-, inter-, or extrasystem stressors. An example of a nursing diagnosis for a geopolitical client system is a potential for normal line of defense system instability related to decreased federal funding, evidenced by hospital bed closures, increased unemployment of health care workers, increased wait lists for hospital admissions, and increased use of emergency rooms. An example of a nursing diagnosis for an aggregate client system is a stable normal line of defense of low-income women related to their empowerment, evidenced by increased lobbying of local and provincial politicians and increased networking among low-income women and with existing community agencies. Examples of primary prevention are networking and activities that support women's empowerment; an example of secondary prevention is lobbying.

COMMUNITY-AS-CLIENT ASSESSMENT GUIDE: A LEARNING EXPERIENCE

One BSN program in the Canadian province of British Columbia is offered at multiple sites in the southern half of the province. Postbasic RN and generic students are enrolled either at the University of Victoria, where both distance and campus courses are offered, or at one of the collaborative partner sites at Okanagan University College, University College of the Cariboo, Langara, Malaspina College, or North Island College. Students at all sites experience the same curriculum, which reflects changes in the health care system and the influence of feminist, phenomenological, and critical social theories. It has a health promotion focus and prepares graduates to work with aggregates and communities as clients as well as individuals and families (Ministry of Advanced Education, 1992).

Students taking the first clinical course are introduced to nursing models and their application to community as client, as well as concepts of epidemiology, demographics, primary health care, and health promotion. Anderson and McFarlane's adaptation of the Neuman Systems Model, *Community as Client: Application of the Nursing Process* (1988) is a popular choice for this course, as students find the detail helps them integrate the above-mentioned concepts and principles with a nursing model as organizing structure. Working in groups of three or four, students assess a geopolitical community, analyze the data, and write nursing diagnoses reflecting the model concepts, followed by written recommendations for primary, secondary, and tertiary interventions to strengthen both the normal and flexible lines of defense. For example, the inability of a community to provide transportation services to isolated citizens has direct implications for the health of the defined system normal line of defense. Nursing diagnoses reflect both strengths and threats to the system and are related to the lines of defense and resistance, such as: "potential problem for intersystem normal line of defense related to inadequate transportation for 40 percent of socially isolated intrasystem and insufficient extrasystem funding for buses." Using a community development approach, recommended interventions might include strategies to empower citizens, such as organizing town hall meetings where citizens identify and prioritize their needs then suggest action plans for reaction to combat the stressors and facilitate reconstitution as needed. Depending on the severity of the problem, this might be considered a primary or tertiary level of intervention, that is, the risk for some clients would be high while others may have some alternative transportation to the existing stressor. An example of secondary level prevention may be nurses working intersectorally to promote healthy public policy.

When students advance to the population-as-client course, they frequently use Beddome's adaptation of the Neuman Systems Model (Beddome, 1989). Students working in groups form partnerships with community individuals and groups to plan and evaluate a program that will influence the health determinants of populations at risk using primary health care principles (WHO, 1978) and health promotion (Epp, 1986; CPHA, 1986) strategies. Students are encouraged to make clinical judgments about what population-specific data are appropriate to collect. Subsystem assessment includes identification of resources, utilization patterns, and community values and attitudes. Like the earlier course, students analyze the data, identify stressors and strengths, write nursing diagnoses that reflects model concepts, and then in collaboration with community partners plan, implement, and evaluate a health promotion program. Populations students have worked with include children, parents, college students, women, smokers, and elders. Sites they have worked in include hospitals, health units, college campuses, seniors' high-rise apartments, low-cost housing complexes, banks, and malls. Programs have included health fairs of every description for a variety of populations, parent education, caregiver support, occupational health, and town hall meetings.

SUMMARY

The purpose of this chapter was to discuss the revised Neuman-based Community-as-Client Assessment Guide for geopolitical and aggregate clients. Although the Community-as-Client Assessment Guide was initially developed to facilitate data collection for geopolitical and aggregate clients by community health nurses, it has been used successfully by students in a BSN educational program. BSN students are able to consistently make high-level clinical judgments about what and how much data to collect for community and aggregate clients followed by analysis and integration of demographic and epidemiological concepts. The Community-as-Client Assessment Guide has proved valuable as a guide for practice and a teaching tool demonstrating critical thinking by students.

FUTURE IMPLICATIONS FOR USE OF THE NEUMAN-BASED COMMUNITY-AS-CLIENT ASSESSMENT GUIDE

Clarification of how to best deal with the increased frequency and complexity of demands on health care systems requires intersectoral collaboration at community and provincial or state levels. Demands characterizing the 21st century relate to societal changes such as increased homelessness, violence, at-risk teenage pregnancies, aging populations, and catastrophic events such as war, AIDS, and poverty. Nurses will assume expanded roles as they participate with other disciplines and agencies to study these and other demands and design effective ways to program for change. The wholistic systems approach of the Community-as-Client Assessment Guide facilitates nurses' collaborative work with other disciplines. The nursing concepts used within the assessment guide provide the framework and create flexibility for collaboration with community partners for broad problem identification and definition, goal setting and exploration, and determination of relevant interventions. These particular features of the Neuman-based Community-as-Client Assessment Guide make it particularly beneficial for nurses and other health disciplines as they move into the 21st century.

ACKNOWLEDGMENT

The author wishes to thank the many BSN students who have used the Community-as-Client Assessment Guide in their course work and who have willingly shared their experiences using it. The author also invites anyone who has used the Community-as-Client Assessment Guide to send their comments to Gail Beddome, Department of Nursing, Okanagan University-College, 333 College Way, Kelowna, B.C., V1V 1V7.

REFERENCES

Anderson, E. T., and McFarlane, J. M. 1988. *Community as Client: Application of Nursing Process.* New York: J. P. Lippincott.

Aroskar, M. A. 1982. Ethical issues in community health nursing. In *Readings in Community Health Nursing,* 2d ed., edited by B. W. Spradley, 80–87. Boston: Little, Brown.

Beddome, G. 1989. Application of the Neuman Systems Model to the assessment of community-as-client. In *The Neuman Systems Model,* 2d ed., edited by B. Neuman. San Mateo: Appleton & Lange.

Beddome, G., Clarke, H. F., and Whyte, N. B. 1993. Vision for the future of public health nursing: A case for primary health care. *Public Health Nursing* 10:13–18.

Berland, A., and Whyte, N. B. 1991. *The Role of the Hospital Nurse in Health Promotion: A Focus Group Approach.* Unpublished research report. Vancouver, B.C.: Registered Nurses Association of B.C.

CPHA. 1986. *Ottawa Charter for Health Promotion.* Ottawa: Canadian Public Health Association.

Clouthier Laffrey, S., and Page, G. 1989. Primary health care in public health nursing. *Journal of Advanced Nursing* 14:1044–1050.

Doucette, S. 1989. The changing role of nurses: The perspective of medical services branch. *Canadian Journal of Public Health* 80:92–94.

Epp, J. 1986. *Achieving Health for All: A Health Promotion Framework.* Ottawa: Health and Welfare Canada.

Goeppinger, J. 1985. Community as client: Using the nursing process to promote health. In *Community Health Nursing: Process and Practice for Promoting Health,* edited by M. Stanhope and J. Lancaster, 379–404. Toronto: Mosby.

Green, L. W., and Kreuter, M. W. 1991. *Health Promotion Planning: An Educational and Environmental Approach,* 2d ed. Toronto: Mayfield.

Labonte, R. 1990. Community and professional empowerment. *Canadian Nurse* 85: 354–361.

Ministry of Advanced Education. 1991. Collaborative nursing curriculum. Unpublished curriculum. Victoria, B.C.: Ministry of Advanced Education.

Neuman, B. 1989. *The Neuman Systems Model.* San Mateo: Appleton & Lange.

Seaton, P. D., Evans, R. G., Ford, M. G., Fyke, K. J., Sinclair, D. R., and Webber, W. A. 1991. *Closer to Home: The Report of the British Columbia Royal Commission of Health Care and Costs.* Victoria, B.C.: Crown.

Stewart, M. 1985. Systematic community health assessment. In *Community Health*

Nursing in Canada, edited by M. Stewart, J. Innes, S. Searl, and C. Smillie, 363–377. Toronto: Gage.

Williams, C. 1982. Community health nursing—What is it? In *Readings in Community Health Nursing,* 2d ed., edited by B. W. Spradley, 73–79. Boston: Little, Brown.

World Health Organization. 1978. *Primary Health Care.* Geneva: World Health Organization.

APPENDIX A ⸻

Community-as-Client Assessment Guide

Aggregate Client	Geopolitical Client
Intrasystem	*Intrasystem*
System—client defined	Same as aggregate client
Physiological	**Physiological**
1. Physical assessment or screening as appropriate 2. Specific maturational stage data, e.g., apgar scores of newborns 3. Health indicators: morbidity, mortality, life expectancy 4. Life-styles, including risk-taking behaviors	Same as aggregate client
Psychological	**Psychological**
1. Emotional health of aggregate members: prevalence of isolation and depression, divorce and crime rates 2. Health beliefs: immunization levels, child-rearing practices	1. Emotional health of community
Developmental	**Developmental**
1. Maturational stage of aggregate 2. Age range and median of aggregate	1. Maturational stage of community 2. Age range and median of population
Sociocultural	**Sociocultural**
1. Demographic characteristics: sex, age, education level, income, and ethnicity 2. Consumer participation in community programs	Same as aggregate client
Spiritual	**Spiritual**
Religious affiliation	Same as aggregate client

Aggregate Client	Geopolitical Client

Client Perceptions
—Perceived problems
—Perceived solutions

Intersystem	*Intersystem*
Primary caregiver system	Geographical or political system

Health and Safety

Health and Safety	Health and Safety
1. Personnel: number, education, and experience	1. Health indicators: morbidity, mortality, life expectancy, etc.
2. Caseload of personnel	2. Resource allocation and utilization
3. Occupational health programs	3. Facilities: hospitals, health department, outpatient clinics
4. Environmental conditions and safety hazards within the building	4. Safety services —Official services, e.g., police, fire —Volunteer services, e.g., block parent, neighborhood watch
	5. Sanitation services, e.g., garbage and sewage disposal
	6. Caseloads of professionals
	7. Environmental conditions and safety hazards: • Air, water, soil inspection • Abandoned or unsafe buildings, trash and garbage, and broken sidewalks

Sociocultural

Sociocultural	Sociocultural
1. Ethnic composition of personnel and languages spoken	1. Cultural composition of population and languages spoken
2. Membership in associations and professional organizations	2. Guiding values
	3. Positions and roles
	4. Associations and clubs
	5. Services to strengthen families, e.g., senior day care
	6. Services for special groups, e.g., handicapped and new immigrant

Education

Education	Education
1. Education level and experience of personnel	1. Personnel: education level of residents
2. Continuing education for employees: journal subscriptions, in-service education	2. Facilities: universities, colleges, schools, libraries
	3. Personnel: number, education, and experience

Communication and Transportation

Communication and Transportation	Communication and Transportation
1. Communication patterns within agencies: formal and informal system	Same as aggregate client

Aggregate Client	Geopolitical Client

Communication and Transportation (cont.)

2. Communication methods to intrasystem and extrasystems: pamphlets, posters, home visits, and mass media
3. Accessibility
   • Location: accessibility and acceptability
   • Hours of service
   • Cultural interpretation and translation services

Recreation

1. Facilities: lunchrooms, lounges, library, etc.
2. Activities: planned and informal

Recreation

1. Facilities: schools, libraries, museums, ice rinks
2. Personnel: number, education, and experience
3. Programs: adult, children, and special needs
4. Accessibility

Economics

1. Resources: funding, personnel, buildings, equipment, supplies
2. Health and welfare benefits for employees: health and dental insurance, pension plans, etc.
3. Paid continuing education programs

Economics

1. Employment: employment status and income levels of residents
2. Income assistance: percentage of the population
3. Education levels, literacy rate
4. Housing: quality and types
5. Industry and occupational health programs

Law and Politics

1. Policy formulation: decision-making and problem-solving patterns
2. Positions and roles
3. Contracts

Law and Politics

1. Power: sanctions and legislation as it relates to health of community

Religion

1. Agency philosophy and mandate, e.g., programs and clientele served
2. Beliefs and values of employees

Religion

1. Number and type of churches
2. Church programs and activities

Client Perceptions
—Perceived problems
—Perceived solutions

Extrasystem
Same as the geopolitical intersystem

Extrasystem

1. Geographical location, climate, urban or rural, topography, square miles
2. Population: number per square mile, mobility

Aggregate Client	Geopolitical Client
Subsystem Data	**Subsystem Data**
Same as the geopolitical intersystem	Collect data selectively about subsystems at a federal level or state or provincial level, or both, as it pertains specifically to the needs of the geopolitical community.

The list of assessment data and the examples given of the type of data to collect serve only as a guide and are not exhaustive.

41

THE SPIRITUAL VARIABLE
A World View

Glenn Curran

The Neuman Systems Model (1989) is a conceptual model that identifies the human spirit as a part of the everyday nursing experience. It is suggested that the spiritual variable is the major influence of a person and the pivot on which the Neuman Systems Model (1989) revolves. This chapter seeks to extend the meaning of the spiritual variable by describing the possible relationships of a highly abstract concept. The context of this work is meant to engender a world view that respects other cultural and religious perspectives.

It is acknowledged that the ideas presented are only one interpretation of the spiritual variable in the Neuman Systems Model (1989). These ideas arise from a personal understanding of Baha'i writings as they relate to spirituality, religion, and God. This humble work is offered as one attempt to expand nursing's description of spirituality and aims to stimulate an ever widening interpretation of this concept.

HUMANISTIC EXISTENTIALISM AND SPIRITUALITY

The ideas of body, mind, and spirit, and their relationship have intrigued and informed human history. Nursing is currently dominated by the philosophies of humanism and existentialism (Bevis, 1982; Cartwright, Davson-Galle and Holden, 1992; Pearson, 1988). Humanistic existentialism identifies and values the

Reviewed by Verna Carson, Lois Lowry, Patricia Hinton Walker, Rosalie Mirenda, and Diane Sampson.

person as a unified whole, greater than the sum of the parts, nothing more, nothing less. The humanist notion suggests that spirituality is a natural expression of a person's need, created by, but limited to human values, as shown in Figure 41–1A. In contrast to this position, it is suggested that spirituality is theocentric in nature, centered in a creative, external force where a person seeks meaning and relationship with God. This transcendent spiritual force is known by differing names throughout the world as represented in Figure 41–1B.

The contrast of a God-centered perspective is important when trying to understand spirituality in the Neuman Systems Model (1989). The description of the spiritual variable is theocentric in purpose and is opposite to that proposed by humanistic existentialism. The difficulty with humanistic existentialism is that it refutes the existence of an external creative God force because the concept lies outside the human frame of reference. It is the very idea of the existence of God as an external force, energy, or entity that is the crux and hallmark to an understanding of the spiritual variable.

THE SPIRITUAL VARIABLE

Spirituality is often described in nursing with the use of concentric circles. Figure 41–2 is a conceptual framework that extends the meaning of the spiritual variable as seen in the client system. The abstract ideas of spirituality presented in this diagram are mainly referenced to Abdu'l-Baha (Barney, 1973). The presentation of the spiritual variable is to be seen as something flexible, dynamic, and interactive. It is acknowledged that a two-dimensional diagram has obvious rigid limitations, that restricts the description of the dynamics involved.

The outer circle. The knowledge of God as a creative force in the universe is known by many names throughout the world. The idea in this outer circle is to show that people know the experience of God in different ways that reflect distinct historical and cultural influences. These descriptions are from Hinduism, Taoism, Judaism, Buddhism, Zoroastrianism, Christianity, Islam and Baha'i. Indigenous cultures particularly in America and Australia also recognize the presence of ancestral spirit beings (Charlesworth, 1984), although they are not adequately represented in this diagram.

Regardless of the many attempts to describe God, there remains an inability to unveil this essential mystery. Allusion and metaphor is frequently used to describe this idea of transcendence. Lao Tzu, in the Tao Te Ching (Lau, 1976), wrote, "[t]he nameless was the beginning of heaven and earth: The named was the mother of the myriad of creatures . . . These two are the same but diverge in name as they issue forth. Mystery upon mystery." The main assumptions about this idea of God are: God is involved in human life, a person seeks to know God, and this spiritual experience highlights the indomitable search for human meaning and purpose.

The Holy Spirit. The Holy Spirit is represented as a solid line. This suggests

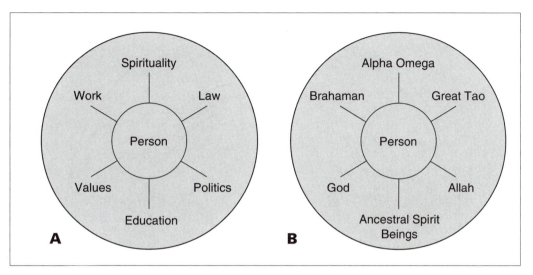

Figure 41–1. (A) Humanistic perspective and (B) theocentric perspective.

that there is a limit to the description about the knowledge of God. In spiritual writings, the Holy Spirit, spirit and soul are frequently interchanged and this multiple use of terms tends to cause some confusion. The term "Holy Spirit" is used here to distinguish between the totality of God and the human spirit or soul. The Holy Spirit that emanates from God, is the mystery of God, but does not represent the totality of God. The Holy Spirit is different from the human spirit and aims to influence and attract the soul to its higher spiritual destiny. It is acknowledged that the Holy Spirit is also identified with a person filled with spiritual perfection, promise, prophecy, and grace.

In simpler terms, the Holy Spirit acts as an intermediary between God and the person in what is regarded as an essential, mystical experience. The Holy Spirit is dynamic, active, and magnetic in its interaction with the human spirit and is ever present and inexhaustible in its power. It is the power of the Holy Spirit that informs and educates the person about God. The connection or communication of a person with God occurs through the Holy Spirit, and the linkage is always present. The Holy Spirit is described by Yogananda (1977) as "the spirit of God that actively sustains every form and force in the universe" (p. 168).

It is to be made clear that the meanings just conveyed are not to be incorrectly seen as anthropomorphic or pantheistic, as neither of these two philosophies are intended or supported by the author or the Neuman Systems Model (1989).

The spirit of faith and the bounty of God. The broken circle is seen as the flexible line of defense and represents the *outermost* extent of the person. The flexible line of defense is the contact of the person with the spiritual world of

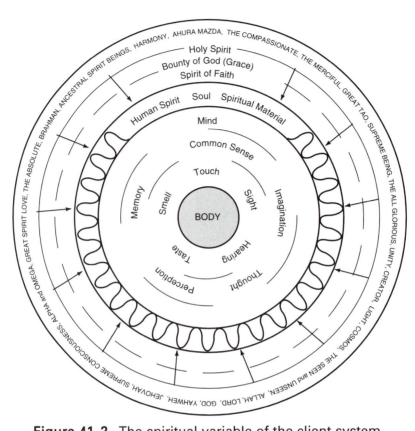

Figure 41–2. The spiritual variable of the client system.

God, as mediated by the Holy Spirit. Abdu'l-Baha (Barney, 1973, 165) commented that "the spirit of faith and the bounty of God comes from the breath of the Holy Spirit." The spirit of faith is accordion-like, in that it increases the strength and protection of the person as it expands outward. The bounty of God also flows through the Holy Spirit as a gift of grace. The flexible line of defense is strengthened by faith and expressed in a person's action. Faith is an active component to well-being. As faith grows, the well-being of a person is strengthened and supported in times of trials.

The human spirit or soul. The human spirit or soul of a person is represented as the normal line of defense. The Neuman Systems Model (1989) describes the preeminent status of the human spirit: "the spirit controls the mind and the mind consciously or unconsciously controls the body" (p. 29). The soul reaches a state of equilibrium that is reflected on the continuum between a person's lower material nature and higher spiritual nature. The material nature of the soul is regressive (it weakens, or is negative in effect); the spiritual nature is progressive (it strengthens, or is positive in effect). While this may appear a Cartesian separation, it is not, as the oscillating wave suggests that a person is sometimes more spiritual, sometimes more material at any given moment, depending on the focus of the person. When the spiritual aspects of life are consciously considered by a person (through prayer, meditation, contemplation, and action), the resulting influence imparts a positive effect on the mind and body. This effect strengthens the person and is beneficial for health.

The human spirit connects with the other variables and the basic structure in a dynamic interrelationship. The aim of the human spirit is to promote optimal health, wellness, happiness, and peace. It must be remembered that the human spirit is within the body as a complex interconnected system. The physical, psychosocial, and spiritual dimensions of a person are interwoven and inseparable during life, and this relationship must always be considered as a whole. It is also accepted that the soul progresses beyond the physical boundary after death.

In religious writings the soul has never been defined in any great detail, except that the essence is spiritual and therefore remains one of the mysteries of God. Religious scripture also suggests that the soul is different from the Holy Spirit, and its primary purpose is to develop and acquire those saintly qualities in life that are reflected or seen as attributes of God.

The mind. The mind is the intermediary between the physical body, senses, and the soul, and is seen as a power rather than as an entity. Ramacharaka (1960) describes this difference: the soul is "independent of the mechanism of the mind, which it uses as an instrument" (p. 70). Abdu'l-Baha (Barney, 1973, 244) uses metaphor to describe this relationship: "spirit is the lamp, mind is the light which shines from the lamp."

The mind responds to the direction of the soul and is seen in the attitude and actions of the person. Some of these spiritual qualities include excellence, love, compassion, selflessness, altruism, detachment, and respect. The opposite to spiritual qualities include mediocrity, hate, cruelty, self, greed, and abuse. Compassion and cruelty, for instance, are at the opposite ends of the continuum in the soul. The action reflects the intention of the person. The power of the mind translates compassion through the sense into a kind action, while cruelty has the opposite physical result. The process also works in reverse to some degree, although the soul is not as dependent on the mind, senses, or body. An example of the higher inclusive nature of the soul may be seen in a person who has had a stroke. The person may lose certain physical and mental capabilities, but the soul remains untouched, or may even be strengthened by the experience.

The body. The body or the physical aspect of a person is represented in a simplistic way. In the diagram the body is in the center and is encapsulated by the spirit as the outer inclusive nature of a person. As the higher levels (body–mind–spirit) of the person emerge, they do so in an order that is congruent with systems thinking. This description suggests that the spiritual is inclusive of the mental and physical. In other words, the person is linked by physical, mental, and spiritual qualities that are seen as higher inclusive levels of development.

The relationship of the spiritual variable to the mind and body is already well described by Neuman (1989). While the material nature of a person is regressive and the spiritual is progressive, this does not suggest that the body is inferior or negative or something to be ignored. The body is the temple in which the human spirit resides. The body is an awe-inspiring, beautiful creation that interacts with the psychosocial and spiritual dimensions of the whole person. This idea suggests that the whole person is to be looked after and sustained to the highest possible degree of health and well-being.

The variables. The physiological, psychological, sociocultural, and developmental variables link with the spiritual variable to create a unique individual person. In the ideal situation there is a balance and harmony in all variables that is seen as optimal wellness.

The Neuman Systems Model (1989) emphasizes the view that the spiritual variable influences and is influenced by all other variables. Nurses are required to thoroughly assess all variables for their influence over health. For instance, when a person is in acute pain, the physical problem must be attended to first before mental, social, family, and spiritual healing can occur. Experienced nurses are well equipped because of their interpersonal and intuitive skills to assess and manage the interrelationship of these variables.

Stressors. The interrelationships of the spiritual variable, stressors, and reactions to stressors are seen as the means to strengthen the spiritual nature of the person. For instance, suffering (physical, mental, and spiritual) that occurs as a result of a stressor may also have a spiritual meaning as a source and motivation to develop and increase understanding and well-being. This notion is slowly being supported by research. Belcher, Dettmore, and Holzemer (1989) explain how a physically ill person nearing death can be stronger than ever in spiritual terms. In the cases they studied, where HIV/AIDS caused great physical, mental, social, and financial stresses, personal well-being increased. Frankl (1962) reflected on this type of experience and suggested that "one is given a last chance to actualize the highest value, to fulfill the deepest meaning, the meaning of suffering, for what matters above all is the attitude we take toward suffering" (p. 112). Nursing studies (Ferrell, Schmidt, Rhiner, Whitehead, Fonbuena, and Forman, 1991; Highfield, 1991; Reed, 1991; Trice, 1990) indicate that well-being can increase despite stressors and that nursing and spirituality are significant to the process.

The environment. The environment remains the same as presented in the Neuman Systems Model (1989). The argument of theodicy that suggests the idea of an "evil" spiritual environment is not supported by this writer, although it is recognized that other cultural perspectives have differing beliefs on this subject.

The created environment appears to act in a similar way to the mind, as an unconscious, dynamic connection between the internal and external environments. The description of the created environment by Neuman (1989, 1990) appears to provide an interesting linkage with the spiritual variable. Both appear to have similar unconscious, unseen processes that buffer the client against stressors and stressor reaction to stimulate client health.

The lines of resistance. The lines of resistance are the known and unknown resources at play within the whole person. These include the five physical senses and the mental or intellectual senses, which combine by the power of the mind to mediate, direct, support, and protect system integrity.

The normal line of defense. The normal line of defense is represented as the human spirit or soul. This comprises a material and spiritual nature and is represented on a continuum at any given moment. The human spirit is an aspect of the whole person that represents and develops the spiritual qualities as part of optimal health. The effects of the human spirit to health are closely linked to the other variables and the environment. These combined factors influence the conscious and unconscious response to stressors.

The flexible line of defense. The flexible line of defense is the spirit of faith of the person, which shields and strengthens the whole person as it extends outwards. Faith is an action that requires constant attention or it begins to weaken.

SUMMARY

The aim of this paper has been to focus attention onto the spiritual variable by extending the conceptual boundaries presented in the Neuman Systems Model (1989). As the title suggests, a world view means that nurses are required to expand functioning to meet the needs of their clients.

Nursing is moving out of its humanistic phase toward the recognition of the spiritual. As indicated at the beginning, this work is one interpretation of the spiritual variable. A schematic framework is presented to indicate possible relationships and connections with the ideas of body, mind, and spirit. The inclusiveness of the spirit over mind and body is congruent with systems thinking.

The spiritual variable interacts in a dynamic relationship with other variables, the basic structure, and the environment. The spiritual variable is also contextually bound to the web of human relationships. Nurses are required to assess and consider these factors as an essential part in the process of providing for the full needs of the client.

FUTURE IMPLICATIONS FOR USE OF THE NEUMAN SYSTEMS MODEL: SPIRITUAL VARIABLE

The nursing profession has a unique opportunity with the Neuman Systems Model (1989). Systems thinking will play an important role in future conceptual presentations of the spiritual variable. Despite the limits imposed by the abstractness of this concept, qualitative methodologies offer a means to explore its relationships. It is also necessary for nurses to continue this exploration with an openness of mind and heart.

The psychic shift occurring throughout the nursing world is focusing nursing practice to a new perception, one based on a world view that seeks unity in diversity, harmony, and optimal wellness. Nursing in an explicit way is taking on board this spiritual perspective. In this arena the Neuman Systems Model (1989) has a preeminent place in nursing history.

ACKNOWLEDGMENTS

The chapter base was first presented as a paper at the Fourth Biennial International Neuman Systems Model Symposium held in April 1993. I wish to acknowledge the guidance and encouragement of Dr. Betty Neuman and Dr. Lois Lowry for their critique in my pursuit of this work. I invite readers to make personal contact.

COMMENTARY by Betty Neuman

This new work by Glenn Curran provides a global perspective of the spiritual variable of the Neuman Systems Model.

Within the United States and some other countries Judeo-Christian interpretations may limit global interpretations for health care. Mr. Curran's work presents a broad interpretation of how the spiritual variable may be viewed with populations from other cultures and religious heritages around the world. His work is not an authoritative or definitive conclusion but rather is offered as one attempt to describe spiritual phenomena with the hope of encouraging others to "investigate and report their own interpretations." He states as "crucial" a unified acceptance of the spirit rather than a secular limited view.

As we move closer to a one-world community requiring expansive thinking and functioning, I hope that readers will be challenged and stimulated to further explore and develop creative ways to use the Neuman spiritual variable worldwide.

REFERENCES

Barney, L. C. 1973. *Some Answered Questions: Collected and Translated from the Persian of Abdu'l-Baha*. New Delhi, India: Baha'i Publishing Trust.

Belcher, A. E., Dettmore, D., and Holzemer, S. P. 1989. Spirituality and sense of well-being in persons with AIDS. *Holistic Nursing Practice* 3(4):16–25.

Bevis, E. O. 1982. *Curriculum Building in Nursing*, 3d ed. Kansas City: C. V. Mosby.

Carson, V. B. 1989. *Spiritual Dimensions of Nursing Practice*. Philadelphia: W. B. Saunders.

Cartwright, T., Davson-Galle, P., and Holden, R. J. 1992. Moral philosophy and nursing curricula: Indoctrination of the new breed. *Journal of Nursing Education* 31(5): 225–228.

Charlesworth, M. 1984. *Religion in Aboriginal Australia: An Anthology,* edited by M. Charlesworth, H. Morphy, D. Bell, and K. Maddock, 1–20. St. Lucia. Queensland. Australia: University of Queensland Press.

Ferrell, B., Schmidt, G. M., Rhiner, M., Whitehead, C. Fonbuena, P., and Forman, S. J. 1992. The meaning of quality of life for bone marrow transplant survivors. *Cancer Nursing* 15(3):153–160.

Frankl, V. E. 1962. *Man's Search for Meaning.* New York: Simon and Schuster.

Highfield, M. F. 1991. Spiritual health of oncology patients: Nurse and patient perspective. *Cancer Nursing* 15(1):1–8.

Lau, D. C. 1976. *Lao Tzu: Tao Te Ching.* Great Britain: Penguin Books.

Neuman, B. 1989. *The Neuman Systems Model,* 2d ed. East Norwalk, Conn.: Appleton & Lange.

Neuman, B. 1990. Health as a continuum: Based on the Neuman Systems Model. *Nursing Science Quarterly* 3(3):129–135.

Pearson, A. 1988. Nursing: From whence to where? In *Searches for Meaning in Nursing 1: Phenomena Encountered in Nursing. Reading 2.1,* 1–17. Faculty of Nursing, Deakin University, Geelong, Victoria.

Ramacharaka, Y. 1960. *The Hindu-Yogi Science of Breath.* London: L. N. Fowler & Co.

Reed, P. G. 1991. Preferences for spiritually related nursing interventions among terminally ill and nonterminally ill hospitalized adults and well adults. *Applied Nursing Research* 4(3):122–128.

Trice, L. B. 1990. Meaningful life experience to the elderly. *Image: Journal of Nursing Scholarship* 22(4):248–251.

Yogananda, P. 1977. *Autobiography of a Yogi.* Los Angeles, Calif.: Self-Realization Fellowship.

42

UTILIZATION OF THE NEUMAN SYSTEMS MODEL
University of South Australia

Sybil Jennifer McCulloch

This chapter describes an undergraduate nursing program at the University of South Australia based on the Neuman Model. The program is successfully conducted at an inner city and a remote area campus. During a sponsored visit by Dr. Neuman in 1991, students, graduates, and staff expressed their satisfaction and success in working with the Neuman Systems Model, both in the classroom and in practice.

BACKGROUND

Australia is a country of some 2,967,909 square miles with a population of 17 million people domiciled mainly in coastal areas where water supplies and climatic conditions make human habitation possible. For the people who live in remote inland areas, the harsh climate, water availability, and isolation are major factors in everyday existence. Australia has a significant indigenous Aboriginal population, many of whom are urbanized. The history of white settlement spans only 200 years.

Importantly, Australia is a multicultural society where, in the process of assimilation, different cultural traditions and practices are increasingly accepted and valued. Major cities of Sydney, Canberra, Brisbane, Melbourne, Adelaide,

Perth, and Darwin evidence a vigorous cosmopolitan environment, yet social problems—particularly unemployment—are increasing as the economy slows in line with worldwide economic trends.

The provision of health services to this diverse and widely dispersed population is complex and expensive and is largely determined and funded by governments of the eight Australian states and territories. Effective distribution of the health care dollar is of paramount importance, and rationalization of services has led to a recent reduction in bed numbers, closure of smaller hospitals, and privatization of others. Health promotion at the government level is largely supported for economic rather than ideological reasons. As the year 2000 approaches, a high percentage of the health budget continues to be spent on inpatient illness-related care, despite recommendations from professional and community groups for greater focus on primary health care.

CHANGES IN NURSE EDUCATION IN AUSTRALIA

The nursing profession in Australia has for many years been advocating a change in emphasis from illness care to a concomitant and increasing focus on illness prevention and wellness promotion. Prior to 1984, however, the majority of nurses were trained in large acute care hospitals, and it is reasonable to conclude that socializing effects increased the tendency toward illness orientation and client dependence. In 1984, as the result of intense political struggle and a relentless national campaign, the federal government agreed to the total transfer of three-year basic nurse education to the higher education system throughout Australia. As a result of subsequent institutional mergers, all preparation of graduate registered nurses is, in the 1990s, within universities, and the first award is at baccalaureate degree level. A second level enrolled nurse continues to be prepared over one year in acute and long-term hospitals, but diminishing numbers will likely be phased into technical and further education colleges in programs that may articulate with three-year baccalaureate programs in the future.

UNIVERSITY PREPARATION OF REGISTERED NURSES

The transfer of nurse education to universities afforded a turning point for change in the preparation of graduates for professional nursing careers. The opportunity to develop totally new programs within a liberal academic context required deep reflection, research, vision, and creativity on the part of nurse leaders. It afforded a unique opportunity to reconsider issues surrounding the purposeful act of nursing, its value orientation, client and nurse roles, and the place of nursing in the wider health care arena. Consideration of past practices, present-day dilemmas, and future opportunities engendered much philosophical debate, analysis, and reordering of principles.

Leaders in education and clinical fields sought to identify the underlying nursing knowledge and principles of practice that would lead to a unifying approach to clinical nursing, research, and education. Adoption of particular models and/or theories as the basis for curriculum development was in many cases supported by active consultation with eminent nurse leaders and careful review of available literature. Following these activities, programs evolved their statements of philosophy and mission, their conceptual frameworks, unifying principles, content, methodologies, anticipated outcomes, and evaluation strategies. Graduates from university programs are now contributing significantly in the delivery of health care in a wide range of settings.

APPLICATION OF THE NEUMAN MODEL IN AUSTRALIA

In 1987 the author was appointed to head one of the largest tertiary nursing programs in Australia, with anticipated intakes of 300 undergraduate students each year. The main program is sited in the central business district of Adelaide, South Australia, with a satellite program in Whyalla (some 480 kilometers away) serving remote communities throughout central Australia. The author in her administrative role was intimately involved in the design of new purpose-built accommodations on both sites; thus curriculum planning and building design occurred in tandem.

In designing a curriculum to meet the needs of two geographically distant and different schools, certain tenets held firm.

1. The curriculum would facilitate the empowerment of students, academic staff, and future clients.
2. The curriculum would be based on a health care model that embraced all aspects of the person in dynamic interaction with the environment.
3. The model chosen would be flexible and adaptable to the diverse environmental contexts of clinical practice.
4. The model would provide the student with an effective tool for assessment, planning, practice, and evaluation in all health care settings.
5. The model would encompass the potential to change the dynamic interaction of nurse/client/health system from one of dependence and alienation to one of independence, interdependence, and personal significance.
6. The model would be acceptable to other academic disciplines that would service some aspects of the program, thus promoting cohesion and articulation between nursing and contributing disciplines.
7. The model would be easily understood by beginning students yet sufficiently sophisticated to support ongoing study at the postdoctoral level.

8. The model would evidence potential to generate further theory development and provide a basis for academic and practice-based research.

The Neuman Systems Model was considered to meet all of these exacting requirements and, as an open systems model, would facilitate consideration of health science theories as the curriculum evolved. The Neuman Model continues to provide the major organizing focus of the curriculum following major review and redevelopment over subsequent years (see Appendix A).

The Neuman Model underpins and illuminates essential concepts used in the learning process, including:

1. Person: application of the Neuman Model to an understanding of the self progressing to an understanding of the other.
2. Process: application of the Neuman Model to primary, secondary, and tertiary nursing intervention.
3. Universality: application of the Neuman Model to an understanding of the individual, the family, the cultural group, organized systems, and complex communities.
4. Outcomes: application of the Neuman Model as a framework for evaluating intervention outcomes and a yardstick for measuring potential and actual response to intrapersonal, interpersonal, and extrapersonal stressors.

TOWARD A DEFINITION OF NURSING

An additional experience for the school has been the way in which the Neuman Model assists in the definition of nursing itself. In Australia, as in other parts of the world, much recent debate has been directed toward a definition of nursing and the identification of professional boundaries. The Neuman Model clearly articulates and advances the role of the nurse as one who promotes system balance through modification of system stressors and strengthens lines of resistance and flexible lines of defense, thus protecting the structural core of the system itself, whether simple and singular or complex and pluralistic. The nurse acts as intermediary, intervening at the primary, secondary, and tertiary level only as the situation requires. Through sharing of nursing knowledge and skill, the client system is able to maintain the locus of control and the core structure remains intact. In all situations there is an opening and a closure of the nursing intervention, thus fulfilling the professional component of nursing yet maintaining the intimacy so essential in the nursing act. Utilization of the Neuman Systems Model also assists in the important process of self-nurture of nurses themselves by providing a self/situational assessment tool that may enhance personal awareness, stressor identification and comfort level, intervention, and future goal setting.

APPLICATION OF THE NEUMAN MODEL IN AUSTRALIA

The visit by Dr. Neuman to Australia elicited wide interest in all states and territories at a time when internal program development and major structural change was occurring in both the health care system and the higher education sector. During her brief stay Dr. Neuman conducted seminars in South Australia, Victoria, and Queensland. Visits to other states were curtailed by distance, time, and cost factors. There is growing evidence, however, that the Neuman Model is widely used in undergraduate and postgraduate nursing programs and is providing a useful framework to support diverse areas of research.

A recent survey of all Australian university programs indicated that in four undergraduate programs the Neuman Model provided the major organizational framework for the curriculum. In 16 others, the Neuman Model was one of several models and theories introduced to undergraduate and postgraduate students. Specific subject areas mentioned were intensive care nursing, theories of nursing, research methodology, and nursing and family health.

Topics of research utilizing the Neuman Model were more difficult to identify but included:

Curran, G., *Spirituality in Nursing*

Neuman, B., Moynehan, L., Gill, D., and Russo, P., *Enhancing Nursing Care of Haemodialysis Patients*

Procter, N., *Application of the Neuman Systems Model to Civil War in the Former Yugoslavia: Implications for Nursing in the 21st Century*

SUMMARY

The Neuman Model provides a unified and in-depth structure for curriculum development, education, and future practice of graduates in a university program serving metropolitan and remote area communities. Students experience the model as rational, descriptive, useful, and stimulating. Utilization of the model in education, practice, and research is evident throughout Australia, and such activity will be documented.

It can be concluded that in developing and sharing her model Dr. Neuman has contributed significantly to the development of nursing in Australia.

REFERENCES

Neuman, B., 1980. The Betty Neuman Health-Care Systems Model. In *Conceptual Models for Nursing Practice,* 2d ed., edited by J. P. Riehl and C. Roy. New York: Appleton-Century-Crofts.

Neuman, B., 1988. *The Neuman Systems Model: Application to Nursing Education and Practice,* Norwalk, Conn.: Appleton-Century-Crofts.

APPENDIX A —————————

Bachelor of Nursing Course Plan

Year 1	Contact Hours
Nursing Practice	150
Nursing Field Experience	60
Professional Studies	63
General Science	108
Anatomy and Physiology	77
Social Studies	144
General Studies	52

Year 2	
Nursing Practice	144
Nursing Field Experience	300
Professional Studies	54
Anatomy and Physiology	72
Microbiology	56
Social Studies	54
Multidisciplinary teamwork	27

Year 3	
Nursing Practice (including electives)	173
Nursing Field Experience	400
Professional Studies	64
Social Studies	27
Physics in the Health Care Environment	10

The Neuman Systems Model is selected as the conceptual framework of the program on the basis of its congruence with philosophical statements of the school on nursing and nursing education. Use of the model gave focus and cohesion to a program that was serviced by experts from a number of disciplines. Utilization of the model ensured that the professional discipline of nursing always remained paramount.

The conceptual framework was sequenced to provide experiences from simple to complex, from self-health to other, and from health to ill health. Students reflect on the health–illness continuum as a progressive and dynamic state of function and dysfunction at social, individual, and cellular levels.

The first year of the program introduces concepts of humanity, health and nursing, the identification and impact of stressors, and the potential for primary intervention and health promotion. Nursing actions are aimed toward strengthening and maintaining the individual's health status. A variety of field experience is offered, including shopping centers, child care services, schools, health centers, and occupational and environmental services.

During the second and third years the program builds on prior experience and focuses on secondary and tertiary intervention with individuals and families experiencing health breakdown. Students apply the nursing process to reduce the effect of stressors and to facilitate the rehabilitation process. Content is organized according to categories of stressors resulting in specific human dysfunction. A wholistic approach to care underpins all curricular endeavors. Students gain field experience in a variety of acute and extended care settings and community agencies. Supporting studies extend the students' understanding of forces that shape society and impinge upon individual and social health and the professional nursing role.

In the third year student experiences are designed to facilitate the synthesis of knowledge and nursing practice with clients at all levels of dependence in a variety of settings. Strands of health teaching and management span the three years, providing the student with the knowledge and skills to fulfill the professional role.

43

USE OF THE NEUMAN SYSTEMS MODEL IN ENGLAND
Abstracts

Barbara Vaughan
Pippa Gough

Health care in the United Kingdom is undergoing radical change at the moment, which is inevitably placing demands on nurses to seriously review the theories from which they work. First, central policies have led to the introduction of market forces where purchasers, representing the local community, identify the services required and commission them from local providers. In such a situation there is an exciting opportunity for nurses to become involved not only in the assessment of need but also within nursing clinics.

Second, there has been a shift from a service that has been largely driven by the need to diagnose and cure disease to one where key health gain targets related to coronary heart disease, cancers, mental illness, HIV/AIDS and sexual health, and accidents have been identified (Department of Health, 1992). Thus there is an increasing emphasis on preventive actions where knowledge is shared with people in order that they can manage their own lives to maximize their health potential and minimize their risk of disease. In line with this there is also an increase in the number of public health nurses. It could be suggested that such a move highlights the critical importance of contextual factors of health as identified in the Neuman Systems Model and reflects the values that underpin many theories of nursing, such as a humanistic belief in person and the right to choice and self-determination. Furthermore, the skills and knowledge that nurses have already identified as critical to good practice, such as teaching, supporting, guiding, and strengthening defenses, place them in an ideal position to respond to such a demand.

A third major change that has occurred is a shift from the traditional apprenticeship-type training sited in hospital-based schools of nursing to a professional education at the diploma or degree level (UKCC, 1986). Thus at last there has been an acknowledgment of the sound knowledge base on which nursing practice is founded, and all students entering nursing have the opportunity to explore theoretical nursing models.

All these changes have led to a need for nurses to draw more heavily on nursing theory in order to be explicit about the knowledge on which they base their practice and the way in which they can contribute to health care in its totality. It is no longer acceptable to rest on the good will of the population in valuing nursing without being clear about the rationale for actions. Goals of practice have to be visible and processes of care based on sound theoretical knowledge. Furthermore, curricula have to withstand the rigor of external scrutiny and offer the opportunity for students to explore the theories that underpin their practice.

Extensive continuing education has exposed many experienced practitioners to the opportunity to study nursing theory and develop their practice further through the use of a model. While there has been a tendency over recent years for some nurses in the United Kingdom to take an inductive approach and begin to develop conceptual models from their own practice (Wright, 1986; Johns, 1991), others have looked to well-established models, such as that described by Betty Neuman, to explore the way in which practice can be guided. In many cases considerable adaptation of the original framework occurs in this process by creative transformation through use and reflection. It can be argued that this use and development of theory in action is entirely appropriate as health care itself is dynamic and cannot be limited to the mere application of theory.

The explicit use of a model in practice is still not widely apparent in many UK settings, and we have a long way to go before it becomes commonplace. Yet the way in which nurses do practice is undoubtedly influenced by the totality of their knowledge and experience. Thus, as the opportunity to explore the Neuman Systems Model through both basic and continuing education increases, so will the influence that it has on practice—a healthy move in the right direction that will ultimately benefit patient care.

PRACTICE NURSING

With a growing emphasis on community nursing in the United Kingdom, the number of practice nurses has rapidly increased. These nurses are based in primary health care teams working with general practitioners, health visitors, and district nurses. They are concerned with assessing the health needs of the population the practice serves and providing direct care for individual patients, which may involve both evaluation and treatment.

Practice nurses recognize that there are many contextual issues that influence the health of the local population, including political, environmental, and economic factors. Sarah Luft has explored the way in which a model of nursing can be used to assist practice nurses is assessing the needs not only of individual patients but also of the population as a whole. She suggests that the Neuman Systems Model lends itself ideally to this situation. For individuals it helps to focus on the intra-, inter- and extrapersonal stressors that they see as important and offers a flexible framework of action that may be initiated by the patient and the nurse. Because of the position of the practice nurse within the community setting, there is also an ideal opportunity to provide continuing support to help people to maintain the optimum health status they have gained.

On a wider basis Luft suggests that using Neuman's model helps to identify the "basic structure" of that population, including such things as the people, environment, housing, culture, and leisure opportunities; the local stressors, such as employment patterns and pollution; and hence the types of intervention that may help to improve health, such as liaison with local housing committees or environmental health services.

This example clearly demonstrates the creative way in which the Neuman Systems Model can be operationalized. Luft suggests that it can help practice nurses to take social, emotional, and environmental issues into consideration along with medical diagnoses. Thus the model allows nurses to offer a broadly based, far-reaching service.
(Contact: Sarah Luft, Senior Lecturer, School of Health Sciences, University of Wolverhampton, 62–68 Lichfield Street, Wolverhampton, WV1 1DJ.)

CONTINUING EDUCATION

Many experienced nurses and midwives in the United Kingdom are enrolling in courses to study their own discipline in greater depth, and in most of these continuing education programs there is an opportunity to explore theories of nursing. Frequently, practitioners undertake these courses on a part-time basis while continuing in their work roles. Unlike initial education in either of these fields, continuing education allows students to test out the application of new knowledge in practice situations with which they are already familiar.

One such course is run at the Sheffield Hallam University with Janet Hargreaves as the tutor. Students from both nursing and midwifery are offered the choice of which model to explore in their own practice setting, and many choose the Neuman Systems Model. The experiences of a few practitioners are described below.

Midwifery

Hilary Camm, an experienced midwife who now works as a manager of a midwifery service, explored the Neuman Systems Model focusing on the assessment and planning processes. She then compared the care plan she had established in conjunction with the client with the computerized care plan that had been used. Not surprisingly, she found there was considerable variation. She suggests that the use of this model is potentially very beneficial in midwifery as it concentrates so clearly on the perceived needs of the client, in this instance the mother, moving away from a physiologically driven approach inherent in so much health care. Through the Neuman Systems Model approach to assessment she was able to gain insight into a more wholistic picture, identifying a range of personal issues for the client that had not previously come to light.

Her only concern is that midwives do have a statutory duty to ensure that some responsibilities are fulfilled that are seen as essential by health care workers but not always recognized as a need by the mothers. As a result, these responsibilities may be excluded from the plan. However, with continuity of care, good interpersonal skills, and some negotiation this difficulty could be easily overcome. Her study has led to a recognition of the need to review the current care planning system in her unit, through peer review and auditing of records with a view to introducing this approach more widely.

Elaine Torrence, also a midwife, used the Neuman Systems Model as a framework for assessing, planning, and delivering midwifery care and has clearly identified the flexibility of this approach in identifying the wide-ranging variation in client needs. She particularly demonstrates the variation in lines of defense arising from the differing social and psychological backgrounds of the mothers.

Her work highlights how the model can bring to light the essential partnership between the midwife and the mother with her partner, ensuring that they have the opportunity to exercise choice in the way their baby is born and that they are truly empowered to participate in decision making. Torrence feels that the Neuman Systems Model can be adapted well to midwifery and finds the humanistic values particularly helpful. She would, however, like to see more work to develop a midwifery model and feels that this could act as a sound basis from which to start.

There is a tendency for midwives to use midwifery in a very different light from nursing, and hence they have difficulty in identifying the way in which theoretical models of nursing can be of use to them. It is therefore encouraging to see how these explorations demonstrate the flexibility of the Neuman Model and the range of situations in which it can be used.

Intensive Care

In contrast to the two studies outlined above, Dawn Adsetts explored the use of the Neuman Systems Model in an Intensive Therapy Unit (ITU). She chose the model because, in her words, "I found the philosophy of the Neuman Systems

Model ideal for use in ITU." With a high demand for responding to patients' physiological needs, she felt that it was easy to ignore other aspects of care, but in using this approach nurses are led towards a much more wholistic approach to care.

Adsetts demonstrated how the use of the Neuman assessment process during a preoperative visit gave her the opportunity to gain a much clearer picture of how one particular patient normally responded to stressors, identifying the physiological and psychosocial mechanisms that he normally employed as defense mechanisms. This information was then drawn on during the postoperative period to assist her in care delivery with particular reference to pain management.

Adsetts experienced some difficulty in finding a practical way of recording information following this structure since the pace of change is so rapid in ITU. However, she feels this could be overcome by the use of simple preset documents that could act as a baseline. She found the experience of using the model an important learning exercise and would like to take the work further.

GENERAL MEDICINE

Paul Swainsbury, who works as a charge nurse on an acute medical ward, explored the use of the Neuman Systems Model and compared it with the activities of living model that is currently in use on the ward. He chose to work with a patient who has suffered from diabetes for a long period of time and is frequently readmitted to the ward as his medical condition is poorly controlled and, despite considerable support from the district nurses, he finds difficulty in managing his own care at home.

Swainsbury recognized that one of the major difficulties for this patient was an unrealistic expectation of his prognosis; he continued to hope that the health care team could rapidly "cure" the ulcers on his feet and that he would be able to return home quickly. To complicate this situation further he was also suffering from severe depression.

What particularly attracted Swainsbury to this model was its flexible approach in the assessment phase and in planning for primary, secondary, and tertiary interventions. He felt that this approach might help him to come to understand the patient's perceptions of his situation more realistically, and indeed this was the outcome. It had been hoped to move him to a "halfway house" to offer additional support during the time his ulcers were healing. What had not come to light previously was the patient's fear of losing his home if he was hospitalized for too long; it was this anxiety that had led to a resistance to the care offered. Once this issue had been dealt with to everyone's satisfaction, it was possible to explore a more realistic care option. Swainsbury feels that this issue would not have been recognized with a less flexible approach to assessment where there was less attention paid to the patient's perceptions of his difficulties.

Swainsbury intends to take his studies further over the forthcoming years and plans to continue exploring ways in which he can use the Neuman Systems Model in both academic and practical work.

CURRICULAR DEVELOPMENT

It became apparent that the model offered scope and a clinical usefulness as well as enhancing the students' ability to make sense of difficult and complex social situations within diverse community-based settings. It was felt that the model, over and above many others, was the one that provided an understanding of environment that was not confined solely to the immediate psychosocial milieu of patients and clients. Donely (1984, cited in Mirenda, 1986) suggests that the model helps prepare nurses who will present a Gestalt of technological, humanistic, and ethical knowledge to meet the demands of the 21st century, and it is this that should be the ultimate goal of all nurse teachers.

(Contact: Carol Clark, Nurse Tutor, Avon and Gloucestershire College of Health, Glenside, Blackberry Hill, Stapleton, Bristol, Avon BS13 1DD.)

COMMUNITY NURSING

The Neuman Systems Model has been used in the Avon and Gloucestershire School of Nursing as the guiding principle behind curriculum development for child care (described above). During their clinical placements students spend time with health visitors, who have a particular responsibility for child health and development. These local practitioners have sought ways of demonstrating in reality the theories the students have studied, including the Neuman Systems Model.

This situation is an excellent example of the interaction that can occur between practice and education. However, introducing model-based practice has not been an easy task for the health visitors leading this work since there was a huge gap in knowledge related to nursing theory among many colleagues and some had difficulty in seeing the need for such a move. Nevertheless, they do recognize the need to be more articulate about the nature of their work and have found that using the Neuman Model helps them to clarify such things as the boundaries of their role, record keeping, evaluation and multidisciplinary communication.

Most importantly, feedback from clients has been very positive, with one commenting that she had "been put in touch with [her] own resources for the first time in [her] life"—a truly powerful example of the value of this model.

A program is also being developed in this area to place all health visiting records on computer so that data can be recorded more efficiently and some analysis of the health needs can be made. Again the Neuman Systems Model has been used as a basis for this work, and it will be exciting to watch the progress. *(Contact: Miriam Wiltshire, Health Visitor, Community Nurse Base, 43A, Nevil Road, Bishopston, Bristol.)*

CONCLUSION

From the information presented above it can be seen that the Neuman Systems Model has been applied in a wide variety of settings within the United Kingdom. It does seem to be particularly favored by nurses working within community settings and midwifery as they find the acknowledgment of environmental issues in terms of the way they impact on the well-being of individuals more easily applicable than many other theoretical models. This may partly be attributed to the fact that most nurses working in these areas are more mature and have had time to develop their understanding of both people and nursing more fully. This does not, however, exclude its suitability for application in other settings.

As the need increases for nurses to become more overtly accountable for their practice in terms of both efficacy and cost-effectiveness, so the need for them to be able to defend their work in practical and theoretical terms will increase. The use of a well-developed theoretical model, such as the one described by Betty Neuman, is undoubtedly of value in our ever-changing health care scene.

REFERENCES

Department of Health. 1992. *Health of the Nation—A Strategy for Health in England.*

Johns, C. 1991. The Burford nursing development unit holistic model of nursing practice. *Journal of Advanced Nursing* 16:1090–1098.

Mirenda, R. 1986. The Neuman Model in practice. *Senior Nurse* 5(3):26–27.

United Kingdom Central Council. 1986. *Project 2000—A New Preparation for Practice.* London: UKCC.

Wright, S. 1986. *Building and Using a Model of Nursing.* London: Edward Arnold.

44

COMMUNITY NURSING IN THE UNITED KINGDOM
A Case for Reconciliation Using the Neuman Systems Model

Margaret Damant

Interest in the inquiry was fostered by my mentor and host for a study program based at Lander University, Greenwood, South Carolina. Walking along a Charleston beach during a period of relaxation, we found a crab experiencing great difficulty in surviving because it could not respond to the environmental stressors and maintain stability. We analyzed the situation with reference to the Neuman Systems Model (Neuman, 1989). What factors are naturally present that enable the crab to maintain a balance between the external and the internal environment? Why is the crab unable to adjust to the present circumstances? How can the stressors be prevented, corrected, or attenuated? As the analysis developed, its relationship with the issue I was seeking to address began to emerge.

This chapter examines the case for change through a reconceptualization of community nursing and a rationalization of the present boundaries as part of a process of reconciliation (harmonization) directed toward an integrated, stable, growth-oriented, and wholistic health care profession.

Reviewed by Janet Sipple, Charlene Beynon, and Patricia Hinton Walker.

THE ISSUE: HOW VIABLE FOR THE FUTURE IS COMMUNITY NURSING IN ITS PRESENT FORM IN THE UNITED KINGDOM?

The 21st century is heralded by the commercialization of health care and a value-for-money ethic. In the closing decade of the 20th century two major influences in this direction can be observed. On the one hand there is a noticeable commitment to consumerism, the promotion of health, and the early detection of impediments. On the other hand the consumer is charged with the responsibility of exercising positive health choices, empowered and advocated by the caring professions. There has been a move toward more egocentric, self-determining values and away from a welfare mentality. For instance, "The Patient's Charter" is a government initiative that sets out the rights and responsibilities of the patient and the standards of care to be expected in the United Kingdom (Department of Health, 1992). In addition, recent legislation has improved clients' access to information, with the right to contribute to decisions regarding their own health and power of choice. In theory this means that clients may consult with the community nurse of choice—the same way in which one relates to the doctor. Are the present boundaries among the different branches of community nursing within the United Kingdom (UK) conducive to this end, or are there more appropriate models?

Community nursing is characterized by a complex relationship among individuals, their immediate environment, and wider socioeconomic forces. The community nurse also lives and practices in the public arena where work can be seen, clients are autonomous, and accountability is readily open to question. "Cure," in some situations, will continue to be an illusive goal, whereas "caring," the therapy of nursing, will become an increasingly important inexact science and resource for the health and well-being of the nation.

Nursing is only one of many disciplines charged with a responsibility to attend to the health needs of clients in the community. Overlaps and gaps among the different disciplines are well documented, particularly in relation to child abuse. It could be argued that there is a need to consider the case for reconciliation not only within community nursing but also between community nursing and other disciplines such as social work, medicine, and the allied professions. However, reconciliation among the different disciplines is part of a much wider debate and one that may not be given the same priority as changes from within. The Neuman Systems Model is used to provide a diagrammatic illustration of the position of community nursing and to conceptualize the case for change.

COMMUNITY NURSING: CONFLICT, CONSENSUS, AND CHANGE

Historically, while sharing a common philosophy rooted in the understanding of cause as well as effect, the various branches of community nursing emerged from different perspectives of health care. The main UK branches are health visiting, founded in the public health orientation, and district nursing, which developed within the tradition of nursing.

The response of community nursing to changing social and political forces over nearly 200 years is characterized by the phenomenon of rise and decline. For instance, district nursing diversified to provide health care in the school and the workplace, but over time each service has developed its identity as a separate branch of community nursing.

Various specialties also emerged from the medical model, for example, diabetic care and the control of communicable diseases. Some specialties developed a functional orientation and have become subsumed within the role of community nursing, such as palliative care. As other professions have developed, this too has had an effect on community nursing, such as the transfer of statutory child life protection duties from health visiting to social work.

The concept of primary health care (PHC) as a first line of defense for health in the community invoked the need for multidisciplinary teamwork and interprofessional collaboration. The establishment of the primary health care team (PHCT) reflected a growing awareness that no one profession could continue to meet the diverse health needs of individuals in their social setting. It has become increasingly apparent that nursing continues to be a major force for health and its facilitation. For instance, community nurses who provide health care within a range of different community settings are active members of the PHCT. The number of registered nurses employed by general (medical) practitioners as practice nurses to provide nursing care in the health center rose quite sharply in the 1980s. This trend continued in the 1990s with the introduction of a new contractual arrangement for doctors that laid greater emphasis on preventive health care and the development of health promotion programs. The potential of an expanding scope for nursing within general practice attracted the interest of community nurses, and within the present decade many have been recruited into these positions (Damant, 1990). Nevertheless, in some circumstances the anticipated opportunities have not been realized, in which case it might be regarded as a "deskilling" process for the community nurse, whose extensive repertoire of skills may be constrained by the medical model and rigid role boundaries. While practice nursing is an important component of PHC, the way in which it has been developed has tended to add to the fragmentation within community nursing, and there is a strong argument to support a more integrated, stable, and wholistic nursing provision for the client.

However, general practice is not alone as a potentially "deskilling" environment for community nursing. For example, a district nurse may possess a health visitor qualification or a health visitor may be qualified in community psychiatric nursing or social work, but employers rarely create opportunities for the practice of such combined roles. There are of course a few exceptions, and the nurse practitioner role is being developed slowly and often reluctantly.

Recent developments in PHC and other community services, together with the impact of social policy, will require the different branches of community nursing to adopt more flexible role boundaries. Community nurses will be expected to engage in shared care with other disciplines while remaining accountable for action, and to accept a broader role in case management. There is some evidence that a more realistic deployment of human resources could be introduced both within and among the different disciplines (Audit Commission, 1992). Although the marketplace has a role in the development of cost-effective care, it is a hard taskmaster and one that may not always acknowledge the lead role of professional education and research in maintaining standards of practice.

There have been notable changes in professional education, particularly in the 1980s, aimed at strengthening the role of community nursing and improving intraprofessional collaboration. Curricula were revised to expand the knowledge base and repertoire of skills in order to give the practitioner the confidence to relate to the increasing complexity of health needs and new methods of working.

Clearly the future will continue the process of rise and decline for community nursing. The survival of a "healthy," growth-oriented profession will depend on its ability to define and energize its primary values, the science of caring, and to recognize and address the forces for change. The next section continues to explore the dynamics of community nursing.

COMMUNITY NURSING: RELATIONSHIPS AND STRESSORS

Community nursing provides direct care to individuals and groups and indirect care through others. Compared to institutional care, where nursing care is a continuous activity, community nursing provides a relatively discontinuous pattern of care. For this reason it can be argued that the primary focus of community care is the informal caregiver (also known as "carer"). Informal caregivers can be divided into several categories according to the contribution they make toward meeting the needs of an individual or a system.

The first category is self-care, which constitutes the largest proportion of all health care in the community. Self-care is usually the responses developed by an individual or group to rebut stressors that threaten health and therefore system stability. These actions relate to the Neuman flexible and normal lines of defense. They may arise from cultural/familial beliefs and practices or from a client's confidence in past coping strategies. The mechanism plays an important part in the validation of self-care decisions, which may include self-medication, the seeking of medical/nursing advice and treatment, health screening, and developmental assessment. The role of nursing intervention is to strengthen the flexible and normal lines of defense by health education, advice, counseling, and hands-on care.

The second category is the informal caregiver network of family, neighbors, and friends. This is a complex network and one that is often threatened by instability through changing roles and values. Care of the caregivers, regardless of age, ability, and relationship, is an essential feature of community nursing and an investment that is crucial for quality care. For example, health visiting intervention might focus on child rearing and family developmental processes. Thus the community nurse acts as both a buffer and a resource by which the flexible and normal lines of defense are strengthened, and so the confidence to draw upon inner personal resources is instilled. Likewise, district nursing intervention is a similar resource where there is distress and conflict associated with illness and disability.

A third category of caregiver is the community itself. A community is the result of a unique cultural, geographical, and historical experience. Communities can provide a caring service through their own voluntary, charitable, and self-help networks. As a potential unit of care, the community exemplifies Neuman's basic assumption about the client system as a dynamic energy source that is in constant exchange with its internal and external environment. Nurses assist in the monitoring, facilitation, and coordination of resources within a community according to the needs of clients. It is a role that involves cooperation and shared care. This may not always be easy. For instance, in some circumstances practitioners may experience a sense of diminished autonomy to the detriment of collaborative, client-centered care (Wilson, 1978). Multiprofessional education was introduced as a process by which to rebut such stressors and reconstitute toward stability.

Schools and residential homes are examples of close-knit communities within a community. Nursing contributes to the healing environment for those with health deficits or risks and intervenes to promote system stability. Community nursing, social work, and the medical and allied professions all have an obligation to cooperate to this end.

The milieu of community care, as illustrated in Figure 44–1, is often characterized by poverty, conflict, loneliness, violence, and discrimination, as well as by consensus and care. Practitioners also have particular need for counsel and support, which can often be unrecognized. Spiritual leaders are an essential resource. The need is great for primary preventive activities to preserve wellness of both client and caregiver.

COMMUNITY NURSING: A CASE FOR RECONCILIATION

The case for reconciliation is complex but easily oversimplified in order to achieve a result. The following investigation is an initial attempt to consider some of the issues and offer a framework for further critical exploration and development.

Several factors have been taken into account, such as the recent changes in UK preregistration programs (United Kingdom Central Council for Nursing, Midwifery and Health Visiting, 1986). These developments aim to create a

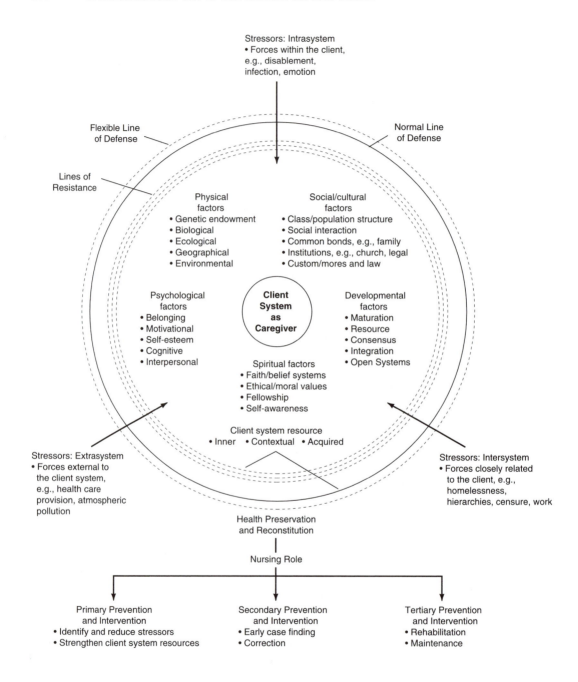

nursing force more responsive to the rapidly changing needs of society. Concepts of health are used to explicate health-limiting processes and intervention strategies for nursing in institutional and noninstitutional settings. Clearly, the time is opportune for a radical and comprehensive review of community nursing.

The far-reaching effect of economic forces and fiscal policies for health within a climate of finite resources and an increasing commitment to skill mix must also be taken into account. Linked with these changes is the abolition of past functional hierarchical management systems in favor of a "flat playing field."

The devolution of decision making, resource management, and strategic planning to those who practice at the interface of care operates within a value-for-money ethic. This can add a new dimension to professional autonomy and collegiality as the primacy of client needs challenge traditional divisions of labor and professional role boundaries. Conditions of employment are likely to undergo fundamental changes with an increase in self-employment and contract working governed by market forces through purchaser/provider mechanisms.

It is inevitable that the present rigid role boundaries within community nursing will be questioned. For example, are the different paradigms of district nursing and health visiting, as they are currently constructed, justifiable? Traditionally there has been an assumption that on the one hand, health visiting interventions target the primary prevention phase of the health/ill health continuum. District nursing on the other hand is seen to engage in secondary and tertiary intervention that facilitate optimum health or a peaceful death. Furthermore, district nursing is characterized by a paradigm of "hands-on" care administered by a team of differently qualified staff, led and supervised by the district nurse. By contrast,

---

Figure 44-1. The caregiver client system, based on Neuman. *Note: The client system* is a unique physical, psychological, social, spiritual, and developmental source for health. The client in this instance is the caregiver, but the concept may be adopted widely to aid definition of family dynamics, clinical problems such as pain, professional issues such as community nursing, and so on. *Health* is a state of equilibrium that is maintained by the client's natural stabilizing mechanisms known as lines of resistance and defense. *Stressors* that threaten the health status of the client can be within the client system (intra) (for example, loss of mobility), between client systems (inter) (for example, racial discrimination), and external systems (extra) (for example, social policy and the poverty trap). *Intervention* is a health-retaining, attaining, and maintaining process directed toward achieving stability within a client system to promote optimum functioning and health.

health visiting is predominently associated with interpersonal skills, which hitherto has not readily accommodated a division of labor approach. Attempts to combine the two roles, in some instances with community midwifery, have been discontinued in most parts of the UK. This decision, influenced by the argument that the demands of acute health care jeopardize primary prevention, is open to challenge. Applying the rigor of the Neuman theory, current distinctions and assumptions that influence community nursing in the United Kingdom might be seen to be flawed for several possible reasons. First, because health is defined as a dynamically changing phenomenon, clients do not necessarily fit neatly into primary, secondary, or tertiary need groups. Second, the process of stability and reconstitution is a wholistic concept that includes primary, secondary, and tertiary prevention and intervention. It is the means by which the multidimensional needs of the client system, within the context of its internal and external environments, are met or assisted toward greater stability by nursing. Third, it becomes clear that communities themselves, as total client systems, need "care" to maintain their integrity and, when necessary, to revive a failing energy source. Community nursing is an integral part of health maintenance and reconstitution as well as prevention related to risk factors. It is a role that needs to operate within a flexible wholistic framework, directed by the nurses accountability to the client.

To potentiate the role of community nursing as a composite entity responsive to the needs of caregivers, would be to construct an integrated model of complementary reconstitutive responses within flexible functional boundaries. The Neuman Model assists the process by which to distinguish between, for example, a gestalt and a reductionist perspective, thereby providing a basis for a different division of labor and skill mix decisions.

To adopt a gestalt, as opposed to a reductionist perspective, would be to develop a model of community nursing for which the primary focus of Figure 44–1 is interpreted from the outer aspect of the client system inwards to the basic structure. This might be seen as a modification of the "public health" orientation strengthened by the growing scientific basis for nursing. The "whole community" approach to care, based on locality or special need groups, would give community nursing a more effective role in strategic planning and the opportunity to influence fiscal policies for health and develop practice through research.

A reductionist approach would focus on the health care needs of individuals/groups within the context of their environment. This broad-based integrated community nursing provision would respond to the diverse needs of client systems. Because of rapidly changing health needs, scientific and technological advances, nursing "specialities," as presently constructed, would not necessarily have a permanent life but they would rise and decline within this broad-based provision according to need. Reconceptualization, within a Neuman framework would achieve controlled fluidity, thus ensuring a close affinity between the different disciplines and safe, sensitive care.

RECONCILIATION—IMPLICATIONS FOR PROFESSIONAL EDUCATION

A long-standing commitment to multiprofessional education in the United Kingdom was created by the evolution of PHCTs in the 1960s. The 1980s were regarded as a watershed in its development as the professions worked together to achieve a common philosophy, standard, and strategy (English National Board for Nursing, Midwifery and Health Visiting, 1983). Although various "shared learning" activities involving different permutations of nursing, social work, medicine, and the allied professions have been developed on an ad hoc basis, the establishment of a "core" curriculum has been an elusive goal.

Very little research has been undertaken to assess the validity of "shared learning" activities. A national study of a 25 percent sample of district nurse and health visitor students in England suggested that shared learning between these two groups was not always a positive experience (Damant, 1991). There was minimal evidence to suggest that the experience promoted positive attitudes toward each other's role and practice, or that it reduced negative stereotypes. Some students expressed negative views about various aspects of shared learning. In particular, tutors were perceived to be ill prepared in its management. Teaching material was often seen to be biased toward one group more than the other, and the individual needs of students were felt to be neglected. In some instances, liaison between the two groups in the clinical setting was a negative experience, thus suggesting a possible incongruence between theory and practice. Health visitor students, in particular, experienced a feeling of camaraderie in shared learning groups but thought academic standards were jeopardized. Many students expressed the belief that shared learning *should* improve practice.

Just as the 1980s were seen as a turning point for educational collaboration in the UK, the European Network for Multiprofessional Education in Health Sciences (EMPE) has made an important contribution in the 1990s. The aim of the EMPE initiative is to promote a truly integrated system of PHC education and practice that optimizes both the collective and unique contribution of family doctors, community nurses, social workers, therapists, administrators, and veterinaries (a hybrid of the UK veterinary and environmental health officer). The richness of such a learning milieu has much to commend as one possible option for the 21st century. Universal recognition of the contribution made by the social, political, and behavioral sciences to quality care aids integration and provides the basis for a core of transferable skills. A shift in the central tenet of curriculum design from that which the practitioner needs to *know* to that which the practitioner needs to *do* requires theory to be distilled from and tested in practice. Figure 44–2 proposes a model utilizing the Neuman theory. It includes a foundation or core curriculum and uses a matrix framework to ensure a balance of objectives and content across a range of disciplines (ENB, 1983). The depth and content of modules can be expanded to meet the needs of advanced or specialized spheres of practice.

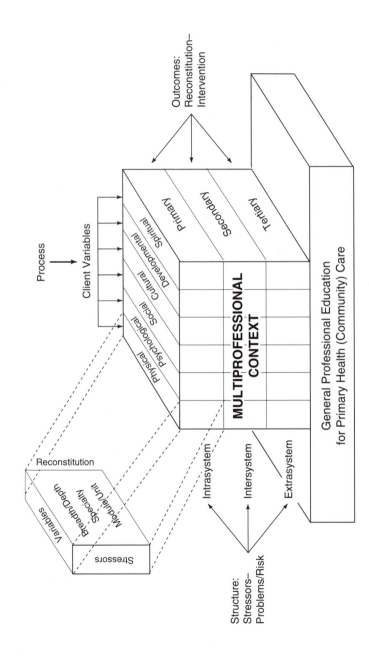

Figure 44–2. A Neuman-based model of multiprofessional community care education. *Note: Stressors* provide the structure for the curriculum design. *Client variables* reflect multidisciplinary knowledge and process of education to underpin practice. The three elements of *reconstitution* steer the intervention process and outcome.

The model should not be seen as a case for a generic practitioner but for an open, interactive system of education and practice in which the whole is more important than its individual components, and where the whole is only as good as its contributing parts. For optimum stability and growth, the academic standard of process and outcome should achieve the level of degree/higher degree. In justification of this assertion there is a strongly held belief that graduate nurses seem more able to recognize, and respond to, "holes in the system." Their decision-making skills are highly developed, they are unlikely to be threatened by the lack of consensus and the presence of conflict, and they have less reliance on other professionals.

THE CHALLENGE OF RECONCILIATION FOR UK COMMUNITY NURSING

The final section will consider the challenge of reconciliation. Damant's research suggests that district nurse and health visitor students valued the autonomy and scope of their respective professions and recognized common elements of their different roles. Students tended to experience a positive identity within the PHCT, and they considered membership in the team and client autonomy to be some of the most attractive features of their role. Market research clearly indicates that community nurses are valued by clients, with many stating that in some instances they would prefer to consult with the nurse rather than the doctor (Cumberlege, 1986). These are important findings for the process of reconciliation. They are the means by which the lines of defense and resistance for stability and growth can be strengthened and provide a buffer for environmental stressors due to change and uncertainty. However, client defense mechanisms can have a negative effect. For instance, a system under threat can reinforce rigid role boundaries and encourage restrictive practices. Under such circumstances a profession can become inward-looking, protective of its own interests, and non-growth-oriented. A loss of identity may be experienced and signs of grieving observed. Such is the challenge of reconciliation, which is diagrammatically presented in Figure 44–3.

FUTURE IMPLICATIONS FOR USE OF THE NEUMAN SYSTEMS MODEL IN COMMUNITY HEALTH NURSING

The Neuman Model provides a tool for the management of change and reconciliation among the different branches of community nursing. One of the primary preventive roles of educators, researchers, and administrators will be to identify and reduce the stressors affecting the practitioner. Consultation and open government will be essential. Their role in secondary prevention will be to respond to symptoms of instability by effective resource management and to generate professional growth-points and opportunities for personal development.

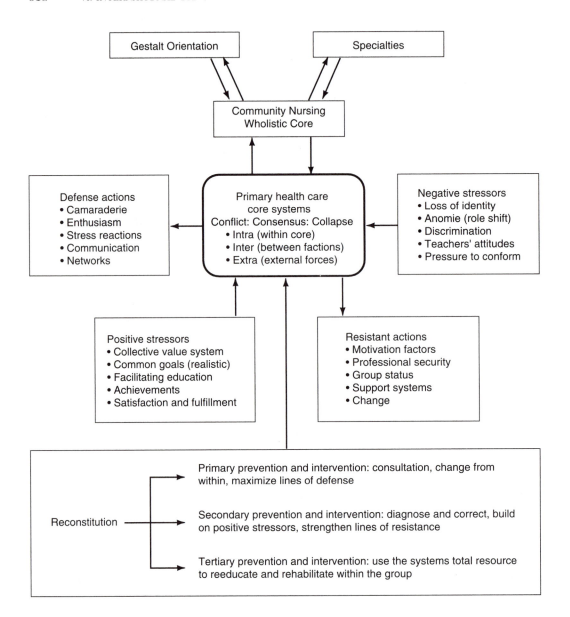

Figure 44–3. A reconciliatory framework based on Neuman.

An aspect of tertiary prevention may include the provision of a safety net to support individual members of the profession through the period of adaptation and toward stability. The personnel role will include counseling and career guidance to preserve self-esteem and opportunities for the redeployment of those who have difficulty in moving toward a more stable position.

A systematic approach is important for the process of reconciliation, which relies on accurate diagnosis and prioritization of need, the negotiation of achievable goals, and evaluation of outcome. Wholistic assessment and audit are the essential elements of the monitoring process.

The point is also made that "it is the preparation of good teachers with positive attitudes and who are well groomed in adult learning that is the starting point of effective multiprofessional education" (Williams, 1980, 11). Research has shown that teachers are in a strong position to influence the stability of a profession in fulfillment of its obligation to care. Teachers in both the classroom and practice setting have the facility to promote an open, growth-oriented system, thus safely permitting continuity and change in the face of uncertainty.

CONCLUSION

The chapter has highlighted some of the issues that influence the case for reconceptualization of the present boundaries between the different branches of community nursing and the need for a renewed commitment to interprofessionalism. In essence, this proposal could be used by all countries to review current health care provision and establish effective practice and education.

As the 21st century approaches, the universal challenge of community care for all practitioners is to seek to significantly reduce, and where possible irradicate, sources of client instability, such as:

- The effect of socioeconomic differences on health
- The misuse and abuse of natural resources essential to life and a healing environment
- The effect of knowledge deficits resulting in health-abusing behavior by empowering clients to make more informed health choices

There is also the challenge of a changing work ethic, coupled with a worldwide specter of unemployment and its health-related concomitants.

Clearly, health is a complex phenomenon, the management of which is influenced by the dominant political ideology and universal trend toward a market economy.

The value of the Neuman Systems Model lies in its flexible structure and appropriate concepts, which are broad enough to encompass the changes ahead in the 21st century. It offers a theoretical perspective that has the capacity to act both as a catalyst for the change process and as an organizational framework for future community nursing and interprofessional collaboration in practice and education. The Neuman Model, at its most pragmatic and powerful, provides a tool that targets the hub of the client system and sets it within a wider context, thereby leading practice toward client-centered goals. The essential role of education is to improve this practice.

ACKNOWLEDGMENTS

Thanks go to Dr. Betty Neuman for her encouragement; Professor Janet Sipple, Academic Dean, Barnes College, St. Louis, Missouri, for her challenging mentorship; the faculties of nursing at Lander University, Greenwood, South Carolina, and University of Wisconsin–Eau Claire for hosting my study program; my colleagues in the UK, particularly Constance Martin, Nurse Adviser, East Sussex Family Services Authority, Loretto Messenger, Director, Community Nursing Courses, St. Martin's College, Lancaster, and Mary Golding, Practice Nurse, Bradford-on-Avon, for commenting on the manuscript.

REFERENCES

Audit Commission for Local Authorities and the National Health Service in England and Wales, 1992, *Homeward Bound: A New Course for Community Health*. London: HMSO.

Cumberlege, J. 1986. *Report of the Community Nursing Review: Neighbourhood Nursing— A Focus for Care*. London: HMSO, 5–6.

Damant, M. 1991. A comparative study of shared learning between health visitors and district nurses. Unpublished MPhil thesis, ENB and University of Plymouth Library.

Damant, M. 1990. *The Report of a Review of Education and Training for Practice Nursing—The Challenges of Primary Health Care in the 1990s*. London: English National Board for Nursing, Midwifery and Health Visiting.

Department of Health. 1992. *The Patient's Charter (National Health Service)*. London: HMSO.

English National Board for Nursing, Midwifery and Health Visiting, 1983, *A Statement on Inter-disciplinary Education,* London: ENB.

Neuman, B. 1989. *The Neuman Systems Model*. Norwalk, Conn.: Appleton & Lange.

United Kingdom Central Council for Nursing, Midwifery and Health Visiting, 1986, *Project 2000: A New Preparation for Practice*. London: UKCC.

Williams, J. 1979. Adult education and inter-professional teaching. In *Education for Co-operation in Health and Social Work,* by H. England. *Journal of the Royal College of General Practitioners*. Occasional Paper 14, 10–11.

Wilson, P. 1978. Linkages among organisations: Considerations and consequences. *Health and Social Work* 134(2):13–33.

45

IN WALES
Using the Model in Community Mental Health Nursing

Patricia Davies
Harold Proctor

In the previous edition, Davies (1989) described the introduction of the Neuman Systems Model within community psychiatric nursing. This included the rationale and objectives for selecting the model. The implementation of the model through the use of the nursing process and evaluation through feedback from clients and nurses was also described. Following discussion of the evaluation, some changes were made to the Neuman generic assessment tool. The community psychiatric nurses (CPNs) were attracted to the model because they hoped it would develop partnership, wholism, and client education.

In this chapter our purpose is to explain how the model has continued to be used in community psychiatric nursing. In particular, we will reflect on how the use of the model has enhanced the quality of nursing practice through the emphasis of partnership, wholism, and client education. Consequently, there is a noticeable differentiation between nursing and medical practice. Finally, there is a short discussion about the model for future practice.

BACKGROUND

The geographical area where most work with the Neuman Systems Model has been undertaken is in the southernmost tip of Powys, known as Ystradgynlais.

Edited and reviewed by Rae Jeanne Memmott.

621

This traditional Welsh mining town has now been affected by national recession and suffers high unemployment. Eight CPNs who work in the area are based either in health centers or the local mental health resource center. The CPNs offer an open referral system, meaning that client referrals can be accepted from anyone. The majority of referrals, however, originate from general practitioners (GPs).

When the CPNs in Ystradgynlais started using the model, first they discussed the assessment with the client and then reviewed it, taking into account the stress areas and model variables (Davies, 1989). This was done rather mechanically by checking the assessment against a list of the intra-, inter-, and extrapersonal factors and physical, psychological, sociocultural, developmental, and spiritual variables that was posted on the agency wall. If they discovered they had failed to gather information related to any elements of the model, they would assess those areas with the client on the next visit.

Now the CPNs are confident enough using the model to be able to check through these elements in their minds as they progress through each assessment and care plan. The more familiar the CPNs are with the model, the easier it is to recall these dimensions without interrupting the flow of the interaction taking place between the CPN and the client.

After initially using the model for assessment and care planning, the CPNs have now started to use the model in indirect activities of client care. For example, they use it as a basis for feedback in supervision sessions and case conferences. The information about clients is communicated based on the structure of the model. The CPNs visualize clients as a system and relate which stress areas they are vulnerable to. They will describe how the client's defense systems are reacting, to what extent the system is compromised, and how they plan to assist the client to regain optimum system stability. Using the model in this context seems to have helped the CPNs provide feedback on clients in a systematic, wholistic way with all information clearly presented in a framework understood by all.

DIFFERENTIATION BETWEEN NURSING AND MEDICAL PRACTICE

When incorporating the Neuman Systems Model into nursing care, it has been noticed that sometimes GPs and CPNs interpret clients' needs and problems differently. A simplified example of this could be a client who is referred to the CPN service by a GP. On the referral form it states that the client is depressed and has been prescribed an antidepressant. Using the model to guide their assessment, the CPNs may find that the client is depressed because of inter- and extrapersonal stressors, such as a poor marital relationship, poor housing, and unemployment. CPNs believe that the requirements for these types of client are not necessarily medication but "talking therapies" such as counseling. The use of other agencies—such as Relate (marriage guidance), social services, and sheltered work organizations—may also be helpful. An understanding of why there is sometimes a difference in managing some clients can be explained by examining the two conceptual frameworks that GPs and CPNs use. The GPs in general base their care on the medical model, that is, diagnosis, treatment, and cure. The CPNs, on the other hand, view care through the Neuman Systems Model, which has been found to generate partnership, wholism, and education.

Clients who present to GPs with emotional problems often have ill-defined and vague symptoms. Such symptoms are notoriously difficult to manage in a medical way because they are hard to diagnose and consequently present problems in treatment and cure. Additionally, these clients require time to sort out their vague and ill-defined problems, which GPs often do not possess (While, 1986; Davies, 1992). Davies (1992) found the following typical responses from GPs:

> "You don't know what is coming through the door and if someone comes in pouring their heart out, you can fall half an hour behind time."

> "Time is a big problem, everyday we see people where I would like to sit down and have an open ended consultation with them, but you just can't, you know we only have 10 minutes." (p. 51)

GP response is often a prescription for drugs. Illing et al. (1991) observed, however, that GPs are under pressure to do something and often want to offer an alternative to medication. It could be argued therefore that referrals of this nature are appropriate for CPNs. It is perhaps understandable that in these circumstances GPs attempt to make a diagnosis (e.g., depression) and then refer to the CPNs. Using the Neuman Model, CPNs, who have more time available, are able to help clients analyze their problems. Through use of preventions as interventions CPNs can develop client partnerships, offer wholistic care, and provide specific education, all of which are integral to the model, thus improving the standard of care. These three areas will be further discussed.

PARTNERSHIP AND EDUCATION

Partnership and education tend to work together and overlap in practice; therefore we considered it important to write about these two areas under the same section. When exploring partnership, Pearson and Vaughan (1986) describe this concept well. They suggest that partnership occurs when nurses work with rather than doing to, for, or at clients. This, of course, has educational implications, because it requires sharing information and knowledge rather than withholding knowledge and telling clients what is best. Clients are then able to make informed choices about their various health care options.

Partnership commences with the assessment. Clients are asked for their opinion on a number of questions that have been adapted from Neuman's generic assessment tool (see Davies, 1989). The questions cover past, present, and future. Clients are asked what is happening at the present time, what happened in the past that led up to the problem, and how they see the future. This gives them many opportunities to express in detail how they feel. It also gives the CPNs a chance to use their listening skills to take in information and help clients feel accepted. It is obviously crucial to partnership formation that clients feel that their thoughts and emotions are being attended to and "taken on board" for what they are. The CPNs can then give their opinion, either by discussing their thoughts on the assessment with clients or, if CPNs are working in a less directive way, by forming a hypothesis.

With the client assessment complete, the parties of this newly established partnership can then go on to negotiate a plan of care. It should be said here that the partnership is not necessarily restricted to clients and CPNs. When appropriate, others can be involved, for example, family members. This is illustrated by the case of a woman who was recently referred to the CPNs with a diagnosis of depression. There were significant intrapersonal difficulties related to both the psychological and physical variables. She felt very sad, had a poor self-image, found it difficult to complete her normal activities of daily living, and was experiencing back pain, sleep disturbance, and appetite loss. Compounding these difficulties were complex interpersonal problems within her immediate family. One of these difficulties was a growing tension between her and her husband. He was involved in a work project that consumed much of his time and was unable to recognize some of the stressors his wife was experiencing. He was included in a number of nursing intervention sessions so that he also became a partner in care. This led to a wider perspective and a greater understanding of the stressors with consequent positive results. He was able to take more time away from work, review some of his own behavior, and offer important suggestions to tackle some of the other difficulties.

This principle of partnership enables clients (and others involved in the system) to feel in control of the process of care rather than being passive recipients, as is often the case with the medical model. Rather than clients being powerless, their power base is maintained within the relationship.

Once a partnership has been established, the educational aspect is incorporated. CPNs can use the model to explain to clients what is happening with their health. Using the Neuman diagrammatic illustration of the model, CPNs can demonstrate to clients the type and nature of stressors affecting their system and how these can best be dealt with. When clients understand what is happening to them, they are usually able to deal with their symptoms. For example, it is very beneficial for clients who suffer panic attacks to understand what is taking place physically during the panic and what could happen. Clients experiencing these symptoms often have catastrophic thoughts that can be allayed somewhat by using a cognitive behavioral approach.

The CPNs have also used the diagram of the Neuman Systems Model as a visual tool to discuss with their clients what is happening. This can be particularly useful when people are dealing with a multiplicity of problems, such as the woman previously described. It can act as a summary of the stressors involved and a useful format to discuss where interventions should be introduced.

In considering the family as the system and looking at interpersonal stressors, another good example of needed client education is in the case of families with a member who suffers from schizophrenia. Much research has been done on how best to alter family patterns of highly expressed emotion to prevent relapse of the family member who has schizophrenia (Brooker, 1990a; Brooker, 1990b; Brooker, 1990c). These are brief examples of how CPNs can use education in secondary and tertiary prevention as intervention.

WHOLISM

Nurses who have had limited contact with the Neuman Systems Model may initially hesitate to incorporate it into their practice. One reason is that they feel it will restrict the way they provide care as they will have to fit clients to the model. In practice, when nurses become familiar with the model, the reverse is true. The model should be seen as a flexible organizing structure on which to base care. It will guide nurses to take into account all environmental stressors (internal and external) that have affected, are affecting, and may affect the client. Indeed, from a wholistic point of view, Neuman (1989) points out that the model is not at all restricting but that "it provides the basis for a broad, comprehensive (umbrellalike) diagnostic statement concerning the entire client condition, from which logically defensible goals are easily or accurately derived" (p. 40).

Wholism has been defined by many. Walsh (1991) from his literature review defined it as an attempt to move away from the conventional mechanistic approach of the mechanical model. Wholism has been described as responding to the person as a whole in their environment and seeing the individual as a combination of spirit, mind, and body. While Neuman reflects this belief, she extends it further as she refers to the five variables (physical, psychological, sociocultural, developmental, and spiritual). She also refers to wholism as being able to "adjust to stress in the internal and external environments" (Neuman, 1989). The idea that wholism reflects the adjustment to stress allows CPNs to explore the past, the present, and the future. As already explained, this aspect is an integral part of the assessment. Using the Neuman Systems Model has helped the CPNs to improve their wholistic approach to care. Clients either present with an idea of where the stress causing their current difficulty has come from, or are unaware of the precipitative factors. Being aware of the key areas where stressors have their influence (intra-, inter-, and extrapersonal) and considering the five Neuman variables, CPNs can help clients examine more clearly the possible causes of their problems. This can be advantageous to clients who believe they are aware of the origin of their stressors as well as those who are not. Those who are not aware are often people who may not yet be able to see clearly the origin of the problem and may be attributing the cause inappropriately. For example, the woman mentioned previously with depression felt initially that she was to blame for many of her feelings. She was able to identify some interpersonal difficulties, but in the early sessions with the CPN intrapersonal factors seemed more significant to her. She felt guilty about how she related to family members and despondent because she did not feel motivated to do her usual household jobs, and she blamed herself for feeling the way she did.

By helping her look at the whole picture, through encouraging her to describe all significant stressors, she was able to identify other reasons for the way she felt. These included interpersonal difficulties with her mother that were longstanding and extrapersonal problems related to early retirement from work due to her back problems. Because of the wholistic nature of assessments based on the Neuman Model, clients usually feel reassured that CPNs have attempted to understand all their difficulties rather than the single problem identified on referral. This gives clients confidence in the CPNs and enhances trust building in the relationship. The model provides a framework for CPNs to work from, and they are able to see how it enhances their wholistic approach. It has also helped CPNs become confident in their work, which in turn is reflected to clients.

IMPLICATIONS FOR THE FUTURE

The Neuman Systems Model (1989) can be used in all areas of nursing practice. For example, a teaching program for student nurses based on the model has been developed by a nurse in Ystradgynlais.

The model elements can provide a framework for resolving complex problems when it is used for the planning of nursing and health services. In this instance the system becomes the community. *Partnership* is incorporated by involving service users and caregivers in the planning process. *Wholism* is incorporated when deciding what service is needed to address any particular stressor experienced by the community, such as a high incidence of unemployment. *Education* (for example, classes on stress management) is needed to maintain the health of the community. The model also helps in determining at which levels of intervention (primary, secondary, or tertiary) services should be targeted.

It is very clear that familiarity with the model does not restrict practice but rather opens up new possibilities for enhancing client care and learning a versatile tool for other nondirect nurse–client activities.

SUMMARY

This chapter has attempted to describe the continued use of the Neuman Systems Model in community psychiatric nursing. We have highlighted the perceived strengths that are produced through using the model: partnership, education, and wholism. These strengths help to improve the quality of nursing care and produce an interesting difference between medical and nursing practice. Finally, we have described briefly how the model will be used in the future.

REFERENCES

Brooker, C. 1990a. Expressed emotion and psychological intervention: A review. *Int J Nurs Stud* 27(3):267–276.

Brooker, C. 1990b. The application of the concept of expressed emotion to the role of the community psychiatric nurse: A research study. *Int J Nurs Stud* 27(3):277–285.

Brooker, C. 1990c. The health education needs of families caring for a schizophrenic relative and the potential role for the community psychiatric nurse. *Journal of Advanced Nursing* 15:1092–1098.

Davies, P. 1989. In Wales: Use of the Neuman Systems Model by community psychiatric nurses. In *The Neuman Systems Model,* 2d ed., edited by B. Neuman. Norwalk, Conn.: Appleton & Lange.

Davies, P. 1992. The community psychiatric nurse and the primary health care team: A study of inter-professional "collaboration." Unpublished thesis, University College of Wales, Swansea.

Illing, J., Drinkwater, C., Rogerson, T., Forster, D., and Rutherford, P. 1990. Evaluation of community psychiatric nursing in general practice. In *Community Psychiatric Nursing,* by C. Brooker. London: Chapman & Hall.

Neuman, B. 1989. The Neuman Systems Model. In *The Neuman Systems Model,* 2d ed., edited by B. Neuman. Norwalk, Conn.: Appleton & Lange.

Pearson, A., and Vaughan, B. 1986. *Nursing Models in Practice.* London: Heinemann.

Walsh, M. 1991. *Models in Clinical Nursing. The Way Forward.* London: Bailliere Tindall.

White, E. 1986. Factors influencing general practitioners to refer clients to community psychiatric nurses. In *Psychiatric Nursing Research,* by J. Brooking. Chichester: Wiley.

46

IN HOLLAND
Application of the Neuman Model in Psychiatric Nursing

Frans Verberk

This chapter describes the contemporary use of theoretical nursing models in psychiatric nursing in the Netherlands. Attention is focused on the way in which the Neuman Model has become recognized in the Netherlands, as well as the attempts made to use it in the subdiscipline of psychiatric nursing. Implications for future utilization of the model are proposed, and advice for future directions in research are offered.

Contact with nursing models in the Netherlands takes place in the course of nursing education. When the first academic nursing program was established at the University of Limburg in Maastricht in 1980, a unique opportunity was provided to study nursing and nursing models in a higher educational setting. Maastricht is in the far southern corner of the Netherlands. A great need was expressed for a similar program located in a more central location, and a number of attempts were made to establish such programs. Initially, the Ministry of Education could not be prevailed upon to support this position. As a result, a cooperative venture came into being with the University of Wales in the United Kingdom. A number of Dutch nursing students were accepted into a course of study for which that university accepted full responsibility.

In 1990 small numbers of students were first given permission to begin their higher education in the more centrally located universities of Utrecht and Groningen. The degree offered by these universities is a "master's in the health

The terms "The Netherlands" and "Holland" are interchangeable as in "The United States" and "America." Persons born in Holland are Dutch.

Translated and reviewed by Raphella Sohier.

sciences" and not a "master's in nursing." This distinction is important in relation to the emphasis placed on theoretical models of nursing. It has been observed by the author that the cooperative program developed by the University of Wales, with its more professional focus on nursing, provides the opportunity to consider the Neuman Systems Model in depth, an opportunity which until now has not presented itself in Dutch universities. It is proposed as a thesis for this article that this advantage will sustain the Welsh master's in nursing program, despite the emergence of the new, essentially less expensive opportunities now available in the Netherlands.

PSYCHIATRIC NURSING IN THE NETHERLANDS

Psychiatric nursing in the Netherlands has evolved in such a way that there is a distinct gulf between the mental health care provided in inpatient and out-patient settings. Distinct forms of psychiatric care have emerged, each with its own set of care modalities. In intramural or inpatient settings, the emphasis has been placed on psychiatric diseases. The medical model has had a great deal of influence on the nature and content of nursing care. In contrast, extramural or outpatient care has been impacted by society's perspectives on behavior, and this view has influenced the content and conduct of care. Inside the profession this has engendered a direction that might be described as social or community psychiatry.

Despite the fact that the two kinds of nursing care are changing and becoming more similar, the distinctions have created a gulf between those nurses providing care in the hospital setting and those functioning in the area of outpatient mental health. As a result the two groups suffer some communication problems. At this moment in history a number of efforts are being made to bridge the gap. It is proposed that widespread utilization of a nursing model by both groups would assist in improving communication. Use of such a model would have positive effects on the psychiatric nursing community in general.

Because the application of nursing models in practice is still a novel idea in the Netherlands, nurses in the psychiatric setting have little experience with them. The models in use at this time are borrowed from other disciplines, a fact that hinders the professionalization of nurses in the psychiatric setting. It is proposed that the use of a nursing model will contribute to this growth and that it will improve the quality of interdisciplinary interactions in the care setting.

GETTING TO KNOW THE NEUMAN SYSTEMS MODEL

The author is a psychiatric nurse in the social psychiatric or outpatient setting who received his master's in nursing degree from the University of Wales. An important objective of his studies was an investigation of nursing models in order to identify the one most suitable for application to psychiatric nursing in the Netherlands. It was considered of great importance to find a model that could accommodate the needs of both the inpatient and outpatient settings and with which nurses, who were as yet unschooled in the use of nursing models, could identify. Another important factor that entered into the choice of Neuman was the systems nature of the model. In Holland systems theory forms an important emphasis in daily practice. This is particularly true of the social or outpatient care setting and is beginning to be true also in the inpatient care setting.

Two criteria emerged that influenced the choice of the Neuman Systems Model. The model had to be one that (1) could be understood in the context of psychiatric nursing in the Netherlands and (2) was based on general systems theory.

Following careful study of diverse nursing models it became clear that the Neuman Systems Model was the most suitable for application in the described setting. Further, the concepts were easy to understand, and the foundation of the model was systematic in nature.

The choice proved to be serendipitous because community psychiatric nurses in Wales were already using the model to direct their practice. Because the author was studying at the University of Wales, he was able to make contact with these nurses, a contact that has since developed into an international exchange.

INTRODUCING THE NEUMAN MODEL IN THE NETHERLANDS

Financial assistance from the National Funds for Community Mental Health made it possible to introduce a pilot project at the Riagg Zuid Hollandse Eilanden (an agency for the care of ambulatory mental health patients). The project has been funded for an initial three-year period.

The primary objective of the project is to improve the quality of nursing care provided to chronically ill psychiatric patients. An important element of the project is to teach and establish the use of the Neuman Systems Model. A team of seven social-psychiatric nurses was formed and made responsible for the change project. The National Fund provided a small budget that enabled the team to take advantage of contacts with the experienced nurses in Wales by way of an international exchange. The seven members of the team met for two hours every second week. They were made responsible for the introduction of the pilot project in their setting. A two-phase process introducing the Neuman Model was developed. Each phase is structured in three steps, detailed below.

Phase 1: Adopting the Model

The objective of the first phase is to gain acceptance for the model. It consists primarily of presenting the model. A visit to Wales is planned to facilitate the exchange of information about the experience of applying the model in practice.

The second step is directed toward a time of experimentation when the

Neuman Model is practiced in order to identify and correct any existing discrepancies between the model and the concrete situations to which it will be applied. Interaction with the Welsh contacts will continue throughout.

The third step constitutes an ongoing evaluation of the progress. One objective of the evaluation is to ascertain whether or not the nurses in the practice setting understand the model sufficiently to put it into practice. At the same time, problems or questions about implementation will be addressed and necessary conditions agreed upon with the management team.

Phase 2: Implementation

The implementation phase is also structured in three steps. The first step is directed toward preparing for the implementation of the model. Instruments and protocols will be developed, and introduction of the clients to the model will occur concomitantly. In this step, as before, the persons responsible for the project will make use of the experience of the Welsh group.

The second step consists of the beginning experience of the model in practice. The instruments and protocols developed earlier will provide support for the nurses during this period. Problems and questions will be addressed as the implementation proceeds, and the leaders will continue to refer to their experienced Welsh colleagues when their own knowledge is insufficient to the task.

The central objective of the third step is evaluation, adjustment, and continuation of the experience with the Neuman Model. Emphasis will be directed toward a determination of its usefulness in practice. Specific problems will be resolved and management concerns addressed in order to continue with the implementation of the model.

NATIONAL DISSEMINATION OF PROJECT INFORMATION

Because of the importance given to psychiatric nursing in the Netherlands and at the request of the funding agency, a number of activities have been incorporated for the purpose of disseminating knowledge about and experience of working with the model. These three activities are designed to introduce the Neuman Model throughout the nursing community in the Netherlands.

The first objective is the publication of a number of articles about the project in national publications. This activity will serve to emphasize the importance of the introduction of the model in the Netherlands. The second activity consists of presentations at symposia. It will be possible by this means to introduce a greater number of interested persons to the project and subsequently to the Neuman Systems Model.

The third objective is the establishment of a support group. Increasing interest in the Neuman Model among nurses who are educators and practitioners, in both inpatient and outpatient psychiatric settings, has suggested this need. As the interest in the model increases, there is constant discussion about the possibility of its being implemented throughout the subdiscipline as the foundation for practice. Difficulties likely to be encountered are under consideration, and it is thought that a support group where clarification of such points could take place would be of help to the psychiatric nursing community as a whole. It will also provide a medium for support of the model's use in educational and practice settings.

INTEREST IN THE NEUMAN MODEL IN THE NETHERLANDS

The Dutch Society of Social-Psychiatric Nurses organized a study day for the purpose of presenting the Neuman Systems Model. Twice as many persons attended the presentation than at any previous study day. Afterwards participants expressed great interest in the content. In addition to the request for more literature about the model, 20 or more persons immediately announced their intention to join the national support group. A second study day produced similar results.

The proof that broad support for and interest in the model exist in the Netherlands can be assumed on the basis of the financial support provided to enable a number of psychiatric nurses from the Netherlands to take part in the Biennial Neuman Symposium in Rochester, New York (1993). The ministry of Welfare, Health, and Culture, the Dutch Society of Social-Psychiatric Nurses, and several psychiatric facilities combined to provide this assistance.

Despite the fact that the Neuman Model is not yet well known in the Netherlands and the activities described here have all taken place within the last 18 months, it is evident that the importance of the model has been recognized.

IMPLICATIONS FOR THE FUTURE

There is a consistent request for literature on the Neuman Model written in Dutch, and there is little question that an important task for the future is a response to this request. It is possible that the Neuman Systems Model text can be translated into Dutch, which would help many Dutch nurses who have difficulty in assimilating texts written in English. While many Dutch nurses speak excellent English, the written language in substantive text form still constitutes a problem for them.

Because the Neuman Model is comparatively unknown in the Netherlands, it will be the task of nurses and especially nurse educators to make it known. It is important that the model become part of nursing education by its inclusion in curricula. Because little is understood of nursing models and theories in contemporary Holland and because other disciplines provide a great variety of theoretical approaches, rehabilitation medicine, case-management approaches, social networking, and theories such as Greunberg's theory of social breakdown have all gained prominence in nursing. In planning the use of the Neuman Model, it will be necessary to consider whether, and how, these and other favored approaches can be incorporated into the model.

Holland is fast becoming a multicultural society. A variety of people call themselves Dutch, and this group has been extended by the emigration of persons from former Dutch colonies as well as numbers of people from the Mediterranean. Despite the fact that the Neuman Systems Model appears to have the capability of incorporating culturally diverse aspects of care (Sohier, 1989), this matter will require consideration in developing the use of the model in Holland. There is also a need for further operational definition of the spiritual variable described by Neuman.

Because the Neuman Model represents a high level of abstraction, it appears that it can be applied in a great many settings and for many purposes. However, greater detail regarding the uses of the model in specific situations is necessary if the model is to live up to its potential. This is particularly true in the psychiatric setting. The model must be applied in a variety of practical situations without impeding its apparent helpfulness in increasing communication among users. Often work is carried out in multidisciplinary teams, and the usefulness of the model in such situations must be demonstrated. It will also be important to clarify the influence the model exerts on the cooperative efforts of the group.

QUALITY ASSURANCE AND THE USE OF THE NEUMAN MODEL

In keeping with the changes occurring in health care financing in the Netherlands, there is a demonstrated need to describe health care outcomes in measurable terms. Measurable criteria form the basis for a systematic evaluation of functional quality in the form of a peer review. Because a single set of reference criteria does not exist at this time, it is almost impossible to develop a common reference within which to evaluate the nursing process. Reviewing the Neuman Model and its accompanying description of the nursing process leads to the conclusion that it may be possible to use it as the foundation for the development of quality standards applicable in psychiatric nursing care.

On the other hand, it is possible that demands coming from directors of client organizations with reference to quality characteristics will provide leadership advice for testing the usefulness of the model. Further, the same demands may provide direction for applying the model in specific practice settings.

RESEARCH ON THE VALUE OF THE NEUMAN MODEL

In order to support the implementation of the Neuman Model in Dutch psychiatric nursing, both implementation and usefulness of the model will need to be evaluated through research. It will be essential to consider whether or not the claims made on behalf of the model are justified.

The following formal propositions are offered:

1. The application of the Neuman Model in psychiatric nursing practice strengthens the professional identity of the nursing profession and facilitates interdisciplinary interaction in the health team.
2. The Neuman Model promotes the interaction between nurse and client by identifying the client's role in the nursing process and supporting accurate assessment of client need.
3. The implementation of the Neuman Model will make it possible to develop explicit criteria with which to evaluate the quality of nursing practice.

Closer scientific examination of the Neuman Model itself will be carried out in conjunction with the master's in nursing course as well as those studies in which the model will be utilized as a theoretical framework.

SUMMARY

Psychiatric nurses in the Netherlands to date have little experience of working with nursing models. While the author was studying for a master's degree in nursing, he concluded that the Neuman Systems Model could be useful for this purpose and, through the medium of the book *Neuman Systems Model* (1989), discovered that a Welsh program had already acquired some experience in applying the model.

Financial assistance from the National Funds for Mental Health together with an interest on the part of a team of nurses working in outpatient psychiatric settings supported the beginnings of a pilot project. The implementation of the Neuman Model in practice depends on the functional outcomes of this pilot project.

The project is planned as an international exchange with nursing colleagues in Wales. The activities are directed toward establishing national familiarity with the model. Thus far, interest across the country is gratifying.

In order to make the model available for use throughout the Netherlands there are some clear implications. For example, there is a need for literature about the model written in Dutch. Further, some research must be carried out to determine whether theories in vogue at this time in the Netherlands can be integrated into the Neuman Systems Model.

It is proposed that nursing practice in the Netherlands will be strengthened by the introduction of the model, that the interaction between nursing need and nursing provision will be facilitated, and that a new nomenclature of criteria for quality assurance can be developed based on the model.

It is proposed that beyond national support nothing is more important than international cooperation in securing extended application of the Neuman Systems Model in psychiatric nursing in the Netherlands.

REFERENCES

Neuman, B., Ed. 1989. *The Neuman Systems Model,* 2d ed. Norwalk, Conn.: Appleton & Lange.

Sohier, R. 1989. Nursing care for the people of a small planet: Culture and the Neuman Systems Model. In *The Neuman Systems Model,* 2d ed., edited by B. Neuman, 139–154. Norwalk, Conn.: Appleton & Lange.

47

A STRUCTURE FOR DOCUMENTING PRIMARY HEALTH CARE IN SWEDEN USING THE NEUMAN SYSTEMS MODEL

Ingegerd Bergbom Engberg
Eva Bjälming
Birgitta Bertilson

The first part of this chapter addresses documentation of nursing care by district nurses and how the Neuman Systems Model was used in the education and supervision of the district nurses in how to best apply the model in their work with clients. The second part illustrates the use of the Neuman Systems Model as a framework for analysis of the district nurses' care of patients with leg ulcers and how the model can contribute to the development of a nursing care protocol and documentation.

Edited and reviewed by Raphella Sohier. Figure 47–3 assistance by Cynthia Capers.

In Sweden registered nurses who have worked for at least two years may continue their education and become district nurses. The 40-week program of study is made up of in-depth courses in social medicine, epidemiology, and public health. Upon completion of the program the district nurse may work in primary health care districts, at child health centers, and as a school nurse. The education of registered nurses and different postbasic specialty programs are under development in Sweden now, and there is an increasing trend toward courses in a more academic tradition.

BACKGROUND

The counties are responsible for health and medical care in Sweden. Usually the county region corresponds to an area that is the center for health and medical care within a specified geographical area. The health and medical care offered to the inhabitants of the county is partly funded by taxes. The general goals for health and medical care are set by the politicians in the board of the county council. The National Social Welfare Board has the responsibility of supervision throughout Sweden.

The district nurses described in this chapter have received a special 40-week primary health care education program. They have private offices located either at a health center or in the community where their clients live. District nurses are employed by the county council or by the community.

Some of the central concepts in public health nursing are wholism, care continuity, consumer availability, and proximity to clients' homes. District nurses have broad functions: they answer questions and give advice by telephone, receive clients in their offices, and make home visits within a limited geographical area with an average population of 1,500. They care for clients of all ages using primary, secondary, and tertiary health prevention and illness care modalities. Some examples of health-related tasks of the district nurse are health care counseling of individuals, child health care, instruction of parents, health check-ups, and providing health information to adults and children individually or in groups. Other functions of the district nurse can include dressings, injections, catheterizations and follow-ups, and home health care, including terminal care. The trend in home health care is toward more advanced nursing care, such as the care of patients on respirators and those receiving dialysis and infusions.

As the district nurses often work in a team, especially when making home visits, it is of great importance that their work be well documented and in accordance with the Swedish patient record legislation. Quality documentation facilitates continuity of care, supports quality of care, and ensures compliance with the law.

I. The District Nurses' Documentation of Nursing Care Application of the Model

Ingegerd Bergbom Engberg and Eva Bjälming

Shared in this chapter is the utility and ability of the Neuman Systems Model in providing a structure for documenting and delivering quality health care in the Sävsjö community. Twenty district nurses are employed in the community, which has a population of 12,100 inhabitants in both towns and rural areas and is 680 square kilometers in size. The district nurses work in teams, and there are a total of six teams in the area. A team consists of a physician, a district nurse, and a practical nurse. The district nurse is responsible for the nursing care, and the physician is responsible for the medical care. The district nurses usually document different treatments, nursing actions, and measures on a patient index card. The card also contains the client's vital statistics, the time and type of treatment, and details about who implemented the treatment plan and/or nursing action. This documentation failed to meet the requirements of the nationally prescribed patient record legislation.

THE SWEDISH PATIENT RECORD LAW

Since 1986 Swedish nurses have been required by law (SFS, 1985:562) to keep written nurses' notes on their patients. The intention of the law is to assure both quality and safety in nursing care. Inadequate documentation has resulted in a number of consequences for nurses that could have been avoided if the documentation of the care had been adequate. According to the legislation, health and medical care institutions prepare and establish protocol for documentation of care.

The aims of the patient record are:

- To be a support for the person or persons responsible for the patient's treatment and to assure that patients receive care that is both safe and of good quality
- To constitute a basis for assessing which actions should be taken by someone who has not previously met the patient, such as an on-call relief physician or nurse

- To be an instrument used in quality assurance
- To constitute the foundation for supervision and control
- To provide information to the patient about the care and treatment received (SOSFS 1990:15)

The patient record is therefore a necessary document in the care of the patient. It is also an important instrument with regard to quality assurance, safety, and follow-up and for the personnel in their work areas.

Further, the law requires that the reasons for taking different nursing care actions and for the medical treatment carried out by the nurse be described in the nursing care record. It is obvious that documentation is inadequate from a nursing perspective if it only consists of a description of the client's condition and circumstances, including the different actions and treatment. The documentation should also constitute an assessment and analysis of the client's total situation from a caring perspective. To accomplish this, a theoretical framework is required that can act as a support so that the caring process is operationalized in daily care. To think and act wholistically is to offer caring.

THE NEUMAN SYSTEMS MODEL

The Neuman Systems Model (1982, 1986, 1989) was assessed as an appropriate structure for the caring process, which identified characteristics of the kinds of care given by the district nurses, especially in terms of their responsibility for primary, secondary, and tertiary prevention as intervention. The Neuman Systems Model emphasizes a wholistic view with both the client and nurse considered part of the immediate system of interaction. Neuman believes that each person is unique and in constant change and flux in relation to environmental influences. The client is thus an open system interacting with the environment and is always in a dynamic condition of wellness, health, or illness in varying degrees. Health and wellness are defined as a condition where all parts are in harmony with the whole person, and a person's environment comprises all the factors that influence and are influenced by the system of which the person is a part. The model is goal-directed, focuses on prevention, and encourages the nurse to learn about the clients' experiences, expectations, and views about their health situation. It also assists in the development of the nurse's knowledge and skills of nursing practice as an art and recognizes the adaptation of continuous changes in the client's health and medical condition. In addition, the model constitutes an analytic tool for skilled nursing care as well as for well-structured documentation according to the intent of the patient record legislation.

PLANNING AND IMPLEMENTATION: APPLICATION OF THE MODEL TO PRIMARY HEALTH CARE

The Program

A study program that included theoretical and practical issues was designed to focus both on interactions among the instructors, supervisors, and district nurses and also on interactions between district nurses and clients (Figure 47–1). The first part of the program consisted of analysis of the group of district nurses as client, planning of interventions, and implementation. The Neuman Systems Model constituted the foundation and framework in this process.

During and after the first meeting with the entire group of district nurses, an assessment of the situation and the needs it represented was undertaken. The group identified stressors, reactions, and the effect on the different lines of defense and resistance (Figure 47–2). After reflection and analysis, diagnosis, goals, and interventions were formulated.

In order to decrease the effects of stressors the proposed intervention was to increase the nurses' knowledge about the requirements stipulated in the patient record legislation, in keeping with concepts of the Neuman Systems Model. Nursing interventions consisted of strategies that they would be encouraged to use to analyze client cases at future meetings. In that way, it was anticipated that the nurses would be engaged as participants and collaborators in the process of developing a client record based on the concepts of the Neuman Systems Model.

Theoretical integration was accomplished through presentation of district nurse practice client case data while simultaneously introducing "stepwise" the Neuman Model content as illustrated in Table 47–1.

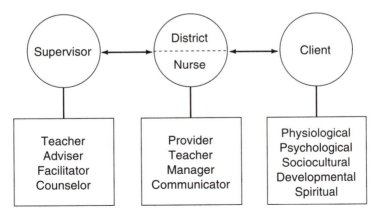

Figure 47–1. The interactions among supervisors, district nurses, and clients.

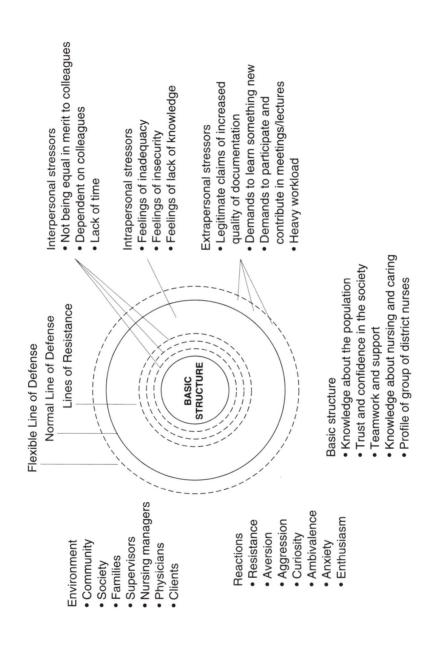

Flexible Line of Defense

Normal Line of Defense

Lines of Resistance

Interpersonal stressors
- Not being equal in merit to colleagues
- Dependent on colleagues
- Lack of time

Intrapersonal stressors
- Feelings of inadequacy
- Feelings of insecurity
- Feelings of lack of knowledge

Extrapersonal stressors
- Legitimate claims of increased quality of documentation
- Demands to learn something new
- Demands to participate and contribute in meetings/lectures
- Heavy workload

BASIC STRUCTURE

Environment
- Community
- Society
- Families
- Supervisors
- Nursing managers
- Physicians
- Clients

Reactions
- Resistance
- Aversion
- Aggression
- Curiosity
- Ambivalence
- Anxiety
- Enthusiasm

Basic structure
- Knowledge about the population
- Trust and confidence in the society
- Teamwork and support
- Knowledge about nursing and caring
- Profile of group of district nurses

Figure 47–2. Analysis of the group of district nurses as a client—an adaptation of the Neuman Systems Model.

TABLE 47–1. THE STEPWISE INTRODUCTION OF THE NEUMAN SYSTEMS MODEL DURING CASE PRESENTATIONS.

Meetings	Topic
Number 1	Presentation of the Neuman Systems Model.
Number 2	Basic structure, stressors, reactions, the five variables, lines of defense, lines of resistance, and identifying these in client cases.
Number 3	Environment, diagnosis, goals, interventions, and identifying these in client cases.
Number 4	Before the meeting every district nurse had sent a client record where stressors, reactions, diagnosis, goals, and interventions were identified. Individual written comments enlightened the supervisors' assessments. Lectures were given about energy flow, wellness, stability, nursing actions, and outcomes.
Number 5	Discussion and evaluation of six client cases.

Proceedings. Each meeting lasted 90 minutes where discussion, questions, and the district nurses' knowledge and experiences were exchanged. District nurse education through case study incorporating model concepts, which facilitated participation of each learner, had the outcome of maintaining the nurses' flexible line of defense in relation to supervision, by expanding the line away from the normal line of defense to reduce the risk of reaction to work-related stressors.

Thus *primary prevention* was focused on education and instruction of nursing theory, and client case data during the first three meetings of the entire group of district nurses. *Secondary prevention* was focused on planned written individual client cases and documentation instructions for one or two client cases carried out in groups of two or three district nurses. The second part of the program was the actual interaction between the district nurse and the client. The goal for the district nurses was to integrate the Neuman Systems Model into their daily work. Thus the chosen strategy was that each district nurse should document the nursing care given with one or more new clients during a six-month period with a supervisory follow-up plan. These interventions were considered tertiary prevention for the purpose of maintaining stability among the district nurses while they were learning the new strategy, thus preventing uncertainty and insecurity in documenting the client care given. For supervision purposes a form was prepared for use in analyzing and discussing the specific documentation.

Outcome

Following the first six months' use of the Neuman Systems Model in the group, it was extended to individual district nurses as client. The supervised individual or small group interventions provided more intimacy and less collegial stress. For example, compared to the group reactions in Figure 47–2, the aversion, aggression, and resistance were very mild under individual supervision. Enthusiasm and motivation for increasing theoretical knowledge, which supported wholistic care of clients, were obvious.

Because of the heavy workload and extra time required for documentation, and in order to reduce stressors, nurses were often encouraged to cooperate in documenting mutual client care. The outcome was one of feeling equal merit in work function. Time and supervision reduced the district nurse's feeling of insecurity in assessment, analysis of client data in this knowledge base, integration factors, and care documentation. The legitimate claims of the increased quality of documentation were not experienced as stress-evoking when the first follow-up evaluation took place after six months of application of the documentation. All district nurses contributed in evaluation of the initial form and its subsequent revision (see Figure 47–3).

Evaluation

At the end of each six-month time period district nurses were asked to respond to an evaluation form. Most of the nurses found that application of the Neuman Systems Model contributed to an increased quality of interaction between the district nurse and client. They also found that the model structure used for documentation made them feel secure, because the essence of caring in the wholistic client approach was evident and satisfying. Further, the client record then fulfilled the requirements in the Swedish patient record legislation; that is, the background and the reasons for nursing care and nursing actions/interventions were fully described. Through the use of nursing diagnosis and client goals the analyses were made explicit.

The documentation form based on Neuman Systems Model was found to be:

1. A support for the district nurse
2. A foundation for good quality and safe care
3. An instrument providing quality assurance
4. A foundation for supervision and control of learning needs
5. A basis for discussion with other colleagues regarding assessment and activity
6. A support and source of information for the client concerning the care and treatment received

Name _____ Civic reg.no. _____

Address _____

Phone: _____

	Background
Date	
Time	
Nurse name	

	Client reactions
Date	
Time	
Nurse name	

Stressors (physiological, psychological, developmental, sociocultural, spiritual; intra-, inter-, extrapersonal factors)

Nursing diagnosis

	Nursing goals (in negotiation with the client)
Date	
Time	
Nurse name	

Nursing interventions (strategies to achieve the goals: primary, secondary, and tertiary prevention)

Flexible Line of Defense
Normal Line of Defense
Lines of Resistance

BASIC STRUCTURE

Figure 47–3. Documentation form.

II. The Model as a Tool for Analyzing District Nurses' Care of Clients with Leg Ulcers

Birgitta Bertilsson

The purpose of this study was to describe how and what district nurses document concerning the treatment and care of clients with leg ulcers. A leg ulcer is defined as an ulcer on the lower part of the leg and/or foot and is considered a symptom of an internal illness. In order to diagnose a leg ulcer, a total history should be taken to identify and assess factors giving rise to the ulcer, including pain, previous ulcers, state of health, mobility, ability to walk, obesity, malnutrition, smoking, other diseases, and current medications taken. Great effort should be made to prevent future leg ulcers. In planning treatment, one must consider the client's entire life situation and try to make the quality of life as good as possible. The goal should be to heal the wound and prevent a recurrence.

THE DISTRICT NURSE AND THE TREATMENT OF LEG ULCERS

In most cases, leg ulcers are the responsibility of the primary health care system. The family practitioner diagnoses the ulcer; the district nurse plans the treatment based on his or her own knowledge and experience and is responsible for continuity of care as he or she carries out the prescribed treatment and changes the dressings. Continuous collaboration with the family practitioner is necessary. The choice of treatment used often depends on the previous experiences of the district nurse and the client. It is important that health care providers inform the patient, as this provides increased understanding and develops the client's motivation and ability to take responsibility for self. This in turn can improve the client's quality of life and the job satisfaction of the caregiver. One way of increasing understanding concerning the ulcer and its treatment is to keep the client informed about the significance of primary, secondary, and tertiary prevention efforts such as use of diuretics, compression, exercise, and diet in regard to both healing of the ulcer and how the foot/leg should be cared for once the ulcer has healed.

USE OF THE NEUMAN SYSTEMS MODEL IN THE TREATMENT OF LEG ULCERS

Nursing care in the treatment of leg ulcers based on the Neuman Systems Model provides the means for identifying, determining, clarifying, and evaluating the dynamic interaction among the five variables, which represent a wholistic view of the client. The model also provides a means for determining the strength of individual reactions to stressors, that is, the ability of the lines of resistance to protect the basic structure. The *physiological variables* considered here are medical diagnosis, vascular changes, diabetes, hypertension, edema, pain analysis, sleep, mobility, overweight, malnourishment, and the appearance, size, and location of the leg ulcer. Examples of *psychological variables* are self-knowledge, ego strength, wellness, uneasiness, fear, disgust, tolerance, acceptance of the situation, and dependence. *Sociocultural variables* are civil status, occupation, job, dwelling, family, home help, activities, leisure-time interest, clubs, hobbies, and life-style. Among the *developmental variables* are age, willingness to change one's pattern of living, flexibility, rigidity, and knowledge about bodily functions. *Spiritual variables* includes the client's system of belief, values, and hope.

SUBJECTS AND METHOD

The Neuman Systems Model was used as a structure for developing four functional evaluative themes used in an interview with a total of eight district nurses as informants from four primary health care districts in Sweden. To repeat, the purpose was to examine the treatment of leg ulcers by district nurses.

Theme 1: *Analyzing the Client's Condition*

The district nurses were asked: When you see a client, how do you analyze/obtain a clear understanding of the client's condition? Physiological condition was determined to cover the general state of health, previous illness, present illness, medications, pain, sleep, diet/dietary habits, overweight, malnourishment, mobility, possible technical aids, smoking, swelling of the leg, and the appearance, size, and location of the ulcer.

Wellness, harmony, anxiety, nervousness, fear, disgust, tolerance, self-knowledge, and acceptance of one's own situation were included in the psychological condition. Sociocultural condition comprised civil status, occupation, job, type of dwelling, home help (including how often and from whom the client receives the help), activities, leisure time, clubs, and hobbies. Developmental condition included age, knowledge about bodily functions, changes in patterns of living, flexibility, and rigidity. Spiritual condition was comprised of religion, values, beliefs, and hope.

Theme 2: *Analyzing the Client's Needs for Nursing Care Interventions*

The interventions were divided into three parts. Primary prevention should focus on wellness related to diet, activity, smoking, education, and presenting underlying illness. Secondary prevention should focus on treatment of the ulcer, symptoms with compression, alleviation of pain, movement, and leg elevation. Tertiary prevention should focus on proper diet, weight reduction, malnourishment related to ulcer, smoking, compression, skin care, movement, and mobilization.

Theme 3: *Analyzing the Client's Reactions to Treatment*

The physical reactions were focused on pain, sleep, the projected healing of the ulcer, movement, and mobilization. The psychological reactions were dependency over slow healing, fatigue due to pain, sleeping difficulties, and confidence in treatment. The developmental reactions were focused on lack of knowledge about the healing process and motivation and support for increasing self-help. Difficulty in handling daily living activities, reactions to advice of family and friends, need for assistance, and dependence were viewed as possible sociocultural reactions.

Theme 4: *Carrying out the Treatment*

The district nurses were asked to comment on how they planned and carried out the required interventions. The consensus was that the method of treatment and planned evaluation chosen should be shared with and accepted by clients. For example, discussion about dressing changes should focus on frequency, result of treatments, and any changes in method of treatment. The district nurses were also asked how they evaluated client progress toward an understanding of tertiary prevention.

FINDINGS

In assessing the clients' physical condition, all district nurses reported that they included previous illness, current medication, and the location and appearance of the leg ulcer in their analysis, and many checked for leg edema, while others asked about the clients' pain. All the district nurses stated that their evaluation of psychological status included the clients' concern and anxiety about their ulcer, while a few considered how clients experienced dressing changes and their entire life situation. For the sociocultural condition all the district nurses referred to the clients' family situation during home visits. A number discussed the possible need for technical or other types of aids and home help when they were making a home visit. Others reported that when clients were of preretirement age they often asked about their work and/or leisure-time interest, and all district nurses stated that they focused primarily on the appearance of the ulcer and how the treatment was to be carried out.

More than half said that they stressed the importance of compression in the form of support stockings or bandaging of the leg after the ulcer had healed in order to prevent the occurrence of new ulcers. Half counseled their clients on dietary habits and weight reduction, while a few stated that they even tried to encourage clients to stop smoking, an intervention that encompassed both primary and tertiary prevention.

More than half the district nurses reported that they analyzed and supported their clients' reactions to slow healing of the ulcer and system reaction to localized treatment of the ulcer, and approximately the same number commented that adequate pain relief was of major importance. Some of the district nurses stated that they encouraged their clients to increase movement. They all indicated being sensitive to their clients' psychological concerns, and most of the nurses listened to their clients, thus reducing anxiety by supporting and encouraging the decisions they made so that their quality of life could be improved. Half the district nurses reported that they encouraged clients to increase self-care and avoid becoming overly dependent. All the district nurses reported that they taught clients about the ulcer healing process and encouraged them to learn how to change dressings. A few said they were sensitive as to whether the client had understood their advice about the treatment or if it had to be reinforced. Slightly more than half the district nurses thought they gave clients sociocultural support by obtaining technical or other types of aids so clients could carry out their daily activities. Some of the district nurses met with home health service when necessary to foster care continuity. Half the nurses felt home visits provided information on total family function, which is an important aspect of wholistic assessment. They noted that family function cannot be assessed when clients are seen in the office setting.

More than half the district nurses stated that they asked clients if they had had an ulcer before, and they also inquired about previous treatments and what treatment the clients had faith in. Most did client teaching while caring for clients, offering them tertiary preventive care while treating the wound.

Although district nurses assessed reactions to treatment such as pain and limited mobility, they did not routinely follow up with the client. Some visited at least once following healing. In the past, priority has not been given to following up on these clients, but nurses are becoming more aware of the need for teaching prevention to increase client quality of life.

DISCUSSION

Much change is needed in wholistic assessment of clients with leg ulcers. At present, documentation reveals that the district nurse records the client's name, address, birth date, and personal registration number; notes underlying illnesses, medication, and responsible physician; and thereafter, concentrates on the ulcer, how it looks, and how it is being treated. The length of time for which treatment was planned, however, was seldom recorded, although a notation was made each time treatment was given. This type of documentation is totally inadequate as we move into the 21st century. Without a common structure to which all nurses can relate, care remains basically focused on physiologic concerns. Little sharing is possible among nurses, as each district nurse practices the art of nursing as he or she has learned it and common understanding of situations is unusual.

The Neuman Systems Model is recommended as the nursing framework for caring for clients with leg ulcers because the model assists in identifying client stressors as well as subsequent measures that help the client to adjust to these stressors and maintain optimal wellness. This evaluative study based on the Neuman Systems Model has illustrated a great need to use a wholistic care perspective in order to improve quality of care and improve documentation.

The model variables should all be considered, as total client function is important to allow the nurse to provide other aspects of care beyond the physiological and to assure optimum level wellness. In identifying all client system stressors, specific nursing measures can be used to facilitate client stressor adjustment toward wellness. The district nurse needs to become more analytic and theoretically based in practice. Consideration of the whole client provides a professional nursing care perspective that will contribute to increased quality of life for the client and higher job satisfaction for the district nurse.

FUTURE IMPLICATIONS FOR MODEL USAGE

The Neuman Systems Model has many advantages. Among them is the construction of a model that encourages continuous assessment and complete care documentation. The model prescribes identification of the nature and analysis of the client's possible and actual reactions to stressors. The district nurse is responsible for identifying stressors, noting reactions, diagnosing the client's general health condition, setting goals, and both evaluating and documenting nursing outcomes of the interventions made.

Important features of the model include not only the nursing process for implementing the model as indicated above, but intervention modalities of primary, secondary, and tertiary prevention, which give a clear sense of direction for both identification of client needs and how to intervene to correct the need. Another important factor is the identification of client strengths, which help the nurse develop a wholistic view and consider the client's resources, thus respecting the uniqueness of every client. This makes it easier to develop appropriate individualized interventions and helps the nurse to be judicious both in nursing activities and in documentation. The negotiation of client goals following clarification of differences between client and nurse perspectives are in keeping with world health care mandates. The two projects clearly indicate the need for the structure that a model provides in order to document nursing care. Based on this finding, and to meet this need, an academic course will be offered at the University College of Health Sciences in Jönköping. The course will focus on nursing models and theories, and a section will deal with documentation based on the Neuman Systems Model. The course will be available to all registered nurses throughout Sweden.

At the end of 1993 a computerized client record based on the Neuman Systems Model was introduced for use by district nurses in the Sävsjö community. We are pleased to be moving in a wholistic manner toward a future of quality client care provided by Sweden's district nurses.

REFERENCES

Neuman, B. 1982. *The Neuman Systems Model*. East Norwalk, Conn.: Appleton & Lange.

Neuman, B. 1989. *The Neuman Systems Model*. East Norwalk, Conn.: Appleton & Lange.

Neuman, B. 1985. The Neuman Systems Model explanation: Its relevance to emerging trends toward wholism in nursing. In *Omvårdnad 1986*, edited by I. Bergbom Engberg and K. Kuld. Omvårdnadsforum HB, Mullsjö, Sweden.

SFS 1985:562 Patientjournallagen. [Patient Record Law]. Svensk författningssamling. Liber, Allmänna förlaget, Stockholm.

SOSF 1990:15 [Book of the National Social Welfare Board]. Socialstyrelsens allmänna råd i omvårdnad inom sluten somatisk vård och primärvård. Författningshandboken. För personal inom hälso- och sjukvård. Sammanställd av Kay Wilow, Almqvist och Wiksell Förlag AB, 1992.

48

BRIEF ABSTRACTS
Use of the Neuman Systems Model in Sweden

Ingegerd Bergbom Engberg

Interest in nursing theories and models among nurses in Sweden is varied. American nurse theorists are often well known among nurse educators, students, and researchers. An increasing number of clinical nurses are also familiar with the different nursing and caring theories. However, there is a reluctance to use and apply theories and models in nursing care practice, since they are often seen as not applicable to the Swedish hospital and health care system. Despite this, the nursing and caring theories have influenced many nurses' thinking in both clinical and educational settings. This increasing interest in nursing theories and models has resulted in the formation of an organization called the Nursing Association for Nursing Theories in Practice, Education, and Research, which is connected to the Swedish Association of Registered Nurses and the Nurses Federation. Nurses who are interested in nursing and caring theories can join this association.

The Neuman Systems Model was introduced to Swedish nurses in 1986 when the first article by Dr. Neuman was published in Swedish. Since then the model has become widely used both in nursing education at different levels and in research. Interest in the model also increased after Dr. Neuman visited Sweden in 1991 and gave lectures in Jönköping, Linköping, and Örebro.

In May 1993 a book about models for nursing and their application in clinical nursing care was published. In this book a comparison made between the Orem, Rogers, and Neuman Systems models. The book, written by Marianne Lindell and Henny Olsson, illustrates the use of the Neuman Systems Model in clinical nursing, based on case studies in obstetrical nursing care. Literature such as this aims to diminish the gap between theory and practice and facilitate the possibilities of widely applying this knowledge in nursing care.

PRIMARY HEALTH CARE MODULES IN BASIC NURSE EDUCATION

At most university colleges throughout Sweden, the Neuman Systems Model is used as a theoretical framework in the module of primary health in nursing education. Two examples are presented here. At the University College in Health and Caring Sciences in Eskilstuna students use the model in the nursing care of clients during their practical training in primary health care. Students observe and analyze clients' stressors and how these influence the flexible line of defense. Students also suggest nursing interventions that aim to maintain the normal line of defense. In this way students are trained in data collection and the making of analyses. In Jönköping the Neuman Systems Model is presented in the primary health care module. The model is also presented by students in different kinds of examination reports, such as theoretical analyses of the model or applications in a practical environment.
(Contact: Kristina Westerberg, University College of Caring Sciences, Drottninggatan 16, S-632 20 Eskilstuna, Tel. +4616125100; Eva Bjälming, University College of Health Sciences, Box 1038, S-551 11 Jönköping, Tel. +4636104889.)

EDUCATION OF DISTRICT NURSES

At the University College of Health Sciences in Jönköping the model is introduced in the education of district nurses. Students have to apply the model during their practical training. Results are given in an examination report. Students may also present theoretical analyses of the model.
(Contact: Eva Bjälming [see above].)

POSTQUALIFICATION STUDIES

In different postqualification studies (i.e., courses in nursing care, preparatory research, and education diploma courses) the Neuman Systems Model is usually presented together with other nursing theories and models. Thus a lot of reports and projects are presented utilizing the Neuman Systems Model. The model is used in both educational and practical settings. One typical example is "The Application of the Neuman Systems Model in Rehabilitation," written by Gunnel Gustavsson, a research student. There are also many theoretical analyses of the model.

(Contact: Gunn Engvall, senior tutor at the University College of Caring Sciences, Uppsala University Children's Hospital, S-751 85 Uppsala, Tel. +4618327223; Gunnel Gustavsson, University College of Health Sciences, Box 1038, S-551 11 Jönköping, Tel. +4636104909.)

RESEARCH IN NURSING CARE

The Neuman Systems Model has been used as a theoretical framework in two research projects by Henny Olsson and Marianne Lindell at the Center for Caring Sciences in Örebro. One of the studies shows how the model can be used in the counseling role of the midwife concerning contraceptive methods. The other study examines bedridden patients' experience of their hygienic situation and cleanliness during their stay at the hospital compared to their usual routines and standards at home.

In a study of herpes zoster patients' experience of postherpetic neuralgia, the wholistic view in the model has led to the design of an interview questionnaire to identify client stressors and reactions.

(Contact: Marianne Lindell and Henny Olsson, Center for Caring Sciences, Box 1324, S-701 13 Örebro, Tel. +4619157111; Ingegerd Bergbom Engberg, University College of Health Sciences, Box 1038, S-551 11 Jönköping, Tel. +4636104871.)

DOCUMENTATION IN PRIMARY HEALTH CARE

Since 1992 district nurses in the Sävsjö community have been using the Neuman Systems Model as a framework for documenting nursing care. The model is applied in the nursing care process, and a format for documentation is based on some of the key concepts in the model. In a meeting with the client at the district nurse's office or a home visit, the client's stressors and reactions are identified. After analysis, the nursing diagnosis is made and aims and interventions are planned. A form is used to record when interventions were carried out and the results of the interventions. For further information see Chapter 47.

(Contact: Annikki Jonsson, Nursing Manager, The Primary Health Care Center, S-576 00 Sävsjö, Tel. +4638211330.)

CONCLUSION

The Neuman Systems Model has inspired many nurses in education, in clinical settings, and in research projects. The examples mentioned here are by no means comprehensive, and hopefully users of the model will give more reports in the future. The model is mostly used in education and primary health care in

Sweden, where it is greatly appreciated because of its wholistic view and clear structure.

REFERENCES

Bergbom Engberg, I., Gröndahl, G-B., and Thibom, K. 1993. The clinical course of herpes zoster—a wholistic view. Submitted.

Lindell, M., and Olsson, H. 1993. Modeller för omvårdnad—teoretiska aspekter och exempel [Models for nursing—theoretical aspects and examples]. Liber, Stockholm.

Lindell, M., and Olsson, H. 1991. Can combined oral contraceptives be made more effective by means of a nursing care model? *Journal of Advanced Nursing* 16:475–479.

Neuman, B. 1986. The Neuman Systems Model explanation: Its relevance to emerging trends toward wholism in nursing. In *Omvårdnad 1986,* edited by I. Bergbom Engberg and K. Kuld. Omvårdnadsforum HB, Mullsjö.

Olsson, H., and Lindell, M. 1993. A pilot study about combining knowledge from caring science and natural science. Submitted.

49

IMPLICATIONS FOR USE OF THE NEUMAN SYSTEMS MODEL IN OCCUPATIONAL HEALTH NURSING

Marian McGee

DEFINITION OF OCCUPATIONAL HEALTH NURSING

Occupational health nursing is a subspecialty of nursing and operates from the dictates of its parent, nursing science. It incorporates concepts from public health sciences and physical sciences. The focus of occupational health nursing practice is on the population of a particular occupation, industry, or work site. The elements of practice include the environment or context, work processes, worker profile and functional patterns, worker encounters with the occupational health nurse (OHN), goals of practice, and actions/behavior (process and dynamics) of the nurse. These elements converge in time in various situations that involve conditions of normalcy, risk, crisis, and/or morbidity.

It follows that occupational health nursing is a situationally derived process of interaction among the occupational nurse, the worker, his or her work, and the workplace. The process proceeds from the basis of assessment of need and function of the worker in the workplace; it is designed to optimize worker health

Reviewed by Barbara Freese.

(i.e., total functioning) through interventions with strategies that include environmental modification or reinforcement, behavioral modification or reinforcement, and biophysical care and maintenance (McGee, 1975, 1981).

This chapter attempts to explicate the rationale and process of occupational health nursing practice using the Neuman Systems Model (NSM) and operating on the assumptions of human function articulated by Neuman (1989). The purpose is to illustrate application of the model in occupational health service.

RELEVANCE OF THE NEUMAN SYSTEMS MODEL TO OCCUPATIONAL HEALTH NURSING

The Neuman Systems Model is relevant to most situations of occupational health practice. Confidence in the model as a grand theory is increasing with documented experiences (Beddome, 1989; Drew, Craig, and Beynon, 1989; Dunn and Trépanier, 1989; Louis, 1989). Empirical testing that establishes "goodness of fit" with middle range theories is strengthening the model's utility for practitioners.

The compatibility of the NSM with the imperatives of public health science is also well established. The model imperatives of primary, secondary, and tertiary prevention are similar to the requisites of public and community health. The model emphasizes problem prevention and health promotion, as does public health practice.

OCCUPATIONAL HEALTH NURSING PROTOCOL USING NEUMAN'S MODEL

Wilson, an educator and consultant in health care administration, makes a critical point regarding the relevance of nursing process to the principal functions of nursing. He states that the implementation element of the nursing process "is not a specific enough term—it is a whole meal in one bite" (1992). Wilson acknowledges the legitimacy of nursing's wish to avoid a list of mastered tasks but argues that to move to a meaningless extreme diminishes the importance of nursing process. Nurses must make every attempt to articulate clearly the intervention strategies for achievement of particular health goals. In order to increase explicitness, this chapter refers to the actions to prevent and control health problems in the workplace as nursing protocol instead of nursing process.

The systems orientation of the Neuman Model facilitates organization of nursing data for assessment and diagnosis. The "systems perspective" of Neuman's latest text (1989) illustrates that in the work setting, the context of worker and work situation can be analyzed readily using systems theory.

PROFILE OF WORK GROUP OR ORGANIZATIONAL RISK

Occupational health nursing assessment includes identification of stressors and their degree of impact on the worker's lines of defense and resistance, along with their source and constancy in the environment. Stressors may be desirable or undesirable as a function of both the worker's relationship with the work and workplace and as a function of the work organization. Analysis of the system's stressors is based on identification of the organization's function and activity flow, its core, lines of resistance, and lines of defense. Within the work situation, identifiable components operate to create stressors and resources to manage stressors. In these strained economic times, the core of the organization and its lines of resistance and defense are as important to worker health as the worker's own set of defenses. Carnevali (1993) supports that view by pointing out that determining the "diagnostic target" for nursing is necessary and involves much more than the individual and the problem/pathology.

It is for that reason that organizational data are considered necessary situational data. As a consequence, the organization and target population (which can be the total personnel employed or a particular work-specific group) must be assessed to establish an organization risk profile (Figure 49–1).

The guidelines for data collection in the form are self-explanatory. It is to be expected that as in any subspecialty of public/community health nursing, the population analysis is aggregate-oriented with a strong imperative to identify risk and pursue risk control, reduction, and prevention. These data also supply evidence of the appropriateness and basis for use of the Neuman Model. Space does not permit further explication of relative and attributable risk; prior publications have addressed population analysis and risk identification (Valanis, 1992), the influence of organizations on collective and individual coping and growth capacity (Argyris, 1993), and use of a conceptual model with an aggregate (Beddome, 1989).

The focus of attention in occupational health nursing practice goes beyond single events associated with an individual client/worker. This aggregate emphasis does not suggest exclusion or deemphasis of the individual and his or her respective patterns and perceptions but rather reinforces the necessity of *total system* assessment and care. It follows that a separate form or guideline for data collection is needed for nursing protocol relevant to the individual client/worker and that both sets of data are necessary for establishing valid diagnostic conclusions and appropriate interventions.

Individual as well as group risk must be established since the NSM dictates problem prevention. Screening strategies can be utilized to detect problems, potential problems, and the level or degree of risk. The worker condition of normalcy, risk, crisis, or morbidity will influence the mode, the items of data collection, and the values assigned to selected variables.

Situational classification:
crisis ( ) normal ( ) risk ( ) morbidity ( )
Client population—Dominant work activity (e.g., truck driving, welding, fiscal manager, human relations manager, critical care nursing, field mining engineer, etc.): _____

_____

Setting (e.g., plant, office building, hospital, field, etc.): _____

_____

Target population size: _____

Organization/employer: _____

Location: rural _____ remote _____ urban _____ suburban _____

Type of organization:
  Goods production: Y( ) N( ) If yes, list: _____

_____

  Goods distribution: Y( ) N( ) If yes, list: _____

_____

  Service production: Y( ) N( ) If yes, list: _____

_____

  Service delivery: Y( ) N( ) If yes, list: _____

_____

Organized health services: Full service: Y( ) N( )
Health professionals: full time, FT / part time PT
  OHN: FT ( ) PT ( )
  Physician: FT( ) PT( )
  H&S officer: FT( ) PT( )
  OT: FT ( ) PT( )
  Physio: FT( ) PT( )
  Other: _____

Stressors Observed/Anticipated by Organization/Work Group

Environmental hazard(s): constant _____ intermittent _____
  Physical (e.g., noise > 85 decibels, air < 10 exchanges / hr.):
    Intra- and extrasystem: _____
    Risk level: high ( ) medium ( ) low ( )
      Lines of defense: flexible _____ normal _____

    Lines of resistance: _____

  Indicators: _____

Social race, gender, status work (promotion/growth opportunity, social/emotional support) intra- and intersystem/group stressors: _____

Figure 49–1. Occupational health nursing risk profile (organization) using the Neuman Model. (Copyright © M. McGee, 1993.)

Risk level: high ( )   medium ( )   low ( )
Lines of defense: flexible _____ normal _____

Lines of resistance: _____

Indicators: _____

Developmental
Organizational growth: Employment by year: _____
Management style (e.g., authoritarian, democratic, oligarchic, etc.):

_____

Diversification: (if yes, identify): _____

Communication pattern: between management/subordinates _____

between peers _____

with the community_____

Indicators: _____

Health status
Health promotion programs: _____

_____

Fitness opportunities: gymnasium _____ eligibility _____
lunch facility _____ adequacy _____ activities _____
rest/am/pm break _____
Participation rate: high _____ medium _____ low _____
Fitness level: high _____ average _____ low _____
Accident rate (reported) _____ per 100 employees_____
type:_____
Workmans compensation claims:_____ by year, '89 _____ '90 _____
'91 _____ '92 _____
Illness rate _____ per 100 employees _____
Impression:
related to work _____
related to life-style _____
related to housing _____
related to other sociocultural factors _____
other_____
Organization population risk status

Risk of: _____ environment related

_____ lifestyle related

_____ work related

_____ event specific

Relative risk: _____

Attributable risk: _____

Collective/population nursing diagnosis: _____

Related to: _____

Figure 49–1. Continued.

PROFILE OF THE INDIVIDUAL WORKER

Nursing assessment of the workforce involves observation of and interaction with individual workers and must take place within the work context (i.e., specific work station or shop floor). Each work activity requires a specific pattern of worker performance; therefore it is mandatory that the OHN have a clear knowledge of the industry for which he or she is a health resource. It is also important to emphasize that the OHN is an advocate of the worker (regardless of rank) and *not* a source of performance appraisal or health information for the company. The protocol for use of the Neuman nursing process format with the individual worker in occupational health nursing is described below.

Assessment

First, the OHN must *identify* cues that reveal client performance (reaction to demands/stressors), cues that identify client perception of demands/stressors, factors that influence client perception, and indicators of screening failure (i.e., penetration of the lines of defense and/or resistance by physical, environmental, or behavioral stressors). Some examples of cues that reveal client performance include how a clerk uses a keyboard, nursing techniques to move a client up in bed, or effort required for a construction worker to use the jackhammer.

Data of client perception range from spontaneous expressions of opinion to subtle behavioral patterns and reactions. Since some people find it difficult to identify or express what they feel, a substrategy to facilitate client self-understanding and articulation may be used. One approach is presented in Gazda's "helping relationship" (1975). Factors that influence client perception may also be revealed in conjunction with collection of organization data (Figure 49–1). The advantage rests with the necessity for concreteness, which links client perception with observable environmental or extrasystem events. Obtaining accurate client perception data may require a series of nurse–worker encounters.

The identification of screening failures is a well-established expectation of occupational health nursing in order to determine the risk of general health problems (e.g., hearing loss, exposure to toxins). In the conceptual focus of the NSM, screening failures can result in stressor penetration of the worker's normal line of defense and lines of resistance. However, OHNs have not adequately observed and documented evidence of penetration of the worker's normal line of defense by workplace stressors. Examples include excessive risk-taking behavior by construction workers and unsafe patterns dictated by the company. Such workplace stressors (actual and potential) can be considered screening failures, but the questions remain of whose failure (organization function or worker function?) and what they mean in terms of risk control or increasing the strength of the lines of defense.

Second, the OHN must *validate* with the client/worker the meaning of stressors. Validation includes evidence of reliability. Are the cues manifested repeatedly over time? When do they vary? How do they vary as the situation changes?

Finally, the OHN must *determine* the degree of stressor penetration with resulting manifestations that will allow inference of a diagnostic statement. For example, a leaking air hose can result in lead toxicity in exposed workers. The specific indicators, such as elevated blood lead level, enable a diagnosis. The OHN determines how these indicators are related to the level of function of lines of defense and/or resistance. Diagnostic indicators must be highly specific in order to rule out competing explanations for the diagnostic statement. To establish the degree of penetration with some observable behavior, the OHN must feel confident that a particular factor (e.g., complaint of headaches) indicates assault on the defense system (e.g., lead leak via air hose).

Diagnosis: Actual and Potential Variance from Wellness/Stability

The OHN must develop a statement that identifies behavioral responses to penetration of flexible and normal lines of defense and/or lines of resistance, and (if possible) identifies the actual or potential stressors. For example, penetration of the normal line of defense could be manifested as "pain and activity intolerance due to wrist and digit compensation related to ergonomic mismatch of typing action and keyboard position."

Planning

The Decision Matrix for Nursing Intervention (Figure 49–2) illustrates one mechanism to facilitate planning. The decision matrix will help demonstrate cost-effectiveness and efficiency in nursing practice; a blank decision matrix form may facilitate documentation. The worker/client should be involved in developing the matrix and making decisions regarding the alternatives identified through its use. Application of the matrix as a planning tool is described below.

First, the OHN must *formulate* nursing goals and, if necessary, subobjectives. Using the example of "pain and activity intolerance" cited earlier, appropriate objectives might include (1) pain/discomfort reduction/elimination, (2) modification of typing pattern, and (3) optimization of ergonomic factors.

Second, the OHN must *identify* all possible alternative methods for goal

Alternatives/Options	Feasibility (space, time)	Client Values	Probable Effectiveness	Choice/ Decision
Medical regimen only (e.g., medication)				
Postural wrist/hand exercises				
Use of Flexguard				
Structural wrist support				
Promotion of general health activities (e.g., exercise, aerobics)				

Figure 49–2. Decision Matrix for Nursing Intervention—Options for Pain Reduction due to Activity Intolerance. (Copyright © M. McGee, 1993.)

achievement. The Decision Matrix for Nursing Intervention (Figure 49–2) illustrates one mechanism to identify and work through the usefulness of alternatives.

Third, the OHN must *negotiate* with the client for preferred goals/objectives and methods. Finally, the OHN must *sequence* the actions required for the method selected. Documentation should include time required, frequency of nursing contact, and expected date of achievement.

Intervention

Primary prevention is most frequently associated with conditions of normalcy and/or risk. The imperative is to reduce encounters, or risk of encounter, with destructive stressors (e.g., physical/verbal abuse, toxins). Examples of occupational health nursing prevention as intervention strategies would include developing self-help groups to strengthen personal coping skills and initiating ergonomic mechanisms for physical stability.

For some occupational health nurses, health promotion is analagous with strengthening the normal line of defense. However, many public/community/ occupational health nurses view health promotion as a fourth level of practice in addition to primary, secondary, and tertiary prevention, rather than being subsumed in primary prevention. One distinction between health promotion and primary prevention lies in the degree of client risk involved, with "health promotion" implying no risk and "primary prevention" implying some level of risk. However, the evidence to distinguish between these two may be circumstantial or obscure and may depend on the provider's belief.

Secondary prevention is usually associated with conditions of crisis and/or morbidity. Prevention as intervention strategies are intended to strengthen normal lines of defense and lines of resistance, to reduce or change client reaction to stressors, and to prevent further penetration by stressors. Examples of nursing strategies would include intervening in physiological crisis (e.g., bleeding), using support in psychic crisis (e.g., bereavement counseling), and intervening in situations of morbidity where care is required to avoid degeneration. This situation is encountered infrequently in occupational health practice, but some medical problems are identified and managed in the work setting. (Examples include corrective positioning in carpal tunnel syndrome and weight loss strategies in workers with heart disease.)

Tertiary prevention is associated with postcrisis and/or morbidity. Prevention as intervention strategies are intended to facilitate reconstitution of the lines of defense and rehabilitation of the functioning client system in order to prevent irreversible complications or degeneration.

Tertiary prevention is an area of client need that is highly relevant to occupational health nursing. The extent to which workers are rehabilitated following morbidity is a crucial aspect of societal health and stability. Degeneration of a capacity has profound impact on the client's self-esteem, on contributions to both the organization and its mission, and on the worker's private life. Nursing prevention as intervention to facilitate worker rehabilitation following morbidity

Evaluation: _____

Anticipated outcomes: _____

_____

Actual outcomes: _____

_____

Discrepancy = _____
Time required = _____ i.e., hours and calendar dates

Actual contact hours _____

Probability of optimum stability = _____ if outcome discrepancy is unacceptable to either OHN
  or worker
Client perception of goal achievement: _____

_____

Coping mechanisms: increased? _____

                    decreased? _____

Indicators:

  Decisional skills: improved? _____

                       no change? _____

  Health behavior skills: increased? _____

                            no change? _____

  Health status: improved? _____

                   no change? _____

  Symptoms/indicators: less? _____

                         worsened? _____

                         no change? _____

  Personal and social support: more secure? _____

                                 less secure? _____

                                 no change? _____

Intervention process acceptability:

  Primary prevention and/or health promotion: _____

  Secondary prevention:_____

  Tertiary prevention: _____

Figure 49–3. Format for evaluation. (Copyright © M. McGee, 1993.)

include *emphasizing* the degree of adaptation or the extent to which preproblem status has been achieved or improved and *employing* strategies to mobilize resources (personal, family, social, industrial, and community).

Throughout rehabilitation, the occupational health nurse must maintain a collaborative, rather than adversarial, relationship with the client/worker and must respect client preferences. Some companies have an adversarial relationship with employees. The extent to which management views subordinates as exaggerating illness and injury claims indicates a system problem and acts as an extrasystem stressor for the worker and an intrasystem stressor for the organization.

Evaluation

Application of the NSM involves evaluation of nursing outcomes as the final step; a form for documentation of the evaluation phase in occupational health nursing is shown in Figure 49–3. As described by Neuman (1989, 20), use of the form involves validation of nursing process and provides feedback for further system input.

REFERENCES

Argyris, C. 1993. *Knowledge for Action: A Guide to Overcoming Barriers to Organizational Change*. San Francisco, Calif.: Jossey-Bass Publishers.

Barnes, M. 1991. Organizational risk profile. Nursing 4402 student assignment, University of Ottawa.

Beddome, G. 1989. Application of the Neuman Systems Model to the assessment of community as client. In *The Neuman Systems Model*, 2d ed., edited by B. Neuman. Norwalk, Conn.: Appleton & Lange.

Carnevali, D., and Thomas, M. D. 1993. *Diagnostic Reasoning and Treatment: Decision Making in Nursing*, 184–185. Philadelphia, Pa.: J. B. Lippincott.

Drew, L., Craig, D., and Beynon, C. 1989. The Neuman Systems Model for community health administration and practice: Provinces of Manitoba and Ontario, Canada. In *The Neuman Systems Model*, 2d ed., edited by B. Neuman. Norwalk, Conn.: Appleton & Lange.

Dunn, S., and Trepanier, M. J. 1989. Application of the Neuman Systems Model to perinatal nursing. In *The Neuman Systems Model*, 2d ed., edited by B. Neuman. Norwalk, Conn.: Appleton & Lange.

Gazda, G., Walters, R. P., and Childers, W. C. 1975. *Human Relations Development: A Manual for Health Sciences*. Boston: Allyn and Bacon, Inc.

Gordon, M. 1987. *Nursing Diagnosis: Process and Application,* 2d ed. Toronto: McGraw-Hill.

Louis, M. 1989. An intervention to reduce anxiety levels for nurses working with long term care clients using Neuman's model. In *Conceptual Models for Nursing Practice,* 3d ed., edited by J. P. Riehl-Sisca. Norwalk, Conn.: Appleton & Lange.

McGee, M. 1975. Determination of family decision making capacity by community health nurses and a measurement of nursing impact. In *Development and Use of Indicators in*

Nursing Research, edited by G. N. Zilm, S. M. Stinson, M. E. Steed, and P. Overton. Edmonton: University of Alberta.

Neuman, B. 1989. *The Neuman Systems Model,* 2d ed. Norwalk, Conn.: Appleton & Lange.

Ontario Occupational Health Nurses Association. 1988. *Standards of Nursing Practice for Occupational Health Nurses.* Etobicoke, Ontario.

Valanis, B. 1992. *Epidemiology in Nursing and Health Care,* 2d ed. Norwalk, Conn.: Appleton & Lange.

Wilson, C. 1992. *QA/CQI: Strategies in Health Care Quality.* Toronto: W. B. Saunders.

Section VII

From the Past to New Beginnings

With love and best wishes to past and future friends of the Neuman Systems Model

—Betty Neuman

50

IN CONCLUSION—
TOWARD NEW
BEGINNINGS

Betty Neuman

Part I of this chapter contains my personal and professional autobiography as it relates to the Neuman Systems Model development. It also fills a need for the many students who request biographical data for course work and personal reasons.

In Part II a chronology of the Neuman Systems Model progress in development and utilization is correlated with the changing trends occurring in the nursing profession, from the model's inception through the fall of 1994. In addition, future perspectives are offered, based on the model's past progression and predictive factors.

Part III includes innovative ideas in model usage to give recognition to both those in the early planning stages of using the model and those who have already implemented the model.

Future major decision making for the Neuman Systems Model is now placed with the Neuman Trustees, a group of professional nurses who are committed to and competent in use of the model. Part IV includes the names of trustees as well as the complete trustee document, which is included as a point of future contact for nursing, emphasizing the importance of trustee functions and availability for assistance. A current list of citations is presented in Appendix A.

I. An Autobiography as History: The Neuman Systems Model Development

I was born in southeastern Ohio in 1924. My birthplace was a 100-acre family farm. My father, a farmer, died at age 37 when I was 11 years old and my brothers were 5 and 16. My mother was a hard-working, enterprising housewife, managing well our limited financial resources.

My older brother, my mother, and I engaged in several summers of hard physical labor to keep the family and farm intact. My younger brother escaped most of the labors, because my mother moved us to a nearby town, Marietta, Ohio, where I completed my final year of high school. My older brother married and continued to maintain the family farm. For many years I have been proud of my early farming heritage, because it taught me the important values of simplicity, humility, and self-reliance.

Because my father had always praised his nurses during six years of intermittent hospitalizations prior to his death from chronic kidney disease, early in life I began to idealize the nursing profession. I developed a strong commitment to become an excellent bedside nurse to repay society a debt of gratitude. Another very important influence was the shared stories of my mother's charity experiences as a self-taught rural midwife. She was often called at night and rode by horse and buggy to perform home deliveries. A favorite memory is stealing away to read her battered general medical book.

When I graduated from high school in the summer of 1942, our country was six months into World War II. Local employment opportunities were limited. Being financially unable to attend nearby Marietta College as I had always wanted, I obtained a position at Wright Airforce Base in Dayton, Ohio, as an aircraft instrument repair technician. It was particularly exciting to install the instruments in fighter warplanes following their repair. I recall refusing an offer of transfer to the New York–based Sperry Rand Company upon receiving the highest test results in the specialty area. Deciding factors were the continuing homesickness, desire to accumulate money toward a nursing education, and charity involvement in the Dayton YWCA as a recreation hostess for servicemen. Later, during evening school classes, I was chosen as a draftsperson by an aircraft contracting agency, where I worked for one year at a higher salary. Concurrent with this position, I often worked evenings as a short-order cook to supplement my income and contribute to my mother and younger brother's needs.

By the time that I had nearly accumulated the necessary funds for entrance into nurse's training, the Cadet Nurse Corps Program became available, expediting my entrance into the three-year diploma nurse program at Peoples Hospital, Akron, Ohio, now renamed General Hospital Medical Center. My goal of becoming an excellent bedside nurse was accomplished as I graduated with honors for two combined graduating classes in the fall of 1947.

Although the diploma program followed the medical model, since the hospital was private in nature and had established a fine reputation, students were required to give complete and total care to clients.

During these years I had saved enough money to purchase from a family friend a 1935 Ford Coupe for $275. Taking our mother with us, my younger brother and I drove south to Florida and west to Los Angeles, where an uncle lived. Three months after arriving, my mother and brother drove back home to Ohio, and I began a position at the Los Angeles General Hospital as a staff communicable disease nurse. At the end of six months, I accepted a promotion to head nurse and remained there another year. Since I was eager to explore other areas of nursing, I assumed a one-year school nurse position followed by a one-year industrial nurse position, both in the greater Los Angeles area.

In 1950 I returned to the Los Angeles General Hospital as a private duty nurse and remained until 1956. During that time I developed broadly based knowledge and skill in critical care for medical, surgical, pediatrics, and many other specialty areas, such as burns, polio, and head injuries. This was long before the development of critical care units. A variety of shift work accommodated the evening classes I was taking preparatory to a one-year, full-time residency to complete the baccalaureate degree in nursing at UCLA. In 1954 I married a beginning resident obstetrician of the Good Samaritan Hospital, helping facilitate both our educational programs. I graduated from UCLA in June 1957 with a major in public health nursing and scholastic honors. The degree was the first from a large extended family of 125 first cousins; to travel so far from home was considered wayward. After helping initiate my husband's private practice, I worked as an office manager and nurse until the birth of a beautiful daughter, Nancy, in 1959.

Between 1964 and 1966, during my UCLA master's program, weekend, evening, and summer nursing activities included special education projects for the Glendale Memorial Hospital, acting as relief psychiatric head nurse at the Queen of Angels Hospital, and volunteer crisis counseling at the Benjamin Rush Clinic, Venice Clinic, and Los Angeles Suicide Prevention Center. Donna Aquilera and I were chosen by UCLA faculty to represent the school of nursing at these clinic facilities to determine the efficacy and relevancy of the nurse role as counselor within early community psychiatric settings. We were fortunate to be the first nurses to validate the nurse counselor role within such settings. We received excellent supervision from agency directors well known in subsequent psychiatric literature. As a result of this experience, I continued to accumulate volunteer counseling hours to become one of the first California Nurse Licensed Clinical Fellows of the American Association of Marriage and Family Therapy.

My master's program was completed in June 1966. It was a federal grant-funded specialty program to prepare public health/mental health nurse consultants to pioneer nurse role development within newly emerging community mental health centers, for which no specific functions or processes were yet developed. In January 1967 I assumed faculty chairmanship of the program from which I graduated, though I had no previous teaching preparation. Initial activities included grant writing to secure funds for expanding the program to become the first in community mental health nurse education. It became a two-quarter postgraduate optional program offering for completed nurse psychiatric master students. It included one semester each in community organization and planning and mental health consultation. The program, which began in the fall of 1967, pioneered the first postmaster-level nurse involvement in role definition with interdisciplinary groups that were beginning to function in the newly emerging community mental health centers in the greater Los Angeles area. Early in the teaching program, an explicit teaching and practice model for mental health consultation was developed by me, validated by students, and published in 1971 in a first faculty coauthored mental health textbook for nurses entitled *Consultation and Community Organization in Community Mental Health Nursing.* It has long been out of print; little interest existed in the area of community mental health for nursing during the late 1960s and very early 1970s. I am indeed grateful for the vital feedback and extraordinary pioneering and cooperative spirit of my students, particularly during the earliest period of this program implementation. They both reinforced and helped me expand my own knowledge and skill as I role-modeled for them the mental health consultation process and nurse role development within a variety of community mental health facilities.

In 1970 I developed the Neuman Systems Model to provide unity, or a focal point, for student learning. Graduate students requested an initial entry class that would provide an overview of the four variables of man (physiological, psychological, sociocultural, and developmental), which they would subsequently study in depth in their clinical specialty programs. I was chosen by the curriculum committee to develop and coordinate such a course, in which guest faculty most knowledgeable in these areas would lecture. Since my major concern was how to provide structure to best integrate student learning in a wholistic manner, I personally developed the model design as it still exists today and received course-teaching faculty approval of its use for student integration of their lecture material. Because of heavy time commitments with the developing community mental health program, I asked for a co-coordinator and chose a young psychiatric faculty, Rae Jeanne Young, (now Memmott), who agreed that we should evaluate the effectiveness of the model design as a teaching tool. It is important to state that neither was I knowledgeable about nursing models nor had a clear trend yet begun in nursing for developing models. The Neuman Systems Model was developed strictly as a teaching aid. However, use of the model proved positive for student learning following a two-year evaluation period; the model was first published in 1972 in the May-June issue of *Nursing Research.* The article, "A Model for Teaching Total Person Approach to Patient Problems," formed the chapter title base for the first book published on nursing models—*The Betty Neuman Health-Care Systems Model: A Total Approach to Patient Problems,* edited by Riehl and Roy in 1974.

The community mental health program continued to expand, with students from throughout the United States and other countries. Two additional faculty were added; one was Kristine Gebbie, a particularly competent program graduate, who contributed significantly to further development of the program. Several articles were coauthored by the program faculty, including a research project on "Measurement of Change in Problem Solving Ability Among Nurses Receiving Mental Health Consultation."

Concurrent with the six-and-one-half-year faculty position, beginning in the winter of 1967 I taught many on- and off-campus credit workshops (some extending through the winter of 1978), conferences, and seminars for the UCLA Extension Division Continuing Education Department and for the Western Interstate Council for Higher Education, Colorado, in states west of the Mississippi River. Teaching areas included group leadership, interviewing, family counseling, crisis intervention, mental health consultation, psychiatric community mental health issues, and curriculum development.

During this same time period, the variety of my professional activities included community-based noncredit course teaching, workshops and conferences, interdisciplinary health care consultation, guest lectures, paper presentations, and various facilitative and leadership functions within nursing and interdisciplinary groups in several states. Mental health consultation activities both fulfilled student learning needs through role-modeling and provided community service to satisfy university requirements. I provided consultation for nursing and interdisciplinary caregiver groups in state mental hospitals, home health agencies, public health agencies, mental health centers, convalescent care centers, penal institutions, hospitals, teen centers, schools, and industries. Facilitating factors for my personal and professional development during these years were both the professional need for creativity and the freedom to be creative. The challenges of continual ambiguity and risk taking, caused by rapid change and lack of mentors, also became motivational in themselves. A tribute must be paid to the UCLA School of Nursing Dean, Lulu Wolfe Hassenplug, and Nurse Continuing Education Director Marjorie Squaires, for providing many opportunities combined with a lack of constraints related to my functioning.

During 1972 increased graduate student interest in the mental health consultation process and the Neuman Systems Model resulted in guest lectures in other UCLA clinical nurse specialist classes. Joan Riehl, a faculty friend and colleague, invited me to coauthor the first book on nursing models, *Conceptual Models for Nursing Practice*. Because of an impending move east, I directed her to Sister Callista Roy, a former UCLA classmate of mine, to coauthor the book. The Neuman Model placed in this book was there first classified as a "systems" model.

The development of the wholistic systemic perspective of the Neuman Systems Model was facilitated by my own basic philosophy of *helping each other live,* many diverse observations and clinical experiences in teaching and encouraging positive aspects of human variables in a wide variety of community settings, and theoretical perspectives of stress related to the interactive, interrelated, interdependent, and wholistic nature of systems theory. The significance of perception and behavioral consequences cannot be overestimated. The preventions adapted from Caplan's work provided an intervention typology for nursing consistent with the systemic perspectives of the model.

In the summer of 1973 we made a permanent move to the East to maintain my mother within her home during her aging years of declining health. Sustaining factors that kept our family viable through many challenges, both personal and professional, were my beautiful daughter Nancy's presence, creativity, spontaneity, joy of life, and many personal talents and achievements, as well as my husband Kree's consistent support, understanding, and love.

From the fall of 1973 through the summer of 1977 a part-time position as the state mental health nurse consultant for the state of West Virginia provided many challenges and professional growth activities in the statewide mental hospital system, such as consultation to and for hospital administrators, interdisciplinary groups, and program development and evaluation. Organizational development activities included conflict resolution, third-party consultation, educational conferences, workshops, seminars, and program planning.

Having been one of the first nurses licensed as a marriage, family, and child counselor in the State of California (in 1970) and also as a clinical member of the American Association of Marriage and Family Therapists and Ohio Social Work Counselors, I have continually maintained a limited private counseling practice since licensure. In 1974 I taught clergy counseling for a local Ohio mental health center. During the same year I helped initiate, develop, and support continuance of a program called "Hope" in a West Virginia state facility for the retarded. The goal was to teach, through a short-term residential program, self-help skills to retarded children so they could be maintained within the home, rather than be institutionalized; to redirect parents in their parenting efforts; and, through counseling and consulting activities for stress reduction and parenting skill development, to stabilize the home environment. This program evolved into a 14-year model program within the state system. I have also had limited involvement in Ohio as a licensed real estate agent, having secured original California licensure in 1971 and Ohio licensure in 1973. Continued love for the land has also led to involvement in securing selected Ohio-based land parcels for private brokerage to oil- and gas-drilling companies. Perhaps because of early work influence at Wright Field, Dayton, Ohio, I acquired a private pilot license while living in California. Another personal interest that has continued through the past few years has been in personal investments and rental housing.

In the fall of 1978, following my mother's death, personal activities focused on rental property management and other investments. These interests coincided with professional activities at nearby Ohio University, Athens, Ohio, including curriculum consultant to the School of Nursing, project planning director for development of a master-level nursing program, and director of nursing and allied health within the University Extension Division to facilitate nursing continuing education workshops.

Following the development of several nursing models during the early 1970s, it was not until the mid-1970s that planning for their implementation began within university settings. From 1976 to the present (1994) my major professional roles have been consultant for Neuman Systems Model implementation, lecturer at conferences, and author. Within the role of consultant for the model, a major function has been that of networking among those using the model or considering its use, clarifying the model's intent, purpose, and components, and supporting implementation plans or existing programs incorporating it. Through international travel, I have enjoyed very much the courtesies, sharing, and comparative views of other nurse professionals, along with important feedback that the model is easily used in diverse cross-cultural settings. Within the lecturer role, I have presented the model to several large international nurse audiences in this country and others, including England, Denmark, Canada, Puerto Rico, Australia, New Zealand, Kuwait and the Far East.

Within the author role, my publications since 1980 include a revised chapter in the second edition of *Conceptual Models for Nursing* (1980), with "tools" developed to further facilitate Neuman Systems Model implementation and for use in nursing practice; the first edition (1982) of *The Neuman Systems Model: Application to Nursing Education and Practice;* a chapter on family use of the model in *Family Health: A Theoretical Approach to Nursing Care* by Clements et al. (1983); an article in *Senior Nurse* (London) (fall 1985); and an invitational chapter on the model in Sweden's annual *Nursing Care Book* (winter 1986). A second book edition entitled *The Neuman Systems Model* was published in the winter of 1989. Since the 1986 First Biennial International Neuman Systems Model Symposium was held at Neumann College, Aston, Pennsylvania, three others, well attended, have been presented by Neuman trustee members. The trustee group was incorporated in 1988. Each symposium has shown increased international participation with an increased level of scholarship. The trustees have introduced and facilitated model implementation throughout the world through paper presentations, publications, and consultation. This third book edition contains sections of newer areas of nursing concern for research, international model use recognition, and nurse administrative protocol.

Following several years of accumulating credit hours toward a doctoral degree at Ohio University, Athens, Ohio, in 1985 I completed a doctoral degree in clinical psychology on transfer to Pacific Western University in Los Angeles.

A few years ago, my husband Kree retired and began to pursue oil painting. We particularly enjoyed walking, reading, music, and gardening. Unfortunately, in the fall of 1992 a major stroke left him aphasic and physically debilitated. Our daughter Nancy, following success in community theater during high school years, was motivated to complete an acting career at UCLA. Now, at age 35, she is a licensed California PhD psychologist in a Monterrey private counseling practice. She is frequently engaged in little theater stage productions and television commercials. She has taught acting and has had roles in both feature and television films. Nancy has recently purchased and personally decorated a beautiful ocean-view home in Pebble Beach and will present me with a first grandchild, Alissa, in fall 1994. Our visits are, indeed, very special occasions.

Since 1980 several important changes have been made that have enhanced the model. A Nursing Process Format was designed, using the model terminology to facilitate its implementation. A major theory for the model has been identified, in cooperation with a colleague and Neuman trustee member, Audrey Koertvelyessy, from Ohio; it has been named *The Theory of Client System Stability*. In the 1989 book edition a new perspective to expand the concept of environment—the *created environment*—was presented, and the spiritual variable was explicitly added to the model diagram as one of the client variables; further explication of the spiritual variable is presented in Chapter 1, Appendix B. A clearer model explanation has been offered by segmenting the model components into the four subcomponents of nursing—client, environment, health, and nursing. The relationship of primary prevention and health promotion has been further qualified.

The initial term *patient* was changed in the 1980 publication to *client* to fulfill the need for a qualifying term that would indicate respect and imply a collaborative-lateral relationship with caregivers. The model title has changed over the years, as the following chronology of publications shows:

- 1972: *A Model for Teaching Total Person Approach to Patient Problems*
- 1980: *The Betty Neuman Health Care Systems Model: A Total Approach to Patient Problems*
- 1982: *The Neuman Health Care Systems Model*
- 1986: *The Neuman Systems Model*

Until and unless research proves the need for change, the original diagram for the Neuman Systems Model will remain the same as when it was developed in 1970, since its structure and concepts are easily understood and implemented.

My hope for the future remains the same as for the past, that through continued nurturance, the Neuman Systems Model will live well into the 21st century to benefit nursing at all levels and across all cultural boundaries.

II. The Neuman Systems Model Utilization: A Chronology

Nursing model implementation began within university nursing education programs in the United States during the 1970s. Planning for use of the Neuman Systems Model for nursing education first began in the early 1970s at Neumann

College, Aston, Pennsylvania. Rosalie Mirenda, Neuman trustee and Neumann College vice president, influenced the model selection and curricular development process; program implementation began in 1980. Other early Neuman Model-based baccalaureate nursing education programs implemented during the late 1970s and early 1980s were at Bob Jones University, Greenville, South Carolina; Delta State University, Cleveland, Mississippi; University of Pittsburgh, Pittsburgh, Pennsylvania; St. Xavier College, Chicago, Illinois; and Union College, Lincoln, Nebraska.

The three Texas Woman's University campuses at Dallas, Houston, and Denton, Texas, and Northwestern State University of Louisiana, Shreveport, Louisiana, implemented the first master-level nursing education programs based on the model in the late 1970s. Though not mandated by the National League of Nursing, Neuman trustee member, Lois Lowry, nursing director, very early implemented the Neuman Model-based associate degree in nursing program at Cecil Community College, North East, Maryland. Interest in conceptual models for theory-based nursing education rapidly began to increase during the late 1970s.

During the early and mid-1980s, as mandated by the National League for Nursing, nursing tended toward both accelerated use of conceptual models for education and early utilization within nursing practice areas and research. Education goal clarification became a priority in relation to new nursing practice role development and expansion. Nursing models became a logical base for validation of the new nurse roles and functions and for communicating who nurses are and what they do, as being different from the past. For example, nurses began to assume roles as coordinators and advocates for client care. The increased development and utilization of the Neuman Model has either led or been concurrent with the emerging trends in nursing toward a broad systemic perspective for wholistic client care. Its relevance should continue well into the 21st century in relation to evolving worldwide health care reform mandates.

To upgrade their diploma nurse education programs, the Methodist Central (four-state) Hospitals in Memphis, Tennessee, and the Altoona Hospital, Altoona, Pennsylvania, implemented the model as a theoretical base. Three additional Neuman Systems Model-based associate degree in nursing programs began at Indiana University–Purdue University at Fort Wayne, Indiana (Elaine Cowan); Sante Fe Community College, Gainesville, Florida (former trustee, Gerry Green); and University of Nevada, Las Vegas, Nevada (Rosemary Witt). Cynthia Capers, Neuman trustee, coordinated the first hospital-based four-year plan for nursing service implementation of the model at the Mercy Catholic Medical Center, Fitzgerald Mercy Division, Darby, Pennsylvania. Other early nursing practice areas using the Neuman Model were at the University of Pennsylvania Hospital, Philadelphia, Neonatal Clinical Care Unit; the University of Maryland, Baltimore, Institute for Emergency Medical Services–Critical Care Unit (Virginia Cardona); and the Boston City Health Department.

The university outside the United States earliest known to utilize the Neuman Systems Model concepts was the University of Puerto Rico, San Juan,

Puerto Rico. The University of Ottawa, Ontario, Canada, also early found the model useful for public health nurse teaching and developed a joint university and community Regional Perinatal Program for Eastern Ontario, Canada (Sandra Dunn). Eugenia Story, a former public health nursing faculty member, University of Ottawa, became an independent consultant for model implementation, contributing to both education and practice settings within Ontario Province, Canada. Her functions also included presentation of workshops for those wanting to learn more about the model and how to apply it. In the early 1980s, the model was implemented for provision of theory-based community health nursing services within the Canadian provinces of Ontario and Manitoba. At Winnipeg, Linda Drew facilitated model-based community health program development for Manitoba, and Dorothy Craig, now a faculty member at the University of Toronto and Neuman trustee, influenced development of standards for Ontario community health nurse practice, incorporating within the standards criteria the Neuman Systems Model.

In the mid-1980s interest in nursing conceptual models accelerated around the world. International nursing model conferences drew large audiences from many countries. The Neuman Systems Model is successfully being used in both education and practice settings in many countries. Hanne Johansen found the model concepts useful in community health nurse teaching for students at Aarhus University, as well as in community health practice areas of Aarhus, Denmark. Community health services sponsored publication of a handbook she authored on use of the Neuman Model in the community for primary prevention for the aged. Ingegerd Harder, also of Aarhus University, and Hanne Seyer-Hansen early authored Neuman Model-based articles and a book interpreting the model for the country of Denmark. In Sweden the model has been used for some time in clinical nurse practice and research. Both England and Wales have found the model particularly useful in community nursing, referred to as "home visiting"; it is also used in a variety of teaching institutions and clinical practice areas within the British Isles. One Australian hospital is known to have incorporated the model concepts, and several schools of nursing in Australia and New Zealand are based on the model. A Lisbon, Portugal, university utilizes the model concepts in public health and critical care nursing courses and community health nursing practice.

During the 1980s requests for consultation, workshops, and conference presentations of the model increased markedly. Several religious-based nurse education programs have found the model particularly suitable and relevant to their curricular needs.

From the mid- to late 1980s nursing literature increasingly reflected the trend toward acceptance of wholistic and systemic concepts as a logical perspective for the field of nursing in its quest as a scientific discipline. The Neuman Systems Model has thus remained relevant and unchanged since its development in 1970. Conceptual models are now viewed as a valid and desirable base for the rapidly accelerating interest and involvement in nursing research studies initiated in both education and practice settings. The research abstracts in Chapter 33, by Margaret Louis, provide information on updated nursing research based on the Neuman Systems Model. The concepts of the model are proving researchable and important for theory development in nursing.

Advances for increased utility of the model are reflected in the following data. A slide presentation explaining the model has been published and marketed by the University of Michigan. At the University of Western Ontario, London, Canada, a self-directed learning package for staff education was developed by Laurie Bernick and Diane Thompson, in addition to their published video presentation of the model, which includes a health assessment and intervention tool. As a result of model implementation for their nursing service, Laura Caramanica and Lorrie Powell have published programmed learning materials available to the public from the Mount Sinai Hospital, Hartford, Connecticut. Jefferson Davis Memorial Hospital, Natchez, Mississippi, where the model has proven its utility since 1984, now has a nursing classification system in place with significant emphasis on primary prevention. The model is fully implemented for psychiatric nursing service at Friends Hospital (see Chapter 26) (Betty Scicchitani and Patricia Maglicco); Philadelphia Whitby Psychiatric Hospital (Corinne Coulter), Whitby, Ontario, Canada (see Chapter 27); and Peterborough Civic Hospital (Wendy Fucile), Peterborough, Ontario, Canada.

The model has become a viable framework for health prevention–promotion activities in a variety of clinical nurse and research areas. For example, Lander University, Greenwood, South Carolina, and Indiana University–Purdue University of Fort Wayne, Indiana, and University of Rochester (see Chapter 29) have developed nurse-managed clinics. Several Canadian hospitals are known to be using the model in general and/or specialized areas of clinical nursing care, including Chedoke-McMaster Hospital, Ottawa Civic Hospital, and Victoria Hospital, all in Ontario, Canada; Juan de Fuca Hospitals, Victoria, British Columbia; and University Hospital of Saskatchewan, Saskatoon, Saskatchewan, Canada.

With the new Ontario, Canada, community health criteria as the Neuman-based standards for nursing, Charlene Beynon, Neuman trustee and supervisor, of the Middlesex Health Unit, London, Ontario, and her highly motivated staff have successfully implemented the Neuman Model for community nursing with workshops offered to other health district nursing units to facilitate use of the model appropriate to criteria used throughout the province. Manitoba is beginning model implementation of their provincewide plan under development since 1982. Though it is difficult to keep an accurate account of model usage, it is widely favored throughout Canada, particularly for community health nursing. Queen's University, Kingston, Ontario, and the University of Saskatchewan, Saskatoon, Saskatchewan, have based their nurse education programs on the Neuman Systems Model; its concepts are also used in faculty programs at both the University of Ottawa and the University of British Columbia.

Since the early 1980s the model has formed the base for multilevel, unilevel, and consortium-type nurse education programs within university settings. These programs have been implemented throughout the United States. Some examples include the California State University Fresno, California (Eleanor Stittich), which has developed a multilevel program for baccalaureate, master's, and nurse practitioner students; Simmons College, Boston, Massachusetts, where Carol Frazier has developed a bilevel nursing program for baccalaureate and master's students; and the University of Nevada, Las Vegas, Nevada, where Rosemary Witt has developed the trilevel associate, baccalaureate, and master's degree programs. Northwestern State University at Shreveport, Louisiana, one of the earliest to implement the model, now has a trilevel nurse education program (Arlene Airhart). The Minnesota Intercollegiate Nursing Consortium, St. Paul, Minnesota, consisting of two schools—St. Olaf College and Gustavus Adolphus—jointly contributed to development of a baccalaureate nurse curriculum based on the Neuman Systems Model, with beginning course computerization. The Tri-County College University nursing consortium program (Lois Nelson) serves baccalaureate students from both the State University of North Dakota, Wells Fargo, North Dakota, and Concordia College, Moorhead, Minnesota. The consortium arrangement is a unique and cost-effective method for curricular development and implementation.

Further advances in model usage are indicated by the report that a large percentage of nursing students from the summer master's program at Portland University, Portland, Oregon (Neuman trustee, Patricia Chadwick), use the Neuman Systems Model for their theory-based nursing research theses. Lander University has progressed from an associate degree in nursing to a baccalaureate degree program, with evolving course computerization. In the Greenwood, South Carolina, community agencies, as well as at some other locations, there is a growing trend for agency use of Neuman Model concepts where students affiliate. This may relate to special education and practice information exchanges, such as those that the Lander University, School of Nursing, facilitates (formerly Neuman trustee Janet Sipple; now Barbara Freese).

Foreign exchange programs are forming a new educational trend in nursing education to reduce cross-cultural differences and incorporate Neuman Model concepts into community agencies where students affiliate. The Seattle Pacific University, Seattle, Washington, where the baccalaureate nurse program is based on the Neuman Systems Model (formerly Margaret Stevenson; now Annalee Oakes), exchanges both students and faculty with the Veterans General Hospital Nursing Program (Bette Wei Wang), Taipei, Taiwan. As a result of direct faculty exchange and ongoing consultation activities, faculty have adapted the model to the Chinese culture at the hospital and developed a new baccalaureate nurse degree program at the Yang Ming Medical College in Taiwan. Seattle Pacific University, School of Nursing, has also implemented the model in Costa Rica.

Significant sharing with other countries, motivating model usage, is further recognized: A Lander University Korean nurse faculty member, Nahn Joo Son Chang, presented a workshop on the Neuman Systems Model at Kyung Hee

University, Seoul, Korea. It was sponsored by the Korean Nurses Academic Society in Seoul and attended by 200 nurse faculty; many indicated they were motivated to use the model in their country. The results of a survey (this joint survey included Neuman trustee Audrey Koertvelyessy) to identify the nature and quality of Neuman Model research was presented by University of Nevada research faculty Margaret Louis (Neuman trustee) at an international nurse research conference in Scotland, where there was much positive feedback and interest in the model's potential for research. During the 1980s Community Health Nursing Standards integrated the Neuman Systems Model concepts as criteria for nurse functions for the province of Ontario, Canada. Dorothy Craig, Neuman trustee, who facilitated original model implementation in Ontario as a base for community health services, also presented her work in London at the Second International Primary Care Conference. Her presentation material was related to a possible new direction and structure for home visiting nurse services and practice in the British Isles. Books, journal publications, paper presentations, and personal visits to other countries by me and others over the years have greatly increased the visibility and utility of the Neuman Systems Model. Model utilization has followed a general pattern of beginning implementation within university settings followed by clinical practice areas and research (see Neuman "citations" by trustee member Jacqueline Fawcett in Appendix A). A listing of Neuman Model implementations identified between 1989 and 1994 follows:

Education

- The University of Tennessee at Martin, Department of Nursing, Baccalaureate Nurse Program, Martin, Tennessee
- Linn-Benton College, Associate Degree in Nursing, Albany, Oregon
- The Los Angeles County USC Medical Center School of Nursing, Associate Degree in Nursing, Los Angeles, California
- Louisiana College, Baccalaureate Nurse Program, Pineville, Louisiana
- Auburn University, Baccalaureate Nurse Program, Auburn, Alabama
- William Rainey Harper College, Associate Degree Nurse Program, Palatine, Illinois

Practice

- The Whitby Psychiatric Hospital Nursing Service, Whitby, Ontario, Canada
- The Collington Care Retirement Community Nursing Service and Clinic, Hyattsville, Maryland
- Centre de Santé, Elizabeth Bruyere Health Center (tertiary care), Ottawa, Ontario, Canada
- Kuakini Health Care System Nursing Service, Honolulu, Hawaii
- Riverside Acute Care Hospital Nursing Service, Ottawa, Ontario, Canada
- Tripler General Army Medical Center, selected nursing service areas, Honolulu, Hawaii
- Oregon State Psychiatric Hospital Nursing Service, Salem, Oregon

- Mansfield University, Baccalaureate Nurse Program, Mansfield, Pennsylvania
- Akureye University, Baccalaureate Nurse Program, Akureye, Iceland
- Maribor University, Baccalaureate Nurse Program, Maribor, Yugoslavia (Slovenia)
- University of Guam, Baccalaureate Nurse Program, Mangilao, Guam
- McNeese State University, Tri-level nurse program and a four-school intercollegiate consortium program for a master of science in nursing, Lake Charles, Louisiana
- Bowie State University, RN–BSN Completion and Master Program, Bowie, Maryland
- South West Medical Center Nursing Service, Oklahoma City, Oklahoma
- Daemen College, RN–BSN Completion Program, Amherst, New York

- Anderson Hospital, Nursing Service, Marysville, Illinois
- St. Luke Hospital, Nursing Service, Fargo, North Dakota
- Mountain View Hospital, Nursing Service, Madras, Oregon
- Oklahoma State Department of Public Health, Public Health Nursing Service, Oklahoma City, Oklahoma
- St. Joseph's Hospital Nursing Service, Reykjavik, Iceland
- Rykov Hospital Nursing Service, Nursing Service, Jonkoping, Sweden
- WHO Collaborative Center for Primary Health Care Nursing, Maribor, Yugoslavia (Slovenia)
- Lake Charles Memorial Hospital Nursing Service, Lake Charles, Louisiana
- West Calcasieu–Cameron Hospital Nursing Service, Sulphur, Louisiana
- St. Patrick's Hospital, Nursing Service, Lake Charles, Louisiana
- Lake Area Medical Center, Lake Charles, Louisiana

THE NEUMAN BIENNIAL INTERNATIONAL SYMPOSIA

All symposia are developed by Neuman trustee members. The First Neuman Systems Model International Symposium, sponsored by and held at Neumann College, Aston, Pennsylvania, in the fall of 1986, was well attended and accepted. The Second Biennial International Symposium, held in Kansas City, Missouri, in the fall of 1988, was sponsored by the newly incorporated Neuman Systems Model Trustees Group, Inc., with success that was luminescent. The 1990 Dayton, Ohio, third symposium was very successful. The 1993 Rochester, New York, fourth symposium represented model maturity by the high professional quality of presentations and increased commitment through participation of trustees and decision making for the future. The symposium resulted in new liaisons with international model users and an associate membership for all users. New proposals for the Neuman Model are beginning to emerge, such as use in outer space and affirmation of identity within the Catholic Franciscan Health System. Model utilization is as unbounded as the imagination; the model contains the concepts to support a futuristic, expanded nursing domain, for example, in the home and larger community. It will move into the 21st century, easily crossing cultural barriers.

FUTURE PERSPECTIVES FOR USE OF THE NEUMAN SYSTEMS MODEL

Based on past patterns of continued escalation in utilization of the Neuman Systems Model and current world usage in the fall of 1994, the author can foresee increasing model utilization well into the 21st century, particularly in large-scale programming (at the state, regional, and even global level). As catastrophic sociopolitical events affect health care in general, multidisciplinary involvement in the human condition will often be required. Its flexible structure for assessment and intervention will increase model relevancy. The model has both preceded and complemented changing trends in nursing, and in health care in general, since its inception. For example, use by the "eclectic" media has, paradoxically, given the Neuman Systems Model major exposure. Its utilization is basically unlimited because of its wholistic systemic base and perspective. I predict continued expansion of the model's utility based on the following factors:

1. With an increasing trend toward home-based and community care, the Neuman Systems-based wholistic model concepts will have continuing relevancy for both nursing education and practice within an expanding nursing domain. The model fits well the new health care reform proposals that emphasize primary prevention for wellness.
2. The model provides potential for resolution of cross-cultural differences and improved health care, since the model's adaptability and utility has been proven in many countries beyond the United States.
3. Contributing to nursing's growth as a scientific discipline, the model concepts have proven researchable for nursing theory development.
4. The model's comprehensiveness contributes to both complex and simply defined areas of nursing concern and interdisciplinary and international involvement. The model concepts support interdisciplinary cooperation—a major trend.
5. The model provides a viable organizing structure within which to process, contain, and retrieve massive amounts of health information. Information overload has become a major social issue.
6. The Neuman Systems Model's developmental potential, visibility, and sustaining factors for the future are assured through the Neuman Model Trustee Group's dedicated membership.

ACKNOWLEDGMENT

I gratefully express my sincere appreciation for all the fine people who in various ways have facilitated the mature status of the Neuman Systems Model. Much time, talent, faith, pioneering spirit, effort, and nurturance of the model was required for it to withstand the test of time in proving its value to the field of nursing. With love and complete confidence, I pay special tribute to each valued Trustee Group member, who will further facilitate development and utilization of the model for the future of nursing.

III. New Initiatives

Part III of this chapter presents a variety of innovative ideas related to new model usage.

The material reflects, in part, nursing trends such as cooperative work with other disciplines. Included are names of contact persons for both recognition and networking.

NEW BEGINNINGS

Nancy Cotton of Colorado has developed an interdisciplinary high-risk assessment tool, based on the Neuman Systems Model, that is designed to predict high risk of falling for elderly rehabilitation clients. Her work is presented in a 1993 publication entitled *An Interdisciplinary High Risk Assessment Tool for Rehabilitation Inpatient Falls,* which is available from University Microfilms International, Ann Arbor, Michigan.
(Contact: Nancy C. Cotton, 700E Drake-K-11, Ft. Collins, Colorado 80525.)

Jullette C. Mitre, through graduate study using the model, identified the purposeful use of "Humor as Primary and Secondary Prevention as Intervention." She describes humor as a "potent" intervention and will be pursuing her research on humor at the doctorate level.
(Contact: Jullette C. Mitre, RA, MSN, MA, 535 North Michigan Avenue, Apt. 1703, Chicago, Illinois 60611.)

Marilyn Schlentz developed "The Minimum Data Set and Levels of Prevention in the Long Term Care Facility," which was published in the March/April 1993 issue of *Geriatric Nursing.* In her work she demonstrated the compatibility of the Neuman Systems Model with the minimum data set, a federal data collection system mandated for long-term care. She is now in the process of negotiating for use of the Neuman Model with board members of the New Jersey chapter of the National Association of Directors of Nursing Administration in Long Term Care. She is also involved with the development of academic management courses specific to long-term care needs.

(Contact: Marilyn Schlentz, EdD, RN, 32 Cannon Road, Freehold, New Jersey 07728.)

At Brigham Young University in Utah, an interdisciplinary faculty group from the College of Nursing and the departments of Religion, Business Administration, and Counseling has elected to study the concept of spirituality. As they apply spiritual principles to their daily functioning, they will determine the effects of spirituality on their professional lives. It has been requested by the Department of Religion that the Neuman Systems Model be interpreted by nursing.

(Contact: Rae Jeanne Memmott, Neuman trustee and Professor, Brigham Young University, 500 SWKT, Provo, Utah 84602.)

Lois Lowry, a Neuman trustee, reports that an interdisciplinary research team consisting of nurses, chaplains, and physicians designed a two-phased study to investigate client reactions, perceptions, and coping mechanisms that affect healing when clients are faced with life-threatening illness. The Neuman Systems Model provides the framework for the study because of its systems approach, breadth, understandable language, and appeal to other disciplines. This study is an outgrowth of the pilot conducted by Clark, Cross, Deane, and Lowry (*Holistic Nursing Practice*, 1991). Data will be gathered through personal interviews and analyzed by qualitative methods to determine categories of commonly used, but probably unconventional, therapies. Based on these findings (phase 1), clinical trials (phase 2) will be designed to test the efficacy and cost-effectiveness of incorporating these modalities into the regimen of care. This proposal has been enthusiastically supported by the hospital administrators and medical staff of a large institution in the Tampa Bay area where the study will be conducted. Funding is being sought to support the study. The university is co-investigator on this study.

(Contact: Dr. Lois Lowry, RN, DNS, Neuman trustee and Professor at the University of South Florida, Tampa, Florida.)

The Neuman Systems Model is the conceptual model chosen by Karen Perrin, RN, MPH, as the theoretical framework for a study to investigate the perception of sexuality in relation to the five variables of person of pregnant adolescents. The purpose of the study is to determine the prevalence of physical and sexual abuse among the pregnant teen population. The relationship of the perpetrator to the victim, the pattern of assault, and demographic characteristics associated with abuse will also be considered. This study will be conducted in the Tampa Bay area.

(Contact: Principal investigator, Karen Perrin, RN, MPH, Adjunct Professor, College of Public Health, University of Southern Florida, Tampa, Florida.)

IMMIGRATION AND NATURALIZATION SERVICE PROJECT

A project is currently in progress to develop a conceptual approach, utilizing the Neuman Systems Model, for the establishment of nurse-managed health care centers in the US Immigration and Naturalization Service (INS) Health Care Program.

The INS maintains nine Service Processing Centers nationwide that operate a medical facility. These medical facilities, which utilize the medical model to provide health care services, currently are under the direction of a medical officer. It is felt that the development of nurse-managed centers will provide for nurse control of practice, direct access by the patient, and wholistic, client-centered service. A goal-directed approach will be utilized to focus on primary, secondary, and tertiary prevention methods to provide health care to this diverse and poorly serviced population. Consistent with the Neuman Systems Model, evaluation of nursing care is based on stated outcomes. Long-term evaluation depends on reassessment of goals and outcomes.

According to Roy C. Lopez, RNC, MSNC, CCHP, initiator of the "centers" program, the development of nurse-managed centers within the INS Health Care Program will provide nursing the opportunity to practice independently in the field of correctional health care, utilizing the Neuman Systems Model to provide client-centered, wholistic health care. Lopez, a commander in the United States Public Health Service, is assigned to the Immigration and Naturalization Service Health Care Program and currently serves as the Western Regional Supervisory Program Management Officer. Commander Lopez is also a graduate student at California State University, Dominguez Hills, Carson, California.
(Contact: Roy Lopez, MSNC, RNC, 12861 Olive Street, Garden Grove, CA 92645. Tel: (714) 897–5914.)

MORE NEUMAN-BASED INITIATIVES

During the past few years the Neuman Systems Model has been used for structuring the World Health Organization Collaborative Center for Primary Health Care Nursing in Maribor, Yugoslavia (Slovenia). The director has recently programmed at the University of Maribor a baccalaureate nurse education curriculum based on Neuman.
(Contact: Majda Slajmer Japelj, International Manager, World Health Organization Collaborative Center for Primary Care Nursing, Slovenia, 62000 Maribor, UL. Talcev 9.)

The Neuman Systems Model is used for **interdisciplinary education** at the East Tennessee State University in the Department of Professional Roles/Mental Health Nursing.

The model serves as an educational cooperative base for nursing, medicine, family therapy, and social work. Clinical education settings used include private practice, mental health centers, therapeutic nursery, inpatient consultation, and public school consultation.

(Contact: Beth Brown, RN, MS, Assistant Professor, College of Nursing, East Tennessee State University, Johnson City, Tennessee 37614. Tel: (615) 929-4476.)

Janet Sipple is a pioneer in the use of nursing theory to develop and guide her rural health practice as a nurse practitioner. Her use of the Neuman Systems Model, a theory-based practice model, both complements and facilitates the course work of her nurse practitioner accelerated seminar learning track series. The learning modules correlate with the American Nursing Association nurse practitioner certification examination criteria. Dr. Sipple views the Neuman Model as forming a comprehensive, flexible base with concepts relevant for establishing important health system collaborative partnerships with clients for increasing the quality of life. The three preventive interventions will be used: primary prevention for health retention and promotion, secondary prevention for acute care support, and tertiary prevention for maintaining optimal client system wellness in chronic care. The model concepts define and give direction for consideration of needs and interventions for one or more clients within a particular community. This implies the identification and consideration of subsystems to benefit the larger rural community as a system and ensures delivery of appropriate health services that are responsive to the needs of all health consumers and clients. Use of the theoretical model supports both program development and evaluation.

(Contact: Janet Sipple, RN, EdD, Professor and Academic Dean, Department of Nursing, Barnes College, St. Louis, Missouri 63108. Tel: (314) 652-7434.)

Glenn Curran is developing a sexual health HIV/AIDS program in the rural northwest region of Tasmania, Australia, within the 1993 criteria of the Australian Community Health Accreditation and Standards Program (CHASP), which incorporates primary health care. The Neuman Systems Model forms the base for the sexual health program as it "accommodates the complexities and dynamics of identified systems (person, group, community, or issue)." Systems thinking is considered particularly relevant to a wholistic, multidisciplinary approach to health care consistent with the above principles of CHASP.

(Contact: Glenn Curran, RN, RMN, B. Nurs. (Hons.), Clinical Nurse Manager, Sexual Health, HIV/AIDS Program, North West Health Region, 11 Jones Street, Burnie, 7320, Tasmania, Australia. Tel: (004) 346315.)

Janice Turner, a clinical nurse specialist, uses the Neuman Systems Model as a base for the new rural health program, a free outreach service of the Lake Charles Memorial Hospital, Lake Charles, Louisiana. From the traveling van she services rural clients, including screening for early risk factors of heart disease and stroke, fetal heart monitoring, and on-site laboratory testing. Major intervention focus at the three Neuman prevention levels is on nutrition, exercise, stress reduction, and medication monitoring. Her self-developed assessment tool is based on the five Neuman Model variables and is used in conjunction with an abbreviated check list. She states, "the most important thing I am doing is looking at the whole person." Following initial screening, contributing stressor effects often become evident, allowing for more in-depth exploration and understanding of the entire client health condition. Once actual and potential stressors are identified, she focuses on the three preventions as interventions, resource referral, and categorizing and correlating types of identified stressors with preventive intervention strategies used across the life span for the rural multiproblem community she serves. Early data suggest clients prefer mobile health services to physician office visits. Her goal is to prove that high-quality wholistic client care is both possible and cost-effective when delivered by an advanced practice nurse. *(Contact: Janice Turner, RN, MSN, Clinical Nurse Specialist, Lake Charles Memorial Hospital, Lake Charles, Louisiana 70601. Tel: (318) 494-3214.)*

The Neuman Systems Model is relevant for **nursing information systems** for practice, research, education, and business. With health care reform on the horizon, there is a critical need for the development of nursing information systems for care of clients in community settings. The shift in the paradigm from illness care to health (health promotion and prevention services) requires the nursing profession to respond with information systems that will track client care, their responses to preventive services, and the costs of these services for managed care.

The Neuman Systems Model, with its delineation of primary prevention, secondary prevention, and tertiary prevention interventions, is well organized for grouping services and tracking cost-effectiveness in the managed care environment. Managed care will require nursing interventions that prevent hospitalizations and/or reduce length of stay, on both the front end (primary prevention) and the back end (tertiary prevention) of health care. However, the need for organizing wholistic assessment, intervention, and outcome data for clinical and health services research is necessary for advancement of the nursing profession. Nursing informatics leaders have identified that the next generation of information systems must be flexible enough to accommodate nursing models of care and must build on the minimum data set established by Harriet Werley. A number of classification systems for organization of the data have been suggested and discussed in the informatics literature. However, many of these are not comprehensive enough to include primary care, community care, community health, and case management.

The Community Nursing Center at the University of Rochester School of Nursing is further developing the Neuman Systems Model as a framework for nursing care and for health services research. In order to evaluate the impact of this innovative community nursing clinic model and the delivery of health care, work is beginning on a clinical information system using the Neuman Systems Model. At this time, the Omaha System, Saba's Home Health Classification System, and evolving nurse practitioner taxonomies are being considered for adaptation with the Neuman Systems Model. Wholistic assessment and nursing interventions are critical additions to development of information systems, which have, in the past, reflected only medical diagnosis and treatment. In order to address social history, functional status assessment, and identification of factors that contribute to barriers and access to care, nursing must work with medicine and other disciplines toward an interdisciplinary computerized patient record that will track clients over time and across settings. However, consistent with the interdisciplinary focus of the Neuman Model, the Neuman system client variables will be used as an overall organizing framework for this new, developing information system.

Categorization of nursing interventions and outcomes across the care continuum are also critical for the future and will position this information system as an important contribution to the need for integrated information systems across care settings. Outcomes measurement, particularly in the areas of cost and quality, include specific clinical outcomes, changes in health status and health risk behaviors, changes in circumstances of living, empowerment of individuals/families, and overall quality of life. Consideration of data elements and structure needed for interdisciplinary practice, financial analysis, and research interests of the Health Care Financing Administration, the Agency for Health Care Policy Research, and the National Institute for Nursing Research is important for practice, education, research, and business purposes. Relevant coding and data collection by nurses about nursing assessment, interventions, and outcomes are necessary for the advancement of the profession during this evolution of health care delivery, where prevention and care outside institutions must be identified and measured.

This information system is being developed for use on a microcomputer (including the laptop), which would eventually allow clinicians to enter data and review client information from remote sites. The design is being carefully considered to facilitate both clinical and health services research with attention to documenting accessible, cost-effective, and quality care outcomes. Additionally, it must be possible to export data into selected formats for further manipulation and statistical analysis for qualitative and quantitative research studies. Funding is being sought to facilitate practice-based research using this Neuman-focused clinical information system in a number of community nursing center sites across the United States.

(Contact: Patricia Hinton Walker, PhD, RN, FAAN, and John M. Walker, MA, Faculty, School of Nursing, University of Rochester, New York 14627. Tel: (716) 275-8902.)

The following shared insights are compiled from teaching experience using the Neuman Systems Model at the Texas Woman's University, Houston campus.

Helping students catch the vision of theory-based nursing practice is an invigorating experience. Especially exciting is introducing the Neuman Systems Model with its inherent characteristics. The Neuman Model forces the planner of health care to move within the client perspective and view both the internal and external environments from the uniqueness of the client position. The concepts within the model require a comprehensive examination of person as an open system and define preventive, therapeutic, and rehabilitative activities in a unique manner. The definitions allow the caregiver to be creative since the operationalization of the concepts does not restrict site or chronological order of use. The model encourages wholism, beginning with a comprehensive assessment, and an insider view. The characteristics of the model and its application in the clinical arena provide invaluable methodologies for futuristic 21st century client care.

Faculty use of the following eclectic collection of teaching–learning principles has yielded much success in guiding students into Neuman theory-based practice:

- Simple to complex: introducing the model with concepts and their definitions; moving from simple relationships to complex relationships, first in an abstract manner and then in applied situations
- Familiar to unknown: introducing those concepts that will be most comfortable for the learner because of past associations
- Ausubel's advance organizers: preparing the learner for both content and process aspects in the learning experience before beginning
- Group process: progressing from the use of small groups to larger groups for assigned tasks that increase in complexity; building upon the diversity (differing clinical perspectives, developmental levels, career trajectories, ethnicities, cultural variations, personal biases, etc.) of the learners within the group; capturing the affective components of responses in student interaction and helping the group deal with their behaviors
- Use of case study: applying the Neuman Model in analysis of clinical cases for theory-based caregiving
- Adult learner: accepting students as learners with much experience upon which knowledge can be built and recognizing that these students learn for future experiences

The uniqueness of utilizing the case study approach in tandem with group process facilitates learning how to use the Neuman Systems Model.
(Contact: Judith Stocks, RN, PhD, Associate Professor, Texas Woman's University, College of Nursing, Houston Center, 1130 M.D. Anderson Boulevard, Houston, Texas 77030.)

The Neuman Systems Model is an excellent wholistic organizing structure for multiservice agencies (MSA). It is being considered for multiservice agency development in one county of Ontario. Long-term care reform was recently introduced into Ontario's health care system in response to economic constraints, an aging population, and consumer demands for a larger role in the planning and delivery of long-term care services. Recent public consultation found existing services to be fragmented and duplicated, with inequitable access and service gaps. The reform promotes greater consumer participation in planning and controlling services they receive. This will be achieved, in part, by restructuring existing services and creating multiservice agencies with a single point of access in each county or local planning area of the province. The Neuman Systems Model was proposed to the MSA Steering Committee of one county as a fitting model for designing the MSA. The model was easily adapted to mirror the following provincial guidelines and principles:

- *Core:* seniors, adults with disabilities, and caregivers
- *Lines of resistance:* emergency response teams, short stay beds in long-term care facilities, and crisis beds
- *Normal lines of defense:* ongoing long-term care services such as in-home services, palliative care, placement coordination, meals, adult day programs, and transportation; provided by case managers, health professionals, personal support workers, and volunteers
- *Flexible line of defense:* MSA board of directors (representing local communities), executive director, education/training, volunteer coordinator, total quality management

The Neuman Model provides a framework for the *structure* and *function* of the MSA and facilitates the planning process, which is essential to the implementation of a new system. It offers a framework for future evaluation and monitoring of the MSA services within communities to ensure that the new system is meeting consumer needs.
(Contact: Nancy Smith, Case Manager, Geriatric Day Hospital, Parkwood Hospital, London, Ontario, N6C 5J1 Canada. Tel: (519) 685-4019.)

For consistently effective articulation among educational programs, the constructs of the Neuman Systems Model serves well as an organizational base for presenting nursing knowledge, nursing process, and nursing roles within the Santa Fe Community College 36-week and 42-week practical nursing (PN) programs, and the associate of science in nursing (ASN) bridge and associate of science in nursing programs (36 weeks and 66 weeks in length, respectively). To facilitate articulation to the ASN bridge program, the PN faculty implemented a Neuman-based curriculum in 1993, using structure similar to the ASN program's Neuman-based curriculum implemented in 1985. Use of the model at the PN level provides structure for assessment and facilitates organization of nursing knowledge to deliver wholistic nursing care. PN graduates who articulate to the ASN bridge program continue to use the constructs of the Neuman Model as they build on nursing knowledge, nursing process, and nursing roles, easily moving from PN roles as caregiver and member of the discipline of nursing to the registered nurse roles as provider of care, manager of care, and member within the discipline of nursing. General education and elective courses (including English composition, college algebra, statistics, general psychology, and humanities) are included in the curriculum, enabling graduates to articulate well to the university setting.
(Contact: Pat Aylward, MSN, RN, CNS, Interim Coordinator for Nursing Programs, Santa Fe Community College, 3000 NW 83 Street W 201, Gainesville,

Florida 32606. Tel: (904) 395-5729 (W), (904) 454-1952 (H); Fax: (904) 395-5711.)

The Neuman Systems Model, currently used for professional nursing practice within a Canadian chronic care hospital, is facilitating policy change in the method of nursing care delivery. Thus a major restructuring of care delivery is taking place on the assumption that through model usage functional status of chronically ill clients will increase with the efficiency of nursing care delivery. Newer approaches to problem solving and decision making will, ideally, support nursing's adaptation to rapidly changing social/environmental forces.

A major goal is to demonstrate the efficacy of the Neuman Model for providing quality client care, effectively containing cost, and optimizing nursing autonomy. The proposed health delivery policy changes, it is anticipated, will foster unification of nursing theory, practice, and research, thus promoting scientific nursing interventions. The Neuman Systems Model is viewed as an alternative policy for developing a more effective efficient health delivery system. The outcome effect should give important future direction for nursing administration and professional nursing practice within health care agencies.

(Contact: Margot Felix, RN, BSc (SocSc), MPA, Nurse Educator/Research and Development, Elisabeth Bruyere Health Centre, Ottawa, Ontario K1N 5C8 Canada. Tel: (613) 562-0050; Fax: (613) 562-6367.)

With great interest and unique experience in international nursing, both Dean Sandra Rogers, DNSc, and Rae Jeanne Memmott, RN, MS, faculty at Brigham University College of Nursing, are exploring various strategies for using the Neuman Systems Model to facilitate reaching the World Health Organization's goal of "Health for all 2000." Many have recognized nursing as the health care profession that could most dramatically impact the achievement of that goal. However, processes by which nurses might most effectively proceed in that direction have remained obscure. It is believed that the Neuman Systems Model can well provide the framework for facilitating the processes required to accomplish World Health Organization goals. These nurse professionals are focusing their exploration on use of the model in schools of nursing, mother–child assessment, community assessment, and health education in underdeveloped countries.

(Contact: Dean Sandra Rogers, DNSc, and Professor Rae Jeanne Memmott, RN, MS, College of Nursing, Brigham Young University, Provo, Utah 84602-5544. Tel: (801) 378-7210; Fax: (801) 378-3198.)

Through use of the Neuman Systems Model to conceptualize retirement as loss, a linkage is made between unresolved grief and illness and client loss of work and perceived health status. Since the literature reflects a dearth of health care emotional support for retirees, a Neuman-based brief-loss counseling tool has been developed with specific guidelines to assist geriatric nurse practitioners in client rehabilitation for cost-effective wholistic care.

(Contact: Mary P. Skowronek, RN, GNP, CRNP, 918 Hawthorne Avenue, Mechanicsburg, PA 17055.)

The Neuman Systems Model was used as a conceptual base for a study that identified self-perceived needs of Vancouver-area families with children with cancer. A dearth of information exists in the literature. An excellent interview tool is now available for gathering intra-, inter-, and extra-family self-perceived needs data that could also be generalized from use in other family illness categories.

(Contact: Heidi Enright, BScN, RN, MSN, Instructor, General Nursing Health Sciences Department, Douglas College, 700 Royal Avenue, New Westminster, B.C. V3L5B2 Canada.)

Following publication of a successful study using the Neuman Model for total care of the hospitalized preschool child with major focus on emotional care, Joan Orr is developing a wholistic Neuman-based inservice training program for child health care for both community and hospital-based interdisciplinary care givers.

(Contact: Joan P. Orr, Lecturer, Child Health, Department of Didactics, The Univeristy of South Africa, 392 Pretoria 0001 RSA.)

A PROPOSAL FOR USE OF THE NEUMAN SYSTEMS MODEL IN NURSING HOMES

The Neuman Systems Model has been proposed for use by directors of nursing in nursing homes to give direction for upgrading long-term client care. As one of the major components in alternative health care delivery systems, nursing homes will experience increasing demands for services in the future and well into the 21st century. Greater numbers of elderly and disabled persons requiring complex care will seek access to nursing home care (Kemper and Murtaugh, 1991). The health care reform movement of the 1990s does not exclude nursing homes from being held accountable for delivery of quality and cost-effective long-term client care. The director of nursing is in the key leadership position for change. An integrated management–Neuman Systems approach is available as an important tool for assessing, diagnosing, strategizing, monitoring, and evaluating the outcomes of care within nursing homes, thus meeting the needs and demands of the client, nursing, and organizational systems (Kelley and Sanders, 1993).

Nursing homes abound with a variety of stressors. One example is an increasing foley catheter infection rate (Laubacher, Robinson, Shipoo, and Hall, 1990). Infections contribute to decreased quality of life for the client and increased cost for care. The stressor of an increased infection rate could affect either or all of the personal, nursing, and organizational systems within the facility.

The use of the Neuman Systems Management Tool (Figure 50–1) in a nursing home to resolve the stressor effect of an increasing foley catheter infection rate evolved from the following scenario: The director of nursing observed a large turnover in all shifts in nursing assistants during the previous six months.

A. Intake Summary:

Who?	What?	Where?	When?	Why?
Personal system	Structure dx	Education	Timing	Goals
Nursing system	Management dx	setting	Timeframe	Short term
Organizational	planning	Practice		Long term
system	organizing	setting		
	directing			
	controlling			
	Outcome dx			

B. Stressors:_____

Environment	Client System		
	Personal	Nursing	Organizational
Internal	_____	_____	_____
External	_____	_____	_____

C. Factors:

	Develop.	Psychol.	Physiol.	Spiritual	Socio/ Cultural
Intrapersonal	_____	_____	_____	_____	_____
Interpersonal	_____	_____	_____	_____	_____
Extrapersonal	_____	_____	_____	_____	_____

D. Organizational orientation to the environment:

Intervention	Environmental dimensions				
	Human Resources	Culture	Socio/ Technical	Structure/ Function	Decision making
Primary	_____	_____	_____	_____	_____
Secondary	_____	_____	_____	_____	_____
Tertiary	_____	_____	_____	_____	_____

E. Problem(s) defined:_____

F. Problem resolution (goal) with rationale:_____

G. Prevention (action plan):_____

H. Outcomes (evaluation):
   Predicted:_____

   Actual:_____

Figure 50–1. Neuman Systems Management Tool for nursing and organizational systems.

The new staff were relatively inexperienced in infection control within the health care environment. The director associated the stressor of increased foley catheter infection as originating from within the nursing system, primarily from a developmental deficit in the agency intrapersonal environment (i.e., hiring new staff). The stressor caused a reaction within the nursing system requiring secondary prevention as intervention from mobilization of internal resources to motivate, educate, and involve nursing assistants in infection control procedures (Neuman, 1989, 21). Following problem definition, a goal was set of reducing the infection rate by 10 percent within three months. This would be achieved through a mandatory in-service program for all nursing assistants containing a cost estimate for the nursing organization, including random monitoring of nursing assistant performance following the in-service and through continuous monitoring of foley catheter-related infections. The predicted outcomes were expected reduction in infection rate, cost savings to consumers, and improvement in the reputation of the nursing home. If the actual outcome showed a continued increase in the infection rate, the director would reassess the nature of the stressor to develop additional strategic choices, such as obtaining the services of an infection control nurse consultant; consumer (client and family) education; and assessment of other organizational components (housekeeping, laundry, and the practices of other health care providers).

The example used here is a single, isolated stressor affecting a relatively limited segment within an agency. However, the Neuman Systems Management Tool can be equally well used more broadly to assess the interrelationships among personal, nursing, and organizational systems within an ever-changing health care environment. The state of health or instability of each interacting system affects and changes relationships among the involved systems. Thus the tool provides a wholistic systems approach to identifying an array of stressors affecting client care that need to be analyzed as a means of determining strategic nursing actions that would retain, achieve, or maintain a desired level of quality nursing and health care. The Neuman Systems Management Tool has great potential for use in a variety of nursing practice and education settings. As community-based nursing centers or academic nursing centers hold the promise of being the nursing practice model for the 21st century, managers must find ways "to identify, document and publish health care outcomes associated with care in the centers" (Gray, 1993, 417). Data gathered from use of the tool are viewed as a powerful means for demonstrating cost savings, justifying expenditures, and negotiating reimbursement for client care. The Neuman Systems Management Tool will prove to be an invaluable resource to health care providers and managers in nursing homes and other health care settings for ensuring quality client care outcomes.

(Contact: Authors and consultants, Connie J. Rowles, DSN, RN, Assistant Professor, School of Nursing, Ball State University, Muncie, Indiana 47306; and Jean A. Kelley, RN, PhD, FAAN, Professor Emeritus, University of Alabama at Birmingham, 4766 Overwood Circle, Birmingham, Alabama 35222.)

For the past two years, the Neuman Systems Model has been used as a curricular base for mental health psychiatric nursing education at the Escola Superior De Enfermagem Maria Fernanda Resende in Lisbon, Portugal. The model was chosen because of "the match in philosophy of approach to client centered care." They have successfully used Neuman-reformulated health assessment questions for school children and have also developed a format to help students identify and relate specific stressors, affecting client behavior, to correspondent client system variables.

(Contact: Marta Lima Basto or Lila Mela Anjos, Escola Superior De Enfermagem De Maria Fernanda Resende, AV. DO Brasil, 53–13 1700 Lisbon, Portugal.)

A research project is underway at the University Hospital, Tromso, Norway, using the Neuman Model to identify stressors that affect the appetites of hospitalized clients. The Model was chosen because it is "both understandable and practical in the work setting." Food has been identified as an important human need in providing wholistic client care. An important nursing responsibility is to create an optimal nutritional state for hospitalized clients, which is accomplished through use of the nursing process as follows:

> This involves obtaining information about the client's eating behavior, assessing the adequacy of their nutritional status, determining the unique goals to be accomplished with regard to individual client nutrition needs, and planning and implementing nursing interventions designed to accomplish these goals. Finally, to complete the nursing process, results of the nursing interventions are evaluated to see if the desired goals have been achieved.

Helping clients respond positively to stressors to maintain system balance is viewed as an important aspect of the Neuman Model's role and function in client health preservation. The current project is based on a 1991 project by the Nordic Council of Ministers on hospital food and its relationship to client well-being in five Nordic countries.

(Contact: Henny M. Olsson, PhD, RNM, BSc in Public Health Nursing, VD in Nursing Education, Associate Professor, Center for Caring Sciences, Uppsala University, Uppsala, Sweden; Tove Forsdahl, RN, Director of Nursing, University Hospital, Tromso, Norway.)

Nursing faculty at Neumann College, Aston, Pennsylvania, believe that a nursing program must prepare nurses to be both accountable and responsible for providing quality health care within a dynamic and pluralistic society. This implies teaching nurses to assume current, dynamic roles and functions that can adapt to rapidly changing health needs and future mandates in a reformed health care system. Based on this philosophy, faculty have developed and implemented a creative baccalaureate nurse curriculum incorporating the following concepts:

- A systems perspective of individuals, health, and nursing
- A view of individuals as complex systems, composed of interdependent variables
- Nursing as dynamic and preventive, therapeutic and rehabilitative

- Nursing as being at the threshold of professional practice
- Nursing as requiring collaboration in multiple and interdisciplinary systems

To provide a theoretical foundation for a wholistic curriculum, the Neuman Systems Model was selected in 1976 for curricular change and will continue its relevancy for 21st century learning needs.

It was recently decided to develop a graduate curriculum at Neumann College to prepare advanced nurse practitioners with a managed care focus. The Neuman Systems Model will again guide the curricular design for a wholistic systematic approach to nursing education.

When the anticipated master of science, physical therapy program is implemented, an interdisciplinary approach to student learning will be programmed with nursing.

Cooperation in interdisciplinary education, practice, and research activity is viewed as both an opportunity and a contribution to ongoing development and use of the Neuman Systems Model well into the 21st century.

(Contact: Rosalie Mirenda, Vice President for Academic Affairs and Professor of Nursing, Neumann College, Aston, Pennsylvania 19014.)

IV. The Neuman Systems Model Trustees Group, Inc.

When the Neuman Systems Model was first published, it was intended for nursing; if it proved valuable, the profession would recognize the fact and further develop, refine, and nurture it. I have refused to market it. Until such time as it either proved or disproved its utility, I considered myself only as a servant of the model, shepherding it during the struggles of its early years. My goal was to provide visibility through attempts to clarify its concepts, develop tools for its use, and motivate and network with those who were using or planned to use it, until it reached maturity. My remaining hope is that the nursing profession, in its continuing efforts to be creative with the Neuman Systems Model, will also commit itself to the preservation of the integrity and identity of the model in the future utilization of its concepts.

Now that the model is fully accepted by those using it and has provided new parameters and terminology for the nursing profession, I joyfully relinquish my former shepherd role. It is now officially placed with personally chosen Neuman Systems Model Trustee Group members, whose competency and dedication offer assurance that the model will surely live on. The Neuman Systems Model Trustees Agreement follows.

THE NEUMAN SYSTEMS MODEL TRUSTEES AGREEMENT

Purpose

The purpose of this Neuman Systems Model Trustees Agreement, established Fall 1988 by the Trustor, Betty M. Neuman, RN, PhD, is to preserve, protect, and perpetuate the integrity of the Model for the future of nursing.

Membership

The membership will be called The Neuman Systems Model Trustees Group, Inc., and will initially include professional nurses from the United States and other countries who for the past two years have been committed to and engaged in the development or use of The Neuman Systems Model. Upon resignation, the current member may appoint a successor with the above qualifications for majority-vote acceptance by the current membership group. A two-thirds vote is required for decision making.

Functions

1. Present or facilitate presentation of the Model and its usage at conferences and meetings.
2. Achieve unanimous agreement on any future permanent changes in the original Neuman Systems Model diagram.
3. Consult or provide consultation activities for nursing education and practice implementation.
4. Provide information, networking, and support to those requiring or requesting it.
5. Trustee member sharing and updating of information and activities related to the model on a continuing basis with a commitment to its further development.
6. Plan, promote, and conduct national and international conferences on the Neuman Systems Model.
7. Establish by-laws or protocol for Trustee Group Membership involvement as required for continued functional relevancy.

Active Membership Effective Fall 1994

Betty Neuman, PhD, FAAN
Founder/Director
Theorist, Author, Consultant, and
Counselor
P.O. Box 488
Beverly, Ohio 45715
Tel: (H) (614) 749-3322

Lois W. Lowry, RN, DNSc[++]
Third and Current President
Associate Professor
College of Nursing
University of South Florida
Tampa, Florida 33612-4799
Tel: (W) (813) 974-2191
        (Fax) (813) 974-5418
        (H) (813) 972-4011

Patricia Hinton Walker, PhD, RN, FAAN
President Elect
Associate Dean and Director of
Community Centered Practice
School of Nursing
University of Rochester
Rochester, New York 14642-8404
Tel: (W) (716) 275-8902
      (Fax) (716) 473-1059
      (H) (716) 392-4041

Janet A. Sipple, RN, PhD⁺
Second President
Professor
Barnes College of Nursing
University of Missouri
St. Louis, Missouri 63110
Tel: (W) (314) 362-4816
      (Fax) (314) 362-1880
      (H) (314) 652-7434

Rosalie M. Mirenda, RN, PhD⁺
First President
Vice President for Academic Affairs
Neumann College
Aston, Pennsylvania 19014-1297
Tel: (W) (215) 459-0905
      (Fax) (215) 459-1370
      (H) (215) 565-2904

Jean A. Kelley, EdD, RN, FAAN
Professor Emeritus,
University of Alabama at Birmingham
Co-Project Director for Faculty
Development for Graduate Nurse
Educators
Southern Regional Education Board
592 Tenth Street, N.W.
Atlanta, Georgia 30318-5790
Tel: (W) (404) 875-9211
      (Fax) (404) 872-1477
      (H) (205) 595-7161

Diane Breckenridge, RN, MSN, PhD candidate
University of Maryland
Abington Memorial Hospital Nursing
School Faculty
Abington, Pennsylvania 19001
Tel: (W) (215) 881-5539
      (Fax) (215) 881-5550
      (H) (215) 836-2193

Dorothy Craig, RN, MScN
Professor
Faculty of Nursing
University of Toronto
Ontario, M5S 1A1 Canada
Tel: (W) (416) 978-2857
      (Fax) (416) 978-8222
      (H) (416) 626-3529

Cynthia Flynn Capers, PhD, RN
Associate Professor and Director
Undergraduate Programs
School of Nursing
LaSalle University
Philadelphia, Pennsylvania 19141
Tel: (W) (215) 951-1430
      (Fax) (215) 951-1896
      (H) (215) 247-0523

Audrey M. Koertvelyessy, MSN, RN, FNP
Captain, USPHS
Nursing Consultant
Division of Nursing
Bureau of Health Professions
Health Resources and Services
Administration
5600 Fishers Lane
Parklawn Building 9-36
Rockville, Maryland 20857
Tel: (W) (301) 443-6333
      (Fax) (301) 443-8586
      (H) (301) 816-2938

Jacqueline Fawcett, RN, PhD
Professor
School of Nursing
University of Pennsylvania
Philadelphia, Pennsylvania 19104
Tel: (W) (215) 898-8289
      (Fax) (215) 573-2114
      (H) (203) 429-9228

**Barbara Fulton Shambaugh,
RN, EdD**
President, Diogenes Ltd.
77 Pond Avenue #1501
Brookline, Massachusetts 02146
Tel: (W) (617) 731-0368
      (Fax) (617) 731-0368
      (H) (617) 566-2596

Rae Jeanne Memmott, RN, MS
Associate Professor
College of Nursing
Brigham Young University
Provo, Utah 84602
Tel: (W) (801) 378-7210
      (Fax) (801) 378-3198
      (H) (801) 225-1886

Jan M. Russell, RN, PhD
Associate Professor
School of Nursing
University of Missouri at Kansas City
Kansas City, Missouri 64131
Tel: (W) (816) 235-1713
      (Fax) (816) 235-1701
      (H) (816) 523-3130

Patricia Aylward, RN, MSN, CNS
Interim Coordinator for Nursing
Programs
Sante Fe Community College
Gainesville, Florida 32606
Tel: (W) (904) 395-5759
      (Fax) (904) 395-5711
      (H) (904) 454-1952

Charlene Beynon, MScN
Assistant Director of Nursing
Middlesex–London Health Unit
Teaching Unit Program
50 King Street
London, Ontario N6A 5L7 Canada
Tel: (W) (519) 663-5317
      (Fax) (519) 663-9581
      (H) (519) 473-1743

Margaret Louis, RN, PhD
Associate Professor
Department of Nursing
University of Nevada at Las Vegas
Las Vegas, Nevada 89154
Tel: (W) (702) 895-3812
      (Fax) (702) 895-4807
      INTERNET: louisrn@Nevada.edu
      (H) (702) 458-7792

Patricia Chadwick, EdD, RN
Professor and Dean
School of Nursing
University of Portland
5000 Willamette Boulevard
Portland, Oregon 97203-5798
Tel: (W) (503) 283-7211
      (Fax) (503) 283-7399
      (H) (503) 645-3741

Raphella Sohier, PhD, RN
Professor of Nursing
Graduate Programs
Massachusetts General Hospital
Institute of Health Professions
Massachusetts General Hospital
101 Merrimac Street
Boston, Massachusetts 02114
Tel: (W) (617) 726-8014
      (Fax) (617) 726-8022
      (H) (617) 524-2667

General Powers*

Items of concern for the Neuman Systems Model will be managed within the Neuman Systems Model Trustee Group Membership.

*The Trustor, Betty M. Neuman, PhD, FAAN, reserves the right to assume any of the functions without consent of the Trustee Group Membership.

⁺Past Presidents

⁺⁺Current President 1993–1995

APPENDIX A

Bibliography

*Citations compiled by Jacqueline Fawcett,
PhD, FAAN*

PRIMARY SOURCES

Neuman, B., and Young, R. J. 1972. A model for teaching total person approach to patient problems. *Nursing Research* 21:264–269.

Neuman, B. 1974. The Betty Neuman Health Care Systems Model: A total person approach to patient problems. In *Conceptual Models for Nursing Practice,* edited by J. P. Riehl and C. Roy, 99–114. New York: Appleton-Century-Crofts.

Neuman, B. 1980. The Betty Neuman Health Care Systems Model: A total person approach to patient problems. In *Conceptual Models for Nursing Practice,* 2d ed., edited by J. P. Riehl and C. Roy, 119–134. New York: Appleton-Century-Crofts.

Neuman, B. 1982. The Neuman Health Care Systems Model: A total approach to client care. In *The Neuman Systems Model: Application to Nursing Education and Practice,* by B. Neuman, 8–29. Norwalk, Conn.: Appleton-Century-Crofts.

Neuman, B. 1982. *The Neuman Systems Model. Application to Nursing Education and Practice.* Norwalk, Conn.: Appleton-Century-Crofts.

Neuman, B. 1982. The systems concept and nursing. In *The Neuman Systems Model: Application to Nursing Education and Practice,* by B. Neuman, 3–7. Norwalk, Conn.: Appleton-Century-Crofts.

Neuman, B. 1983. Family intervention using the Betty Neuman Health Care Systems Model. In *Family Health: A Theoretical Approach to Nursing Care,* by I. W. Clements and F. B. Roberts, 239–254. New York: John Wiley & Sons.

Neuman, B. 1983. The family experiencing emotional crisis. Analysis and application of Neuman's Health Care Systems Model. In *Family Health: A Theoretical Approach to Nursing Care,* by I. W. Clements and F. B. Roberts, 353–367. New York: John Wiley & Sons.

Neuman, B. 1985. The Neuman Systems Model. *Senior Nurse* 5(3):20–23.

Neuman, B. 1989. The Neuman nursing process format: Family. In *Conceptual Models for Nursing Practice,* 3d ed., by J. P. Riehl-Sisca, 49–62. Norwalk, Conn.: Appleton & Lange.

Neuman, B. 1989. In conclusion—in transition. In *The Neuman Systems Model,* 2d ed., by B. Neuman, 453–470. Norwalk, Conn.: Appleton & Lange.

Neuman, B. 1989. *The Neuman Systems Model,* 2d ed. Norwalk, Conn.: Appleton & Lange.

Neuman, B. 1989. The Neuman Systems Model. In *The Neuman Systems Model,* 2d ed., by B. Neuman, 3–63. Norwalk, Conn.: Appleton & Lange.

Neuman, B. 1990. The Neuman Systems Model: A theory for practice. In *Nursing Theories in Practice,* edited by M. E. Parker, 241–261. New York: National League for Nursing.

Neuman, B. M. 1990. Health as a continuum based on the Neuman Systems Model. *Nursing Science Quarterly* 3:129–135.

COMMENTARY

Aggleton, P., and Chalmers, H. 1989. Neuman's Systems Model. *Nursing Times* 85(51): 27–29.

Barrett, M. 1991. A thesis is born. *Image: Journal of Nursing Scholarship* 23:261–262.

Beckman, S. J., Boxley-Harges, S., Bruick-Sorge, C., Harris, S. M., Hermiz, M. E., Meininger, M., and Steinkeler, S. E. 1994. Betty Neuman: Systems Model. In *Nursing Theorists and Their Work,* 3d ed., by A. Marriner-Tomey, 269–304. St. Louis: C. V. Mosby.

Bigbee, J. 1984. The changing role of rural women: Nursing and health implications. *Health Care of Women International* 5:307–322.

Biley, F. 1990. The Neuman Model: An analysis. *Nursing (London)* 4(4):25–28.

Burney, M. A. 1992. King and Newman: In search of the nursing paradigm. *Journal of Advanced Nursing* 17:601–603.

Campbell, V. 1989. The Betty Neuman Health Care Systems Model. An analysis. In *Conceptual Models for Nursing Practice,* 3d ed., by J. P. Riehl-Sisca, 63–72. Norwalk, Conn.: Appleton & Lange.

Christensen, P. J., and Kenney, J. W., eds. *Nursing Process: Application of Conceptual Models.* St. Louis: C. V. Mosby.

Cross, J. R. 1985. Betty Neuman. In *Nursing Theories Conference Group, Nursing Theories. The Base for Professional Nursing Practice,* 258–286. Englewood Cliffs, N.J.: Prentice-Hall.

Cross, J. R. 1990. Betty Neuman. In *Nursing Theories. The Base for Professional Nursing Practice,* 3d ed., edited by J. B. George, 259–278. Norwalk, Conn.: Appleton & Lange.

Fawcett, J. 1989. Analysis and evaluation of the Neuman Systems Model. In *The Neuman Systems Model,* 2d ed., by B. Neuman, 65–92. Norwalk, Conn.: Appleton & Lange.

Fawcett, J. 1994. *Analysis and evaluation of conceptual models of nursing* 3d ed. Philadelphia: F. A. Davis.

Fawcett, J., Carpenito, J. J., Efinger, J., Goldblum-Graff, D., Groesbeck, M. J. V., Lowry, L. W., McCreary, C. S., and Wolf, Z. R. 1982. A framework for analysis and evaluation of conceptual models of nursing with an analysis and evaluation of the Neuman Systems Model: In *The Neuman Systems Model: Application to Nursing Education and Practice,* by B. Neuman, 30–43. Norwalk, Conn.: Appleton-Century-Crofts.

Haggart, M. 1993. A critical analysis of Neuman's Systems Model in relation to public health nursing. *Journal of Advanced Nursing* 18:1917–1922.

Harris, S. M., Hermiz, M. E., Meininger, M., and Steinkeler, S. E. 1989. Betty Neuman: Systems Model. In *Nursing Theorists and Their Work,* 2d ed., by A. Marriner-Tomey, 361–388. St. Louis: C. V. Mosby.

Hermiz, M. E., and Meininger, M. 1986. Betty Neuman. Systems Model. In *Nursing Theorists and Their Work,* by A. Marriner, 313–331. St. Louis: C. V. Mosby.

Hinton Walker, P. 1993. Care of the chronically ill: Paradigm shifts and directions for the future. *Holistic Nursing Practice* 8(1):56–66.

Hoffman, M. K. 1982. From model to theory construction: An analysis of the Neuman Health-Care Systems Model: In *The Neuman Systems Model: Application to Nursing Education and Practice,* by B. Neuman, 44–54. Norwalk, Conn.: Appleton-Century-Crofts.

Huch, M. H. 1991. Perspectives on health. *Nursing Science Quarterly* 4:33–40.

Lancaster, D. R., and Whall, A. L. 1989. The Neuman Systems Model. In *Conceptual Models of Nursing. Analysis and Application,* 2d ed., by J. J. Fitzpatrick and A. L. Whall, 255–270. Bowie, Md.: Brady.

Meleis, A. I. 1991. *Theoretical Nursing: Development and Progress,* 2d ed. Philadelphia: J. B. Lippincott.

Mirenda, R. M., and Wright, C. 1987. Using nursing model to affirm Catholic identity. *Health Progress* 68(2):63–67, 94.

Reed, K. S. 1993. *Betty Neuman. The Neuman Systems Model.* Newbury Park, Calif.: Sage.

Salvage, J., and Turner, C. 1989. Brief abstracts: The Neuman Model use in England. In *The Neuman Systems Model,* 2d ed., by B. Neuman, 445–450. Norwalk, Conn.: Appleton & Lange.

Stevens, B. J. 1982. Forward. In *The Neuman Systems Model: Application to Nursing Education and Practice,* by B. Neuman xiii–xiv. Norwalk, Conn.: Appleton-Century-Crofts.

Thibodeau, J. A. 1983. *Nursing Models: Analysis and Evaluation.* Monterey, Calif.: Wadsworth.

Venable, J. F. 1974. The Neuman Health Care Systems Model: An analysis. In *Conceptual Models for Nursing Practice,* by J. P. Riehl and C. Roy, 115–122. New York: Appleton-Century-Crofts. Reprinted 1980 in *Conceptual Models for Nursing Practice,* 2d ed., by J. P. Riehl and C. Roy, 135–141. New York: Appleton-Century-Crofts.

Walker, L. O., and Avant, K. C. 1983. *Strategies for Theory Construction in Nursing.* Norwalk, Conn.: Appleton-Century-Crofts.

Whall, A. L. 1983. The Betty Neuman Health Care Systems Model. In *Conceptual Models of Nursing. Analysis and Application,* by J. J. Fitzpatrick and A. L. Whall, 203–219. Bowie, Md.: Brady.

RESEARCH

Ali, N. S., and Khalil, H. Z. 1989. Effect of psychoeducational intervention on anxiety among Egyptian bladder cancer patients. *Cancer Nursing* 12:236–242.

Bass, L. S. 1991. What do parents need when their infant is a patient in the NICU? *Neonatal Network* 10(4):25–33.

Beynon, C., and Laschinger, H. K. 1993. Theory-based practice: Attitudes of nursing managers before and after educational sessions. *Public Health Nursing* 10:183–188.

Blank, J. J., Clark, L., Longman, A. J., and Atwood, J. R. 1989. Perceived home care needs of cancer patients and their caregivers. *Cancer Nursing* 12:78–84.

Bowdler, J. E., and Barrell, L. M. 1987. Health needs of homeless persons. *Public Health Nursing* 4:135–140.

Bueno, M. N., Redeker, N., and Norman, E. M. Analysis of motor vehicle crash data in an urban trauma center: Implications for nursing practice and research. *Heart and Lung* 21:558–567.

Burke, S. O., and Maloney, R. 1986. The Women's Value Orientation Questionnaire: An instrument revision study. *Nursing Papers* 18(1):32–44.

Cantin, B., and Mitchell, M. 1989. Nurses' smoking behavior. *The Canadian Nurse* 85(1):20–21.

Capers, C. F. 1991. Nurses' and lay African Americans' views about behavior. *Western Journal of Nursing Research* 13:123–135.

Carroll, T. L. 1989. Role deprivation in baccalaureate nursing students pre- and post-curriculum revision. *Journal of Nursing Education* 28:134–139.

Cava, M. A. 1992. An examination of coping strategies used by long-term cancer survivors. *Canadian Oncology Nursing Journal* 2:99–102.

Clark, C. C., Cross, J. R., Deane, D. M., and Lowry, L. W. 1991. Spirituality: Integral to quality care. *Holistic Nursing Practice* 5:67–76.

Courchene, V. S., Patalski, E., and Martin, J. 1991. A study of the health of pediatric nurses administering Cyclosporine A. *Pediatric Nursing* 17:497–500.

Decker, S. D., and Young, E. 1991. Self-perceived needs of primary caregivers of home-hospice clients. *Journal of Community Health Nursing* 8:147–154.

Freiberger, D., Bryant, J., and Marino, B. 1992. The effects of different central venous line dressing changes on bacterial growth in a pediatric oncology population. *Journal of Pediatric Oncology Nursing* 9:3–7.

Gavigan, M., Kline-O'Sullivan, C., and Klumpp-Lybrand, B. 1990. The effects of regular turning on CABG patients. *Critical Care Nursing Quarterly* 12(4):69–76.

Grant, J. S., and Bean, C. A. 1993. Self-identified needs of informal caregivers of head-injured adults. *Family and Community Health* 15(2):49–58.

Grant, J. S., Kinney, M. R., and Davis, L. L. 1993. Using conceptual frameworks of models to guide nursing research. *Journal of Neuroscience Nursing* 25:52–56.

Gries, M., and Fernsler, J. 1988. Patient perceptions of the mechanical ventilation experience. *Focus on Critical Care* 15:52–59.

Heffline, M. S. 1991. A comparative study of pharmacological versus nursing interventions in the treatment of postanesthesia shivering. *Journal of Post Anesthesia Nursing* 6:311–320.

Hinds, C. 1990. Personal and contextual factors predicting patients' reported quality of life: Exploring congruency with Betty Neuman's assumptions. *Journal of Advanced Nursing* 15:456–462.

Hoch, C. C. 1987. Assessing delivery of nursing care. *Journal of Gerontological Nursing* 13:1–17.

Johnson, P. 1983. Black hypertension: A transcultural case study using the Betty Neuman model of nursing care. *Issues in Health Care of Women* 4:191–210.

Kahn, E. C. 1992. A comparison of family needs based on the presence or absence of DNR orders. *Dimensions of Critical Care Nursing* 11:286–292.

Koku, R. V. 1992. Severity of low back pain: A comparison between participants who did and did not receive counseling. *American Association of Occupational Health Nurses Journal* 40:84–89.

Leja, A. M. 1989. Using guided imagery to combat postsurgical depression. *Journal of Gerontological Nursing* 15(4):6–11.

Loescher, L. J., Clark, L., Atwood, J. R., Leigh, S., and Lamb, G. 1990. The impact of the cancer experience on long-term survivors. *Oncology Nursing Forum* 17:223–229.

Louis, M. 1989. An intervention to reduce anxiety levels for nursing working with long-term care clients using Neuman's Model. In *Conceptual Models for Nursing Practice,* 3d ed., by J. P. Riehl-Sisca, 95–103. Norwalk, Conn.: Appleton & Lange.

Louis, M., and Koertvelyessy, A. 1989. The Neuman Model in research. In *The Neuman Systems Model,* 2d ed., by B. Neuman, 93–114. Norwalk, Conn.: Appleton & Lange.

Lowry, L. W., and Jopp, M. C. 1989. An evaluation instrument for assessing an associate degree nursing curriculum based on the Neuman Systems Model. In *Conceptual Models for Nursing Practice,* 3d ed., by J. P. Riehl-Sisca, 73–85. Norwalk, Conn.: Appleton & Lange.

Lowry, L. W., and Anderson, B. 1993. Neuman's framework and ventilator dependency: A pilot study. *Nursing Science Quarterly* 6:195–200.

Nortridge, J. A., Mayeux, V., Anderson, S. J., and Bell, M. L. 1992. The use of cognitive style mapping as a predictor for academic success of first semester diploma nursing students. *Journal of Nursing Education* 31:352–356.

Radwanski, M. 1992. Self-medicating practices for managing chronic pain after spinal cord injury. *Rehabilitation Nursing* 17:312–318.

Sirles, A. T., Brown, K., and Hilyer, J. C. 1991. Effects of back school education and exercise in back injured municipal workers. *American Association of Occupational Health Nursing Journal* 39:7–12.

Speck, B. J. 1990. The effect of guided imagery upon first semester nursing students performing their first injections. *Journal of Nursing Education* 29:346–350.

Vaughn, M., Cheatwood, S., Sirles, A. T., and Brown, K. C. 1989. The effect of progressive muscle relaxation on stress among clerical workers. *American Association of Occupational Health Nurses Journal* 37:302–306.

Waddell, K. L., and Demi, A. S. 1993. Effectiveness of an intensive partial hospitalization program for treatment of anxiety disorders. *Archives of Psychiatric Nursing* 7:2–10.

Wilson, V. S. 1987. Identification of stressors related to patients' psychological responses to the surgical intensive care unit. *Heart and Lung* 16:267–273.

Ziegler, S. M. 1982. Taxonomy for nursing diagnosis derived from the Neuman Systems Model. In *The Neuman Systems Model: Application to Nursing Education and Practice,* by B. Neuman, 55–68. Norwalk, Conn.: Appleton-Century-Crofts.

Ziemer, M. M. 1983. Effects of information on postsurgical coping. *Nursing Research* 32:282–287.

DOCTORAL DISSERTATIONS

Burritt, J. E. 1988. The effects of perceived social support on the relationship between job stress and job satisfaction and job performance among registered nurses employed in acute care facilities. *Dissertation Abstracts International* 49:2123B.

Capers, C. F. 1987. Perceptions of problematic behavior as held by lay black adults and registered nurses. *Dissertation Abstracts International* 47:4467B.

Collins, A. S. 1992. Effects of positional changes on selected physiological and psychological measurements in clients with atrial fibrillation. *Dissertation Abstracts International* 53:200B.

Flannery, J. C. 1988. Validity and reliability of Levels of Cognitive Functioning Assessment Scale for adults with closed head injuries. *Dissertation Abstracts International* 48:3248B.

Goble, D. S. 1991. A curriculum framework for the prevention of child sexual abuse. *Dissertation Abstracts International* 52:2004A.

Harbin, P. D. O. 1990. A Q-analysis of the stressors of adult female nursing students enrolled in baccalaureate schools of nursing. *Dissertation Abstracts International* 50:3919B.

Heaman, D. J. 1992. Perceived stressors and coping strategies of parents with developmentally disabled children. *Dissertation Abstracts International* 52:6316B.

Lancaster, D. R. N. 1992. Coping with appraised threat of breast cancer: Primary prevention coping behaviors utilized by women at increased risk. *Dissertation Abstracts International* 53:202B.

McDaniel, G. M. S. 1990. The effects of two methods of dangling on heart rate and blood pressure in postoperative abdominal hysterectomy patients. *Dissertation Abstracts International* 50:3923B.

Moody, N. B. 1991. Selected demographic variables, organizational characteristics, role orientation, and job satisfaction among nurse faculty. *Dissertation Abstracts International* 52:1356B.

Norman, S. E. 1991. The relationship between hardiness and sleep disturbances in HIV-infected men. *Dissertation Abstracts International* 51:4780B.

Norris, E. W. 1990. Physiologic response to exercise in clients with mitral valve prolapse syndrome. *Dissertation Abstracts International* 50:5549B.

Peoples, L. T. 1991. The relationship between selected client, provider, and agency variables and the utilization of home care services. *Dissertation Abstracts International* 51:3782B.

Poole, V. L. 1992. Pregnancy wantedness, attitude toward pregnancy, and use of alcohol, tobacco, and street drugs during pregnancy. *Dissertation Abstracts International* 52:5193B.

Rowe, M. L. 1990. The relationship of commitment and social support to the life satisfaction of caregivers to patients with Alzheimer's disease. *Dissertation Abstracts International* 51:1747B.

Schlosser, S. P. 1985. The effect of anticipatory guidance on mood state in primiparas experiencing unplanned cesarean delivery (metropolitan area, Southeast). *Dissertation Abstracts International* 46:2627B.

Sipple, J. E. A. 1989. A model for curriculum change based on retrospective analysis. *Dissertation Abstracts International* 50:1927A.

Tennyson, M. G. 1992. Becoming pregnant: Perceptions of black adolescents. *Dissertation Abstracts International* 52:5196B.

Terhaar, M. F. 1989. The influence of physiological stability, behavioral stability and family stability on the preterm infant's length of stay in the neonatal intensive care unit. *Dissertation Abstracts International* 50:1328B.

Vincent, J. L. M. 1988. A Q-analysis of the stressors of fathers with an infant in an intensive care unit. *Dissertation Abstracts International* 49:3111B.

Watson, L. A. 1991. Comparison of the effects of usual, support, and informational nursing interventions on the extent to which families of critically ill patients perceived their needs were met. *Dissertation Abstracts International* 52:2999B.

Webb, C. A. 1988. A cross-sectional study of hope, physical status, cognitions and meaning and purpose of pre- and post-retirement adults. *Dissertation Abstracts International* 49:1922A.

Whatley, J. H. 1989. Effects of health locus of control and social network on risk-taking in adolescents. *Dissertation Abstracts International* 50:129B.

MASTER'S THESES

Anderson, R. R. 1992. Indicators of nutritional status as a predictor of pressure ulcer development in the critically ill adult. *Masters Abstracts International* 30:92.

Averill, J. B. 1989. The impact of primary prevention as an intervention strategy. *Masters Abstracts International* 27:89.

Baskin-Nedzelski, J. 1992. Job stressors among visiting nurses. *Masters Abstracts International* 30:79.

Besseghini, C. 1990. Stressful life events and angina in individuals undergoing exercise stress testing. *Masters Abstracts International* 28:569.

Blount, K. R. 1989. The relationship between the parent's and five to six-year-old child's perception of life events as stressors within the Neuman Health Care Systems framework. *Masters Abstracts International* 27:487.

Elgar, S. J. 1992. The influence of companion animals on perceived social support and perceived stress among family caregivers. *Masters Abstracts International* 30:732.

Fields, W. L. 1988. The effects of the 12-hour shift on fatigue and critical thinking performance in critical care nurses. *Masters Abstracts International* 26:237.

Finney, G. A. H. 1990. Spiritual needs of patients. *Masters Abstracts International* 28:272.

Goldstein, L. A. 1988. Needs of spouses of hospitalized cancer patients. *Masters Abstracts International* 26:105.

Haskill, K. M. 1988. Sources of occupational stress of the community health nurse. *Masters Abstracts International* 26:106.

Morris, D. C. 1991. Occupational stress among home care first line managers. *Masters Abstracts International* 29:443.

Murphy, N. G. 1990. Factors associated with breastfeeding success and failure: A systematic integrative review (Infant nutrition). *Masters Abstracts International* 28:275.

Petock, A. M. 1991. Decubitus ulcers and physiological stressors. *Masters Abstracts International* 29:267.

Sammarco, C. C. A. 1990. The study of stressors of the operating room nurse versus those of the intensive care unit nurse. *Masters Abstracts International* 28:276.

Scarpino, L. L. 1988. Family caregivers' perception associated with the chemotherapy treatment setting for the oncology client. *Masters Abstracts International* 26:424.

Sullivan, M. M. 1991. Comparisons of job satisfaction scores of school nurses with job satisfaction normative scores of hospital nurses. *Masters Abstracts International* 29:652.

Wilkey, S. F. 1990. The effects of an eight-hour continuing education course on the death anxiety levels of registered nurses. *Masters Abstracts International* 28:480.

EDUCATION

Arndt, C. 1982. Systems theory and educational programs for nursing service administration. In *The Neuman Systems Model: Application to Nursing Education and Practice,* by B. Neuman, 182–187. Norwalk, Conn.: Appleton-Century-Crofts.

Baker, N. A. 1982. The Neuman Systems Model as a conceptual framework for continuing education in the work place. In *The Neuman Systems Model: Application to Nursing Education and Practice,* by B. Neuman, 260–264. Norwalk, Conn.: Appleton-Century-Crofts.

Bourbonnais, F. F., and Ross, M. M. 1985. The Neuman Systems Model in nursing education: Course development and implementation. *Journal of Advanced Nursing* 10:117–123.

Bower, F. L. 1982. Curriculum development and the Neuman Model. In *The Neuman Systems Model: Application to Nursing Education and Practice,* by B. Neuman, 94–99. Norwalk, Conn.: Appleton-Century-Crofts.

Bruton, M. R., and Matzo, M. 1989. Curriculum revisions at Saint Anselm College: Focus on the older adult. In *The Neuman Systems Model,* 2d ed., by B. Neuman, 201–210. Norwalk, Conn.: Appleton & Lange.

Capers, C. F. 1986. Some basic facts about models, nursing conceptualizations, and nursing theories. *Journal of Continuing Education* 16:149–154.

Conners, V. L. 1982. Teaching the Neuman Systems Model: An approach to student and faculty development. In *The Neuman Systems Model: Application to Nursing Education and Practice,* by B. Neuman, 176–181. Norwalk, Conn.: Appleton-Century-Crofts.

Conners, V. L. 1989. An empirical evaluation of the Neuman Systems Model: The University of Missouri–Kansas City. In *The Neuman Systems Model,* 2d ed., by B. Neuman, 249–258. Norwalk, Conn.: Appleton & Lange.

Conners, V., Harmon, V. M., and Langford, R. W. 1982. Course development and implementation using the Neuman Systems Model as a framework: Texas Woman's University (Houston Campus). In *The Neuman Systems Model: Application to Nursing Education and Practice,* by B. Neuman, 153–158. Norwalk, Conn.: Appleton-Century Crofts.

Dale, M. L., and Savala, S. M. 1990. A new approach to the senior practicum. *Nursing Connections* 3(1):45–51.

Dyck, S. M., Innes, J. E., Rae, D. I., and Sawatzky, J. E. 1989. The Neuman Systems Model in curriculum revision: A baccalaureate program, University of Saskatchewan. In *The Neuman Systems Model,* 2d ed., by B. Neuman, 225–236. Norwalk, Conn.: Appleton & Lange.

Edwards, P. A., and Kittler, A. W. 1991. Integrating rehabilitation content in nursing curricula. *Rehabilitation Nursing* 16:70–73.

Harty, M. B. 1982. Continuing education in nursing and the Neuman Model. In *The Neuman Systems Model: Application to Nursing Education and Practice,* by B. Neuman, 100–106. Norwalk, Conn.: Appleton-Century-Crofts.

Johansen, H. 1989. Neuman Model concepts in joint use—community health practice and student teaching—School of Advanced Nursing Education, Aarhus University, Aarhus, Denmark. In *The Neuman Systems Model,* 2d ed., by B. Neuman, 334–362. Norwalk, Conn.: Appleton & Lange.

Johnson, M. N., Vaughn-Wrobel, B., Ziegler, S., Hough, L., Bush, H. A., and Kurtz, P. 1982. Use of the Neuman Health Care Systems Model in the master's curriculum: Texas Woman's University. In *The Neuman Systems Model: Application to Nursing Education and Practice,* by B. Neuman, 130–152. Norwalk, Conn.: Appleton-Century-Crofts.

Johnson, S. E. 1989. A picture is worth a thousand words: Helping students visualize a conceptual model. *Nurse Educator* 14(3):21–24.

Karnels, P. 1993. Conundrum game for nursing theorists: Newman, King, and Johnson. *Nurse Educator* 18(6):8–9.

Kilchenstein, L., and Yakulis, I. 1984. The birth of a curriculum: Utilization of the Betty Neuman Health Care Systems Model in an integrated baccalaureate program. *Journal of Nursing Education* 23:126–127.

Knox, J. E., Kilchenstein, L., and Yakulis, I. M. 1982. Utilization of the Neuman Model in an integrated baccalaureate program: University of Pittsburgh. In *The Neuman Systems Model: Application to Nursing Education and Practice,* by B. Neuman, 117–123. Norwalk, Conn.: Appleton-Century-Crofts.

Laschinger, S. J., Maloney, R., and Tranmer, J. E. 1989. An evaluation of student use of the Neuman Systems Model: Queen's University, Canada. In *The Neuman Systems Model,* 2d ed., by B. Neuman, 211–224. Norwalk, Conn.: Appleton & Lange.

Lebold, M., and Davis, L. 1980. A baccalaureate nursing curriculum based on the Neuman Health Care Systems Model. In *Conceptual Models for Nursing Practice,* 2d ed., by J. P. Riehl and C. Roy, 151–158. New York: Appleton-Century-Crofts.

Lebold, M. M., and Davis, L. H. 1982. A baccalaureate nursing curriculum based on the Neuman Systems Model: Saint Xavier College. In *The Neuman Systems Model: Application to Nursing Education and Practice,* by B. Neuman, 124–129. Norwalk, Conn.: Appleton-Century-Crofts.

Louis, M., Witt, R., and LaMancusa, M. 1989. The Neuman Systems Model in multilevel nurse education programs: University of Nevada, Las Vegas. In *The Neuman Systems Model,* 2d ed., by B. Neuman, 237–248. Norwalk, Conn.: Appleton & Lange.

Lowry, L. 1985. Adapted by degrees. *Senior Nurse* 5(3):25–26.

Lowry, L. W. 1988. Operationalizing the Neuman Systems Model: A course in concepts and process. *Nurse Educator* 13(3):19–22.

Lowry, L. W., and Green, G. H. 1989. Four Neuman-based associate degree programs: Brief description and evaluation. In *The Neuman Systems Model,* 2d ed., by B. Neuman, 283–312. Norwalk, Conn.: Appleton & Lange.

Mirenda, R. M. 1986. The Neuman Systems Model: Description and application. In *Case Studies in Nursing Theory,* edited by P. Winstead-Fry, 127–166. New York: National League for Nursing.

Moxley, P. A., and Allen, L. M. H. 1982. The Neuman Systems Model approach in a master's degree program: Northwestern State University. In *The Neuman Systems Model: Application to Nursing Education and Practice,* by B. Neuman, 168–175. Norwalk, Conn.: Appleton-Century-Crofts.

Mrkonich, D. E., Hessian, M., and Miller, M. W. 1989. A cooperative process in curriculum development using the Neuman Health Care Systems Model. In *Conceptual Models for Nursing Practice,* 3d ed., by J. P. Riehl-Sisca, 87–94. Norwalk, Conn.: Appleton & Lange.

Mrkonich, D., Miller, M., and Hessian, M. 1989. Cooperative baccalaureate education: The Minnesota intercollegiate nursing consortium. In *The Neuman Systems Model,* 2d ed., by B. Neuman, 175–182. Norwalk, Conn.: Appleton & Lange.

Nelson, L. F., Hansen, M., and McCullagh, M. 1989. A new baccalaureate North Dakota–Minnesota nursing education consortium. In *The Neuman Systems Model,* 2d ed., by B. Neuman, 183–192. Norwalk, Conn.: Appleton & Lange.

Nichols, E. G., Dale, M. L., and Turley, J. 1989. The University of Wyoming evaluation of a Neuman-based curriculum. In *The Neuman Systems Model,* 2d ed., by B. Neuman, 259–282. Norwalk, Conn.: Appleton & Lange.

Reed-Sorrow, K., Harmon, R. L., and Kitundu, M. E. 1989. Computer-assisted learning and the Neuman Systems Model. In *The Neuman Systems Model,* 2d ed., by B. Neuman, 155–160. Norwalk, Conn.: Appleton & Lange.

Ross, M. M., Bourbonnais, F. F., and Carroll, G. 1987. Curricular design and the Betty Neuman Systems Model: A new approach to learning. *International Nursing Review* 34:75–79.

Sipple, J. A., and Freese, B. T. 1989. Transition from technical to professional-level nursing education. In *The Neuman Systems Model,* 2d ed., by B. Neuman, 193–200. Norwalk, Conn.: Appleton & Lange.

Stittich, E. M., Avent, C. L., and Patterson, K. 1989. Neuman-based baccalaureate and graduate nursing programs, California State University, Fresno. In *The Neuman Systems Model,* 2d ed., by B. Neuman, 163–174. Norwalk, Conn.: Appleton & Lange.

Story, E. L., and DuGas, B. W. 1988. A teaching strategy to facilitate conceptual model implementation in practice. *Journal of Continuing Education in Nursing* 19:244–247.

Story, E. L., and Ross, M. M. 1986. Family centered community health nursing and the Betty Neuman Systems Model. *Nursing Papers* 18(2):77–88.

Tollett, S. M. 1982. Teaching geriatrics and gerontology: Use of the Neuman Systems Model. In *The Neuman Systems Model: Application to Nursing Education and Practice,* by B. Neuman, 159–164. Norwalk, Conn.: Appleton-Century-Crofts.

ADMINISTRATION

Arndt, C. 1982. Systems concepts for management of stress in complex health-care organizations. In *The Neuman Systems Model: Application to Nursing Education and Practice,* by B. Neuman, 97–114. Norwalk, Conn.: Appleton-Century-Crofts.

Bowman, G. E. 1982. The Neuman assessment tool adapted for child day-care centers. In *The Neuman Systems Model: Application to Nursing Education and Practice,* by B. Neuman, 324–334. Norwalk, Conn.: Appleton-Century-Crofts.

Breckenridge, D. M., Cupit, M. C., and Raimondo, J. M. 1982. Systematic nursing assessment tool for the CAPD client. *Nephrology Nurse* 24(January/February):26–27, 30–31.

Burke, Sr., M. E., Capers, C. F., O'Connell, R. K., Quinn, R. M., and Sinnott, M. 1989. Neuman-based nursing practice in a hospital setting. In *The Neuman Systems Model,* 2d ed., by B. Neuman, 423–444. Norwalk, Conn.: Appleton & Lange.

Capers, C. F., and Kelly, R. 1987. Neuman nursing process: A model of holistic care. *Holistic Nursing Practice* 1(3):19–26.

Capers, C. F., O'Brien, C., Quinn, R., Kelly, R., and Fenerty, A. 1985. The Neuman Systems Model in practice. Planning phase. *Journal of Nursing Administration* 15(5):29–39.

Caramanica, L., and Thibodeau, J. 1987. Nursing philosophy and the selection of a model for practice. *Nursing Management* 10(10):71.

Davies, P. 1989. In Wales: Use of the Neuman Systems Model by community psychiatric nurses. In *The Neuman Systems Model,* 2d ed., by B. Neuman, 375–384. Norwalk, Conn.: Appleton & Lange.

Drew, L. L., Craig, D. M., and Beynon, C. E. 1989. The Neuman Systems Model for community health administration and practice: Provinces of Manitoba and Ontario, Canada. In *The Neuman Systems Model,* 2d ed., by B. Neuman, 315–342. Norwalk, Conn.: Appleton & Lange.

Fawcett, J., Botter, M. L., Burritt, J., Crossley, J. D., and Fink, B. B. 1989. Conceptual models of nursing and organization theories. In *Dimensions of Nursing Administration. Theory, Research, Education, and Practice,* edited by B. Henry, M. Di Vincenti, C. Arndt, and A. Marriner, 143–154. Boston: Blackwell Scientific Publications.

Flannery, J. 1991. FAMLI-RESCUE: A family assessment tool for use by neuroscience nurses in the actue care setting. *Journal of Neuroscience Nursing* 23:111–115.

Hinton Walker, P., and Raborn, M. 1989. Application of the Neuman Model in nursing administration and practice. In *Dimensions of Nursing Administration. Theory, Research, Education, and Practice,* edited by B. Henry, C. Arndt, M. Di Vincenti, and A. Marriner-Tomey, 711–723. Boston: Blackwell Scientific Publications.

Johns, C. 1991. The Burford Nursing Development Unit holistic model of nursing practice. *Journal of Advanced Nursing* 16:1090–1098.

Kelly, J. A., Sanders, N. F., and Pierce. J. D. 1989. A systems approach to the role of the nurse administrator in education and practice. In *The Neuman Systems Model,* 2d ed., by B. Neuman, 115–138. Norwalk, Conn.: Appleton & Lange.

Mann, A. H., Hazel, C., Geer, C., Hurley, C. M., and Podrapovic, T. 1993. Development of an orthopaedic case manager role. *Orthopaedic Nursing* 12(4):23–27, 62.

Mayers, M. A., and Watson, A. B. 1982. Nursing care plans and the Neuman Systems Model: In *The Neuman Systems Model: Application to Nursing Education and Practice,* by B. Neuman, 69–84. Norwalk, Conn.: Appleton-Century-Crofts.

Mischke-Berkey, K., and Hanson, S. M. H. 1991. *Pocket Guide to Family Assessment and Intervention.* St. Louis: Mosby Year Book.

Mischke-Berkey, K., Warner, P., and Hanson, S. 1989. Family health assessment and intervention. In *Nurses and Family Health Promotion: Concepts, Assessment, and Interventions,* edited by P. J. Bomar, 115–154. Baltimore: Williams and Wilkins.

Moynihan, M. M. 1991. Implementation of the Neuman Systems Model in an acute care nursing department. In *Nursing Theories in Practice,* edited by M. E. Parker, 263–273. New York: National League for Nursing.

Neal, M. C. 1982. Nursing care plans and the Neuman Systems Model: II. In *The Neuman Systems Model: Application to Nursing Education and Practice,* by B. Neuman, 85–93. Norwalk, Conn.: Appleton-Century-Crofts.

Neuman, B., and Wyatt, M. 1980. The Neuman Stress/Adaptation systems approach to education for nurse administrators. In *Conceptual Models for Nursing Practice* 2d ed., by J. P. Riehl and C. Roy, 142–150. New York: Appleton-Century-Crofts.

Pinkerton, A. 1974. Use of the Neuman Model in a home health-care agency. In *Conceptual Models for Nursing Practice,* by J. P. Riehl and C. Roy, 122–129. New York: Appleton-Century-Crofts.

Quayhagen, M. P., and Roth, P. A. 1989. From models to measures in assessment of mature families. *Journal of Professional Nursing* 5:144–151.

Schlentz, M. D. 1993. The minimum data set and the levels of prevention in the long-term care facility. *Geriatric Nursing* 14:79–83.

Simmons, L., and Borgdon, C. 1991. The clinical nurse specialist in HIV care. *The Kansas Nurse* 66(1):6–7.

Vokaty, D. A. 1982. The Neuman Systems Model applied to the clinical nurse specialist role. In *The Neuman Systems Model: Application to Nursing Education and Practice,* by B. Neuman, 165–167. Norwalk, Conn.: Appleton-Century-Crofts.

PRACTICE

Anderson, E., McFarlane, J., and Helton, A. 1986. Community-as-client: A model for practice. *Nursing Outlook* 34:220–224.

Baerg, K. L. 1991. Using Neuman's model to analyze a clinical situation. *Rehabilitation Nursing* 16:38–39.

Baker, N. A. 1982. Use of the Neuman Model in planning for the psychological needs of the respiratory disease patient. In *The Neuman Systems Model: Application to Nursing Education and Practice,* by B. Neuman, 241–251. Norwalk, Conn.: Appleton-Century-Crofts.

Balch, C. 1974. Breaking the lines of resistance. In *Conceptual Models for Nursing Practice,* by J. P. Riehl and C. Roy, 130–134. New York: Appleton-Century-Crofts.

Beckingham, A. C., and Baumann, A. 1990. The ageing family in crisis: Assessment and decision-making models. *Journal of Advanced Nursing* 15:782–787.

Beddome, G. 1989. Application of the Neuman Systems Model to the assessment of community-as-client. In *The Neuman Systems Model,* 2d ed., by B. Neuman, 363–374. Norwalk, Conn.: Appleton & Lange.

Beitler, B., Tkachuck, B., and Aamodt, D. 1980. The Neuman Model applied to mental health, community health, and medical-surgical nursing. In *Conceptual Models for Nursing Practice,* 2d ed., by J. P. Riehl and C. Roy, 170–178. New York: Appleton-Century-Crofts.

Benedict, M. B., and Sproles, J. B. 1982. Application of the Neuman Model to public health nursing practice. In *The Neuman Systems Model: Application to Nursing Education and Practice,* by B. Neuman, 223–240. Norwalk, Conn.: Appleton-Century-Crofts.

Bergstrom, D. 1992. Hypermetabolism in multisystem organ failure: A Neuman systems perspective. *Critical Care Nursing Quarterly* 15(3):63–70.

Beyea, S., and Matzo, M. 1989. Assessing elders using the functional health pattern assessment model. *Nurse Educator* 14(5):32–37.

Biley, F. C. 1989. Stress in high dependency units. *Intensive Care Nursing* 5:134–141.

Breckenridge, D. M. 1982. Adaptation of the Neuman Systems Model for the renal client. In *The Neuman Systems Model: Application to Nursing Education and Practice,* by B. Neuman, 267–277. Norwalk, Conn.: Appleton-Century-Crofts.

Breckenridge, D. M. 1989. Primary prevention as an intervention modality for the renal client. In *The Neuman Systems Model,* 2d ed., by B. Neuman, 397–406. Norwalk, Conn.: Appleton & Lange.

Brown, M. W. 1988. Neuman's systems model in risk factor reduction. *Cardiovascular Nursing* 24(6):43.

Buchanan, B. F. 1987. Human-environment interaction: A modification of the Neuman Systems Model for aggregates, families, and the community. *Public Health Nursing* 4:52–64.

Bullock, L. F. C. 1993. Nursing interventions for abused women on obstetrical units. *AWHONN's Clinical Issues in Perinatal and Women's Health Nursing* 4(3):371–377.

Cardona, V. D. 1982. Client rehabilitation and the Neuman Model. In *The Neuman Systems Model: Application to Nursing Education and Practice,* by B. Neuman, 278–290. Norwalk, Conn.: Appleton-Century-Crofts.

Clark, F. 1982. The Neuman Systems Model: A clinical application for psychiatric nurse practitioners. In *The Neuman Systems Model: Application to Nursing Education and Practice,* by B. Neuman, 335–353. Norwalk, Conn.: Appleton-Century-Crofts.

Clark, J. 1982. Development of models and theories on the concept of nursing. *Journal of Advanced Nursing* 7:129–134.

Craddock, R. B., and Stanhope, M. K. 1980. The Neuman Health Care Systems Model: Recommended adaptation. In *Conceptual Models for Nursing Practice,* 2d ed., by J. P. Riehl and C. Roy, 159–169. New York: Appleton-Century-Crofts.

Cunningham, S. G. 1982. The Neuman Model applied to an acute care setting: Pain. In *The Neuman Systems Model: Application to Nursing Education and Practice,* by B. Neuman, 291–296. Norwalk, Conn.: Appleton-Century-Crofts.

Cunningham, S. G. 1983. The Neuman Systems Model applied to a rehabilitation setting. *Rehabilitation Nursing* 8(4):20–22.

Davis, L. H. 1982. Aging: A social and preventive perspective. In *The Neuman Systems Model: Application to Nursing Education and Practice,* by B. Neuman, 211–214. Norwalk, Conn.: Appleton-Century-Crofts.

Delunas, L. R. 1990. Prevention of elder abuse: Betty Neuman health care systems approach. *Clinical Nurse Specialist* 4:54–58.

Dunbar, S. B. 1982. Critical care and the Neuman Model. In *The Neuman Systems Model: Application to Nursing Education and Practice,* by B. Neuman, 297–307. Norwalk, Conn.: Appleton-Century-Crofts.

Dunn, S. I., and Trépanier, M. J. 1989. Application of the Neuman Model to perinatal nursing. In *The Neuman Systems Model,* 2d ed., by B. Neuman, 407–422. Norwalk, Conn.: Appleton & Lange.

Eclin, D. J. 1982. Palliative care and the Neuman Model. In *The Neuman Systems Model: Application to Nursing Education and Practice,* by B. Neuman, 257–259. Norwalk, Conn.: Appleton-Century-Crofts.

Fawcett, J., Archer, C. L., Becker, D., Brown, K. K., Gann, S., Wong, M. J., and Wurster, A. B. 1992. Guidelines for selecting a conceptual model of nursing: Focus on the individual patient. *Dimensions of Critical Care Nursing* 11:268–277.

Fawcett, J., Cariello, F. P., Davis, D. A., Farley, J., Zimmaro, D. M., and Watts, R. J. 1987. Conceptual models of nursing: Application to critical care nursing practice. *Dimensions of Critical Care Nursing* 6:202–213.

Foote, A. W., Piazza, D., and Schultz, M. 1990. The Neuman Systems Model: Application to a patient with a cervical spinal cord injury. *Journal of Neuroscience Nursing* 22:302–306.

Fulbrook, P. R. 1991. The application of the Neuman Systems Model to intensive care. *Intensive Care Nursing* 7:28–39.

Galloway, D. A. 1993. Coping with a mentally and physically impaired infant: A self-analysis. *Rehabilitation Nursing* 18:34–36.

Gavan, C. A. S., Hastings-Tolsma, M. T., and Troyan, P. J. 1988. Explication of Neuman's model: A holistic systems approach to nutrition for health promotion in the life process. *Holistic Nursing Practice* 3(1):26–38.

Goldblum-Graff, D., and Graff, H. 1982. The Neuman Model adapted to family therapy. In *The Neuman Systems Model: Application to Nursing Education and Practice,* by B. Neuman, 217–222. Norwalk, Conn.: Appleton-Century-Crofts.

Gunter, L. M. 1982. Application of the Neuman Systems Model to gerontic nursing. In *The Neuman Systems Model: Application to Nursing Education and Practice,* by B. Neuman, 196–210. Norwalk, Conn.: Appleton-Century-Crofts.

Herrick, C. A., and Goodykoontz, L. 1989. Neuman's Systems Model for nursing practice as a conceptual framework for a family assessment. *Journal of Child and Adolescent Psychiatric and Mental Health Nursing* 2:61–67.

Herrick, C. A., Goodykoontz, L., Herrick, R. H., and Hackett, B. 1991. Planning a continuum of care in child psychiatric nursing: A collaborative effort. *Journal of Child and Adolescent Psychiatric and Mental Health Nursing* 4:41–48.

Hiltz, D. 1990. The Neuman Systems Model: An analysis of a clinical situation. *Rehabilitation Nursing* 15:330–332.

Hoeman, S. P., and Winters, D. M. 1990. Theory-based case management; High cervical spinal cord injury. *Home Healthcare Nurse* 8:25–33.

Kido, L. M. Sleep deprivation and intensive care unit psychosis. *Emphasis: Nursing* 4(1):23–33.

Knight, J. B. 1990. The Betty Neuman Systems Model applied to practice: A client with multiple sclerosis. *Journal of Advanced Nursing* 15:447–455.

Lindell, M., and Olsson, H. 1991. Can combined oral contraceptives be made more effective by means of a nursing care model? *Journal of Advanced Nursing* 16:475–479.

McInerney, K. A. 1982. The Neuman Systems Model applied to critical care nursing of cardiac surgery clients. In *The Neuman Systems Model: Application to Nursing Education and Practice,* by B. Neuman, 308–315. Norwalk, Conn.: Appleton-Century-Crofts.

Millard, J. 1992. Health visiting an elderly couple. *British Journal of Nursing* 1:769–773.

Mirenda, R. M. 1986. The Neuman Model in practice. *Senior Nurse* 5(3):26–27.

Mirenda, R. M. 1986. The Neuman Systems Model: Description and application. In *Case Studies in Nursing Theory,* edited by P. Winstead-Fry, 127–166. New York: National League for Nursing.

Moore, S. L., and Munro, M. F. 1990. The Neuman Systems Model applied to mental health nursing of older adults. *Journal of Advanced Nursing* 15:293–299.

Orr, J. P. 1993. An adaptation of the Neuman Systems Model to the care of the hospitalized preschool child. *Curationis* 16(3): 37–44.

Piazza, D., Foote, A., Wright, P., and Holcombe, J. 1992. Neuman Systems Model used as a guide for the nursing care of an 8-year-old child with leukemia. *Journal of Pediatric Oncology Nursing* 9(1):17–24.

Pierce, J. D., and Hutton, E. 1992. Applying the new concepts of the Neuman Systems Model. *Nursing Forum* 27:15–18.

Redheffer, G. 1985. Application of Betty Neuman's Health Care Systems Model to emergency nursing practice: Case review. *Point of View* 22(2):4–6.

Reed, K. 1982. The Neuman Systems Model: A basis for family psychosocial assessment. In *The Neuman Systems Model: Application to Nursing Education and Practice,* by B. Neuman, 188–195. Norwalk, Conn.: Appleton-Century-Crofts.

Reed, K. S. 1989. Family theory related to the Neuman Systems Model. In *The Neuman Systems Model,* 2d ed., by B. Neuman, 385–396. Norwalk, Conn.: Appleton & Lange.

Reed, K. S. 1993. Adapting the Neuman Systems Model for family nursing. *Nursing Science Quarterly* 6:93–97.

Rice, M. J. 1982. The Neuman Systems Model applied in a hospital medical unit. *The Neuman Systems Model: Application to Nursing Education and Practice,* by B. Neuman, 316–323. Norwalk, Conn.: Appleton-Century-Crofts.

Robichaud-Ekstrand, S., and Delisle, L. 1989. Neuman en médecine-chirurgie [The Neuman Model in medical-surgical settings]. *The Canadian Nurse* 85(6):32–35.

Rodrigues-Fisher, L., Bourguignon, C., and Good, B. V. 1993. Dietary fiber nursing intervention: Prevention of constipation in older adults. *Clinical Nursing Research* 2:464–477.

Ross, M., and Bourbonnais, F. 1985. The Betty Neuman Systems Model in nursing practice: A case study approach. *Journal of Advanced Nursing* 10:199–207.

Ross, M. M., and Helmer, H. 1988. A comparative analysis of Neuman's Model using the individual and family as the units of care. *Public Health Nursing* 5:30–36.

Shaw, M. C. 1991. A theoretical base for orthopaedic nursing practice: The Neuman Systems Model. *Canadian Orthopaedic Nurses Association Journal* 13(2):19–21.

Smith, M. C. 1989. Neuman's model in practice. *Nursing Science Quarterly* 2:116–117.

Sohier, R. 1989. Nursing care for the people of a small planet: Culture and the Neuman Systems Model. In *The Neuman Systems Model,* 2d ed., by B. Neuman, 139–154. Norwalk, Conn.: Appleton & Lange.

Spradley, B. W. 1990. *Community Health Nursing: Concepts and Practice.* Glenview, Ill.: Scott, Foresman/Little, Brown Higher Education.

Sullivan, J. 1986. Using Neuman's model in the acute phase of spinal cord injury. *Focus on Critical Care* 13(5):34–41.

Torkington, S. 1988. Nourishing the infant. *Senior Nurse* 8(2):24–25.

Utz, S. W. 1980. Applying the Neuman Model to nursing practice with hypertensive clients. *Cardio-Vascular Nursing* 16:29–34.

Wallingford, P. 1989. The neurologically impaired and dying child: Applying the Neuman Systems Model. *Issues in Comprehensive Pediatric Nursing* 12:139–157.

Weinberger, S. L. 1991. Analysis of a clinical situation using the Neuman Systems Model. *Rehabilitation Nursing* 16:278, 280–281.

INDEX